The Complete Q&A for the NCLEX-RN Exam

FIFTH EDITION

AUTHOR
PATRICIA A. HOEFLER, M.S.N., R.N.

CONTRIBUTING AUTHORS
Lois Walker, Ph.D., R.N.
Carol Kozik, M.S.N., R.N.
Sandra Bailey, M.S.N., R.N.
Susan W. Dockers, Ph.D., R.N.
Barbara J. Galvin, M.S.N., R.N.
Marianne Markowitz, M.S.N., R.N.
Marian L. Kovatchitch, M.S.N., R.N.

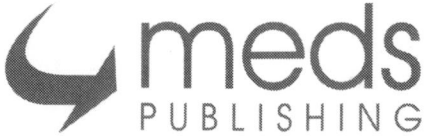

MEDICAL EDUCATION DEVELOPMENT SERVICES

4000 BLACKBURN LANE, SUITE 260

BURTONSVILLE, MARYLAND 20866

www.medspub.com

Editor: Mark Williams-Abrams

FIFTH EDITION 2004

Copies of this book may be obtained from:
MEDICAL EDUCATION DEVELOPMENT SERVICES
4000 Blackburn Lane, Suite 260
Burtonsville, Maryland 20866
www.medspub.com

ISBN: 1-56533-502-3
Printed in the United States of America.

TABLE OF CONTENTS

NCLEX-RN

INTRODUCTION

SECTION I

PREPARING FOR THE EXAM

A. What You Should Know About the NCLEX-RN Exam

1. General information
    a. The first integrated exam was given in July 1982
    b. The purpose of the exam is to determine that a candidate is prepared to practice entry-level nursing safely
    c. The exam is designed to test essential knowledge of nursing and a candidate's ability to apply that knowledge to clinical situations
    d. The purpose of the new test plan is to bring the exam in line with current nursing behaviors (the nursing process and decision making)
    e. Exam is "pass/fail," and no other score is given

2. Computerized Adaptive Testing
    a. Computer program continuously scores answers and selects questions suitable for each candidate's competency level for a more precise measurement of competency
    b. A higher weight is assigned to difficult questions so a passing score can be obtained by answering a lot of easier questions-or a smaller number of more difficult questions
    c. Special screen design is used (see SCREEN DESIGN below)
    d. Use the mouse to move the cursor on the screen to the desired location.

Single-click your mouse to select an option as your answer.
    e. A drop-down calculator also is featured. Double-click your mouse on the calculator icon, and the drop-down calculator will appear.
    f. After you have confirmed your selection, click on "next" to input your answer and proceed to the next screen
    g. After you proceed to the next screen, you CANNOT go back to a previous question to change your answer.

3. Exam schedule
    a. Given year-round
    b. Retake policy: The exam can only be repeated every 90 days

4. Number of questions and time allowed
    a. No minimum amount of time; however, a candidate must answer a minimum of 75 test questions
    b. Maximum time is five hours, with a maximum of 265 test questions
    c. About one out of three candidates completes the exam in less than two hours; one in three will use the complete five hours
    d. The computer will automatically stop as soon as one of the following occurs:
        1) Candidate's measure of competency is determined to be above or below the passing standard
        2) Candidate has answered all 265 test questions
        3) Maximum amount of time (five hours) has expired

5. A candidate will pass by either:

Case Scenario and Stem

SCREEN DESIGN

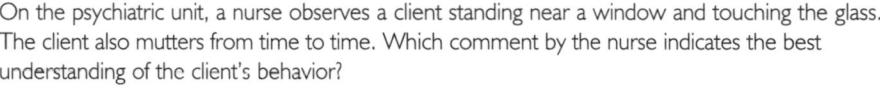

On the psychiatric unit, a nurse observes a client standing near a window and touching the glass. The client also mutters from time to time. Which comment by the nurse indicates the best understanding of the client's behavior?

   1. "Why are you standing by the window and touching the glass?"

   2. "There you are. I came to see if you wanted to see the video we are showing on the unit?"

   3. What are you looking at through the window?"

   4. "Are you hearing voices or seeing things?"

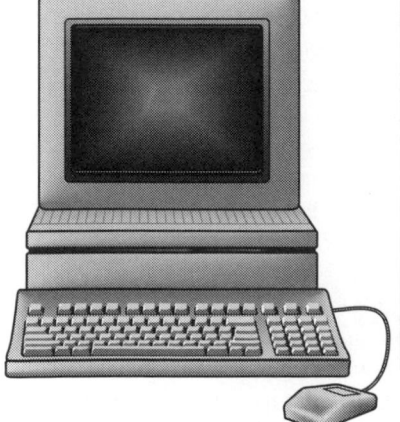

Choices 1, 2, 3, and 4

   a. Answering 75 to 265 questions above the passing standard (the required weighted score) for all questions answered, within the time allowed; or

   b. Answering at least 75 questions within the time allowed and achieving the passing standard for the last 60 questions answered

6. Types of questions
   a. The majority of the questions are standard multiple choice
     1) Each question has four options
     2) The best option is the only correct answer
   b. Exam includes 15 unmarked experimental or "try-out" questions
   c. A small percentage of the questions are alternative format questions including:
     1) Fill-in-the-blank items
     2) Calculation items
     3) Ordered response (sequencing) items
     4) Hot Spot (point and click) items
     5) Multiple Response items
     6) Items with graphs, tables, or charts

7. Exam procedure:
   a. Look for the BEST answer to each question
   b. It is not possible to skip questions or return to previous questions
   c. Mandatory 10-minute break after first two hours and after another one-and-one-half hours
   d. Scratch paper provided for calculations must be returned at end of exam

8. Structure of the test plan *
   a. Safe, Effective Care Environment

1) Management of Care	13 - 19%
2) Safety and Infection Control	8 - 14%

   b. Health Promotion and Maintenance   6 - 12%
   c. Psychosocial Integrity   6 - 12%
   d. Physiological Integrity

1) Basic Care and Comfort	6 - 12%
2) Pharmacological and Parenteral Therapies	13 - 19%
3) Reduction of Risk Potential	13 - 19%
4) Physiological Adaptation	11 - 17%

Information courtesy of the National Council of State Boards of Nursing, Inc., Test Plan April 2004.

B. Schedule Your Study Time
1. The minimum time for preparation is two hours a day for six to eight weeks
   a. Spend 1/3 of your time reviewing content
   b. Spend 2/3 of your time answering test questions

2. For content review, use an NCLEX-RN exam review book such as this one, which outlines content
3. Begin with areas that are most difficult for you, or the areas that are least familiar
4. For more detailed information on your difficult or less familiar areas, use a good nursing reference manual
5. Review medical-surgical, pediatric, women's health, and psychiatric nursing, as well as nursing management and alternate test item formats
6. Use a body systems approach for medical-surgical and pediatric nursing areas
7. When studying body systems and the associated diseases, remember to:
   a. Define the disease in terms of the pathophysiological process that is occurring
   b. Identify the client's early and late manifestations
   c. Identify the most important or life-threatening complications
   d. Define the medical treatment
   e. Identify and prioritize the nursing interventions associated with early and late manifestations
   f. Identify what the nurse teaches the client/family to prevent or adapt to disease
8. To schedule your study time:
   a. List the areas you need to review
   b. Count the number of days you have available to study
   c. Estimate the amount of time needed for each area
   d. On your calendar, write the area to review, the number of questions to answer, and the amount of time needed for each study day

C. Answer Many Questions
1. Answering questions will develop your test-taking skills
2. Use questions similar to those on the NCLEX exam
3. Answer a minimum of 3,000 test questions
4. Include answering test questions in your study plan. For example, answer 100 questions each day for a month.
5. If you are at high risk, answer 5,000 test questions
6. Use at least three different question-and-answer books, including MEDS Publishing's *Complete Q&A for the NCLEX-RN Exam* with CD-ROM
7. Using a variety of books provides a more comprehensive preparation
8. An online question and answer program which mimics the NCLEX exam such as MEDS StarNurse Exam-A-Day™ will give you more realistic experience with answering alternative item format questions

D. Assess Your Progress

1. Each time you answer questions, check the number of questions you answered correctly
   a. If you answer less than 65% correctly, this is a warning signal! Spend lots of time reviewing content and answering more questions in this area of nursing.
   b. If you answer 65 to 75% correctly, your performance is average. Success in this area is uncertain. Continue working with this content until your score is above 75%. Work on building your confidence by answering more questions in this area.
   c. If you answer 75 to 85% correctly, your performance is very good. Only return to this area after you have at least 75% in all other areas. Feel confident.
   d. If you answer 85 to 95% correctly, your performance is superior. Don't waste time on this. Feel very confident.

2. For each wrong answer, identify why you answered wrong
   a. You may have answered a question wrong because you did not know the facts or got confused about the information
      1) Identify this as a content weakness
      2) Review the content again
   b. You may have answered a question wrong because you misread the question, did not understand what it was asking, or did not know how to select the best answer
      1) Identify this as a test-taking deficiency
      2) For further assistance with test-taking deficiencies, we recommend MEDS test-taking book, *Successful Problem Solving & Test Taking for Nursing and NCLEX-RN Exams*.

3. Check the number of questions that you identified as difficult and went back to answer later. See how many of them you answered correctly.

SECTION II

ANSWERING QUESTIONS

A. Identify the Critical Elements in the Question

1. Identify the issue in the question
   a. The issue is the problem about which the question is asking
   b. The issue may be a:
      1) Drug: for example, digoxin (*Lanoxin*), furosemide (*Lasix*)
      2) Nursing problem: for example, alteration in comfort, potential for infection
      3) Behavior: for example, restlessness, agitation

   4) Disorder: for example, diabetes mellitus, ulcerative colitis
   5) Procedure: for example, glucose tolerance test, cardiac catheterization

2. Identify the client in the question
   a. The client in the question is usually the person with the health problem
   b. The client in a test question may also be a relative or significant other or another member of the health care team with whom the nurse is interacting
   c. The correct answer to the question must relate to the client in the question

3. Look for the key words
   a. Key words focus attention on what is important
   b. Key words may appear in bold print
   c. Examples:
      1) During the early period, which of the following nursing procedures would be **best**?
      2) The nurse would expect to find which of the following characteristics in an **adult** diabetic?
      3) Which of the following nursing actions is **vital**?
      4) Which of the following nursing actions would be best **initially**?

4. Identify what the stem is asking and determine whether the question has a true response stem, a false response stem or a priority stem
   a. Be clear about what the stem is asking before you look at the options
   b. If the question is not clear to you, rephrase it using your own words
   c. Determine whether the question has a true response stem, a false response stem or a priority stem
      1) True response stem
         a) Definition: A true response stem requires an answer that is a true statement
         b) Examples:
            (1) The nurse would assign the nursing assistant to:
            (2) Which manifestation would the nurse expect to assess?
            (3) The therapeutic response by the nurse would be:
            (4) The nurse evaluates that the client has a positive response to the medication when the client has:
      2) False response stem
         a) Definition: A false response stem requires an answer that is a false statement

b) Examples:
(1) Which of the following nursing actions would be inappropriate?
(2) Which of the following statements by the client would indicate a need for further instruction?
(3) Which of the following describes incorrect placement of the hands during CPR?
(4) Which of the following actions would place the client at risk?

3) Priority response stem
a) Definition: A priority response stem requires the candidate to select the best answer from four plausible responses
b) Examples:
(1) Which client would the nurse assess first?
(2) The nurse's initial action would be to:
(3) The nurse should give immediate consideration to which of the following findings?
(4) The task that the nurse has the nursing assistant complete first would be:

B. Use a Selection Procedure to Eliminate Incorrect Options

1. Most NCLEX questions are standard multiple choice questions which have four options. The correct answer is the BEST answer. The other three options are "distractors."
2. Distractors are options made to look like correct answers. They are intended to distract you from answering correctly.
3. As you read each of the four options, make a decision about it.
   a. This option is true (+)
   b. This option is false (−)
   c. I am not sure about this option (?)
4. If the stem is a true response stem:
   a. An option that is true (+) might be the correct answer
   b. An option that is false (−) is a distractor. Eliminate this option
   c. An option that you are not sure about (?) is possibly the correct answer
5. If the stem is a false response stem:
   a. An option that is true (+) is a distractor. Eliminate this option.
   b. An option that is false (−) may be the correct answer
   c. An option that you are not sure about (?) is

possibly the correct answer
6. Do not return to options you have eliminated
7. If you are left with one option, that is your answer
8. If you are left with one (+) option and one (?) option, select the (+) option as your answer
9. If you are left with two (+) options, use strategies to select the best answer

C. Use Test-Taking Strategies When You Are Unable to Select the Best Option

1. The Global Response Strategy
   a. A global response is a general statement that may include ideas of other options within it
   b. Look for a global response when more than one option appears to be correct
   c. The global response option will probably be the correct answer
2. The Similar Distractors Strategy
   a. Similar distractors say basically the same thing using different words
   b. Since there is only one correct answer in a question, similar distractors must be wrong
   c. Eliminate similar distractors. Select for your answer an option that is different.
3. The Similar Word or Phrase Strategy
   a. When more than one option appears to be correct, look for a similar word or phrase in the stem of the question and in one of the four options
   b. The option that contains the similar word or phrase may be the correct answer
   c. Use this strategy after you have tried to identify a global response option and eliminated similar distractors
4. The Absolute Word Strategy
   a. Absolute words include words such as "only", "every", "always", and "never"
   b. When a response includes an absolute word it is unlikely to be the correct answer

D. Answering Communication Questions

1. The NCLEX exam includes many communication questions because the ability to communicate therapeutically is essential for safe practice
2. Identify the critical elements as in all questions. Pay particular attention to identification of the client in the question. Remember that the answer must relate to the client.
3. Learn to identify communication tools that enhance communication.
   a. Being silent: Nonverbal communication
   b. Offering self: "Let me sit with you."
   c. Showing empathy: "You are upset."
   d. Focusing: "You say that . . ."
   e. Restatement: "You feel anxious?"

   f.   Validation/clarification: "What you are saying is . . .?"

   g.   Giving information: "Your room is 423."

   h.   Dealing with the here and now: "At this time, the problem is . . ."

4. Learn to identify non-therapeutic communication blocks.

   a.   Giving advice: "If I were you, I would . . ."

   b.   Showing approval/disapproval: "You did the right thing."

   c.   Using clichés and false reassurances: "Don't worry. It will be all right."

   d.   Requesting an explanation: "Why did you do that?"

   e.   Devaluing client feelings: "Don't be concerned. It's not a problem."

   f.   Being defensive: "Every nurse on this unit is exceptional."

   g.   Focusing on inappropriate issues or persons: "Have I said something wrong?"

   h.   Placing the client's issues "on hold": "Talk to your doctor about that."

5. When answering communication questions, select an option that illustrates a therapeutic communication tool. Eliminate options that illustrate non-therapeutic communication blocks.

E. Answering Questions that Focus on Setting Priorities

1. Priority-setting questions ask the test taker to identify either what comes first, is most important, or gets the highest priority

2. Examples:

   a.   What is the nurse's initial response?

   b.   The nurse should give immediate consideration to which of the following?

   c.   Which nursing action receives the highest priority?

   d.   What should the nurse do first?

3. Use guidelines to help you to answer priority setting questions

   a.   Maslow's Hierarchy of Needs indicates that physiological needs come first

   b.   Maslow's Hierarchy of Needs indicates that when no physiological need is identified, safety needs come first

   c.   Nursing Process indicates that assessment comes first

   d.   Communication Theory indicates focusing on feelings first

   e.   Teaching/Learning Theory indicates focusing on motivation first

PREPARING FOR EXAM TIME

A. Plan for Everything

1. Assemble everything you will need for the exam the night before:

   a.   Identification: two IDs with signatures, including one with recent photograph

   b.   Watch

   c.   Several sharpened pencils (with erasers) for calculations

2. Plan to arrive at the test site early:

   a.   Know the route to the exam site

   b.   Know how long it will take to get there

   c.   Know where you will park and if you will need coins for a parking meter

3. Pay close attention to your own physiological needs:

   a.   Dress in layers

   b.   Get a good night's sleep the night before the exam

   c.   Eat a good breakfast

   d.   Avoid stimulants and depressants

   e.   Use the bathroom just before the exam

4. During the exam:

   a.   Listen to the instructions

   b.   Pace yourself; don't spend too long on any one question

   c.   Don't let yourself become distracted. Focus your attention on answering the questions.

   d.   Go with your first choice. Use test-taking strategies only when you cannot decide between close options.

   e.   Keep your thoughts positive!

B. Manage Your Anxiety Level

1. Moderate levels of anxiety increase your effectiveness

2. Don't cram the night before the exam

3. Do something enjoyable and relaxing the night before the exam

4. Learn and practice measures to manage your anxiety level during the exam as needed

   a.   Take a few deep breaths

   b.   Tense and relax muscles

   c.   Tell yourself positive affirmations

   d.   Visualize a peaceful scene

   e.   Visualize your success

C. Test-Taking Tips

1. Prepare comprehensively and be sure to be well rested for the exam

2. Read each question carefully, identifying the critical elements. Each question must be answered in sequence, and you may not skip or go back to change your answers to any questions.

3. Don't panic if the computer stops after a short time! It does not mean that you failed. The computer stops when the exam is able to determine with at least 95% certainty that you have demonstrated the ability, or inability, to practice safely at the minimal level of nursing competency.

4. It is helpful to know that most students pass by answering a maximum of 119 questions. However, you can still pass the exam even if you answered all 265 questions.

5. If you are having difficulty choosing between the best two options, use the test taking strategies you have learned in this review.

6. You should anticipate that the test questions will increase in difficulty

7. Use your scratch paper wisely. Since you cannot review earlier questions to help recall previous facts, use the scratch paper provided for calculations to remember facts from previous questions. Sometimes, information from one question is helpful in answering another question.

8. Don't panic if someone finishes before you! The test adapts to each candidate's level of ability, and it means that you may take longer to prove that you are capable of practicing competently at the beginning level of nursing.

9. Keep a positive attitude! Remember that you have learned a great amount of nursing knowledge, and the exam is only designed to determine whether you are able to practice safely at the entry level.

NOTES

NCLEX-RN

Test 1

NCLEX-RN TEST 1

1. A client, 88 years old, is being discharged from the hospital after treatment for poor circulation to her lower extremities. Which of the following actions, if taken by the client, would indicate that the pre-discharge teaching by the nurse may have been unsuccessful?

   1. The client puts on stockings with elastic tops and tells the nurse that she does not like other kinds of hosiery.
   2. The client tells the nurse that she will get a thermometer to measure the temperature of the bath water.
   3. The client asks her husband to take her sandals home, and bring a pair of shoes to the hospital for her to wear home.
   4. The client tells the nurse that she is going to have to remember to keep her legs uncrossed.

2. Restraints may be used to immobilize a client, or the client's extremity. The nurse understands that the least appropriate rationale for using restraints on a client would be:

   1. To prevent a client from pulling out an IV or other type of therapy.
   2. To reduce the risk to all elderly clients from falling out of bed or off a chair.
   3. To prevent removal of life support equipment.
   4. To prevent injury to health care personnel by combative clients.

3. A client is being discharged after the diagnosis of a peptic ulcer. Which of the following nutritional measures should the nurse emphasize to help decrease the acid secretions of the stomach?

   1. Increase intake of milk and cream products.
   2. Limit alcohol consumption.
   3. Avoid high fiber foods.
   4. Eat a bland diet; decaffeinated coffee only.

4. A 35-year-old client has the following laboratory values reported on his chart: hematocrit 35%, hemoglobin 13 g/dL, platelet count 150,000/mm³, white blood cell count, 6,000/mm³. The nurse would analyze which of the following laboratory reports as an indication that the client's condition has improved?

   1. Hematocrit 42%.
   2. Hemoglobin 12.8 g/dL.
   3. Platelet count 180,000/mm³.
   4. White blood cell count 8,000/mm³.

5. After a series of nine ECT treatments, a client reports his depressive symptoms are gone. He now complains of short-term memory loss. The most appropriate nursing action is to:

   1. Immediately report the problem to his psychiatrist.
   2. Encourage him to ventilate his feelings about the problem.
   3. Explain that this memory loss is temporary, and his memory will return to normal in four to eight weeks.
   4. Tell him this is a side effect of the treatment, and he can expect his memory to return to normal in five to 10 days.

6. A client is receiving verapamil hydrochloride (Calan) and propranolol (Inderal). The nurse should monitor the client closely for signs of:

   1. Hypertension.
   2. Increased peripheral resistance.
   3. Bradycardia and heart failure.
   4. Diarrhea.

7. The physician has prescribed high dose erythromycin lactobionate (Erythrocin Lactobionate-IV) IV for a client with acute pelvic inflammatory disease (PID) caused by Neisseria gonorrhea. Because of the high dose therapy, the nurse should monitor the client for which of the following reactions?

   1. Seizures.
   2. Atrial fibrillation.
   3. Acute renal failure.
   4. Hearing loss.

8. While observing a two-year-old girl recently admitted to the hospital, the nurse becomes concerned by which of the following characteristics?

   1. The child is not yet potty trained.
   2. The child replies "no" to every question.
   3. The child cannot share toys.

(4.) The child recognizes four to six words.

9. **A client is in the hospital with renal failure. She is on fluid restrictions. The nurse would avoid:**

  (1.) Providing a variety of fluids in small containers.
  2. Informing the client and family about the restriction.
  3. Allowing the client to help keep a record of oral intake.
  4. Providing fluids only during meal times.

10. **A male college student, age 19, is admitted to the psychiatric unit with complaints of suicidal thoughts and plans to hang himself. Which action should the nurse avoid?**

  1. Remove his clothing, dress him in a hospital gown, and have him restrained in a seclusion room until a complete assessment of suicide risk can be done.
  2. Contact a family member to ask if he has made any prior suicide attempts.
  3. Place the client on suicide precautions.
  (4.) Encourage the client to discuss recent events that led him to feel so hopeless.

11. **A three-year-old girl is brought to the physician's office with persistent otitis media. In order to assess factors that may be contributing to the unresolved illness, the nurse should ask the parents which question?**

  1. "Does anyone smoke around, or in the same house as, the child?"
  2. "Is the child playing with other children with otitis media?"
  3. "Does the child get water in her ears during the bath?"
  (4.) "Has the child had a fever recently?"

12. **A client asks if she may have an occasional alcoholic beverage during her pregnancy. The nurse should advise her that, in relation to alcohol consumption during pregnancy, she should do which of the following?**

  1. Limit drinking to beer or wine.
  (2.) Abstain from consuming all alcoholic beverages.
  3. Drink no more than one ounce of liquor each day.
  4. Dilute liquor well with water or soda before drinking it.

13. **A client has died unexpectedly. His family arrives immediately after his death. The best initial nursing action is to:**

  (1.) Pull the curtain to provide privacy for the grieving family.
  2. Perform postmortem care so that the body is prepared properly for the funeral home.
  3. Notify the minister so he can be present when the family first sees the client.
  4. Ask the family to return in 30 minutes while you clean the body and straighten the room and bedding.

14. **A daughter has come to take her mother home from the hospital. Her mother has had a colostomy. The daughter tells the nurse that she doesn't know how she is going to care for her mother's colostomy. The best response by the nurse is:**

  1. "Your mother can take care of her colostomy without difficulty."
  2. "What part of your mother's care concerns you?"
  (3.) "A home health nurse will be stopping by tomorrow. If you have any questions, you can ask her."
  4. "It is quite simple. I'll make sure that her colostomy bag is clean before she leaves."

15. **A 53-year-old client is scheduled for a cardiac catheterization. When he arrives for the procedure, he reports he awoke that morning with "butterflies in his stomach," a sense of restlessness, urinary frequency, and some difficulty concentrating as he drove to the hospital. The admitting nurse assesses his anxiety level as:**

  1. Mild.
  2. Moderate.
  (3.) Severe.
  4. Panic.

16. **Six days after starting antihypertensive therapy that includes spironolactone (Aldactone), a client calls the Health Clinic to tell the nurse that he is having "palpitations" and "skipped heart beats." Initially, the nurse should tell the client to:**

  (1.) Stop taking the medication.
  2. Lie down and rest when these side effects occur.
  3. Report to the Clinic for a visit with his physician.
  4. Eat a diet high in potassium-rich foods.

17. **Which of the following diagnostic studies should the nurse monitor most closely while the client is taking captopril (Capoten)?**

  1. Creatinine.
  (2.) Hemoglobin and hematocrit.

3. Urinalysis.
4. Serum glucose.

18. **A client is admitted to the hospital and is in the terminal stages of cancer. The nurse goes into his room to give him some medicine and finds him crying. The most appropriate nursing action is to:**

    1. Sit with the client and hold his hand.
    2. Tell the client that someone will call his minister, so that the minister can comfort him.
    3. Notify the family to come to the hospital and stay with him.
    4. Give the client his medication and allow him to cry in private.

19. **The nurse's goal in positioning a client for a vaginal examination is to:**

    1. Provide for the client's comfort.
    2. Provide a position that promotes access for examination by the physician.
    3. Provide for a position of comfort for the physician.
    4. Provide the correct position while ensuring the client's comfort and privacy.

20. **A client receiving cisplatin (Platinol) for his cancer develops a WBC count of 1,000 cells/mm³. What fact is important for the nurse to consider?**

    1. The client has an increased chance of infection.
    2. The client needs more foods high in iron.
    3. The client needs additional fluids.
    4. The family should be called to the bedside.

21. **Which statement by a client indicates to the nurse an accurate understanding of pregnancy induced hypertension?**

    1. "I should not get pregnant again, since pregnancy induced hypertension is likely to occur in subsequent pregnancies."
    2. "I will have to be on a high protein diet for at least six months when I go home after delivery."
    3. "As soon as the baby is delivered, I will not have any more hypertension, proteinuria, or edema."
    4. "I will see my doctor regularly after I am discharged, because I may have an elevated blood pressure for a while."

22. **A 51-year-old man is admitted to an alcohol treatment unit. His wife reports that he has been drinking daily for 20 years and recently lost his driver's license for driving while intoxicated. During the** admission interview, the client tells the nurse that he is only there because his wife has threatened to leave him if he does not get treatment. He states, "I only have one drink after work each evening." What is the most appropriate response for the nurse to make to his statement?

    1. "What is your definition of "one" drink?"
    2. "Are you feeling angry with your wife for insisting you get treatment?"
    3. "If you only have one drink, how did you get a DWI?"
    4. "Do you use any other drugs besides alcohol?"

23. **A client is scheduled for a mastectomy in the morning. Her daughter is visiting and says to the nurse, "I should call my brothers and sisters and have them here in the morning just in case something goes wrong." The best response by the nurse would be:**

    1. To ask the mother if she would like her children there in the morning.
    2. To suggest that the daughter ask her mother how she feels about that.
    3. To say to the daughter, "If your brothers and sisters want to be here, they are welcome."
    4. To ask the daughter what she knows about her mother's surgery and diagnosis.

24. **A client's psychiatrist orders lithium carbonate, 300 mg q.i.d. After five days, the nurse notes that the client's laboratory report indicates a serum lithium level of 1.0 mEq/liter. Based on this report, what nursing action is most appropriate at this time?**

    1. Withhold the next dose of lithium and notify the psychiatrist.
    2. Ask that the laboratory test be repeated.
    3. Assess the client for possible toxic effects.
    4. Administer the next dose of lithium as ordered.

25. **An 18-month-old girl is admitted for a surgical repair of the cleft palate. She returns from the operating room, supine, with an IV, and a mist tent on room air. What is the priority nursing action?**

    1. Medicate for pain.
    2. Check the IV for signs of infiltration.
    3. Turn the child on her side.
    4. Review the postoperative orders.

26. **A client has just returned to her room after abdominal surgery. She has a nasogastric tube in place and a drain attached to a hemovac. A**

Foley catheter is draining <u>clear yellow urine</u>. The best rationale for the nurse ensuring that the side rails are up on the bed is which of the following?

1. To prevent the urine collection bag and tubing from getting tangled up in the side rails when the client is turned in bed.
2. To prevent the client from falling out of bed after receiving an anesthetic.
3. To provide a place to attach the nasogastric tubing to prevent it from being dislodged.
4. To attach the call light so it is within easy reach.

27. While starting an intravenous infusion (IV), the nurse's gloved hands become contaminated with blood. The client has not been diagnosed with any organisms that are transmitted by way of the blood stream. Immediately upon completion of the task, the nurse should:

1. Remove the gloves carefully and complete a thorough handwashing.
2. Wash the gloved hands, and then throw the gloves away.
3. Prepare an incident report so that this occurrence will be documented, in case a health care problem develops at a later date.
4. Ask the client to have a blood test to determine if a bloodborne pathogen is present in the client's blood.

√ 28. A 92-year-old client is admitted to the hospital with abdominal pain. During the initial assessment, the nurse notes that the client is not giving appropriate answers to questions. The client just nods and smiles while the nurse is talking to him. The nurse is probably dealing with what developmental problem?

1. The client is experiencing so much pain that he cannot focus on the nurse's questions.
2. It must be assumed that the client is probably confused due to his age.
3. The client is probably hard of hearing.
4. Most elderly live in a fantasy world and are unable to comprehend what others say to them.

29. A client calls the prenatal clinic at 39 weeks of gestation to report that she just had a gush of fluid from the vagina. Which of the following is the best response by the nurse at this time?

1. "Your contractions will probably begin within the next 24 hours. If they do not, call back."
2. "You should not introduce anything into the vagina because rupture of membranes places you at risk for sepsis."

3. "You should come to the clinic for a short visit so we can assess you and the fetus."
4. "You should go to the labor unit at the hospital for admission."

30. In planning care for a four-year-old admitted to the hospital, the nurse would include providing which toy?

1. A plastic stethoscope.
2. A brightly colored mobile.
3. A jigsaw puzzle.
4. A helium balloon.

31. The nurse knows that which of the following conditions would ineffectively be treated by aspirin?

1. Arthritis.
2. A 102° F fever.
3. An ulcer.
4. A headache.

√ 32. The nurse working in a geriatric facility understands that an inaccurate generalization about the elderly is that:

1. Their primary focus turns more inward, with a narrowing of outside interests.
2. They have the capacity to enjoy life and seek new experiences.
3. Their interest in sexual activity continues into old age as long as they enjoy good health and the availability of a partner.
4. They need a sense of being useful and activities that support this view.

33. The nurse tells a client that she needs to be catheterized for a urine specimen. The client pulls the covers to her neck. She glances at the open door and says, "Someone might see me out there!" The best action by the nurse to alleviate the client's concern is:

1. Explain the procedure to the client.
2. Obtain some assistance, since the client does not appear to be comfortable and may be resistant to the procedure.
3. Close the door and assure the client that you will cover her as much as possible during the procedure.
4. Gather all of the needed equipment before starting the procedure.

34. A client taking lithium is discharged from the hospital after being taught to recognize the signs

and symptoms of lithium toxicity. The nurse knows learning has occurred when the client calls the unit to report that she is experiencing which of the following?

1. Vomiting and diarrhea.
2. Fine hand tremor.
3. Polyuria.
4. Drowsiness and lethargy.

35. A client returns from surgery for her fractured hip. Her family is waiting anxiously to see her. What is the most important parameter for the nurse to assess immediately after the client is transferred to her bed?

1. The client's ability to deep breathe and cough.
2. The client's vital signs.
3. The surgical dressing.
4. Turn the client on the unaffected side.

36. An ambulatory client is being readied for bed. The nursing action that promotes safety for this client is which of the following?

1. Turning off all of the lights to help promote sleep and rest.
2. Instructing the client in the use of the call bell.
3. Putting the side rail up.
4. Placing the bed in the high position.

37. As a health care professional caring for sick clients, it is imperative that the nurse practice good personal hygiene. Good personal hygiene includes all of the following except:

1. Clean, well groomed hair.
2. A light, fragrant cologne.
3. Good oral hygiene.
4. Absence of body odor.

38. A 25-year-old female client is taking ampicillin (Omnipen) and birth control pills containing estrogen. What information should the nurse provide?

1. Take both medications with breakfast to avoid gastric upset.
2. When used together, serum potassium levels may rise.
3. The effect of the birth control pills may be reduced while the client is taking ampicillin.
4. Urticaria is much more common when antibiotics are given with other drugs.

39. An elderly client is admitted to a long-term care facility. Which of the following measures would

be most important in planning his care?

1. An explanation of the roles of the registered nurse, practical nurse and the nursing assistant.
2. An understanding of his routine for his own care at home.
3. An assessment of his mobility.
4. An introduction to his health care team members.

40. The nurse understands that prednisone is used in treating cancers because of which effect?

1. Antimicrobial.
2. Anticoagulant.
3. Anti-inflammatory.
4. Anti-infective.

41. A client is admitted to the hospital with abdominal pain. She overhears her doctor and nurse discussing cancer of the liver. Later, she says to her nurse, "Having cancer of the liver must be a terrible thing." Which of the following statements would be the best response by the nurse?

1. "Yes, it is a terrible disease."
2. "What made you think about cancer of the liver?"
3. "Any kind of cancer is terrible, but you can't live without a liver."
4. "Yes it is. A client on this floor has it, and it's sad for everyone."

42. When the mother of a five-year-old boy expresses concern over her son's stuttering, which response by the nurse is least appropriate?

1. Vocal hesitancy is common in children younger than age seven.
2. It may help if you stop your son and encourage him to begin the word over.
3. Singing songs or nursery rhymes may ease stuttering.
4. Look directly at your son while he is speaking.

43. A 72-year-old client was admitted to the hospital for pneumonia. He is receiving oxygen at six liters by mask. The nurse would avoid which action, when obtaining his vital signs?

1. Take an axillary temperature.
2. Listen to his lungs when counting respirations.
3. Listen to an apical heart rate.
4. Take an oral temperature.

44. When administering the first dose of enalapril (Vasotec) to a client, it is most important for the nurse to closely monitor the client's:

1. Pulse rate.
2. Blood pressure.
3. Urine output.
4. Level of consciousness.

45. **Before she is discharged from the hospital, a client and her husband attend a client education class on the topic of depression. The nurse instructs them about behaviors that could indicate a recurrence of depression. Which symptom would the nurse avoid including in the instruction?**

    1. Psychomotor retardation.
    2. Grandiosity.
    3. Self-devaluation.
    4. Insomnia.

46. **The nurse is teaching a client about self breast exams. The client tells the nurse that she doesn't understand why she is being taught this since she doesn't plan on doing it anyway. The best response by the nurse would be:**

    1. "Self breast exam is taught to women to detect any lumps or changes in the breast that can be an early sign of cancer, and early treatment has a higher rate of cure."
    2. "You're right. If you don't plan on doing the exam, then I don't need to show you how to do it."
    3. "If you don't plan on doing the exam yourself, then you should have your doctor do it at your annual check up."
    4. "It is your body and you have the right to do whatever you choose."

47. **A two-year-old girl is admitted to the hospital with croup. She has been placed in a mist tent with room air. Which statement by the parents indicates effective client teaching?**

    1. "The mist will give my child extra fluids."
    2. "My child must remain in the mist tent at all times."
    3. "My child may have toys inside the mist tent."
    4. "The mist tent will provide the extra oxygen my child needs."

48. **A client, age 23, is currently taking oral amoxicillin and clavulanate (Augmentin) for otitis media. She also takes birth control pills containing estrogen. Which of the following instructions should the client be given?**

    1. Take both medicines as prescribed.
    2. An alternate method of birth control should be used while taking Augmentin.

3. There is an increased risk of hypersensitivity when both these medications are taken at the same time.
4. Drink extra fluids while taking the Augmentin to prevent kidney damage.

49. **An emergency room nurse is assessing a client for cocaine intoxication. The nurse knows that all of the following symptoms are associated with cocaine intoxication except:**

    1. Seizures.
    2. Hyperactivity.
    3. Paranoid behavior.
    4. Nystagmus.

50. **A client uses tamoxifen (Nolvadex) for her cancer. The nurse knows that tamoxifen has which of the following actions?**

    1. Antimicrobial.
    2. Anti-estrogenic.
    3. Androgenic.
    4. Anti-inflammatory.

51. **A confused elderly client has wet herself and is standing in the hospital corridor in a puddle of urine. She has trouble getting to the bathroom in time. She looks ashamed. She says to the nurse, "I want to go outside for a walk now." Which of the following statements would be the most therapeutic response by the nurse?**

    1. "Before we go for a walk, perhaps we can make a list that will help you make your bathroom trips easier."
    2. "Right now, let me wipe up the urine on the floor, and let's get a change of clothing for you. I am sure that this problem is upsetting for you."
    3. "This has been a problem for you. Let's see if we can find a solution together."
    4. "Wetting yourself is very upsetting. Yes, let's take a walk."

52. **A 98-year-old client was admitted to the hospital with a cerebral vascular accident with left-sided paralysis. He is placed on an air mattress, and anticoagulant therapy is ordered. The best nursing rationale for turning this client every two hours is which of the following?**

    1. To prevent sensory deprivation by varying what the client sees in his environment.
    2. To prevent skin breakdown, which is a common problem in the elderly.
    3. To prevent stasis of blood in the lower extremities.

4. To increase blood supply to the affected side.

53. **A one-year-old boy is brought to the physician's office with fever, irritability, and loss of appetite. A diagnosis of otitis media is made, and the child is placed on p.o. amoxicillin with clavulanate (Augmentin) 150 mg t.i.d. for 10 days. Which nursing instruction must be included in the child's plan of care?**

1. "Drink clear fluids while on the medication."
2. "Take an extra nap, since amoxicillin may cause drowsiness."
3. "Stay indoors until the medication is finished."
4. "Take the medication for the full length of time."

54. **A two-year-old boy is receiving bleomycin (Blenoxane) IV. His mother tells the nurse that it is time for her son to have his polio immunization. What is the best response by the nurse?**

1. "We will schedule it for next week."
2. "The cancer drug will delay any possibility of polio."
3. "Your son's immunizations will need to be delayed until a later time."
4. "I'll call the doctor later today."

55. **What foods does the nurse recommend that a pregnant client with iron-deficiency anemia include in her diet to increase iron intake?**

1. Green leafy vegetables, dried fruits, and beans.
2. Milk and cheese.
3. Coffee and bran.
4. Snack foods, mid morning and afternoon.

56. **The psychiatrist orders tranylcypromine (Parnate) for a depressed client who has not responded to tricyclics. The nurse knows that dietary teaching is essential. The nurse's instructions to the client advise her to avoid all of the following except:**

1. Beer and red wine.
2. Cheddar cheese and sausage.
3. Cottage cheese and canned peaches.
4. Liver and Italian green beans.

57. **A client is admitted to the hospital with active tuberculosis. She is placed in respiratory isolation and started on medication. A chest x-ray is ordered. While transporting the client to x-ray, the nurse should do which of the following?**

1. Wear a mask and gown for protection from the client's organisms.
2. Have the client wear a mask and protect the wheel chair with a clean bath blanket or sheet.
3. Have x-ray come to the client's room to do the x-ray.
4. No special precautions need to be taken.

58. **A client is in the hospital because of severe weight loss and refusal to eat. The physician orders the insertion of a nasogastric tube for feeding. The nurse finds the client with the tube removed. The client tells that nurse that he "doesn't need that thing." Which of the following is the most appropriate response by the nurse?**

1. "You shouldn't have done that! Now I have to put it down again."
2. "Why did you pull that tube out? Do you want to die?"
3. "Tell me what you don't like about the tube."
4. "Your doctor is going to be very upset with you for doing this."

59. **A client is admitted with anorexia nervosa. A nasogastric tube is to be inserted. The best nursing approach to prepare the client for the procedure would include which action?**

1. Assist the client to a sitting position.
2. Explain the procedure to the client.
3. Make sure that any dentures are securely in place in the client's mouth.
4. Have a stethoscope available to listen for proper placement.

✓60. **An elderly client expresses feelings of grief for his earlier life. Which nursing action is most appropriate to best help the client cope with this stage in his life?**

1. Listening attentively and allowing the client to talk about the past.
2. Giving the client some activities to perform so he won't have time to dwell on the past.
3. Let the client know that this is a common problem of the aging population.
4. Tell the client about some of the younger clients in the hospital who are in worse shape than he is.

61. **A 52-year-old client is scheduled for coronary artery bypass surgery in the morning. Before the surgery she states to the nurse, "I don't think I'm going to have the surgery. Everybody has to die sometime." The best nursing response would be?**

1. "If you don't have the surgery, you will most likely die sooner."
2. "There are always risks involved with surgery. Why have you changed your mind about the operation?"
3. "Bypass surgery must be very frightening for you. Tell me how you feel about the surgery."
4. "I will call your doctor and have him come in and talk to you."

62. **The nurse is teaching a class of expectant mothers. A woman asks if the fluid surrounding the fetus in utero is important. The nurse's explanation to the group is based on an understanding that all of the following are functions of amniotic fluid except?**

1. Cushion the fetus against injury.
2. Control the fetus's body temperature.
3. Provide nutritional exchange for the fetus.
4. Allow freedom of movement for the fetus.

63. **A 66-year-old man is an out-patient taking tricyclic antidepressants. The client's wife telephones the clinic and tells the nurse that she has just found her husband lying unconscious and his empty bottle of medication on the nightstand. Overdoses of tricyclic antidepressants are:**

1. Medical emergencies.
2. Serious but rarely fatal.
3. Dangerous for clients in poor health.
4. Easily treated by inducing vomiting.

64. **During postoperative recovery, a client develops a tachyarrhythmia. The physician prescribes propranolol (Inderal) 1 mg by slow IV push, not to exceed 1 mg/minute. The nurse should monitor the client for which of the following adverse reactions?**

1. Congestive heart failure (CHF).
2. Hypertensive crisis.
3. Intestinal obstruction.
4. Seizures.

65. **A client fell at home and fractured her hip. She is to have surgery in the morning. In preparing the client for surgery, what is outside the scope of the nurse's responsibility?**

1. Assessing the health status of the client.
2. Explaining the operative procedure and any risks that may be involved with the procedure.
3. Determining that the history, physical, and spe-

cific laboratory tests have been ordered or completed according to hospital protocol.
4. Determine that a signed surgical consent form is completed.

66. **Which of the following assessments made by the nurse could be considered a manifestation of the most potentially life-threatening side effect of captopril (Capoten)?**

1. Rash.
2. Fever.
3. Dry cough.
4. Tachycardia.

67. **A client is to receive his first injection of interferon, alfa-2a, recombinant (Roferon-A) for his hairy cell leukemia. What side effects would the nurse advise the client to expect?**

1. Reduced urine output.
2. Severe vomiting.
3. Flu-like symptoms.
4. Weight gain.

68. **During the assessment of an elderly client, which of the following effects of the aging process would the nurse be most likely to find?**

1. Decline in physiological and sensory systems of the body.
2. Decreased skin resilience.
3. Diminished hearing acuity.
4. Absent sexual activity.

69. **A client is six weeks pregnant with her first baby. She asks the nurse when she will experience quickening. The nurse tells her that most clients feel quickening:**

1. During the last weeks of pregnancy.
2. Between the second and third months of pregnancy.
3. Between the fourth and fifth months of pregnancy.
4. Soon after implantation, once the uterus begins to rise out of the pelvis.

70. **In prescribing medication for an elderly psychiatric client, the nurse knows which of the following statements about elderly clients is most accurate?**

1. The elderly cannot be safely treated with tricyclic antidepressants.
2. The elderly require lower doses of antidepressants than younger clients.

3. The elderly respond more quickly to the therapeutic effects of antidepressants than younger clients.
4. The elderly can be treated safely and effectively with all antidepressants.

71. **A client, 65 years old, is admitted to the hospital for surgery after finding a lump in his right testicle. He asks the nurse, "Do you think the doctor will find cancer?" Which of the following statements would be the most appropriate nursing response?**

1. "Most lumps found in the testicles are benign."
2. "It must be difficult for you not to know what the doctor will find."
3. "I think that you should discuss this with your doctor."
4. "It might be, but the doctor won't know until the surgery is performed."

72. **A client is in the intensive care unit and is in a coma as a result of a head injury. The most important action in performing mouth care on this client is to:**

1. Turn the client to her side before starting mouth care.
2. Use a soft toothbrush.
3. Use a mouth bite to keep her mouth open.
4. Wear gloves.

73. **A client has been admitted to the hospital with vomiting, diarrhea and extreme weakness. Her husband has stayed at her bedside since admission. She is on bed rest and is receiving IV therapy. A nursing intervention that will best promote rest and comfort for the client would be:**

1. Having the client's husband leave the room for a while so she can sleep.
2. Keeping the emesis basin and bedpan empty and clean for her use.
3. Leaving the bedpan on the bedside stand so it is within easy reach.
4. Closing the door to the client's room.

74. **A client is very confused and combative. The physician orders the client to be placed in a jacket restraint and wrist restraints. In order to prevent injury to the client with restraints, the most important nursing action would be to:**

1. Explain the procedure and reason for the restraints to the client and the family.
2. Remove the restraints and observe the extremities

for circulation at least every four hours.
3. Tell the client that if he is more cooperative the restraints will not be necessary.
4. Document the use of restraints in the chart.

75. **An eight-year-old girl is admitted to the hospital in vaso-occlusive crisis from sickle cell anemia. After recovery, discharge teaching should include which of the following?**

1. Drink eight to 10 glasses of fluid per day.
2. Avoid playground activities at school.
3. Maintain an updated HIB immunization.
4. Assume postural drainage positions every six hours.

76. **A client is placed on ferrous sulfate tablets twice a day as an iron supplement for anemia. The doctor tells her to take the medication with orange juice. Which of the following is the most important reason for drinking orange juice when taking the medication is?**

1. The medication has an unpleasant taste, and the orange juice will help disguise the taste.
2. The orange juice will help avoid constipation, which is a side effect of the medication.
3. The orange juice will help the gastrointestinal tract absorb the medication more efficiently.
4. The medication can cause nausea, and the orange juice will help alleviate this problem.

77. **A client is admitted to the hospital with abdominal pain. She tells the nurse that her father died recently and that she misses him. She begins crying while talking about her father. The nurse's assessment reveals that the client's temperature is 102.6° F and her abdomen is soft without tenderness. To which of the following observations should the nurse give immediate attention?**

1. The client is crying.
2. The temperature of 102.6° F.
3. A soft, non-tender abdomen.
4. The client is grieving.

78. **When the nurse is doing discharge teaching for a client taking captopril (Capoten), which of the following interventions should receive highest priority?**

1. Do not drive while taking this medication.
2. Blood pressure should be monitored daily when home.

3. Limit the intake of coffee, tea, and cola drinks.
4. Notify the physician if a cough or sore throat develops.

79. **A client is taking nadolol (Corgard) 80 mg p.o. daily for treatment of hypertension. During a follow-up appointment six months later, the client exhibits hypertension, agitation, and tachycardia. The nurse may suspect:**

    1. A drug interaction.
    2. Nadolol toxicity.
    3. An allergic reaction.
    4. Nadolol withdrawal.

80. **A client is to begin taking lithium. Before administering the first dose, the nurse could avoid checking to see that which of the following tests have been completed?**

    1. BUN, creatinine, 24-hour creatinine clearance.
    2. TSH, T4, T3RU, T4I.
    3. Electroencephalogram (EEG).
    4. Electrocardiogram (ECG).

81. **While getting an elderly client who is very weak out of bed, the best nursing approach initially is:**

    1. Locking the wheels of the bed.
    2. Placing the equipment to provide the safest transfer that is possible for the client.
    3. Aligning the wheel chair is as close to the bed as possible, to prevent the client from falling to the floor.
    4. Removing the leg support on the wheel chair on the side closest to the bed.

82. **Which of the following outcomes can the nurse anticipate when a client is taking lisinopril (Zestril)?**

    1. Decreased pulse rate.
    2. Decreased chest pain.
    3. Diuresis.
    4. Increased peripheral resistance.

83. **A client is admitted with back pain. During the assessment the nurse notes his vital signs to be: temperature 103.2° F, pulse 90, respirations 30, and blood pressure 128/88. The initial nursing action should be:**

    1. Give the client some medication such as Tylenol for his temperature.

2. Notify the physician of the vital signs.
3. Apply heat to the area of pain in his back.
4. Have the client lie flat in bed to help alleviate the pain.

84. **A client is brought to the hospital by her husband. The admitting nurse notes the presence of pressured speech, irritable mood, and high distractibility. Her husband reports that she has not slept for the past three nights and was hyperactive at home. In addition to prescribing lithium for the client, the nurse anticipates that the psychiatrist will most likely order:**

    1. A sedative-hypnotic.
    2. An anti-anxiety agent.
    3. An antipsychotic.
    4. An antihistamine sedative.

85. **A client is seen in the clinic with complaints of vomiting, diarrhea, headache, and dizziness, and says she has the flu. The nurse takes her vital signs and obtains the following: Blood pressure of 198/110, pulse of 82, respirations of 24 and temperature of 100.8° F. The nurse should give immediate consideration to which of the following?**

    1. Complaints of vomiting.
    2. Complaints of diarrhea.
    3. Complaints of headache and dizziness.
    4. Temperature of 100.8° F.

86. **A 60-year-old client is scheduled for surgery tomorrow. Upon entering the client's room, the nurse notices that flames are coming out of the waste basket. The first action to take is which of the following:**

    1. Place the folded blanket from the client's bed over the entire opening of the waste basket.
    2. Find the nearest fire extinguisher to put the fire out.
    3. Tell the client that he is not supposed to be smoking.
    4. Pull the nearest fire alarm.

87. **In obtaining a blood pressure measurement, the most appropriate nursing action is:**

    1. Obtain the proper equipment, place the client in a comfortable position, and record the appropriate information in the client's chart.
    2. Measure the client's arm, if you are uncertain of the size of cuff to use.

3. Have the client recline or sit comfortably in a chair with the forearm at the level of the heart.
4. Document the measurement, which extremity was used, and the position that the client was in during the measurement.

88. **A client tells the nurse that his name is not spelled right on his identification bracelet. The best action by the nurse is:**

    1. Tell the client that as long as his medical record numbers are correct, the mistake is not a problem.
    2. Ask the client for the correct spelling and change his medical records.
    3. Notify the admitting office of the error and obtain a correct identification bracelet for the client.
    4. Notify the physician.

89. **A 45-year-old business executive was diagnosed with a gastric ulcer two years ago. At that time he was advised to scale down his activities and learn to relax. He returns to the HMO with increased epigastric pain. Upon questioning, he tells the nurse that he has been busier than ever. Which of the following short-term goals for dealing with stress would be the most realistic for the nurse to advise to the client?**

    1. Express his emotions more directly.
    2. Decrease his workload.
    3. Use relaxation techniques each day.
    4. Decrease social activities.

90. **An obese client has been placed on a high protein, low calorie diet by his physician. What nursing action is most appropriate?**

    1. Explain to the client that he will have to change his eating habits.
    2. Explain the importance of exercise when dieting.
    3. Explain to the client what types of foods are permitted on a low calorie, high protein diet.
    4. Tell the client that if he doesn't stay on this diet he will continue to gain weight.

91. **Admitted to the hospital with pulmonary emphysema, a client is extremely short of breath and is receiving oxygen per nasal cannula. The most important nursing action for this client receiving oxygen therapy is to:**

    1. Make sure the client is receiving at least six liters per minute to alleviate his respiratory distress.
    2. Provide low oxygen percentages to prevent respiratory arrest.

3. Provide oral hygiene.
4. Clean the nostrils around the cannula as needed.

92. **A client with chronic obstructive pulmonary disease (COPD) is admitted for management of hypertension. The physician orders propranolol (Inderal) 40 mg p.o. twice a day. The nurse's most appropriate response is to:**

    1. Administer the Inderal one hour before or two hours after meals.
    2. Withhold the Inderal if the pulse is less than 60 beats per minute.
    3. Question the physician regarding the order for Inderal.
    4. Monitor the blood pressure prior to administration of the Inderal.

93. **A three-year-old boy is admitted with laryngotracheobronchitis. His parents seem extremely anxious and the child is crying. Which nursing diagnosis has the highest priority?**

    1. Potential for infection.
    2. Ineffective airway clearance.
    3. Altered parenting.
    4. Impaired tissue perfusion.

94. **After surgery the client requires one unit of blood because of a hemorrhage that occurred during surgery. Within 30 minutes of hanging the unit of blood, the client complains of itching and headache. Her blood pressure is 80/64. The first nursing action should be to:**

    1. Notify the physician.
    2. Obtain a urine specimen.
    3. Notify the laboratory.
    4. Stop the infusion of blood.

95. **An elderly client is receiving care at the clinic because of weight loss. Which of the following nursing actions is most appropriate for the care of this individual?**

    1. Have the client keep a seven day diet log.
    2. Weigh the client at each office visit.
    3. Develop a diet that will improve the nutritional intake of the client.
    4. Discuss the client's appetite and eating habits.

96. **A male client has been taking atenolol (Tenormin) for two months for treatment of hypertension. He tells the nurse at the Health Clinic that he "has no energy or enthusiasm" like he used to. He states**

"I just want to sleep all the time—life holds no interest for me." The nurse recognizes these statements to be indicative of which side effect of Tenormin?

1. Depression.
2. Diminished libido.
3. Drowsiness.
4. Mental changes.

97. A client is admitted to the hospital with decreased circulation in her left leg. During her admission assessment, which is the most important nursing action initially?

1. Obtain the past medical history.
2. Assess for circulation to her left leg by obtaining pedal pulses.
3. Obtain the client's vital signs.
4. Ask the client if she has had a recent injury to her leg.

98. An elderly client is on bed rest. While administering an intramuscular injection, the most important action to prevent introduction of the medication into the venous system is which of the following?

1. Inject the medication slowly to allow for slow absorption.
2. Insert the needle at a 45-degree angle where there are fewer blood vessels.

3. Use the Z track method of injection.
4. Aspirate the drug after insertion of needle.

99. A four-month-old infant is admitted with a ventricular septal defect, and undergoes a cardiac catheterization. Post-catheterization, which sign would alert the nurse to a potential complication?

1. Pedal pulses palpable bilaterally.
2. Apical pulse 140 beats/minute.
3. Blood pressure 96/40.
4. Groin dressing intact with small amount of blood noted.

100. A client with right-sided weakness needs to be transferred from his bed to a wheel chair. When transferring the client, the nurse must remember which the following?

1. Keep the client at arm's length while transferring him.
2. Bend at the waist to get down to his level.
3. Maintain a straight back and bend at the knees.
4. Attempt to transfer the client alone, before determining that help is needed.

NCLEX-RN

Test 1

Questions with
Rationales

NCLEX-RN TEST 1 WITH RATIONALES

1. **A client, 88 years old, is being discharged from the hospital after treatment for poor circulation to her lower extremities. Which of the following actions, if taken by the client, would indicate that the pre-discharge teaching by the nurse may have been unsuccessful?**

   1. The client puts on stockings with elastic tops and tells the nurse that she does not like other kinds of hosiery.
   2. The client tells the nurse that she will get a thermometer to measure the temperature of the bath water.
   3. The client asks her husband to take her sandals home, and bring a pair of shoes to the hospital for her to wear home.
   4. The client tells the nurse that she is going to have to remember to keep her legs uncrossed.

   1. *Correct choice! Elastic tops on stockings decrease circulation and should be avoided by clients with circulation problems. This action and statement by the client indicate that the teaching by the nurse has not been successful. The cause for the failure should be assessed and addressed by the nurse prior to discharge.*
   2. *This statement indicates that the client has successfully learned that poor circulation can impair the client's ability to sense temperature. Because this question has a false response stem, this option cannot be the correct answer.*
   3. *Clients with poor circulation need to wear shoes that protect their feet from injury. This action by the client indicates to the nurse that learning has taken place. Because this question has a false response stem, this option cannot be the correct answer.*
   4. *Crossing the legs at the knees impairs circulation and should be avoided by the client. This statement by the client indicates to the nurse that the client understands the discharge instructions. Because this question has a false response stem, this option cannot be the correct answer.*

2. **Restraints may be used to immobilize a client, or the client's extremity. The nurse understands that the least appropriate rationale for using restraints on a client would be:**

   1. To prevent a client from pulling out an IV or other type of therapy.
   2. To reduce the risk to all elderly clients from falling out of bed or off a chair.

   3. To prevent removal of life support equipment.
   4. To prevent injury to health care personnel by combative clients.

   1. *Wrong. A confused client may pull out an IV or nasogastric tube because of discomfort or inability to understand the purpose of the therapy. This question has a false response stem and is asking you to identify the option that is NOT an appropriate rationale for using restraints on a client.*
   2. *Very good! This option implies that all elderly clients should be restrained in order to reduce the risk of falls. Many elderly clients can care for themselves without falling. Each individual should be assessed for their risk for falling. This inappropriate rationale is the answer because this question has a false response stem.*
   3. *Wrong. Some clients may become combative or confused while on life support equipment and may cause that equipment to become dislodged. This question is asking you to identify the option that is NOT an appropriate rationale for using restraints on a client.*
   4. *Incorrect. Occasionally a client can become combative, and restraints can be the only means of protecting the health care worker while providing care. The stem of the question asks you to identify the option that is NOT an appropriate rationale for using restraints on a client.*

3. **A client is being discharged after the diagnosis of a peptic ulcer. Which of the following nutritional measures should the nurse emphasize to help decrease the acid secretions of the stomach?**

   1. Increase intake of milk and cream products.
   2. Limit alcohol consumption.
   3. Avoid high fiber foods.
   4. Eat a bland diet; decaffeinated coffee only.

   1. *No! A diet rich in milk and cream is not going to benefit the client with an ulcer and, over time, it will increase serum lipids, which can lead to atherosclerosis.*
   2. *Correct choice! Overstimulation by alcohol and coffee can cause over secretion of gastric acids, leading to delayed healing.*
   3. *There is no evidence to suggest that high fiber foods lead to over-secretion of gastric acids. The client should include some of these foods in his diet to prevent constipation.*

4. *Not the correct choice. There is little evidence to support the theory that bland diets are more beneficial than regular meals. Clients are encouraged to eat whatever agrees with them, but they should avoid all forms of coffee, even decaffeinated coffee, during the early stages of ulcer healing.*

4. A 35-year-old client has the following laboratory values reported on his chart: hematocrit 35%, hemoglobin 13 g/dL, platelet count 150,000/mm³, white blood cell count, 6,000/mm³. The nurse would analyze which of the following laboratory reports as an indication that the client's condition has improved?

1. Hematocrit 42%.
2. Hemoglobin 12.8 g/dL.
3. Platelet count 180,000/mm³.
4. White blood cell count 8,000/mm³.

1. *Good choice! This choice shows a hematocrit within the normal limits of 42% to 50% for an adult male. This indicates that the client's condition has improved since the original laboratory report, which indicated a low hematocrit.*
2. *A normal hemoglobin for an adult male is 13 to 16 grams/dL. The original laboratory value was on the low side of normal. A decrease in hemoglobin would not be an improvement for this client.*
3. *Normal platelet counts range from 130,000 to 370,000/mm³. The original laboratory values indicated a platelet count that is within normal limits. This option shows a platelet count that is also within normal limits. This would not be an indication that the client's condition has improved.*
4. *Normal white blood cell counts range from 4,100 to 10,900mm³. The original laboratory values indicated a white blood cell count that is within normal limits, as is the white blood cell count reported in this option. This would not be an indication that the client's condition has improved.*

5. After a series of nine ECT treatments, a client reports his depressive symptoms are gone. He now complains of short-term memory loss. The most appropriate nursing action is to:

1. Immediately report the problem to his psychiatrist.
2. Encourage him to ventilate his feelings about the problem.
3. Explain that this memory loss is temporary, and his memory will return to normal in four to eight weeks.
4. Tell him this is a side effect of the treatment, and he can expect his memory to return to normal in five to 10 days.

1. *The nurse should chart this symptom but it does not need to be reported immediately to the psychiatrist because it is an expected outcome of the ECT treatments.*
2. *This option is appropriate but it is not the most appropriate nursing action because the client has not been given important information about his memory problems.*
3. *Correct. Research indicates that short-term memory problems are temporary outcomes of ECT treatment. While the duration of these memory problems may differ among individuals, it usually does not last longer than two months.*
4. *This response is only partially true. Memory problems that are temporary are common side effects of ECT. The length of time the client experiences these memory problems may differ among individuals, however, most often it is for more than five to 10 days.*

> **TEST-TAKING TIP:** *Note that, although Options 3 & 4 both express the similar idea that the side effect is temporary, there is a significant difference in the duration described in each option. When using the test-taking strategy of eliminating similar options, be careful to identify and compare any key words in the options to be certain that the options are, in fact, similar.*

6. A client is receiving verapamil hydrochloride (Calan) and propranolol (Inderal). The nurse should monitor the client closely for signs of:

1. Hypertension.
2. Increased peripheral resistance.
3. Bradycardia and heart failure.
4. Diarrhea.

1. *No! The client should be monitored for hypotension, not hypertension. Hypotension occurs as both drugs decrease myocardial contractions and lower peripheral resistance.*
2. *Not this choice! Increased peripheral resistance is the same as hypertension.*

> **STRATEGY ALERT!** *When two options are this similar, neither can be the correct answer.*

3. *Right! Bradycardia and heart failure can occur when these drugs are used together.*
4. *Wrong choice! Nausea and constipation are reported, but not diarrhea.*

7. The physician has prescribed high dose erythromycin lactobionate (Erythrocin Lactobionate-IV) IV for a client with acute pelvic inflammatory disease (PID) caused by Neisseria gonorrhea. Because of the high dose therapy, the nurse should monitor the client for which of the following reactions?

1. Seizures.
2. Atrial fibrillation.
3. Acute renal failure.
4. Hearing loss.

1. *Wrong choice. Seizures are not an adverse effect that would be likely, even with high dose therapy of erythromycin.*
2. *Wrong choice! Cardiac arrhythmias are not an adverse reaction to erythromycin therapy.*
3. *Wrong! Clients who receive erythromycin, even high dose IV therapy, are not at risk for renal failure. Recall that 95% of erythromycin is excreted via the liver and bile. The major concern would be for hepatic failure.*
4. ***Excellent! You obviously know your meds! Hearing loss can occur with high IV doses of erythromycin. The client should be instructed to notify the nurse of any hearing changes.***

8. **While observing a two-year-old girl recently admitted to the hospital, the nurse becomes concerned by which of the following characteristics?**

   1. The child is not yet potty trained.
   2. The child replies "no" to every question.
   3. The child cannot share toys.
   4. The child recognizes four to six words.

   1. *Wrong choice! Although toilet training may begin as early as 18 months, toddlers achieve control at varying ages. Usually this is around three years.*
   2. *Wrong! Negativism is a normal characteristic in toddlers. It is considered an expression of developing autonomy.*
   3. *Wrong choice! Two-year-olds may play alongside another child in parallel play, but they are not ready to share and play cooperatively.*
   4. ***Great choice! A two-year-old should have a 300 word vocabulary. A four to six word vocabulary may indicate health problems, such as hearing loss.***

9. **A client is in the hospital with renal failure. She is on fluid restrictions. The nurse would avoid:**

   1. Providing a variety of fluids in small containers.
   2. Informing the client and family about the restriction.
   3. Allowing the client to help keep a record of oral intake.
   4. Providing fluids only during meal times.

   1. *This nursing measure allows for choices and variety. This is something the nurse would want to include in the nursing care plan for this client. The stem of the question is asking for an action the nurse should AVOID.*

2. *Informing the client and the family of the restriction is an appropriate nursing action that will make compliance with the restriction more likely. This question has a false response stem, so look for something the nurse should NOT do.*
3. *This nursing action promotes participation of the client in her own care. This is an appropriate nursing action. The question has a negative response stem. Look for something the nurse should NOT do.*
4. ***Good, you recognized that this is something that the nurse should not do! The client may become thirsty at other than meal times, so this nursing measure can lead to noncompliance on the part of the client and family. This inappropriate action is the correct answer because the question has a false response stem.***

10. **A male college student, age 19, is admitted to the psychiatric unit with complaints of suicidal thoughts and plans to hang himself. Which action should the nurse avoid?**

    1. Remove his clothing, dress him in a hospital gown, and have him restrained in a seclusion room until a complete assessment of suicide risk can be done.
    2. Contact a family member to ask if he has made any prior suicide attempts.
    3. Place the client on suicide precautions.
    4. Encourage the client to discuss recent events that led him to feel so hopeless.

    1. ***Correct. There is no data to indicate that this level of suicide precautions is needed. Remember, legally the client is entitled to receive care in the least restrictive setting. In hospitals, this means the client cannot be restrained or confined in the seclusion room without documentation that he or she is dangerous to himself or others. This inappropriate action is the correct answer because this question has a negative response stem.***
    2. *Wrong choice. Persons who have made a previous suicide attempt are 20 times more likely to succeed at suicide than those who have not. Since this is a major risk factor for suicide, the nurse should obtain information about prior suicide attempts from both the client and his family. This cannot be the correct option because the stem is asking for a false response.*
    3. *This is an appropriate action, so it cannot be the correct response. The suicidal client's behavior must be supervised until he has sufficient self-control to ensure his safety. The level of supervision, as well as other suicide precautions, that will be needed to ensure his safety have to be assessed for each client.*

4. *This action is appropriate, so it cannot be the correct response. Suicidal crisis is usually precipitated by specific recent events that the client is not able to cope with effectively. Before the nurse can intervene therapeutically, an assessment must be done to determine what events or factors have led to the suicidal crisis.*

11. **A three-year-old girl is brought to the physician's office with persistent otitis media. In order to assess factors that may be contributing to the unresolved illness, the nurse should ask the parents which question?**

    1. "Does anyone smoke around, or in the same house as, the child?"
    2. "Is the child playing with other children with otitis media?"
    3. "Does the child get water in her ears during the bath?"
    4. "Has the child had a fever recently?"

    1. *Correct choice! Allergies to common irritants such as smoke can cause congestion and chronic otitis media.*
    2. *Wrong. Otitis media itself is not contagious. A better question might be whether the child had been exposed to children with colds.*
    3. *Incorrect. Water in the ears may cause "swimmer's ear." This is generally not a concern unless the child has had a myringotomy.*
    4. *Incorrect. A fever may indicate acute otitis media but it will not provide information about what factors are contributing to a chronic state.*

12. **A client asks if she may have an occasional alcoholic beverage during her pregnancy. The nurse should advise her that, in relation to alcohol consumption during pregnancy, she should do which of the following?**

    1. Limit drinking to beer or wine.
    2. Abstain from consuming all alcoholic beverages.
    3. Drink no more than one ounce of liquor each day.
    4. Dilute liquor well with water or soda before drinking it.

    1. *No. The best response the nurse can give to the client is total abstinence of all forms of alcohol in pregnancy.*
    2. *Correct answer. This may seen a little strict, but there is no documented safe alcohol level in pregnancy; therefore, total abstinence is recommended.*
    3. *No safe level of alcohol has been established. The best response the nurse can give to the client is total abstinence of all forms of alcohol in pregnancy.*

4. *Incorrect. Diluting the liquor does not reduce the total amount of alcohol consumed. Total abstinence is recommended because there is no documented safe alcohol level in pregnancy.*

13. **A client has died unexpectedly. His family arrives immediately after his death. The best initial nursing action is to:**

    1. Pull the curtain to provide privacy for the grieving family.
    2. Perform postmortem care so that the body is prepared properly for the funeral home.
    3. Notify the minister so he can be present when the family first sees the client.
    4. Ask the family to return in 30 minutes while you clean the body and straighten the room and bedding.

    1. *Excellent! The family members are the clients in this question. Their immediate needs concern confirming the death by viewing the body. Privacy is important at this time. This nursing action addresses the clients' present needs.*
    2. *The family members are the clients in this question. This option does not address the family's present needs.*
    3. *The family members are the clients in this question. The minister may be called after the family's immediate needs are addressed. The initial action should focus on the clients' needs.*
    4. *The family members are the clients in this question. Although the client's body should be made presentable for viewing, 30 minutes is an unreasonable amount of time to make the clients wait to see their deceased family member.*

14. **A daughter has come to take her mother home from the hospital. Her mother has had a colostomy. The daughter tells the nurse that she doesn't know how she is going to care for her mother's colostomy. The best response by the nurse is:**

    1. "Your mother can take care of her colostomy without difficulty."
    2. "What part of your mother's care concerns you?"
    3. "A home health nurse will be stopping by tomorrow. If you have any questions, you can ask her."
    4. "It is quite simple. I'll make sure that her colostomy bag is clean before she leaves."

    1. *This statement may be true but it does not allow the client to express her concerns. The daughter is the client in this question, and the nurse's response should always be therapeutic for the client.*

2. *Excellent! The daughter is the client in this question. This response is therapeutic for the daughter because it uses the communication tool of clarification to allow her to express her concerns.*

3. *No. The daughter is the client in this question, and the nurse's response should be therapeutic for the client. This response is not therapeutic because it uses the communication block of putting the client's concerns "on hold."*

4. *The daughter is the client in this question, and the nurse's response should be therapeutic for the client. This response uses the communication block of false reassurance and it is not therapeutic because it fails to address the client's concerns.*

15. **A 53-year-old client is scheduled for a cardiac catheterization. When he arrives for the procedure, he reports he awoke that morning with "butterflies in his stomach," a sense of restlessness, urinary frequency, and some difficulty concentrating as he drove to the hospital. The admitting nurse assesses his anxiety level as:**

   1. Mild.
   2. Moderate.
   3. Severe.
   4. Panic.

   1. *No. In mild anxiety, the client is alert and able to concentrate closely on the task at hand. This client reported having some difficulty with concentration. He also has several physical symptoms that indicate his anxiety level is more than mild.*

   2. *Good work! The combination of physical symptoms and some difficulty concentrating indicates that his level of anxiety is moderate. This is not unusual considering the intrusive medical procedure he is about to undergo.*

   3. *Wrong. In severe anxiety the person is only able to focus on small details or scattered details and has a great deal of discomfort. The client was able to drive and reported only some difficulty concentrating, so his anxiety is not severe.*

   4. *Wrong. At the panic level the client is disorganized and may appear either paralyzed (unable to act) or hyperactive and agitated. The client's anxiety is not this high.*

16. **Six days after starting antihypertensive therapy that includes spironolactone (Aldactone), a client calls the Health Clinic to tell the nurse that he is having "palpitations" and "skipped heart beats." Initially, the nurse should tell the client to:**

   1. Stop taking the medication.

   2. Lie down and rest when these side effects occur.
   3. Report to the Clinic for a visit with his physician.
   4. Eat a diet high in potassium-rich foods.

   1. *Incorrect. This would not be appropriate information to give the client. It would be important for the client to have follow-up care to determine the cause of the symptomatology. Discontinuing antihypertensive therapy could be life-threatening to the client.*

   2. *Wrong. Cardiac arrhythmias are not "expected" side effects of Aldactone therapy and should not be ignored or tolerated. Another intervention is more appropriate at this time.*

   3. *Yes! Because Aldactone is a potassium-sparing diuretic used in the management of hypertension, the nurse must be alert for signs and symptoms of hyperkalemia: fatigue, muscle weakness, paresthesia, and cardiac arrhythmias. The client is advised to notify the physician if any of these signs/symptoms occur.*

   4. *No. This is not accurate information to give a client who is taking Aldactone. This action could exacerbate the problem with "palpitations and skipped heart beats."*

17. **Which of the following diagnostic studies should the nurse monitor most closely while the client is taking captopril (Capoten)?**

   1. Creatinine.
   2. Hemoglobin and hematocrit.
   3. Urinalysis.
   4. Serum glucose.

   1. *Right! Capoten should be used cautiously in clients with renal impairment because of the frequent side effect of proteinuria. Renal failure can also occur: creatinine, BUN, and electrolyte levels should be monitored periodically.*

   2. *Incorrect. Leukopenia can occur as a side effect: the white blood cell count (WBC) with differential should be monitored prior to initiation of therapy, every two weeks for the first three months, and periodically thereafter during the course of Capoten therapy.*

   3. *Wrong choice. A urinalysis will not give the most accurate assessment of renal function, although it is a good screening test. Make another selection.*

   4. *No. Capoten, an ACE inhibitor, does not affect the blood glucose level. Choose again.*

18. **A client is admitted to the hospital and is in the terminal stages of cancer. The nurse goes into his room to give him some medicine and finds him crying. The most appropriate nursing action is to:**

1. Sit with the client and hold his hand.
2. Tell the client that someone will call his minister, so that the minister can comfort him.
3. Notify the family to come to the hospital and stay with him.
4. Give the client his medication and allow him to cry in private.

*1. **Excellent! In this option, the nurse uses the communication tool of being silent, which conveys to the client that he is important. Holding the client's hand is a nonverbal way for the nurse to express understanding of the client's feelings. This response by the nurse is therapeutic.***
2. This response by the nurse uses the communication block of putting the client's needs on hold. Also, there is no information in the case scenario to indicate that he wishes to see the minister at this time. Do not read into the question! The nurse should respond therapeutically to the client's immediate needs.
3. In this action, the nurse does not respond to the client's immediate needs. Also, there is no information in the case situation to indicate that the client wishes to see his family at this time. Do not "read into" the question! The nurse should respond therapeutically to the client's immediate needs.
4. This is not an appropriate nursing action, since it ignores the fact that the client is crying. The nurse's response must be therapeutic for the client.

19. **The nurse's goal in positioning a client for a vaginal examination is to:**

1. Provide for the client's comfort.
2. Provide a position that promotes access for examination by the physician.
3. Provide for a position of comfort for the physician.
4. Provide the correct position while ensuring the client's comfort and privacy.

1. Providing for client's comfort is one aim of positioning. There is a more complete option.
2. Access to the examination site is important, but this is not a complete statement of the nurse's goal in positioning a client.
3. Although the physician's comfort during a procedure is important, it is not the nurse's goal in positioning a client.
*4. **Excellent! This is the only complete statement of the nurse's goal, which includes providing for the comfort and privacy needs of the client.***

20. **A client receiving cisplatin (Platinol) for his cancer develops a WBC count of 1,000 cells/mm³. What fact is important for the nurse to consider?**

1. The client has an increased chance of infection.
2. The client needs more foods high in iron.
3. The client needs additional fluids.
4. The family should be called to the bedside.

*1. **Correct! The normal white cell count should be 5-10,000 cells/mm³. A count this low puts the client at risk for an infection.***
2. Wrong. Foods high in iron will help anemia (a low red blood cell count) but not leukopenia (a low white cell count).
3. Wrong. Fluids will not help the client's WBC count.
4. Wrong choice! A low count is dangerous, but not a reason to call a family to the bedside. Treatment may need to be suspended for a while until the counts go higher.

21. **Which statement by a client indicates to the nurse an accurate understanding of pregnancy induced hypertension?**

1. "I should not get pregnant again, since pregnancy induced hypertension is likely to occur in subsequent pregnancies."
2. "I will have to be on a high protein diet for at least six months when I go home after delivery."
3. "As soon as the baby is delivered, I will not have any more hypertension, proteinuria, or edema."
4. "I will see my doctor regularly after I am discharged, because I may have an elevated blood pressure for a while."

1. Wrong! Pregnancy induced hypertension is most commonly seen in young primigravid clients. It is not a contraindication for future pregnancies.
2. No. The client will not require a high protein diet after delivery. Increased protein in the diet is required for pregnancy. Following delivery, the dietary need for protein will return to the usual level.
3. Not quite. Symptoms of pregnancy induced hypertension, including hypertension, proteinuria, and edema, may continue for up to 48 hours after delivery.
*4. **You are correct! The client should see her doctor regularly after discharge.***

> **TEST-TAKING TIP:** The word "may" in this option makes it appear more correct. Words like "may," "sometimes," "often," and "at least" — which are imprecise expressions — can actually make a statement correct. These words are clues that an option may be the correct answer.

22. **A 51-year-old man is admitted to an alcohol treatment unit. His wife reports that he has been drinking daily for 20 years and recently lost his driver's license for driving while intoxicated. During the**

admission interview, the client tells the nurse that he is only there because his wife has threatened to leave him if he does not get treatment. He states, "I only have one drink after work each evening." What is the most appropriate response for the nurse to make to his statement?

1. "What is your definition of "one" drink?"
2. "Are you feeling angry with your wife for insisting you get treatment?"
3. "If you only have one drink, how did you get a DWI?"
4. "Do you use any other drugs besides alcohol?"

1. *Correct. Estimating the client's alcohol consumption is necessary to determine how to best manage his withdrawal. The admitting nurse must ask the details of his alcohol use, including what he drinks, how much, how often, and does he use other substances besides alcohol. Some individuals could define one drink as a 12-ounce glass of bourbon.*
2. *This is not incorrect, but it is not the most appropriate response to the client's statement. The client is denying that he needs treatment.*
3. *No, this statement is provocative and most likely would elicit a defensive or argumentative response from the client that would not be therapeutic. The question asks for a response to the client's statement.*
4. *This is a good question to ask while taking a substance abuse history, but it is not the best response at this point in time, nor does it respond to the client's statement.*

23. A client is scheduled for a mastectomy in the morning. Her daughter is visiting and says to the nurse, "I should call my brothers and sisters and have them here in the morning just in case something goes wrong." The best response by the nurse would be:

1. To ask the mother if she would like her children there in the morning.
2. To suggest that the daughter ask her mother how she feels about that.
3. To say to the daughter, "If your brothers and sisters want to be here, they are welcome."
4. To ask the daughter what she knows about her mother's surgery and diagnosis.

1. *Wrong. Although the mother is the person with the health care problem, the client in the question is her daughter. The nursing response should be addressed to the daughter.*
2. *Wrong. The daughter is the client in this question. This response is not therapeutic for the daughter*

because it does not address her concern about her mother's impending surgery.
3. *Wrong. The daughter is the client in this question. This response is not therapeutic because it focuses on the needs of the brothers and sisters, not on the daughter's concerns about her mother's surgery. This response might also appear to the daughter to validate her fears about the surgery.*
4. *You are correct. The daughter is the client in this question, and the nurse is addressing the daughter's needs by clarifying the daughter's understanding of her mother's health problems. This response is therapeutic for the daughter.*

24. A client's psychiatrist orders lithium carbonate, 300 mg q.i.d. After five days, the nurse notes that the client's laboratory report indicates a serum lithium level of 1.0 mEq/liter. Based on this report, what nursing action is most appropriate at this time?

1. Withhold the next dose of lithium and notify the psychiatrist.
2. Ask that the laboratory test be repeated.
3. Assess the client for possible toxic effects.
4. Administer the next dose of lithium as ordered.

1. *This is not correct because the lithium level is within the therapeutic range. Identify a better option.*
2. *This is not necessary. The lithium level is within the therapeutic range.*
3. *Good try. The nurse should continuously assess the client's responses to medication. The question, however, is specific. What action is appropriate based on the laboratory report?*
4. *Correct. The lithium level is within the therapeutic range and therefore the next dose should be administered as ordered.*

25. An 18-month-old girl is admitted for a surgical repair of the cleft palate. She returns from the operating room, supine, with an IV, and a mist tent on room air. What is the priority nursing action?

1. Medicate for pain.
2. Check the IV for signs of infiltration.
3. Turn the child on her side.
4. Review the postoperative orders.

1. *Wrong. The child may need medication for pain at some point; however, this is not of immediate concern.*
2. *Wrong! The IV site should be checked frequently to assure patency and placement; however, this is not of immediate concern.*
3. *Great choice! Airway is always an immediate pri-*

ority. Turning the child on her side will protect the child from aspiration.

4. *Wrong choice! The postoperative orders should be reviewed when the child is admitted to the acute care floor. This would not take precedence, however, over establishing a patent airway in a child at risk for aspiration.*

26. **A client has just returned to her room after abdominal surgery. She has a nasogastric tube in place and a drain attached to a hemovac. A Foley catheter is draining clear yellow urine. The best rationale for the nurse ensuring that the side rails are up on the bed is which of the following?**

    1. To prevent the urine collection bag and tubing from getting tangled up in the side rails when the client is turned in bed.
    2. To prevent the client from falling out of bed after receiving an anesthetic.
    3. To provide a place to attach the nasogastric tubing to prevent it from being dislodged.
    4. To attach the call light so it is within easy reach.

    1. *This option might be a possibility. The urine collection bag and tubing can be attached to the side rails even if the side rails are lowered, so this is not a reason for having the side rails up on the bed.*
    2. **This is the correct answer. Postoperative clients who have received anesthesia usually are very sleepy and not aware of their surroundings. The client may fall out of bed if the side rails are not raised. This is the best option because it provides for the safety of the client. Good work!**
    3. *No! It is an incorrect nursing action to attach the nasogastric tube to the side rail, because it may become dislodged when the side rail is lowered or raised.*
    4. *This option might be a possibility. The call light can be attached to the side rail even if the side rails are lowered, so this is not the reason for having the side rails up on the bed.*

27. **While starting an intravenous infusion (IV), the nurse's gloved hands become contaminated with blood. The client has not been diagnosed with any organisms that are transmitted by way of the blood stream. Immediately upon completion of the task, the nurse should:**

    1. Remove the gloves carefully and complete a thorough handwashing.
    2. Wash the gloved hands, and then throw the gloves away.
    3. Prepare an incident report so that this occurrence will be documented, in case a health care problem develops at a later date.

    4. Ask the client to have a blood test to determine if a bloodborne pathogen is present in the client's blood.

    1. **Very good. Universal precautions require the use of gloves and hand washing in the care of all clients. This response addresses the issue in the question.**
    2. *Washing the gloves while still on the nurse's hands does not result in clean hands for the nurse. Handwashing is still required for infection control.*
    3. *Unless there is a break in the nurse's skin, there is no need for an incident report or further investigation.*
    4. *This is not a nursing action. If there is a concern about transmission of a disease, the nurse should follow the hospital protocol.*

28. **A 92-year-old client is admitted to the hospital with abdominal pain. During the initial assessment, the nurse notes that the client is not giving appropriate answers to questions. The client just nods and smiles while the nurse is talking to him. The nurse is probably dealing with what developmental problem?**

    1. The client is experiencing so much pain that he cannot focus on the nurse's questions.
    2. It must be assumed that the client is probably confused due to his age.
    3. The client is probably hard of hearing.
    4. Most elderly live in a fantasy world and are unable to comprehend what others say to them.

    1. *This is not correct. Clients in severe pain may not be able to focus on a conversation, but they would usually not be smiling. Also, the stem of the question asks you to identify a developmental issue.*
    2. *It is possible that the client is confused, however, the stem of the question asks you to identify a possible developmental problem. Confusion is not a developmental problem of the aging!*
    3. **Very good. The senses often diminish in the aged population. Therefore, it would not be unusual for the client to be hard of hearing. If he is hard of hearing, this could explain why the nurse is not receiving appropriate responses.**
    4. *This is not an accurate statement about the aging population! This cannot be the answer.*

29. **A client calls the prenatal clinic at 39 weeks of gestation to report that she just had a gush of fluid from the vagina. Which of the following is the best response by the nurse at this time?**

    1. "Your contractions will probably begin within the next 24 hours. If they do not, call back."

2. "You should not introduce anything into the vagina because rupture of membranes places you at risk for sepsis."

3. "You should come to the clinic for a short visit so we can assess you and the fetus."

4. "You should go to the labor unit at the hospital for admission."

1. *Wrong. Although this statement is correct, it is not the best response. Additional information needs to be given to a client with ruptured membranes who is not in labor.*

2. *Wrong. This statement is correct but not the best response because there is no attempt to evaluate the fetus in this option.*

3. *This is the best response because the risk of a prolapsed cord is greatest at the time of rupture of membranes. Evaluation of the fetal heart rate and the color of the amniotic fluid can provide the health care provider with valuable information regarding fetal well-being. This can only be done by seeing the client.*

4. *Incorrect. A client with ruptured membranes, who is not in labor, needs an evaluation of fetal well-being and teaching regarding the risk of sepsis, but this does not require hospitalization. An outpatient visit will suffice.*

30. **In planning care for a four-year-old admitted to the hospital, the nurse would include providing which toy?**

1. A plastic stethoscope.
2. A brightly colored mobile.
3. A jigsaw puzzle.
4. A helium balloon.

1. *You are correct! Pre-school play centers on imitation of adults. Providing a stethoscope allows the child to imitate the health personnel and to ease the fear of unfamiliar equipment.*

2. *Wrong! A brightly colored mobile is appropriate for a very young infant. It would not meet the activity needs of a pre-school child.*

3. *Wrong choice! A jigsaw puzzle is too difficult for most pre-school children and will frustrate them, rather than entertain them.*

4. *Wrong choice! Helium balloons might entertain the child, but the rubber in a deflated balloon presents a choking hazard.*

31. **The nurse knows that which of the following conditions would ineffectively be treated with aspirin?**

1. Arthritis.
2. A 102° F fever.

3. An ulcer.
4. A headache.

1. *Not this option. Aspirin and other NSAIDs are used for mild to moderate pain relief and to relieve the pain of arthritis. Remember, this question has a false response stem. You are looking for an INCORRECT statement.*

2. *Wrong choice. Fever is reduced by a peripheral vasodilatation effect, which results in sweating and heat loss. You are looking for an INCORRECT statement for this false response question.*

3. *Right choice! Aspirin is irritating to the stomach and causes bleeding; therefore, it would not be used for ulcers.*

4. *Aspirin and other NSAIDs are indeed used for mild to moderate pain relief. You are looking for something that should NOT be treated with aspirin.*

32. **The nurse working in a geriatric facility understands that an inaccurate generalization about the elderly is that:**

1. Their primary focus turns more inward, with a narrowing of outside interests.
2. They have the capacity to enjoy life and seek new experiences.
3. Their interest in sexual activity continues into old age as long as they enjoy good health and the availability of a partner.
4. They need a sense of being useful and activities that support this view.

1. *Correct. This is not an accurate statement about old age. As persons age, they continue to maintain outside interests and an active involvement in life. Those elders who do not are most likely suffering from a physical or emotional problem.*

2. *This is accurate, so it cannot be the correct option.*

3. *This is accurate, so it cannot be the correct option. One of the many myths about aging is that all interest in sexual activity disappears. The truth is that sexuality remains important for individuals of all ages.*

4. *This is accurate, so it cannot be the correct option. Research indicates that elders who continue to pursue useful activities into late life enjoy a happier and longer life than those who do not.*

33. **The nurse tells a client that she needs to be catheterized for a urine specimen. The client pulls the covers to her neck. She glances at the open door and says, "Someone might see me out there!" The best action by the nurse to alleviate the client's concern is:**

1. Explain the procedure to the client.
2. Obtain some assistance, since the client does not appear to be comfortable and may be resistant to the procedure.
3. Close the door and assure the client that you will cover her as much as possible during the procedure.
4. Gather all of the needed equipment before starting the procedure.

1. *Explaining the procedure is an appropriate nursing action, but it doesn't address the client's concern.*
2. *Although the client exhibits concern about privacy, the case situation does not indicate that she will be uncooperative. Do not "read into" the question! The client is communicating non-verbally to the nurse and indicating a concern for privacy. The nurse should respond therapeutically and address the client's concern.*
3. ***Very good! The client has expressed her concern for privacy. The nurse uses both verbal and non-verbal communication to respond therapeutically, addressing the client's concern.***

4. *This is an appropriate nursing action, but it does not address the client's concern.*

34. **A client taking lithium is discharged from the hospital after being taught to recognize the signs and symptoms of lithium toxicity. The nurse knows learning has occurred when the client calls the unit to report that she is experiencing which of the following?**

1. Vomiting and diarrhea.
2. Fine hand tremor.
3. Polyuria.
4. Drowsiness and lethargy.

1. ***Correct. Vomiting and diarrhea are early signs of lithium toxicity. The client should omit the next dose of lithium and notify the physician for instructions.***
2. *Fine hand tremor is a common side effect reported by about half of the clients on lithium. It is not a sign of impending toxicity.*
3. *Polyuria is a common side effect reported by about 60% of the clients on lithium. It is not a sign of impending toxicity.*
4. *Drowsiness and lethargy are common side effects of lithium and are not signs of impending toxicity.*

35. **A client returns from surgery for her fractured hip. Her family is waiting anxiously to see her. What is the most important parameter for the nurse to assess immediately after the client is transferred to her bed?**

1. The client's ability to deep breathe and cough.
2. The client's vital signs.
3. The surgical dressing.
4. Turn the client on the unaffected side.

1. *Incorrect choice. Having the client cough and deep breathe is an important measure, but it is not the most important assessment parameter at this time.*
2. ***A change in vital signs can provide the earliest indication that a complication of surgery is occurring. This is a vital assessment and the most important parameter for initial assessment after surgery.***
3. *The dressing should be observed for unusual bleeding or drainage, however, this assessment is not the most important initially.*
4. *Although this is an appropriate action for this client, it is not an assessment parameter. This is an implementation action. This option does not answer the question asked in the stem.*

36. **An ambulatory client is being readied for bed. The nursing action that promotes safety for this client is which of the following?**

1. Turning off all of the lights to help promote sleep and rest.
2. Instructing the client in the use of the call bell.
3. Putting the side rail up.
4. Placing the bed in the high position.

1. *No. Don't turn off all the lights. A small light should remain on in the event that the client wakes up to go to the bathroom and becomes disoriented to place.*
2. ***Right! The client should be instructed in the use of the call bell in the event that help is needed.***
3. *No! Putting the side rails up on a client that is ambulatory could cause a fall if the client attempted to climb over them to get out of bed.*
4. *No! A client who is ambulatory should have the bed in a low position to prevent a fall when getting out of bed.*

37. **As a health care professional caring for sick clients, it is imperative that the nurse practice good personal hygiene. Good personal hygiene includes all of the following except:**

1. Clean, well groomed hair.
2. A light, fragrant cologne.
3. Good oral hygiene.
4. Absence of body odor.

1. *Clean, well groomed hair helps to prevent transmission of bacteria and is important in personal hygiene. This is not the answer, because this question has a false response stem.*
2. ***Very good! Many sick clients have a heightened awareness of odors, and even mild colognes can be nauseating.***
3. *Fresh smelling breath is important, since the nurse spends much time talking with clients. This is not the answer, because this question has a false response stem.*
4. *Body odor is offensive to most people. Since the nurse works closely with clients, good body hygiene is very important. This is not the answer, because this question has a false response stem.*

38. **A 25-year-old female client is taking ampicillin (Omnipen) and birth control pills containing estrogen. What information should the nurse provide?**

1. Take both medications with breakfast to avoid gastric upset.
2. When used together, serum potassium levels may rise.
3. The effect of the birth control pills may be reduced while the client is taking ampicillin.
4. Urticaria is much more common when antibiotics are given with other drugs.

1. *Wrong! Taking ampicillin with food may interfere with its effectiveness, so this would not be advisable.*
2. *No. Potassium levels are only monitored with IV penicillins that contain high amounts of potassium, such as penicillin G potassium.*
3. ***Good choice! Estrogen metabolism is increased, or there is a reduction of enterohepatic circulation of estrogens, when ampicillin is taken by a woman using birth control pills. Another form of birth control should be used while a client is on ampicillin.***
4. *This is not correct. Urticaria can occur with a sensitivity penicillin, regardless of whether another medication is being used.*

39. **An elderly client is admitted to a long-term care facility. Which of the following measures would be most important in planning his care?**

1. An explanation of the roles of the registered nurse, practical nurse and the nursing assistant.
2. An understanding of his routine for his own care at home.
3. An assessment of his mobility.
4. An introduction to his health care team members.

1. *The question focuses on the most important nursing measure. Explanations to the client are necessary to help the client feel comfortable in the new surroundings, however, this is not the most important action. This is an implementation action. The question is directed to what is needed in planning care.*
2. ***Congratulations! This is a difficult question! It is most important that the nurse find out and understand the client's routines at home so that these routines may be integrated in his present care. The goal of the nurse is to create a safe environment for the client. Following pre-existing routines will help the client feel more secure and less threatened. This question requires the ability to plan nursing care for an elderly client.***
3. *This is a good choice, but not the best answer. The ability of the client to move and care for himself is important. It just isn't the most important measure among the listed options.*
4. *Like Option 1, this option involves giving information to the client. Since these options are similar, both are incorrect. The question focuses on the most important nursing measure. Introducing the members of the health care team is important to help the client feel safe and comfortable in his new surroundings but it is not the most important action among the listed alternatives.*

40. **The nurse understands that prednisone is used in treating cancers because of which effect?**

1. Antimicrobial.
2. Anticoagulant.
3. Anti-inflammatory.
4. Anti-infective.

1. *Incorrect. Prednisone does not have an antimicrobial effect. Antimicrobials are antibiotics, like penicillin.*
2. *No, heparin and coumadin are anticoagulants, which prevent blood clotting.*
3. ***Correct. Prednisone has a wide variety of effects, but its anti-inflammatory properties help with the treatment of cancers by suppressing swelling.***
4. *No, anti-infectives include antibiotics or antimicrobials.*

41. **A client is admitted to the hospital with abdominal pain. She overhears her doctor and nurse discussing cancer of the liver. Later, she says to her nurse, "Having cancer of the liver must be a terrible thing." Which of the following statements would be the best response by the nurse?**

1. "Yes, it is a terrible disease."
2. "What made you think about cancer of the liver?"
3. "Any kind of cancer is terrible, but you can't live

without a liver."
4. "Yes it is. A client on this floor has it, and it's sad for everyone."

1. This response is a factual statement but it doesn't encourage further communication between the nurse and the client. The client has an obvious concern or she wouldn't have mentioned the subject. Her need for more information should be addressed by the nurse.
2. **Correct! This question clarifies for the nurse why the client is concerned about cancer of the liver. The case situation tells you that the client overheard her doctor and nurse talking about a client. The client may think that the conversation concerned her. This response by the nurse enhances therapeutic communication through clarification.**

> **STRATEGY ALERT!** Note that the phrase "cancer of the liver" appears in both the question and this option. This is a clue that this might be the correct answer.

3. This response by the nurse does not identify or clarify why the client is talking about this particular illness. The nurse needs more information, and this response deters the client from pursuing this topic any further.
4. This response does not address the client in the question. It addresses the other client and "everyone" who is sad. This response can also be interpreted as a breach in confidentiality for the client who has the cancer. This is an inappropriate response.

42. **When the mother of a five-year-old boy expresses concern over her son's stuttering, which response by the nurse is least appropriate?**

1. Vocal hesitancy is common in children younger than age seven.
2. It may help if you stop your son and encourage him to begin the word over.
3. Singing songs or nursery rhymes may ease stuttering.
4. Look directly at your son while he is speaking.

1. Wrong choice, this response could be quite appropriate. Vocal hesitancy is common in young children and often corrects itself. The mother may feel reassured that her son is not yet at an age where stuttering is of concern.
2. **Correct! It would not be appropriate to advise stopping the child mid-word or mid-sentence. Such an intervention often draws attention to the stuttering and may actually worsen it.**
3. No, this response is very appropriate! The repetition of songs and nursery rhymes may help the child speak more smoothly.

4. Wrong choice, this is a very appropriate response! Offering the child full attention, without rushing the child or drawing attention to the stuttering, will assist the child in speaking clearly.

43. **A 72-year-old client was admitted to the hospital for pneumonia. He is receiving oxygen at six liters by mask. The nurse would avoid which action, when obtaining his vital signs?**

1. Take an axillary temperature.
2. Listen to his lungs when counting respirations.
3. Listen to an apical heart rate.
4. Take an oral temperature.

1. No, the nurse does not have to avoid this action. An oral temperature of a client receiving oxygen therapy via nasal cannula or mask is not a reliable measurement. Axillary temperature would be unaffected by the O_2 therapy. The stem of the question asks for an action the nurse should AVOID.
2. Not a correct choice. The nurse should auscultate the lungs because the client has pneumonia. The stem of the question asks for a false statement, so look for an action the nurse should AVOID.
3. Incorrect choice. Auscultating an apical heart rate in an elderly client is important because it allows the nurse to assess for any abnormal heart sounds. This question has a false response stem. Look for an action the nurse should AVOID.
4. **Very good! This is an action the nurse should avoid because the oral temperature of a client receiving oxygen therapy via nasal cannula or mask is not a reliable measurement.**

44. **When administering the first dose of enalapril (Vasotec) to a client, it is most important for the nurse to closely monitor the client's:**

1. Pulse rate.
2. Blood pressure.
3. Urine output.
4. Level of consciousness.

1. Incorrect. Tachycardia can occur with administration of Vasotec, but is not that common. The physician should be notified of any significant changes in the pulse during the course of drug therapy.
2. **Absolutely. A common side effect of Vasotec is hypotension: the blood pressure should be monitored frequently during initial dosage adjustment. A precipitous drop in blood pressure during the first one to three hours following the first dose may require volume expansion with normal saline, but is not normally considered an indication for stopping therapy. The client must be monitored closely for at least one hour after blood pressure has stabilized.**

3. *Wrong choice. Renal failure or oliguria are rare side effects in the absence of preexisting renal disease. The nurse would want to monitor urine output but under the facts given in this question, the nurse would more closely monitor another parameter.*

4. *Not indicated. The central nervous system (CNS) side effects that commonly occur are dizziness, headache, and fatigue not change in level of consciousness.*

45. **Before she is discharged from the hospital, a client and her husband attend a client education class on the topic of depression. The nurse instructs them about behaviors that could indicate a recurrence of depression. Which symptom would the nurse avoid including in the instruction?**

    1. Psychomotor retardation.
    2. Grandiosity.
    3. Self-devaluation.
    4. Insomnia.

    1. *Wrong choice. This behavior could indicate a recurrence of depression, so it cannot be the correct option.*
    2. **Correct. Grandiosity is not associated with depression; it is associated with the manic phase of bipolar depression. The nurse would not include grandiosity in an instruction about signs and symptoms of depression.**
    3. *Wrong. This behavior could indicate a recurrence of depression, so it cannot be the correct option.*
    4. *Insomnia or hypersomnia are two interrupted sleep patterns that are associated with depression. This is not correct because this negative response question asks for an option that describes a behavior the nurse would NOT include in an instruction about signs and symptoms of depression.*

46. **The nurse is teaching a client about self breast exams. The client tells the nurse that she doesn't understand why she is being taught this since she doesn't plan on doing it anyway. The best response by the nurse would be:**

    1. "Self breast exam is taught to women to detect any lumps or changes in the breast that can be an early sign of cancer, and early treatment has a higher rate of cure."
    2. "You're right. If you don't plan on doing the exam, then I don't need to show you how to do it."
    3. "If you don't plan on doing the exam yourself, then you should have your doctor do it at your annual check up."
    4. "It is your body and you have the right to do whatever you choose."

    1. **Correct! This response by the nurse gives the cli-**

ent information concerning the rationale for self breast exams. This response provides information that will allow the client to make an informed choice. The communication strategy is to give information.*

STRATEGY ALERT! *Note that Options 2 and 4 are similar in that they both support the client's decision not to do the self exams. Similar distractors should be eliminated.*

2. *This response indicates that the nurse has become defensive, which is a block to communication because it places the client also on the defensive. This approach does not promote therapeutic communication.*

3. *Having a physician perform an exam annually is a good validation action but it should not replace monthly self exams. This is not an appropriate response, since it does not address the need for regular breast exams to detect early changes and it implies that this is an acceptable recommendation. It does not provide for further explanation of the client's statement.*

4. *Although it is true that clients should have choices concerning their health care, the choices should be informed choices. This client has made a decision without the benefit of an explanation of the rationale for the intervention. This response does not encourage any further communication and is not therapeutic.*

47. **A two-year-old girl is admitted to the hospital with croup. She has been placed in a mist tent with room air. Which statement by the parents indicates effective client teaching?**

    1. "The mist will give my child extra fluids."
    2. "My child must remain in the mist tent at all times."
    3. "My child may have toys inside the mist tent."
    4. "The mist tent will provide the extra oxygen my child needs."

    1. *Wrong! The amount of moisture that the child breathes in will not add to her fluid intake.*
    2. *Incorrect! While the mist tent will benefit the child, the child may be removed for short periods of time, particularly if the child is upset and needs to be held.*
    3. **Correct! A goal of treatment is to keep the child quiet and calm to reduce oxygen demand. Toys may help achieve this goal.**
    4. *Wrong! The mist tent on room air only provides cool humidity, not oxygen.*

48. **A client, age 23, is currently taking oral amoxicillin and clavulanate (Augmentin) for otitis media. She also takes birth control pills containing estrogen. Which of the following instruc-**

tions should the client be given?

1. Take both medicines as prescribed.
2. An alternate method of birth control should be used while taking Augmentin.
3. There is an increased risk of hypersensitivity when both these medications are taken at the same time.
4. Drink extra fluids while taking the Augmentin to prevent kidney damage.

1. *Exactly! You remembered that an alternate method of birth control is only required when a client is taking ampicillin, bacampicillin, or penicillin V.*
2. *Incorrect. Recall that there are only three antibiotics that require this action: ampicillin, bacampicillin, or penicillin V. With this information, now make the correct choice.*
3. *No. Although hypersensitivity is always a concern when antibiotics are given, there is no evidence that these two medications are synergistic in that regard.*
4. *Not necessary. Augmentin should be taken with food to minimize GI distress and an adequate fluid intake is important for general good health, but extra fluids are not indicated. This drug should be used cautiously in clients with renal impairment because it is excreted by the kidneys.*

49. **An emergency room nurse is assessing a client for cocaine intoxication. The nurse knows that all of the following symptoms are associated with cocaine intoxication except?**

1. Seizures.
2. Hyperactivity.
3. Paranoid behavior.
4. Nystagmus.

1. *Wrong choice. Higher doses of cocaine, and the use of "crack," can cause seizures.*
2. *No. This false response question asks for a symptom NOT associated with cocaine use. Hyperactivity and hyper alertness are common effects of cocaine intoxication.*
3. *This is not the correct option because paranoid behavior can be a symptom associated with cocaine intoxication. Look for a symptom the nurse would NOT expect to find.*
4. *Correct. Nystagmus frequently occurs with the use of PCP, NOT cocaine.*

50. **A client uses tamoxifen (Nolvadex) for her cancer. The nurse knows that tamoxifen has which of the following actions?**

1. Antimicrobial.
2. Anti-estrogenic.
3. Androgenic.

4. Anti-inflammatory.

1. *Wrong. Tamoxifen does not have an antimicrobial effect.*
2. *Right choice! Tamoxifen is used to treat cancer of the breast in both pre- and post menopausal women. It has been shown to delay recurrences.*
3. *Wrong choice! Androgens are the male hormones and are used to treat breast cancer. Tamoxifen is an anti-estrogen and does not increase male hormone production.*
4. *Incorrect! Tamoxifen does not have an anti-inflammatory effect.*

51. **A confused elderly client has wet herself and is standing in the hospital corridor in a puddle of urine. She has trouble getting to the bathroom in time. She looks ashamed. She says to the nurse, "I want to go outside for a walk now." Which of the following statements would be the most therapeutic response by the nurse?**

1. "Before we go for a walk, perhaps we can make a list that will help you make your bathroom trips easier."
2. "Right now, let me wipe up the urine on the floor, and let's get a change of clothing for you. I am sure that this problem is upsetting for you."
3. "This has been a problem for you. Let's see if we can find a solution together."
4. "Wetting yourself is very upsetting. Yes, let's take a walk."

1. *The issue in this question is a wet client standing in a puddle of urine. This response does not address the current problem. Also, the client is confused, so making a list is not an appropriate action.*
2. *Right! This response deals with the here and now by helping the client focus on her current need, which is dry clothes, and is informing the client that she is going to wipe up the urine off the floor. The nurse is also showing empathy. This response is therapeutic for the client.*

> **STRATEGY ALERT!** The words "urine on the floor" in this option are similar to the words "puddle of urine" in the question. This is a clue that this may be the correct answer.

3. *The client is feeling uncomfortable, and her basic needs for dry clothes and a safe environment must be met. The client is also confused, and she is feeling ashamed. Discussing possible solutions to the problem of not being able to get to the bathroom in time will not be helpful.*
4. *In this response, the nurse is showing empathy, however, the response does not address the client's basic need at this time for dry clothes, or the nurs-*

ing priority of wiping up the urine off the floor.

52. **A 98-year-old client was admitted to the hospital with a cerebral vascular accident with left-sided paralysis. He is placed on an air mattress, and anticoagulant therapy is ordered. The best nursing rationale for turning this client every two hours is which of the following?**

    1. To prevent sensory deprivation by varying what the client sees in his environment.
    2. To prevent skin breakdown, which is a common problem in the elderly.
    3. To prevent stasis of blood in the lower extremities.
    4. To increase blood supply to the affected side.

    1. *Although this is accomplished by turning a client, it is not the best rationale for turning this client. Read the other options, and try to identify a better rationale.*
    2. **Correct. The elderly have very thin, fragile skin that breaks down very easily. Therefore, in order to prevent bed sores, the client should be turned every two hours.**
    3. *This is not a rationale for turning the client, because turning the client does not prevent stasis of blood. Contraction of the muscles or support stockings are measures that help prevent stasis of blood in the lower extremities. This cannot be the answer.*
    4. *No. Increased blood supply may reach the affected side by turning the client, but only every other two hours! This is not the best reason for turning this client. Read the other options, and try to identify a better rationale.*

53. **A one-year-old boy is brought to the physician's office with fever, irritability, and loss of appetite. A diagnosis of otitis media is made, and the child is placed on p.o. amoxicillin with clavulanate (Augmentin) 150 mg t.i.d. for 10 days. Which nursing instruction must be included in the child's plan of care?**

    1. "Drink clear fluids while on the medication."
    2. "Take an extra nap, since amoxicillin may cause drowsiness."
    3. "Stay indoors until the medication is finished."
    4. "Take the medication for the full length of time."

    1. *Wrong! It is not necessary to be on clear fluids only, and clear fluids may not offer complete nutrition.*
    2. *Wrong! Amoxicillin does not cause drowsiness. The child may need extra sleep while recovering, but this is not a priority.*
    3. *Wrong! There is no reason why the child should stay indoors, provided the child is adequately*

dressed for the weather. Keeping the child indoors for 10 days may limit his activity unnecessarily.

    4. ***Congratulations! A full course of an antibiotic must be given to ensure that the medication is completely effective. Incomplete courses may result in recurrent and/or resistant infections.***

54. **A two-year-old boy is receiving bleomycin (Blenoxane) IV. His mother tells the nurse that it is time for her son to have his polio immunization. What is the best response by the nurse?**

    1. "We will schedule it for next week."
    2. "The cancer drug will delay any possibility of polio."
    3. "Your son's immunizations will need to be delayed until a later time."
    4. "I'll call the doctor later today."

    1. *Wrong! This in not an appropriate response because the vaccine cannot be given at this time.*
    2. *This is an incorrect statement. In addition, it is inadvisable to tell parents not to worry.*
    3. ***Excellent choice! You remembered it was unsafe to give a live virus vaccine while the client was being treated for cancer. The vaccine will need to be given at a later date.***
    4. *Incorrect choice! It is inappropriate to cause the mother to worry more about the situation. The immunizations will be given later.*

55. **What foods does the nurse recommend that a pregnant client with iron-deficiency anemia include in her diet to increase iron intake?**

    1. Green leafy vegetables, dried fruits, and beans.
    2. Milk and cheese.
    3. Coffee and bran.
    4. Snack foods, mid morning and afternoon.

    1. ***Correct. Green leafy vegetables, dried fruits and beans are rich in iron.***
    2. *No, although milk and dairy products provide important nutrients, including calcium, they actually interfere with absorption of iron.*
    3. *No, coffee and foods high in fiber will retard absorption.*
    4. *No, snack foods are high in fat content and would not be recommended.*

56. **The psychiatrist orders tranylcypromine (Parnate) for a depressed client who has not responded to tricyclics. The nurse knows that dietary teaching is essential. The nurse's instructions to the client advise her to avoid all of the following except:**

1. Beer and red wine.
2. Cheddar cheese and sausage.
3. Cottage cheese and canned peaches.
4. Liver and Italian green beans.

1. Beer and red wine should be avoided, but this stem is asking for a false response. Read the options to identify the substances that the client does NOT have to avoid.

2. Cheddar, or other aged cheeses, and sausage, or other cured or aged meats, should be avoided. This stem is asking which substances the client does NOT have to avoid. Read the options again.

3. *Correct. Cottage cheese and cream cheese are two cheeses that can be safely eaten because they are not aged. Also, most fresh fruits are allowed.*

4. Liver and Italian green beans (fava beans) should be avoided. Read the other options to identify the substances that do NOT have to be avoided.

57. **A client is admitted to the hospital with active tuberculosis. She is placed in respiratory isolation and started on medication. A chest x-ray is ordered. While transporting the client to x-ray, the nurse should do which of the following?**

1. Wear a mask and gown for protection from the client's organisms.
2. Have the client wear a mask and protect the wheel chair with a clean bath blanket or sheet.
3. Have x-ray come to the client's room to do the x-ray.
4. No special precautions need to be taken.

1. When a client with a communicable disease is being transported to another department in the hospital, it is important to protect everyone with whom the client may come in contact — not just the nurse!

2. *Very good! This answer addresses what the nurse should do while transporting the client, to provide protection for anyone who may come in contact with the client.*

3. The case scenario does not state that a portable x-ray was ordered. The stem of the question very specifically asks what the nurse should do while transporting the client to x-ray. This option does not address the issue of the question!

4. The case scenario states that the client is in respiratory isolation, which indicates that something should be done to prevent the spread of the disease to others in the hospital.

58. **A client is in the hospital because of severe weight loss and refusal to eat. The physician orders the insertion of a nasogastric tube for feeding. The** nurse finds the client with the tube removed. The client tells that nurse that he "doesn't need that thing." Which of the following is the most appropriate response by the nurse?

1. "You shouldn't have done that! Now I have to put it down again."
2. "Why did you pull that tube out? Do you want to die?"
3. "Tell me what you don't like about the tube."
4. "Your doctor is going to be very upset with you for doing this."

1. Wrong! This response implies that the nurse is inconvenienced by the client's actions. "You shouldn't have done that!" is a judgmental statement that is non-therapeutic and therefore not an appropriate response.

2. This response is judgmental because it implies that the client did something wrong and that he did it because he wants to die. The response also puts the client on the defensive by requesting an explanation with a "why" question, which is a block to therapeutic communication.

3. *Correct. This response allows the client to tell the nurse how he feels about the tube and what it means to him. It promotes therapeutic communication and doesn't judge the client's actions.*

4. This response focuses not on the client but on the doctor. It also expresses the opinion of the nurse, which is not important. This response is judgmental in that it implies that the client did something that is wrong because his doctor is not going to be happy with him. Therapeutic communication promotes the expression of the client's feelings. This option does not promote communication.

59. **A client is admitted with anorexia nervosa. A nasogastric tube is to be inserted. The best nursing approach to prepare the client for the procedure would include which action?**

1. Assist the client to a sitting position.
2. Explain the procedure to the client.
3. Make sure that any dentures are securely in place in the client's mouth.
4. Have a stethoscope available to listen for proper placement.

1. This is an appropriate position, but it is not the best nursing approach. The word "best" is a key word in the stem of the question.

2. *Excellent! Having the client well-informed reduces fear and is helpful in gaining the cooperation of the client, which is necessary for implementation of this procedure.*

3. *This is an inappropriate action. Insertion of an NG tube may induce gagging. Dentures could become dislodged and cause the client to choke. Dentures should be removed before this procedure.*

4. *The stem asks for "the best nursing approach to prepare the client" for insertion of an NG tube. Although a stethoscope is necessary to allow the nurse to hear air that might be instilled into the stomach, this measure does not prepare the client for the procedure.*

60. An elderly client expresses feelings of grief for his earlier life. Which nursing action is most appropriate to best help the client cope with this stage in his life?

1. Listening attentively and allowing the client to talk about the past.
2. Giving the client some activities to perform so he won't have time to dwell on the past.
3. Let the client know that this is a common problem of the aging population.
4. Tell the client about some of the younger clients in the hospital who are in worse shape than he is.

1. ***Excellent. Listening to the client allows for ventilation of the client's feelings about the loss of a healthy, active life. This facilitation is the best nursing intervention to help the client cope.***

2. *Providing the client with activities will help pass time, but will not help the client cope with the loss that he is experiencing. The client's feelings of loss are the issue in this question. The answer must address the issue. The nurse should help the client deal with his feelings.*

3. *This is not therapeutic because this kind of generalization devalues the client's feelings. The client's feelings of loss are the issue in this question. The nurse should help the client cope with his feelings.*

4. *This is not therapeutic because it devalues the client's feelings. The client's feelings of loss are the issue in this question. The nurse should help the client cope with his feelings.*

61. A 52-year-old client is scheduled for coronary artery bypass surgery in the morning. Before the surgery she states to the nurse, "I don't think I'm going to have the surgery. Everybody has to die sometime." The best nursing response would be?

1. "If you don't have the surgery, you will most likely die sooner."
2. "There are always risks involved with surgery. Why have you changed your mind about the operation?"
3. "Bypass surgery must be very frightening for you. Tell me how you feel about the surgery."

4. "I will call your doctor and have him come in and talk to you."

1. *Wrong! This response devalues the client's feelings and is a block to any further communication!*

2. *The first part of this response addresses the procedure but not the client's fear. The second part is an illustration of requesting an explanation. The nurse has asked a question beginning with the word "why." This can be intimidating and is a communication block. To be therapeutic, the response should address the client's feelings.*

3. ***Very good! The nurse's response shows empathy and focuses on the client's feelings in a nonthreatening way by using the communication tool of clarification.***

4. *This response does not address the client's feelings and puts the issue of the client's feelings on hold. This is not the best response.*

62. The nurse is teaching a class of expectant mothers. A woman asks if the fluid surrounding the fetus in utero is important. The nurse's explanation to the group is based on an understanding that all of the following are functions of amniotic fluid except?

1. Cushion the fetus against injury.
2. Control the fetus's body temperature.
3. Provide nutritional exchange for the fetus.
4. Allow freedom of movement for the fetus.

1. *Wrong, this is an accurate statement. The fluid surrounding the fetus serves as a cushion against injury. Remember, this question has a false response stem and is asking for an inaccurate statement.*

2. *Wrong, this is an accurate statement. This false response stem is looking for a statement that is inaccurate. The fetal body temperature is related to the temperature of the amniotic fluid.*

3. ***Correct choice. Although the fetus does swallow the amniotic fluid, it has no nutritional value. The only source of nutrition and oxygenation for the fetus is through the placenta.***

4. *Wrong. If there is not sufficient fluid, the ability of the fetus to move is impeded. Remember, this question has a false response stem and is asking for a statement that is incorrect.*

63. A 66-year-old man is an out-patient taking tricyclic antidepressants. The client's wife telephones the clinic and tells the nurse that she has just found her husband lying unconscious and his empty bottle of medication on the nightstand. Overdoses of tricyclic antidepressants are:

1. Medical emergencies.
2. Serious but rarely fatal.
3. Dangerous for clients in poor health.
4. Easily treated by inducing vomiting.

1.   Correct! Tricyclics are among the most dangerous substances available when taken in overdose. Emergency medical attention and hospitalization should be sought for any client who has over-dosed, regardless of the amount ingested. Serious, life threatening symptoms can develop over the three to five days following the overdose.

2.   This is not an accurate statement. Tricyclics are extremely dangerous and often fatal if emergency medical care is not obtained. This cannot be the correct answer.

3.   This is not accurate because overdoses are equally dangerous for all clients, regardless of their health status.

4.   Although the ingested drug should be removed by gastric lavage or emesis, overdoses require additional medical treatment, including close electro-cardiogram monitoring.

64.   **During postoperative recovery, a client develops a tachyarrhythmia. The physician prescribes pro-pranolol (Inderal) 1 mg by slow IV push, not to exceed 1 mg/minute. The nurse should monitor the client for which of the following adverse reactions?**

1. Congestive heart failure (CHF).
2. Hypertensive crisis.
3. Intestinal obstruction.
4. Seizures.

1.   Correct. Inderal is a beta-adrenergic blocker that decreases heart rate and blood pressure, along with AV conduction. Life-threatening side effects are congestive heart failure, pulmonary edema, and bradycardia. The client should be assessed routinely for evidence of CHF (peripheral edema, dyspnea, rales/crackles, fatigue, weight gain, jugular venous distention).

2.   No. Inderal is a beta-adrenergic blocker that decreases heart rate and blood pressure. The side effect would be hypotension--not hypertension.

3.   Wrong. Frequent side effects of Inderal are nausea, vomiting, and diarrhea. Although constipation may occur, it is not common nor does it lead to intestinal obstruction.

4.   Incorrect. Inderal may cause central nervous system side effects of fatigue, depression, weakness, and insomnia, but seizures are not seen. Choose again.

65.   **A client fell at home and fractured her hip. She is to have surgery in the morning. In preparing the client for surgery, what is outside the scope of the nurse's responsibility?**

1. Assessing the health status of the client.
2. Explaining the operative procedure and any risks that may be involved with the procedure.
3. Determining that the history, physical, and specific laboratory tests have been ordered or completed according to hospital protocol.
4. Determine that a signed surgical consent form is completed.

1.   This is an expected standard of care for the preoperative client. However, the question has a false response stem so this is not the correct answer.

2.   Excellent! Explaining the procedure and risks is a physician responsibility. This is not a nursing responsibility. Since this question has a false response stem, this is the only correct option and the answer.

3.   This action is a nursing responsibility that is part of record keeping and helps assure the safety of the client. However, the question has a false response stem so this is not the correct answer.

4.   A signed surgical consent is necessary for this case situation. It is a nursing responsibility to assure that the signed consent form is on the client's chart prior to surgery. This accurate statement is not the answer, however, since this question has a false response stem.

66.   **Which of the following assessments made by the nurse could be considered a manifestation of the most potentially life-threatening side effect of captopril (Capoten)?**

1. Rash.
2. Fever.
3. Dry cough.
4. Tachycardia.

1.   Incorrect. Rashes are common side effects of Capoten therapy and are not considered life-threatening. Make another selection.

2.   Absolutely right! Fever is an indication of an inflammatory/infectious process somewhere in the body. A life-threatening side effect of Capoten therapy is neutropenia, which means that a client can die from a simple respiratory infection without neutrophils present to fight the causative organisms. The client's WBC with differential should be monitored prior to initiation of therapy, every two weeks for the first three months, and periodically thereafter during the course of drug therapy.

3. *Wrong. Dry cough is not a common side effect of Capoten therapy (although it can occur). A productive cough should be reported immediately to the physician because of the risk of respiratory infection, which can be life-threatening if the client's WBC count is decreased.*
4. ***No. Tachycardia is not a frequently occurring side effect and is not as life-threatening as that of another option.***

67. **A client is to receive his first injection of interferon, alfa-2a, recombinant (Roferon-A) for his hairy cell leukemia. What side effects would the nurse advise the client to expect?**

1. Reduced urine output.
2. Severe vomiting.
3. Flu-like symptoms.
4. Weight gain.

1. *Wrong. Interferon is a natural body protein and does not affect the kidneys.*
2. *No, severe vomiting would be an unexpected side effect.*
3. ***Correct. The symptoms from interferon are usually mild and include malaise, fever, nausea and some vomiting.***
4. *Wrong choice! Weight gain is not a problem with interferon. Nausea and vomiting are more likely to occur.*

68. **During the assessment of an elderly client, which of the following effects of the aging process would the nurse be most likely to find?**

1. Decline in physiological and sensory systems of the body.
2. Decreased skin resilience.
3. Diminished hearing acuity.
4. Absent sexual activity.

1. ***Good! This is a general statement about the effects of aging.***
2. *Loss of skin resilience is a normal finding in the elderly. However, this is not the best option.*
3. *Many elderly clients experience some hearing loss. This is an expected finding in the elderly. However, this is not the best option.*
4. *Wrong. Sexual activity does not cease in the elderly.*

69. **A client is six weeks pregnant with her first baby. She asks the nurse when she will experience quickening. The nurse tells her that most clients feel quickening:**

1. During the last weeks of pregnancy.
2. Between the second and third months of pregnancy.
3. Between the fourth and fifth months of pregnancy.
4. Soon after implantation, once the uterus begins to rise out of the pelvis.

1. *Quickening is the perception of fetal movement and should certainly be felt earlier than the last weeks of pregnancy.*
2. *Incorrect, since this is too early for the client to feel fetal movement.*
3. ***Correct, most women will feel fetal movement between 16 and 20 weeks. It is wise to give them this range so that the woman does not worry when she doesn't feel movement by the fourth month or 16 weeks.***
4. *Incorrect, since this is too early for the client to feel fetal movement.*

70. **In prescribing medication for an elderly psychiatric client, the nurse knows which of the following statements about elderly clients is most accurate?**

1. The elderly cannot be safely treated with tricyclic antidepressants.
2. The elderly require lower doses of antidepressants than younger clients.
3. The elderly respond more quickly to the therapeutic effects of antidepressants than younger clients.
4. The elderly can be treated safely and effectively with all antidepressants.

1. *This is not accurate. A careful assessment must be done to rule out clients with cardiac problems or glaucoma. If an elderly client does not have these medical problems, she can safely be treated with antidepressants, especially those that have a lower incidence of anticholinergic side effects.*
2. ***Correct. Elderly clients are treated with lower doses because of their increased sensitivity to the anticholinergic and cardiovascular side effects.***
3. *This is not accurate. Response rates can take up to three to four weeks for all clients, regardless of age.*
4. *This is not accurate. It is best to avoid treating elderly clients with those antidepressants that have a higher incidence of anticholinergic or orthostatic hypotensive side effects.*

71. **A client, 65 years old, is admitted to the hospital for surgery after finding a lump in his right testicle. He asks the nurse, "Do you think the doctor will find cancer?" Which of the following statements would be the most appropriate nursing response?**

1. "Most lumps found in the testicles are benign."
2. "It must be difficult for you not to know what the doctor will find."
3. "I think that you should discuss this with your doctor."
4. "It might be, but the doctor won't know until the surgery is performed."

1. *This may be an accurate statement, but it does not allow the client to express his fears concerning cancer. This response blocks communication between the client and the nurse.*
2. ***Very good! This response promotes communication by allowing the client to express his feelings.***
3. *Referring the client's concern to the doctor puts the client's concern on hold and is not a therapeutic nursing response. The client's feelings and concerns need to be addressed by the nurse.*
4. *This response does not help the client to explore his feelings and is not a therapeutic nursing response.*

72. **A client is in the intensive care unit and is in a coma as a result of a head injury. The most important action in performing mouth care on this client is to:**

1. Turn the client to her side before starting mouth care.
2. Use a soft toothbrush.
3. Use a mouth bite to keep her mouth open.
4. Wear gloves.

1. ***Very good! Turning the client on her side is the most important intervention, since it will help prevent aspiration of the fluids used for cleaning the mouth.***
2. *A soft toothbrush is preferred, but this is not the most important action in this procedure.*
3. *This intervention is helpful while cleaning the mouth, but this is not the most important action in this procedure.*
4. *The nurse should wear gloves, but is it not the most important action in this procedure.*

73. **A client has been admitted to the hospital with vomiting, diarrhea and extreme weakness. Her husband has stayed at her bedside since admission. She is on bed rest and is receiving IV therapy. A nursing intervention that will best promote rest and comfort for the client would be:**

1. Having the client's husband leave the room for a while so she can sleep.
2. Keeping the emesis basin and bedpan empty and clean for her use.
3. Leaving the bedpan on the bedside stand so it is within easy reach.
4. Closing the door to the client's room.

1. *The case scenario does not state that the client's husband is not allowing her to rest. Do not "read into" the question!*
2. ***Very good. Since vomitus and stool are a source of odor, it is important for the nurse to eliminate any odors that can cause discomfort for the client. It is also important to have these utensils available for the client's use.***
3. *This is an inappropriate action. Remember that the bedpan is a dirty utensil, and should not be placed in a clean area.*
4. *While closing the door may provide some privacy and decreased noise, the issue of the question is vomiting and diarrhea. The stem asks for an intervention that will promote rest and comfort for this client. This is not the best response.*

74. **A client is very confused and combative. The physician orders the client to be placed in a jacket restraint and wrist restraints. In order to prevent injury to the client with restraints, the most important nursing action would be to:**

1. Explain the procedure and reason for the restraints to the client and the family.
2. Remove the restraints and observe the extremities for circulation at least every four hours.
3. Tell the client that if he is more cooperative the restraints will not be necessary.
4. Document the use of restraints in the chart.

1. *This is an important part of nursing care. However, this action will not prevent injury to the client. This is not the answer.*
2. ***Very good. This nursing action will help prevent nerve and musculoskeletal injuries to the client as a result of poor circulation potentially caused by the restraints.***
3. *The case scenario tells you that the client is confused. Giving him this choice is inappropriate.*
4. *Documentation of the use of restraints and the client's behavior that warranted their use for the client's safety is very important. However, this action will not prevent injury to the client. This is not the answer.*

75. **An eight-year-old girl is admitted to the hospital in vaso-occlusive crisis from sickle cell anemia. After recovery, discharge teaching should include which of the following?**

1. Drink eight to 10 glasses of fluid per day.
2. Avoid playground activities at school.
3. Maintain an updated HIB immunization.
4. Assume postural drainage positions every six hours.

1. *Great choice! Hydration will decrease the viscosity of the blood. An increased viscosity is caused by the thick, sickled cells.*
2. *Wrong. While strenuous activity should be avoided, mild activity is encouraged to maintain muscle tone and build activity tolerance.*
3. *Wrong! An immunization for hemophilus influenza B is given to infants. HIB immunizations are not given after age six.*
4. *Wrong! Sickle cell anemia results in chronic anemia, but not in airway impairment. Postural drainage will not benefit the child with sickle cell anemia.*

76. **A client is placed on ferrous sulfate tablets twice a day as an iron supplement for anemia. The doctor tells her to take the medication with orange juice. Which of the following is the most important reason for drinking orange juice when taking the medication is?**

    1. The medication has an unpleasant taste, and the orange juice will help disguise the taste.
    2. The orange juice will help avoid constipation, which is a side effect of the medication.
    3. The orange juice will help the gastrointestinal tract absorb the medication more efficiently.
    4. The medication can cause nausea, and the orange juice will help alleviate this problem.

    1. *This is not correct. The medication is a tablet. Nothing is needed to disguise the taste.*
    2. *Constipation can be a side effect of ferrous sulfate. Drinking orange juice with the tablets is not adequate to prevent constipation, so this cannot be the most important reason for drinking orange juice with the medication.*
    3. *Excellent! The vitamin C in the orange juice will help with the absorption of the iron. This is the most important reason.*
    4. *Some clients experience nausea when taking ferrous sulfate. However, orange juice will not alleviate this symptom. This cannot be the answer.*

77. **A client is admitted to the hospital with abdominal pain. She tells the nurse that her father died recently and that she misses him. She begins crying while talking about her father. The nurse's assessment reveals that the client's temperature is 102.6° F and her abdomen is soft without tenderness. To which of the following observations should the nurse give immediate attention?**

    1. The client is crying.
    2. The temperature of 102.6° F.
    3. A soft, non-tender abdomen.
    4. The client is grieving.

1. *The case scenario tells you that the client is crying when she talks about her father, who died recently. Crying is a normal part of the grieving process, and the client's grief is a psychological consideration. However, the stem of the question asks you to identify an observation that requires the nurse's immediate attention. It must first be determined if there is a physiological cause related to the client's behavior.*
2. *Very good! An elevated temperature may be a sign of an infection or disease. A client with a temperature of 102.6° F is not well. This can affect her behavior, which may or may not be related to the death of her father.*
3. *This is an important assessment finding because of the client's complaint for admission to the hospital. However, a soft non-tender abdomen is a normal finding, and should not be a cause of concern for the nurse. The stem of the question asks you to identify an observation that requires the nurse's immediate attention. Can you identify a physiological need?*
4. *The client's grief is important, and the nurse will need to address the client's feelings. However, this is not the priority in this situation. The stem of the question asks you to identify an observation that requires the nurse's immediate attention. It must first be determined if there is a physiological cause related to the client's behavior.*

78. **When the nurse is doing discharge teaching for a client taking captopril (Capoten), which of the following interventions should receive highest priority?**

    1. Do not drive while taking this medication.
    2. Blood pressure should be monitored daily when home.
    3. Limit the intake of coffee, tea, and cola drinks.
    4. Notify the physician if a cough or sore throat develops.

    1. *Incorrect. Capoten may cause dizziness: the client is cautioned to avoid driving and other activities requiring alertness until response to medication is known; however, the client may return to driving once the dizziness resolves.*
    2. *Wrong. The client and family should be instructed on the proper technique for blood pressure monitoring and should be advised to check blood pressure at least weekly and report significant changes to the physician. Daily monitoring is not required.*
    3. *No. The client should avoid excessive amounts of these products, but this is not the priority instruction. Products containing caffeine, such as coffee, tea, chocolate, and cola drinks may potentially increase blood pressure.*
    4. *Correct choice. You remembered that the more serious side effects of ACE inhibitors (such as Capoten) are renal damage and neutropenia.*

Neutropenia can be life-threatening: because of the risk of infection, the client should notify the physician if a cough, sore throat, or fever develops.

79. A client is taking nadolol (Corgard) 80 mg p.o. daily for treatment of hypertension. During a follow-up appointment six months later, the client exhibits hypertension, agitation, and tachycardia. The nurse may suspect:

    1. A drug interaction.
    2. Nadolol toxicity.
    3. An allergic reaction.
    4. Nadolol withdrawal.

    1. Wrong. There is no information given in the question to suggest that a drug interaction has occurred. It would not be realistic to make this assumption without more data.

    2. No. Nadolol toxicity would be evidenced by bradycardia (pulse less than 50 beats per minute). This client has tachycardia.

    3. Incorrect. An allergic reaction would be manifested by pharyngitis, erythematous rash, fever, sore throat, laryngospasms, or respiratory distress. These symptoms are not present in this client. Make another selection.

    4. Yes! The nurse may suspect nadolol withdrawal if the client has been taking a beta-adrenergic blocker (like Corgard) and experiences rebound hypertension, tachycardia, or angina. The client is instructed not to discontinue the drug abruptly after chronic therapy; hypersensitivity to catecholamines may have developed, causing exacerbation of angina, MI, and ventricular dysrhythmias.

80. A client is to begin taking lithium. Before administering the first dose, the nurse could avoid checking to see that which of the following tests have been completed?

    1. BUN, creatinine, 24-hour creatinine clearance.
    2. TSH, T4, T3RU, T4I.
    3. Electroencephalogram (EEG).
    4. Electrocardiogram (ECG).

    1. Lithium is excreted by the kidneys, so a pre-treatment assessment of kidney function is essential. However, the question is asking which testing is not needed. Read over the other options to identify the one that is unnecessary.

    2. Thyroid testing is important because long-term use of lithium may lead to thyroid dysfunction. This question has a false response stem, so this cannot be the correct answer.

    3. Excellent! Pretreatment testing is necessary to rule

out medical problems that may predispose the client to lithium toxicity. Cardiovascular disease, renal disease and thyroid dysfunction are such medical problems. An EEG is not needed.

    4. A pretreatment ECG is necessary to rule out cardiovascular problems. This cannot be the correct answer because this question has a false response stem.

81. While getting an elderly client who is very weak out of bed, the best nursing approach initially is:

    1. Locking the wheels of the bed.
    2. Placing the equipment to provide the safest transfer that is possible for the client.
    3. Aligning the wheel chair is as close to the bed as possible, to prevent the client from falling to the floor.
    4. Removing the leg support on the wheel chair on the side closest to the bed.

    1. The wheels of the bed should be in the locked position to prevent it from moving. There is another option that is a more comprehensive or inclusive statement of the best nursing approach. Read all of the options before selecting the best one!

    2. Good work! This option is the best because it emphasizes assuring the client's safety and is a comprehensive statement about the initial nursing approach in transferring a client.

    3. This is an appropriate action that provides for the client's safety. However, there is another option that is a more comprehensive or general statement of the best nursing approach initially. Read all of the options before selecting the best one!

    4. This an appropriate action, since it provides unobstructed access to the wheel chair. However, this is not the best approach initially. There is another option that is a more comprehensive or general statement of the best nursing approach.

82. Which of the following outcomes can the nurse anticipate when a client is taking lisinopril (Zestril)?

    1. Decreased pulse rate.
    2. Decreased chest pain.
    3. Diuresis.
    4. Increased peripheral resistance.

    1. Wrong. Zestril, an antihypertensive ACE inhibitor, is used alone or in combination with other antihypertensives in the management of hypertension. A side effect of this drug is tachycardia, not bradycardia.

    2. No. Zestril, an antihypertensive ACE inhibitor, may cause angina pectoris (chest pain) as a side effect.

    3. Correct! Zestril is an antihypertensive ACE inhibitor: it's action is to block the formation of

angiotensin II. When this happens, diuresis and vasodilation occur, which will decrease blood volume and peripheral resistance—causing lowered blood pressure.

4. *Wrong. Zestril, an antihypertensive ACE inhibitor, will cause vasodilation and decreased peripheral resistance. Blood pressure rises if the client experiences INCREASED peripheral resistance.*

83. **A client is admitted with back pain. During the assessment the nurse notes his vital signs to be: temperature 103.2° F, pulse 90, respirations 30, and blood pressure 128/88. The initial nursing action should be:**

1. Give the client some medication such as Tylenol for his temperature.
2. Notify the physician of the vital signs.
3. Apply heat to the area of pain in his back.
4. Have the client lie flat in bed to help alleviate the pain.

1. *The case scenario does not indicate that there is an order for this medication. You cannot assume that one has been written! What is the issue in this question? The answer must be related to the issue.*
2. ***You are right. Because the vital signs are not within normal limits, vital signs are the issue in this question. The answer must be related to the issue. The key word in the stem is "initial." The first thing the nurse should do is to notify the physician of the abnormal findings. It is very important to know your vital signs!***
3. *The most significant data obtained during the assessment does not concern back pain. Back pain is the admitting diagnosis, but it is not the issue in this question. The answer must address the issue.*
4. *The most significant data obtained during the assessment does not concern back pain. Back pain is the admitting diagnosis, but it is not the issue in this question. The answer must address the issue. Also, since the cause of the pain has not been identified, lying flat in bed may not be appropriate or helpful.*

84. **A client is brought to the hospital by her husband. The admitting nurse notes the presence of pressured speech, irritable mood, and high distractibility. Her husband reports that she has not slept for the past three nights and was hyperactive at home. In addition to prescribing lithium for the client, the nurse anticipates that the psychiatrist will most likely order:**

1. A sedative-hypnotic.
2. An anti-anxiety agent.
3. An antipsychotic.
4. An antihistamine sedative.

1. *This is not the correct medication. A sedative at bedtime might help her sleep, but most psychiatrists would avoid using these drugs because of their abuse potential. There are other medications that would be tried first.*
2. *This is not the correct medication. There is a better choice. Read the other options again.*
3. ***Correct. Antipsychotics are often given early in the course of treatment with lithium to control behavior until the lithium level is within the therapeutic range.***
4. *Antihistamines are mild sedatives and would not be an appropriate choice for the client. Identify a better answer from the other options.*

85. **A client is seen in the clinic with complaints of vomiting, diarrhea, headache, and dizziness, and says she has the flu. The nurse takes her vital signs and obtains the following: Blood pressure of 198/110, pulse of 82, respirations of 24 and temperature of 100.8° F. The nurse should give immediate consideration to which of the following?**

1. Complaints of vomiting.
2. Complaints of diarrhea.
3. Complaints of headache and dizziness.
4. Temperature of 100.8° F.

1. *Vomiting is a symptom that should be evaluated with further assessment of signs of dehydration and weight loss. This option identifies the physiological needs of hydration and nutrition. However, all of the options in this question address physiological needs! Which need is most critical for the client?*
2. *Diarrhea is a symptom that should be evaluated with further assessment of signs of dehydration and weight loss. Diarrhea may also have several different causes that may need to be explored, depending on the severity of the problem. The severity is not indicated in the case situation. This option identifies the physiological needs of hydration and nutrition. However, all of the options in this question address physiological needs.*
3. ***Excellent! The complaints of headache and dizziness are very important symptoms for a client with a blood pressure of 198/110, since they may indicate poor circulation to the brain. This can be life-threatening to the client, and should receive immediate attention.***
4. *An elevated temperature identifies a physiological need of the client. However, this temperature elevation is not a threat to the client's safety. Since all of the options are physiological needs, the need that most threatens the client's life or well being is the most important.*

86. **A 60-year-old client is scheduled for surgery tomorrow. Upon entering the client's room, the**

nurse notices that flames are coming out of the waste basket. **The first action to take is which of the following:**

1. Place the folded blanket from the client's bed over the entire opening of the waste basket.
2. Find the nearest fire extinguisher to put the fire out.
3. Tell the client that he is not supposed to be smoking.
4. Pull the nearest fire alarm.

1. *Excellent! Placing the blanket over the waste basket will eliminate the source of oxygen, which is an element needed for a fire to burn. This is the fastest method in this scenario for putting out a small fire.*
2. *While a fire extinguisher will put out this small fire, it is not the best first action in this situation. While the nurse is getting the extinguisher, the fire will increase.*
3. *This is not an appropriate first action during this situation. Providing for the immediate safety of the client is most important.*

> **TEST-TAKING TIP:** *The case scenario in this question does not tell you that the client has been smoking, and it is incorrect to assume this. Do not "read into" the question!*

4. *An attempt should be made to quickly extinguish a small fire at the time it is found, since it can become out of control within ten minutes. The fire alarm should be pulled as soon as initial measures to extinguish the fire have been implemented.*

87. **In obtaining a blood pressure measurement, the most appropriate nursing action is:**

1. Obtain the proper equipment, place the client in a comfortable position, and record the appropriate information in the client's chart.
2. Measure the client's arm, if you are uncertain of the size of cuff to use.
3. Have the client recline or sit comfortably in a chair with the forearm at the level of the heart.
4. Document the measurement, which extremity was used, and the position that the client was in during the measurement.

1. *Very good! This is a general or comprehensive statement about the correct procedure, and it includes the basic ideas that are found in the other options.*
2. *This option is a possibility. The correct size cuff is necessary in order to obtain a reliable measurement. However, this is not the best option. Try to restate the question in your own words, and reread the other options.*

3. *This is an appropriate nursing action. The client should be relaxed and comfortable for a reliable reading. However, this is not the best option.*
4. *Documentation of these parameters is essential. However, this is not the best option.*

88. **A client tells the nurse that his name is not spelled right on his identification bracelet. The best action by the nurse is:**

1. Tell the client that as long as his medical record numbers are correct, the mistake is not a problem.
2. Ask the client for the correct spelling and change his medical records.
3. Notify the admitting office of the error and obtain a correct identification bracelet for the client.
4. Notify the physician.

1. *The client's identification bracelet should be corrected. It is possible that his name also appears incorrectly in his medical chart and other hospital records as well, and these records will have to be checked.*
2. *The client's records will have to be corrected. However, this is not the correct procedure, since the hospital has other records in addition to the chart. The client's identification bracelet should also be corrected.*
3. *Good choice! The admitting office must be informed of the error, and the client's identification bracelet should show his name correctly.*
4. *The spelling of the client's name is not a medical problem. This in an inappropriate nursing action.*

89. **A 45-year-old business executive was diagnosed with a gastric ulcer two years ago. At that time he was advised to scale down his activities and learn to relax. He returns to the HMO with increased epigastric pain. Upon questioning, he tells the nurse that he has been busier than ever. Which of the following short-term goals for dealing with stress would be the most realistic for the nurse to advise to the client?**

1. Express his emotions more directly.
2. Decrease his workload.
3. Use relaxation techniques each day.
4. Decrease social activities.

1. *Incorrect choice! This goal is important, but will take time to implement. The stem is looking for the best short-term goal.*
2. *Incorrect! This is an important goal, but it is not the most realistic option.*
3. *Correct. The nurse can demonstrate relaxation techniques and instruct him to begin performing them immediately. This is the most realistic short-term goal.*

4. *This could be an important goal. If, however, social activities are a form of relaxation for the client, this would not be a good goal for him.*

90. **An obese client has been placed on a high protein, low calorie diet by his physician. What nursing action is most appropriate?**

    1. Explain to the client that he will have to change his eating habits.
    2. Explain the importance of exercise when dieting.
    3. Explain to the client what types of foods are permitted on a low calorie, high protein diet.
    4. Tell the client that if he doesn't stay on this diet he will continue to gain weight.

    1. *This statement may be true, but it does not provide much useful information for the client. Consider the other options before selecting the best one.*
    2. *Exercise enhances the diet process by burning up calories. However, this option does not address the issue of the question, which is a high protein, low calorie diet. There is also no indication that exercise is included in this client's care plan. Do not "read into" the question!*
    3. ***Very good. Providing the client with knowledge concerning the types of foods that he can eat will help him to be more compliant.***
    4. *Although this may be a true statement, it is nontherapeutic. Also, the nurse does not know that the client is gaining weight at this time. Do not "read into" the question!*

91. **Admitted to the hospital with pulmonary emphysema, a client is extremely short of breath and is receiving oxygen per nasal cannula. The most important nursing action for this client receiving oxygen therapy is to:**

    1. Make sure the client is receiving at least six liters per minute to alleviate his respiratory distress.
    2. Provide low oxygen percentages to prevent respiratory arrest.
    3. Provide oral hygiene.
    4. Clean the nostrils around the cannula as needed.

    1. *This is an inappropriate action for a client who has emphysema. High levels of oxygen can cause respiratory distress.*
    2. ***Very good. This is the most important nursing action for this client, because it provides for his safety.***
    3. *This is an appropriate nursing action. However, it is not the most important action.*
    4. *This is an appropriate nursing action, but it is not the most important action.*

92. **A client with chronic obstructive pulmonary disease (COPD) is admitted for management of hypertension. The physician orders propranolol (Inderal) 40 mg p.o. twice a day. The nurse's most appropriate response is to:**

    1. Administer the Inderal one hour before or two hours after meals.
    2. Withhold the Inderal if the pulse is less than 60 beats per minute.
    3. Question the physician regarding the order for Inderal.
    4. Monitor the blood pressure prior to administration of the Inderal.

    1. *No. Inderal can be given with meals or immediately after eating. Tablets may be crushed and mixed with food or fluids for clients who have difficulty swallowing.*
    2. *Incorrect. Inderal can frequently cause bradycardia and the client should be advised to withhold the dose and contact the physician if the pulse is less than 50 beats per minute or if the blood pressure changes significantly.*
    3. ***Good choice! Inderal, a beta-adrenergic blocker, will block the sympathetic response in the bronchioles, causing bronchospasms in the client with COPD. These clients would do better with a Beta-1 selective blocker such as atenolol (Tenormin).***
    4. *Wrong. The client should be instructed to take the blood pressure at least weekly and to report any significant changes. Taking the blood pressure prior to each medication administration would not be necessary.*

93. **A three-year-old boy is admitted with laryngotracheobronchitis. His parents seem extremely anxious and the child is crying. Which nursing diagnosis has the highest priority?**

    1. Potential for infection.
    2. Ineffective airway clearance.
    3. Altered parenting.
    4. Impaired tissue perfusion.

    1. *Not the priority. The child already has an infection. While this places him at risk, it does not place him in immediate danger.*
    2. ***Good work! ABC's. Laryngotracheobronchitis can result in impaired airway clearance because of upper airway swelling. Maintenance of an open airway is of immediate concern.***
    3. *Wrong! There may be a need to calm and reassure the parents, however, this is not of immediate concern.*

4.   *Wrong! There may eventually be impaired tissue perfusion if the child does not receive enough oxygen. Maintaining airway clearance, which is the correct option, will eliminate the need for this diagnosis.*

94.   **After surgery the client requires one unit of blood because of a hemorrhage that occurred during surgery. Within 30 minutes of hanging the unit of blood, the client complains of itching and headache. Her blood pressure is 80/64. The first nursing action should be to:**

1.   Notify the physician.
2.   Obtain a urine specimen.
3.   Notify the laboratory.
4.   Stop the infusion of blood.

1.   *The key word in the stem of the question is "first." This action does not provide for the immediate safety of the client. The action should be done, but is it not the first thing to do.*
2.   *This intervention will be necessary, but it is not the first thing the nurse should do. The key word in the stem of the question is "first." This action does not provide for the immediate safety of the client.*
3.   *The laboratory will need to be notified, but not immediately. What is the first action to be done by the nurse?*
4.   ***This is the proper first response to symptoms of a blood reaction. All of the other measures will be done, but they should occur after the blood is stopped. This action provides for the immediate safety of the client.***

95.   **An elderly client is receiving care at the clinic because of weight loss. Which of the following nursing actions is most appropriate for the care of this individual?**

1.   Have the client keep a seven day diet log.
2.   Weigh the client at each office visit.
3.   Develop a diet that will improve the nutritional intake of the client.
4.   Discuss the client's appetite and eating habits.

1.   *Keeping a diet log is a useful tool in evaluating diet habits and obtaining baseline data. This is an excellent intervention, however, it is not the best answer to this test question.*
2.   *Weighing the client at each visit provides for a means of evaluating the client's progress. This is an appropriate nursing action to include in the plan of care for this client, but there is another option that is better.*

3.   *Developing a diet to improve nutritional intake may be appropriate, however, the nurse does not have enough information to accomplish it at this time. Look for a better option.*
4.   ***In this option, the nurse will assess the client's appetite and eating habits. This is the most appropriate nursing action because it may reveal why the client is losing weight. This assessment will also give the nurse important information to use in developing a plan to improve the client's nutritional intake. The nurse should always assess first.***

96.   **A male client has been taking atenolol (Tenormin) for two months for treatment of hypertension. He tells the nurse at the Health Clinic that he "has no energy or enthusiasm" like he used to. He states "I just want to sleep all the time—life holds no interest for me." The nurse recognizes these statements to be indicative of which side effect of Tenormin?**

1.   Depression.
2.   Diminished libido.
3.   Drowsiness.
4.   Mental changes.

1.   ***Correct. Depression is a side effect of Tenormin therapy and can be manifested by a sense of sadness, dejection, despair, or melancholy. When depressed, clients are likely to isolate themselves and avoid social contact with others; sleep becomes one mechanism of escape. Other central nervous system side effects of Tenormin include memory loss, mental changes, nightmares, drowsiness, dizziness, fatigue, and weakness.***
2.   *Wrong. Diminished libido (decreased sexual desire) is a side effect of Tenormin therapy, but would not be manifested by lack of energy or enthusiasm for life with a desire to "sleep all the time."*
3.   *Incorrect. Drowsiness, a side effect of Tenormin, is manifested by decreased mental alertness and acuity. It would not be evidenced by statements of despair or dejection.*
4.   *Mental changes, a side effect of Tenormin, would be evidenced by hallucinations and/or disorientation. The client's stated symptoms do not suggest these problems.*

97.   **A client is admitted to the hospital with decreased circulation in her left leg. During her admission assessment, which is the most important nursing action initially?**

1.   Obtain the past medical history.

2. Assess for circulation to her left leg by obtaining pedal pulses.
3. Obtain the client's vital signs.
4. Ask the client if she has had a recent injury to her leg.

1. *A client's past medical history is important and provides baseline information for planning of care. This option is a possible answer. However, it is important to identify the key words in this question before selecting the best option. Is this the "most important" nursing action "initially"?*
2. ***Excellent! Assessing the reason for the client's admission is very important — and the most important initially. "Initially" is the key word.***
3. *Baseline data is important. This is an appropriate nursing action and a possible answer. However, the reason for the client's admittance should be addressed before the routine head to toe assessment is performed. The stem of the question asks you to select the action that is most important initially. Be sure to identify key words in the question before selecting your answer!*
4. *Although this is important information, it can be obtained after the initial assessment of the client's specific problem is completed. It is important to identify the key words in this question before selecting the best option. This not the most important nursing action initially.*

98. **An elderly client is on bed rest. While administering an intramuscular injection, the most important action to prevent introduction of the medication into the venous system is which of the following?**

1. Inject the medication slowly to allow for slow absorption.
2. Insert the needle at a 45-degree angle where there are fewer blood vessels.
3. Use the Z track method of injection.
4. Aspirate the drug after insertion of needle.

1. *No. Injecting the medication slowly decreases trauma at the site and minimizes discomfort for the client. It does not prevent medication from entering the venous system.*
2. *No. An intramuscular injection is administered at a 90-degree angle. A subcutaneous injection is administered at a 45-degree angle. Neither position will prevent the medication from entering the venous system.*
3. *Wrong. The Z track method is used for irritating medications. It does not prevent medication from entering the venous system.*

4. ***Right! The drug is aspirated to determine if any blood is in the syringe. If blood is seen, the medication will enter the venous system if it is injected. Many intramuscular medications are not safe for intravenous administration.***

99. **A four-month-old infant is admitted with a ventricular septal defect, and undergoes a cardiac catheterization. Post-catheterization, which sign would alert the nurse to a potential complication?**

1. Pedal pulses palpable bilaterally.
2. Apical pulse 140 beats/minute.
3. Blood pressure 96/40.
4. Groin dressing intact with small amount of blood noted.

1. *Wrong! Palpable pedal pulses indicate circulation to the lower extremities. This is an expected finding.*
2. *Wrong! Normal range for a four-month-old can go as high as 140. This would not be cause for alarm.*
3. *Wrong! A blood pressure of 96/40 is an expected reading for a four-month-old infant.*
4. ***Correct answer! Any bleeding from the entry site of the cardiac catheter could indicate potential hemorrhage.***

100. **A client with right-sided weakness needs to be transferred from his bed to a wheel chair. When transferring the client, the nurse must remember which the following?**

1. Keep the client at arm's length while transferring him.
2. Bend at the waist to get down to his level.
3. Maintain a straight back and bend at the knees.
4. Attempt to transfer the client alone, before determining that help is needed.

1. *This is incorrect. When lifting an object or a client, it is important to hold the object or person close to the body, where there is the base of support.*
2. *The nurse should not bend at the waist, since all weight of the person will be placed on the back muscles and possibly cause injury to the nurse.*
3. ***Excellent. A straight back usually limits the amount of weight that is placed on the back muscles. Good body mechanics are essential in preventing injury to the nurse.***
4. *If a client or object appears to be too heavy for one person, the nurse should always get help first rather than attempt the lift alone and risk a back injury.*

NOTES

NCLEX-RN

Test 2

NCLEX-RN TEST 2

1. **A client, admitted with a tentative diagnosis of pernicious anemia, is scheduled for a Schilling test. The nurse would avoid which action, likely to jeopardize the accuracy of the test results?**

   1. Tell the client that she must fast for 12 hours prior to the test.
   2. Give an IM injection of vitamin B12 one hour after an oral dose of vitamin B12 tagged with radioactive cobalt.
   3. Start a 24-hour urine specimen after the client receives the oral dose of radioactive vitamin B12.
   4. Allow the client to eat breakfast after the IM injection of vitamin B12 is given.

2. **A 15-year-old client is being seen in the family planning clinic. She says to the nurse that she is nervous and has never had a pelvic examination before. Which of the following is the best nursing response?**

   1. "All you have to do is relax."
   2. "It is only slightly uncomfortable."
   3. "What part of the exam makes you nervous?"
   4. "If you want birth control pills, then a pelvic exam is required."

3. **Immediately after delivery, what is the priority nursing action in the care of the newborn?**

   1. Confirm identification and apply bracelet.
   2. Examine the infant to rule out any birth defects.
   3. Dry the infant, and place in a warm environment.
   4. Instill silver nitrate solution into the infant's eyes.

4. **A couple brought their 20-month-old child to the emergency room with second and third degree burns on her legs and feet. She is admitted for treatment of the burns and investigation into the possibility of abuse. The client has three sisters. She is admitted with a teddy bear and old blanket, and has dirty fingernails. Her parents state that she climbed into the bathtub alone. Which of the following is most important for the nurse to include in the documentation?**

   1. Treatment for the burns, parental visiting patterns and observations of the mother-child relationship.
   2. Parental visiting patterns, parents' comments to nurses and a description of the burns.

   3. Observation of the mother-child relationship, the types of toys the child has and whether the child is clean.
   4. Observation of relationship between parents and the client's siblings, treatment of the burns and the types of toys the child has.

5. **Which of the following actions, if taken by a nurse to prepare a client for an electroencephalogram (EEG), is one that should be questioned?**

   1. The client is given a mild sedative the evening prior to the procedure.
   2. The client's intake of coffee and alcohol is restricted for 48 hours prior to the procedure.
   3. The client is told that the procedure is painless.
   4. The nurse washes and dries the client's hair prior to the procedure.

6. **A client was treated four weeks previously for a streptococcal pharyngitis and is seeking treatment for recurrent symptoms. The nurse understands that the most likely cause of the client's recurring symptoms is which of the following?**

   1. Enlarged cervical lymph node involvement.
   2. Failure to complete his oral antibiotic therapy.
   3. Contact with his co-workers.
   4. Failure to change his toothbrush.

7. **The home health nurse knows to assess a client for what additional complications as a result of long-term morphine use?**

   1. Diuresis.
   2. Diarrhea.
   3. Constipation.
   4. Mydriasis.

8. **A client complains of a throbbing headache after a lumbar puncture. Which action by the nurse would be most appropriate at this time?**

   1. Darken the client's room and close the door.
   2. Keep the client flat in bed for six to eight hours after the procedure.
   3. Encourage the client to limit fluid intake for eight hours after the procedure.
   4. Report the headache to the nurse in charge.

9. A discharged client will continue taking lithium and will be seen in the clinic on a regular basis after discharge. The nurse's discharge teaching would include information on which of the following behaviors, likely to lead to the occurrence of dose-related lithium toxicity?

1. Fasting.
2. Mild exercise.
3. Increasing sodium intake.
4. Receiving Carbamazepine (Tegretol) therapy.

10. A client is to undergo various diagnostic tests and procedures for evaluation of neurologic function. When the client asks the nurse which test uses a gas as a contrast medium, the nurse responds that the appropriate test is the:

1. Pneumoencephalogram.
2. Echoencephalogram.
3. Brain scan.
4. Electroencephalogram.

11. The nurse learns a client is a college sophomore who recently transferred to the local university from another school in his home state. He reports he has been feeling depressed since he arrived and tells the nurse, "I can't seem to get with it...I don't know anyone here and can't get interested in my classes." The nurse diagnoses one of his nursing problems as which of the following?

1. Guilt related to failure to achieve his goals.
2. Inability to cope related to loss or separation from loved ones.
3. Feelings of hopelessness related to change of residence.
4. Low self-esteem related to lack of trust.

12. Following spinal cord injury at or above T6, the nurse should watch the client closely for signs of autonomic dysreflexia. The nurse is aware that this potentially dangerous response could be triggered by:

1. Elevated blood pressure.
2. Severe headache.
3. Distended bladder.
4. Edema of the spinal cord.

13. A client in the oliguric phase of acute renal failure has a serum potassium level of 5.5 mEq/L. If the client's potassium level continues to rise, the nurse will expect to observe which of the following on the EKG?

1. Depressed ST segments.
2. Peaked tall T waves.
3. Prolonged QT interval.
4. Presence of U waves.

14. A 12-year-old with a myelomeningocele at L2 is being seen at the clinic. Which statement by the child would indicate the need for more client teaching?

1. "I always drink three extra glasses of water every day."
2. "My teacher says I need remedial reading."
3. "I only need to catheterize myself twice a day, now."
4. "I do wheelchair exercises while watching TV."

15. A 76-year-old client was admitted to the hospital for surgery for a fractured hip. The client says to the nurse, "I guess I've lived long enough, and my number's up". Which of the following is the most therapeutic response by the nurse?

1. "You are in really good shape for your age."
2. "This is just a minor setback. You will be on your feet in no time."
3. "You feel that your life is ending?"
4. "The doctors and nurses are going to take good care of you while you are here. There's nothing to worry about."

16. A client who had surgery 24 hours earlier is experiencing dyspnea and tachycardia, and has developed a fever. The nurse suspects atelectasis. If this complication is present, the nurse's auscultation of the client's lung sounds would reveal:

1. Diminished breath sounds.
2. Rhonchi.
3. A pleural friction rub.
4. Absent breath sounds.

17. When beginning ampicillin (Omnipen) 250 mg p.o. q six hours for a client's infection, the nurse should monitor which of the following?

1. Urine output.
2. Urticaria or skin rash.
3. Potassium level.
4. Heart rate.

18. The client's last menstrual period began on April 2nd. She is certain that she conceived on April 16th. According to Nagele's rule, which of the following would be her expected date of confinement?

1. January 23rd.
2. January 9th.
3. July 9th.
4. July 23rd.

19. In planning care for a newborn with a surgical repair of a myelomeningocele, the nurse should be aware that this child is prone to developing which of the following?

1. Osteomyelitis.
2. Decubitus.
3. Otitis media.
4. Hydrocephalus.

20. Before giving preoperative medication to a client going to surgery, the nurse must make sure that:

1. The client has an empty bladder.
2. Vital signs are documented on the preoperative check list.
3. Dentures are removed.
4. The consent form has been signed.

21. A nurse working in an adolescent clinic should know which of the following about obesity?

1. In teenagers, it is commonly due to hypothyroidism, hypopituitarism, or other endocrine problem.
2. Obesity is no more likely to be associated with emotional conflicts in teenagers who are not obese, than in teenagers who are obese.
3. During adolescence, obesity is highly correlated with significant psychopathology.
4. Obesity is often associated with poor recognition of either hunger or satiation.

22. A client was told that her doctor found a lump in her breast and that a biopsy would have to be done. The client asks the nurse, "Do you think it is cancer?" Which of the following would be the best initial response by the nurse?

1. "You seem to be worried about what the doctor may find."
2. "Do you have a family history of breast cancer?"
3. "We won't know anything until the biopsy is done."
4. "Most lumps are not cancerous, so you really shouldn't worry."

23. A three-month-old client is being admitted with pyloric stenosis. She has an IV of D5 & 0.2 N/S at 22 mL/hour. She is NPO awaiting surgery. Which nursing assessment takes priority?

1. Urine output of 30 mL in two hours.
2. IV site red.
3. Skin turgor elastic.
4. Baby acts slightly irritable.

24. A client who is seven weeks pregnant is complaining of urinary frequency. She asks the nurse if this will continue throughout the pregnancy. Which of the following is the best response by the nurse?

1. "Yes, it will, but if you decrease your fluid intake it won't be so bothersome."
2. "No, it should only last until 12 weeks of gestation, but it will return near the end of the pregnancy."
3. "No, it should only last until 28 weeks of gestation unless you have poor bladder tone."
4. "There is no way to predict how long it will last, we'll just have to wait and see."

25. A client is hypertensive. The nurse is preparing to do client teaching. Which of the following goals is least appropriate?

1. The client eliminates sodium from the diet.
2. The client exercises moderately each day.
3. The client maintains weight appropriate for height.
4. The client discontinues use of birth control pills.

26. A client's behavior becomes a problem on the unit because he talks incessantly with everyone he sees. He also tends to intrude on private conversations as well as constantly interrupt others when they are speaking. During a team conference, various ways of handling the client's behavior are discussed. Which of the following is the best course of action to follow?

1. Escort the client back to his room each time the staff observe him talking with other clients.
2. Discuss this problem in a community meeting with all the clients on the unit present.
3. Discuss the problem with the client and identify specific limits or consequences that the staff will apply if he is not able to control his behavior.
4. Wait until his lithium levels are in the therapeutic range, when he will have better self-control.

27. A client is admitted to the hospital after complaining of chest pain. The client's history reveals congestive heart failure. He has been receiving digoxin (Lanoxin). The nurse understands that the purpose of giving the client digoxin is to:

1. Increase cardiac size.
2. Decrease cardiac output.
3. Increase the force of cardiac contraction.
4. Slow the pulse rate.

28. **A client is an insulin dependent diabetic. He is scheduled for a gall bladder x-ray in the Outpatient Department. He was given medication to take as a prep for this test. Which of the following nursing actions is most important when preparing the client for this test?**

    1. Explain the procedure to the client, and ask if he has any questions.
    2. Give the client directions to the Outpatient Department and the parking lot.
    3. Explain to the client that he should not take his insulin before the x-ray.
    4. Tell the client to take his insulin and eat breakfast before leaving home.

29. **When doing a physical assessment on a client with early common bile duct obstruction, the nurse would expect to see which clinical manifestation?**

    1. Dark yellow urine.
    2. Ascites.
    3. Clay-colored feces.
    4. Petechiae.

30. **The nurse is speaking to a group of young couples regarding the process of conception. Some of them are interested in preventing conception, and others are trying to achieve conception. Which of the following information should be related to these couples who wish to plan the timing of pregnancy?**

    1. The female ovum is only capable of fertilization for 48 hours after ovulation.
    2. The male sperm is capable of fertilization for up to three days after ejaculation.
    3. Abstinence of intercourse for 48 hours after a rise in basal body temperature will prevent pregnancy.
    4. The ideal time for fertilization to occur is day 12-16 of the menstrual cycle.

31. **The nursing assistant says to the nurse, "This client is incontinent of stool three or four times a day. I get angry when I think that he is doing it just to get attention. I think adult diapers should be used for him." Which of the following is the best initial nursing response?**

    1. "You are probably right. Soiling the bed is one way of getting attention from the nursing staff."

2. "Changing his bed and cleaning him must be tiresome for you. Next time it happens, I'll help you."
3. "It's upsetting to see an adult regress."
4. "Why don't you spend more time with him if you think that he is behaving this way to get more attention?"

32. **When transferring a client from a bed to a chair, the nurse should use which of the following techniques to avoid a back injury?**

    1. Bend at the waist while maintaining a wide stance, lift the client to a standing position, and then pivot the client toward the chair.
    2. Have the client lock his or her hands around the nurse's neck, so that the client will feel more secure during the transfer.
    3. Place the bed in an elevated position so that the client's hips are at the same level as the nurse's hip, resulting in the center of gravity being the same for both individuals.
    4. Bend at the knees, while maintaining a wide stance and straight back, with the client's hands on the nurse's shoulders and the nurse's hands at the client's axillae.

33. **A six-month-old infant is one day postoperative after receiving a colostomy. When the nurse positions him on his side, he stiffens and begins to cry. Which initial nursing action would the nurse take?**

    1. Leave the baby to rest, as infants' pain perception is not the same as older children.
    2. Check when the last pain medication was given to see if able to give it now.
    3. Check the abdominal dressing, as this may indicate an infection.
    4. Call the mother in, as this is a sign of decreased attachment.

34. **The nurse administering digoxin (Lanoxin) to a client notices that his breakfast is untouched. He also is complaining of nausea. The nurse checks his vitals, which are BP 118/72, P 60, R 22. How would the nurse interpret the data?**

    1. The client is anxious and fearful.
    2. The client needs a change in diet.
    3. This is a normal reaction to the hospital.
    4. He may be exhibiting a drug reaction.

35. **A physician has prescribed oral neomycin as well as a neomycin enema for a client with cirrhosis who is having central nervous system changes. The nurse would know that the neomycin has been effective if which of these laboratory values are decreased?**

1. White blood cell count.
2. Ammonia.
3. Creatinine.
4. Serum albumin.

36. **A client has been incontinent of loose stool and is complaining of a painful perineum. The most appropriate nursing action initially is to:**

    1. Notify the physician to obtain an order for the loose stools.
    2. Check the client's perineum.
    3. Turn the client every two hours.
    4. Increase the client's fluid intake to prevent dehydration.

37. **A client with advanced cirrhosis is admitted with bleeding esophageal varices. A Sengstaken-Blakemore tube has been inserted. In planning care for this client, the nurse knows that the primary purpose of the Sengstaken-Blakemore tube is to:**

    1. Coagulate the bleeding varices.
    2. Prevent the aspiration of blood into the lungs.
    3. Apply direct pressure to the bleeding varices.
    4. Provide a means for removing blood from the stomach.

38. **A pregnant client on iron supplements for iron-deficiency anemia calls and reports that her stools are black. She has no abdominal pain or cramping. What is the best response by the nurse?**

    1. "Come right in and we will check things out."
    2. "Go to the emergency room and your doctor will meet you there."
    3. "This is normal because of the way that iron is broken down during digestion."
    4. "What else have you been eating? This is unusual."

39. **The nurse finds an elderly client with her IV pulled out, standing next to her bed with the side rails in the up position. The client is confused, does not have an identification bracelet on, and cannot remember her name. What should the nurse do first?**

    1. Help the client into bed, and remind her to call the nurse when she wants to get out of bed.
    2. Help the client into bed, and then restart the IV.
    3. Place a restraining vest on the client.
    4. Put an identification bracelet on the client and help her back to bed.

40. **A client's husband asks to speak to the nurse about what effects he and his wife should expect after she is treated with electroconvulsive therapy.**
    He says, "I know it will improve her depression but couldn't it also turn her into a vegetable?" After explaining that ECT will not cause any brain damage, what additional information can the nurse ethically give him?

    1. "The main side effects, which are only temporary, are mild confusion, a slight headache, and short-term memory problems."
    2. "Most clients have no adverse effects to this treatment. In rare cases it has been known to cause fractures resulting from the induced seizure."
    3. "Some clients with cardiac problems have been known to have a heart attack, but we will monitor her closely to be certain this does not happen."
    4. "There are no permanent adverse effects associated with this treatment. The only common side effect is short-term memory problems, which can last for a few weeks."

41. **A 39-year-old client is having surgery on his bowel. The doctor orders a cleansing enema for the morning of surgery. Which of the following nursing interventions is most appropriate?**

    1. Wear gloves to insert the tubing.
    2. Use universal precautions and provide comfort measures to help the client relax during the procedure.
    3. Lubricate the tubing well prior to insertion.
    4. Position the client on his side and drape the client for warmth and privacy.

42. **A client, admitted with ascites and an elevated serum ammonia level secondary to cirrhosis, is receiving dietary instructions. The nurse will know that the client has accurate understanding of his dietary needs if he selects a menu that is:**

    1. High in protein, low in salt.
    2. High in calories, moderate in protein.
    3. Low in carbohydrates, high in fat.
    4. Low in calcium, low in potassium.

43. **A 14-month-old girl is admitted to the hospital with a fractured femur. Which of the following lunches would be most appropriate for the nurse to provide?**

    1. Infant formula.
    2. Chicken fingers and string beans.
    3. Strained chicken and strained beans.
    4. Hamburger and french fries.

44. **An 82-year-old client is diagnosed with colon cancer. She asks the nurse several questions about what the doctor might be planning to do. The nurse does not know which options the physician may**

have decided to recommend to the client. The physician will be making rounds within the hour. Which of the following nursing actions is most appropriate?

1. Help the client write down the questions to ask her physician, so that she doesn't forget when the doctor rounds in 30 minutes.
2. Assure the client that the doctor will tell her what has been planned.
3. Tell the client to have her daughter call the doctor to ask what options the doctor plans to recommend.
4. Provide the client with articles from several medical journals that discuss colon cancer.

45. A 16-year-old, 5'4" high school student is admitted to an eating disorders program by her psychiatrist. She tells the admitting nurse she has lost 25 pounds over the past month and now weighs 85 pounds. The nursing assessment identifies several behaviors that are characteristic of clients in the beginning stages of anorexia nervosa, which could include:

1. Appetite loss, amenorrhea, bradycardia, loss of 15% of pre-illness body weight.
2. Appetite loss, amenorrhea, tachycardia, hyperactivity.
3. Tachycardia, insomnia, fear of obesity, bulimia.
4. Amenorrhea, bradycardia, disturbed body image, loss of 15% of pre-illness body weight.

46. The nurse is assisting a frail elderly client to eat. The client begins to choke and indicates to the nurse that she cannot talk. The first nursing action is to:

1. Perform the Heimlich maneuver to obtain a patent airway.
2. Begin mouth to mouth resuscitation.
3. Place an oxygen mask on the client.
4. Go to the nurses' station to get some help.

47. A client is discharged from the hospital. She will continue taking lithium and will be seen in the clinic on a regular basis after discharge. The nurse knows that the client on long-term lithium therapy risks developing which condition?

1. Hyperthyroidism.
2. Hypoglycemia.
3. Impaired kidney function.
4. Gall stones.

48. A client is gravida 5 para 4. During admission, the nurse assesses that contractions are occurring every two minutes and lasting approximately

45 seconds. The client says she has been in labor for approximately 10 hours. The priority assessment the nurse needs to make at this time is which of the following?

1. Time the client last ate.
2. Cervical dilatation.
3. Allergies to medications.
4. Vital signs.

49. The physician has ordered a client to be discharged on a 2000 calorie diabetic diet. What is the most important nursing action in developing a teaching plan for this client's diet?

1. Obtaining sample menus from the dietitian to give to the client.
2. Asking the client to identify the types of foods that she usually eats and prefers.
3. Telling the client that she will have to change all of her previous eating habits.
4. Advising the client to buy only dietetic foods.

50. While changing a surgical dressing, the nurse notes green, foul-smelling drainage at the incision site. Another postoperative client is sharing the same room with this client. The most appropriate nursing action is to:

1. Place the client with the drainage in a private room.
2. Institute drainage and secretion precautions.
3. Move the other client to another room.
4. Place the client in strict isolation until the organism has been cultured and identified.

51. The nurse walked into the room to assess a four-year-old admitted with croup. The mother says, "He never wets the bed at home, I am so embarrassed." The nurse helps the mother and then invites her into the hall. Which of the following statements is the nurse's most appropriate response to the mother's statement?

1. "I know this can really be embarrassing, but I have kids myself, so I understand and it doesn't bother me."
2. "It is not uncommon for children to regress during a hospitalization. His toileting skills will return when he is feeling better."
3. "It's probably due to the medication we are giving him for his infection."
4. "I plan to discuss your child's incontinency with the physician as this may require further investigation."

52. The nurse would expect to make which of the following observations about a client to relate to a

diagnosis of myocardial infarction rather than angina?

1. A feeling of an intermittent strangling sensation.
2. Complaints of sudden substernal pain after an argument.
3. Feelings of numbness or weakness in arms and wrists.
4. Profuse perspiration with nausea and vomiting.

53. **A 22-year-old client has had surgery on his foot and has just been returned to his room from the recovery room. The initial assessment indicates that he is stable. An hour later, his roommate turns on the call light and tells the nurse that the client has gotten up and hopped on one foot to the bathroom, using his IV pole for support. Which of the following actions would the nurse do first?**

1. Open the bathroom door to assess if the client is okay.
2. Help the client back to bed and get him a urinal.
3. Explain to the client that it is not safe for him to be hopping around on one foot.
4. Get a wheelchair and help the client back to bed when he is done in the bathroom.

54. **A client who is incontinent of stool has been placed on a bowel training program. The nurse understands that the goal of bowel training is:**

1. To prevent soiling of the bed.
2. To prevent cancer of the colon.
3. To prevent loose stools.
4. To provide the client with control over his bowels.

55. **A client is sitting by his food tray and pushing the food around on his plate. He says to the nurse, "I hate hospital food. Is this the only thing that I can get to eat?" Which of the following responses would be the best initial response by the nurse?**

1. "What is it about the food that you dislike?"
2. "Well, the other clients haven't complained about the food. Is something else bothering you?"
3. "I'll call the kitchen and order something else for you."
4. "Is there something special that you would like to eat?"

56. **The alcoholic client tells the nurse he has not had anything to drink for 24 hours prior to admission. He complains of feeling anxious and shaky. Based on a knowledge of alcohol withdrawal, what other behaviors could the nurse expect him to display during the early phase of alcohol withdrawal?**

1. Coarse tremors, tachycardia, insomnia.
2. Confusion, visual hallucinations, delusions.
3. Disorientation, confabulation, memory deficits.
4. Incoordination, impaired thinking, irregular eye movements.

57. **A client diagnosed with schizophrenia says, "They lied about me and are trying to poison my food." Which of the following statements is the nurse's best response to the client?**

1. "You are mistaken. Nobody has told lies about you or tried to poison you."
2. "You're having very frightening thoughts."
3. "Tell me more about your concerns about being poisoned."
4. "Tell me who would do such things to you?"

58. **A client delivers a six-pound 12-ounce male infant at 39 weeks of gestation. She experienced an unremarkable labor and delivery. The nurse caring for the client 14 hours after delivery, assesses the following: Breasts soft; fundus firm, U +1, slightly deviated to the right; lochia moderate rubra; T 100° F, P 88, R 18. Which of the following nursing actions should be initiated?**

1. Ask her to empty her bladder.
2. Report her temperature elevation.
3. Suggest that she begin to nurse more frequently so her milk will come in.
4. Nothing, these are normal assessments for 14 hours after delivery.

59. **A client, age 63, is being discharged after insertion of a pacemaker for a persistent dysrhythmia. Which of the following statements made by the client indicates the need for further teaching?**

1. "I know that I have to check my pulse every day, preferably in the morning."
2. "I sure will miss being able to continue with my bowling league. I guess I'll take up walking as a sport!"
3. "I'll stay away from my wife's microwave oven so that it doesn't interfere with my pacemaker."
4. "If I start having any palpitations or dizziness, I'll call my doctor right away."

60. **An ASO titer is drawn on an 11-year-old in the hospital with acute glomerulonephritis. The mother asks the nurse why the titer was drawn. Which response by the nurse is most justifiable?**

1. "This will tell us if he's ever had the measles."
2. "This will tell us if he's had a recent strep infection."

3. "This lab work is done routinely on all patients."
4. "This is done to determine the level of antibiotic is his blood."

61. **An 88-year-old client is admitted to the hospital with chest pain. His daughter tells the nurse that he has certain routines for his personal hygiene and for taking his medicine. She is concerned that he will be uncooperative while in the hospital. Which of the following would be the best initial response by the nurse?**

    1. Assure the daughter that everything possible will be done to accommodate her father's needs.
    2. Ask the daughter what routines and medicines her father uses at home.
    3. Inform the daughter that the hospital has policies that have to be followed, and that the best care will be provided for her father.
    4. Tell the daughter that she should inform the doctor about her father's routines so that orders can be written to meet the client's needs.

62. **The client is to receive a medication for control of tachycardia and an irregular heart rate. The nurse obtains the following vital signs prior to administering this medication: BP 98/54, P 48, R 30, T 98° F. The client's skin is cool, with cyanosis of the fingers and lips. Which of the following is the priority nursing action?**

    1. Administer the medication as ordered by the physician.
    2. Omit the medication for a day or two, depending on the client's response and symptoms.
    3. Notify the physician concerning the client's status before administering the medication.
    4. Give the client one half of the ordered dose.

63. **A client is receiving an intravenous infusion. The nurse observes the client for signs of infiltration of the IV solution. Which symptom, if noted by the nurse, is associated with a complication other than infiltration?**

    1. The infusion rate slows or stops while the tubing is not kinked.
    2. The area around the injection site feels warm to the touch.
    3. Swelling, hardness or pain located around the needle site.
    4. Blood fails to return in the tubing when the bottle is lowered.

64. **A client is admitted to the hospital with respiratory difficulty, wheezing on expiration, coughing, and diaphoresis. An intravenous infusion of ami-** nophylline is ordered. **The nurse knows that which of the following best describes the purpose of giving this medication?**

    1. To relax the bronchial smooth muscles.
    2. To increase the tone in the respiratory passages.
    3. To cause bronchoconstriction.
    4. To decrease the inflammatory reaction.

65. **The first, most important nursing action when a nurse discovers a fire in a client's room is which of the following?**

    1. Pull the fire alarm and notify the hospital operator.
    2. Close fire doors and client room doors.
    3. Remove the client from the room.
    4. Place moist towels or blankets at the threshold of the door of the room with the fire.

66. **A 74-year-old client is admitted with respiratory acidosis as a complication of chronic COPD. Her blood gases reveal she is in primary respiratory acidosis. The nurse knows that this probably results from which of the following?**

    1. Decreased exhalation of carbon dioxide.
    2. Increased mucous secretion.
    3. Long-term theophylline administration.
    4. Recent vomiting and diarrhea.

67. **A client is readmitted to the hospital. After two weeks, her lithium level is within the therapeutic range and she no longer has manic symptoms. Before discharge, what information should the nurse give to the client about diet when taking lithium?**

    1. Sodium intake should be restricted.
    2. Fluid intake should be restricted to 1000 mL per day.
    3. An adequate daily intake of sodium and fluids should be maintained.
    4. Sodium and fluid intake should be increased.

68. **In providing care to a client who is hyperventilating, the nurse knows that which of the following conditions is most likely to be associated with hyperventilation?**

    1. Fatigue.
    2. Opiate withdrawal.
    3. Anxiety.
    4. Petit mal epilepsy.

69. **A client asks the nurse how much weight is safe for her to gain during her pregnancy. The nurse**

appropriately teaches the client, that in relation to gaining weight during pregnancy, which of the following is recommended?

1. A maximum weight gain of about 15 pounds (6.8 kg).
2. A weight gain of about 12 pounds (5.5 kg) each trimester.
3. As long as the client does not feel hungry, the actual amount of weight gain has little significance.
4. A range of about 20 to 30 pounds (9 to 14.5 kg).

70. **The nurse is caring for a client who had abdominal surgery two days ago. Which of the following assessment data requires immediate action by the nurse?**

1. A urinary drainage bag with 100 cc's of straw colored urine.
2. A wound dressing with thick light green drainage.
3. A blood pressure reading of 98/66.
4. Shallow respirations, with a rate of 30.

71. **A nine-year-old is admitted for surgery for slipped capital femoral epiphysis. Aware of the main concerns of a child of this age, the nurse would want to plan to do which of the following?**

1. Arrange for his parents to be with him continuously.
2. Obtain a telephone to be at his bedside.
3. Plan with the physician to obtain Patient Controlled Analgesia postoperatively.
4. Provide special hospital pajamas.

72. **Two weeks after a client started taking amitriptyline (Elavil) she reported that she was sleeping better and her appetite had improved. She said, however, that she still felt hopeless and sad. In response to this, the best action for the nurse to take is to:**

1. Notify her physician so that she can be switched to another drug.
2. Ask her physician to increase her dose of Elavil.
3. Explain that antidepressants often take three to four weeks to be fully effective.
4. Chart her complaints in the nursing notes.

73. **In the middle of making morning rounds, a client says to the nurse, "I almost died last night." Which of the following is the most therapeutic nursing response?**

1. "You made it through the night."
2. "Patients do have dreams that they die when they

are hospitalized."
3. "Are you feeling okay now?"
4. "That must have been frightening for you. Tell me more about it."

74. **A client returns from surgery with two penrose drains in place. In anticipation of frequent dressing changes, what should the nurse use to most effectively reduce skin irritation around the incision area?**

1. Montgomery straps.
2. Silicone spray.
3. Hypoallergenic tape.
4. Large, bulky absorbent pads.

75. **A client has congestive heart failure and is on digoxin (Lanoxin). In response to this client's question, the nurse explains that digoxin affects cardiac function through which of the following mechanisms?**

1. Decreasing the strength of cardiac contractions and increasing the heart rate and conduction time.
2. Increasing the strength of cardiac contractions, the heart rate and conduction time.
3. Increasing the strength of contractions while decreasing the conduction time and heart rate.
4. Decreasing the strength of cardiac contractions, the heart rate and conduction time.

76. **During administration of medications to a client, the priority nursing assessment is which of the following?**

1. Help the client swallow medications without aspirating by keeping the head in a neutral position.
2. Identify the client by checking the client's identification bracelet and asking for his name.
3. Keep all prepared medications in sight.
4. Check the client for desired or undesired drug effects within an hour after administration of the medication.

77. **A 78-year-old diabetic who is blind was admitted to the hospital for an infected leg ulcer. The nurse would avoid which nursing intervention in caring for this client?**

1. Place her food tray directly in front of her on the overbed table and remind her that the tea is hot.
2. Speak to the client when entering her room, and identify oneself.
3. Show her where everything is in the room.
4. Place her belongings within easy reach.

78. A four-year-old is brought into the emergency room with burns to her neck and face. Which of the following has the highest nursing priority for this child at this time?

    1. Potential for infection.
    2. Ineffective individual coping.
    3. Fluid volume deficit.
    4. Potential for ineffective airway clearance.

79. When administering ear drops with a dropper, which of the following actions taken by the nurse best prevents contamination of the bottle of medication?

    1. Washing hands prior to preparing the medication.
    2. Holding the dropper with the tip above the ear canal.
    3. Washing the client's ear prior to instilling the medication.
    4. Filling the dropper with only the prescribed number of drops.

80. The primary nurse learns that an obsessive-compulsive client has a full set of dentures because he eroded all his tooth enamel with his brushing rituals. He also brushes his tongue several times a day, and has developed several ulcerations on it. His nursing care plan should set the highest initial priority for which of the following?

    1. Eliminating his brushing and mouth care rituals.
    2. Verbalizing the underlying cause of his behavior.
    3. Seeking out the nurse when he is feeling anxious.
    4. Reestablishing healthy tissue in his mouth and tongue.

81. The nurse caring for a client with a history of congestive heart failure is aware that which condition is likely to contribute to digoxin (Lanoxin) toxicity?

    1. Hypokalemia.
    2. Hypocalcemia.
    3. Obesity.
    4. Hyponatremia.

82. A 77-year-old client was hospitalized for observation after a fall that he experienced when he was walking for exercise. He is to ambulate for the first time since his fall. He tells the nurse that he is afraid to get up. Which of the following statements would be the best response by the nurse?

    1. "There is nothing to be afraid of. Your doctor

wouldn't have written the order if the doctor didn't think that you were ready."
    2. "Tell me what concerns you about getting up today?"
    3. "I will have another person here to help you when you get up."
    4. "Are you afraid of falling again?"

83. After six months, the physician determines that the client is no longer responding well to lithium. After discontinuing the lithium, the physician prescribes valproic acid (Myproic Acid), an anticonvulsant that is also effective in bipolar disorders. What special instructions should the nurse give the client about valproic acid?

    1. A pretreatment EEG must be done and repeated in six months.
    2. Liver function and hematology levels must be monitored.
    3. Thyroid function tests must be done every six months.
    4. The white blood count must be monitored regularly.

84. The nurse would instruct an antepartum client to call the physician if she experiences which of the following symptoms in her pregnancy?

    1. Facial edema.
    2. Urinary frequency.
    3. Nausea and vomiting.
    4. Breast leakage.

85. A client is to be transferred from her bed to a stretcher, in order to be transported to surgery for a fractured hip. The first most important nursing action is to:

    1. Provide for the client's privacy with a blanket.
    2. Lock the wheels on the stretcher and the bed.
    3. Have four people available for lifting the client.
    4. Provide a lifting device to assist with moving the client.

86. After a bronchoscopy, which assessment, if made by the nurse, would require immediate action by the nurse?

    1. Blood-tinged mucous.
    2. Complaints of hoarseness when speaking.
    3. Irritation and discomfort when swallowing.
    4. Difficulty breathing.

87. A 38-year-old client is admitted with PIH (pregnancy induced hypertension). The physician or-

ders a urinalysis. When the nurse collects the urine specimen, which of the following measures taken by the nurse is the most important?

1. Labeling the container with the client's room number.
2. Checking the identification of the client.
3. Using sterile gloves when handling a urine specimen.
4. Instructing the client to put the specimen on the counter at the nurses' station for pick-up.

88. A client is hospitalized for a closed reduction of a fractured femur and application of a cast. A vital nursing action in the care of this client is to:

1. Perform neurovascular checks of the extremities.
2. Use the palms of the hands when moving an extremity with a wet cast.
3. Provide an instrument for the client to scratch the itching areas of skin under the cast.
4. Petal the edges of the cast to provide smooth edges.

89. In planning preoperative care for a client, the nurse is aware that obtaining legal, informed consent to perform surgery is the responsibility of:

1. The nurse.
2. The surgeon.
3. The client's family physician.
4. The client.

90. A 21-year-old client is admitted to the hospital because of extreme weight loss. It is noted on the admission assessment that the client believes that she is overweight at 88 pounds. What aspect of care should the nurse consider the patient's first priority?

1. Assessing the client's nutritional status.
2. Obtaining a psychiatric consult.
3. Planning a therapeutic diet for the client.
4. Talking to the family members to find out more about the client's self-concept.

91. A client has an intravenous fluid infusing per gravity at 125 mL/hour. Which of the following assessment findings indicates to the nurse that the IV site needs to be changed?

1. The IV is infusing at 75 mL/hour regardless of the height of the IV bag.
2. The area around the IV site is reddened but not tender.
3. There is fluid leaking at the connecting site.
4. There is blood backing up in the IV tubing.

92. A post-mastectomy client returns to the surgical unit with a closed-wound suction device (Hemovac)

in place. Which action by the nurse will ensure proper operation of the device?

1. Irrigate the tubing with sterile normal saline once each shift.
2. Empty the device when it's full.
3. Keep the tubing above the level of the surgical incision.
4. Recollapse the device whenever it's one-half to two-thirds full of air.

93. An antepartum client's lab work reveals that she has a negative rubella titer. The nurse knows that the result of the test:

1. Means that the client does not have rubella at this time.
2. Means that the client is immune to rubella and need not worry about exposure in this pregnancy. She does not need to be immunized.
3. Means that the client is not immune to rubella and needs to be immunized as soon as possible.
4. Means the client is not immune to rubella and will need an immunization following delivery.

94. A two-year-old boy is brought to the emergency room with nausea and diarrhea. Which statement by the parents would cause the nurse to be most concerned?

1. "His last wet diaper smelled very strong."
2. "He is very quiet when he is playing."
3. "His lips are dry and crusty."
4. "He cries whenever I put him down."

95. A four-year-old who had hydrocephalus as an infant is admitted with a malfunctioning ventriculo-peritoneal shunt. Following new shunt placement, the nurse conducts a postoperative check. Which assessment would demand an immediate response from the nurse?

1. Sleepy, very difficult to arouse.
2. Pupils equal and reactive to light.
3. BP 100/60, apical pulse of 90.
4. Urine output 33 mL in two hours.

96. A client is admitted to the hospital for cataract surgery of the left eye. The physician has ordered eye drops to be administered to both eyes at frequent intervals prior to surgery. Which of the following nursing actions is most appropriate?

1. Use aseptic technique and avoid dropping the medication onto the cornea.
2. Gently wash away any crust along the eyelid margin with warm water.

3. Have the client look up toward the ceiling prior to instillation of drops.
4. Drop prescribed number of drops into the conjunctival sac.

97. **The nurse can evaluate the agoraphobic client's progress as improving when the client is able to attend which of the following activities?**

1. Daily community/milieu meetings.
2. Occupational therapy on the unit.
3. The hospital gift shop.
4. A unit picnic in a local park.

98. **A client is seen in the emergency room for abdominal pain, and is scheduled for emergency surgery. Which of the following is most important for the nurse to include in preoperative teaching for the client?**

1. An explanation of the hospital billing process for clients receiving surgery.
2. Instruction about deep breathing and coughing, with abdominal splinting.
3. Having the client sign the surgical consent.
4. An explanation of where the incision will be and how much drainage to expect on the dressing after surgery.

99. **A 75-year-old man is a psychiatric client who is taking lithium for a bipolar mood disorder. The nurse knows that elderly clients:**

1. Cannot be safely treated with lithium.
2. Take the same dosage of lithium as younger adults.
3. Treated with lithium have a therapeutic range of 0.6-0.8 mEq/L.
4. Treated with lithium have a therapeutic range of 0.6-1.4 mEq/L.

100. **The nurse enters a client's room. The client's son tells the nurse, "You people can't do anything right. Ever since my father was admitted to this hospital, it has been one mistake after another. I am taking him out of here before you kill him." The most therapeutic response by the nurse is which of the following?**

1. "You feel that your father is not being well taken care of?"
2. "We have the best intentions for the clients."
3. "I'll get the supervisor for you."
4. "Your father hasn't complained about the care. What specifically is the problem?"

NCLEX-RN

Test 2

Questions with Rationales

NCLEX-RN TEST 2 WITH RATIONALES

1. **A client, admitted with a tentative diagnosis of pernicious anemia, is scheduled for a Schilling test. The nurse would avoid which action, likely to jeopardize the accuracy of the test results?**

   1. Tell the client that she must fast for 12 hours prior to the test.
   2. Give an IM injection of vitamin B12 one hour after an oral dose of vitamin B12 tagged with radioactive cobalt.
   3. Start a 24-hour urine specimen after the client receives the oral dose of radioactive vitamin B12.
   4. Allow the client to eat breakfast after the IM injection of vitamin B12 is given.

   1. *No, this is correct procedure. You are asked to select the action the nurse would AVOID.*
   2. *No, this is standard procedure for the Schilling test. Look for an action that the nurse would AVOID.*
   3. **Correct! In a Schilling test, the 24-hour urine collection begins from the time the client receives the injection of vitamin B12 — not the oral dose.**
   4. *No, this is correct procedure. You are to choose an action the nurse would AVOID.*

2. **A 15-year-old client is being seen in the family planning clinic. She says to the nurse that she is nervous and has never had a pelvic examination before. Which of the following is the best nursing response?**

   1. "All you have to do is relax."
   2. "It is only slightly uncomfortable."
   3. "What part of the exam makes you nervous?"
   4. "If you want birth control pills, then a pelvic exam is required."

   1. *No. This statement does not address the client's concerns, and it blocks communication by using a cliché and false reassurance.*
   2. *Incorrect! This response does not address the client's concerns and does not encourage further expression of feelings by the client. This response blocks communication.*
   3. **Excellent choice! This response recognizes the client's feelings and uses the tool of clarification to encourage the client to share her concerns. This response is therapeutic.**
   4. *Wrong! This statement is true in its literal sense, but the scenario does not indicate that the client has requested birth control pills. This statement could easily be interpreted as expressing the nurse's disapproval. This response is also not therapeutic because it does not address the feelings that the client has shared with the nurse.*

3. **Immediately after delivery, what is the priority nursing action in the care of the newborn?**

   1. Confirm identification and apply bracelet.
   2. Examine the infant to rule out any birth defects.
   3. Dry the infant, and place in a warm environment.
   4. Instill silver nitrate solution into the infant's eyes.

   1. *Wrong! Correct identification of the newborn is important, but it will not be detrimental to the health of the infant if it is delayed until the mother holds the infant. There is another, more important, action.*
   2. *No. A careful assessment of the newborn is done soon after birth but often only gross or obvious birth defects are identified in the delivery room. A thorough assessment is completed as part of admission to newborn nursery.*
   3. **Congratulations! Best choice! Failure to dry the infant and keep it warm could result in unnecessary use of oxygen by the infant and resultant respiratory distress. Keeping the infant dry and warm will prevent such complications.**
   4. *Not the best choice. Installation of silver nitrate after birth may be important, but it can be delayed until the infant goes to the newborn nursery. The drops interfere with newborn visual acuity and can affect the bonding process, so delaying until the mother has held the infant is routine.*

4. **A couple brought their 20-month-old child to the emergency room with second and third degree burns on her legs and feet. She is admitted for treatment of the burns and investigation into the possibility of abuse. The client has three sisters. She is admitted with a teddy bear and old blanket, and has dirty fingernails. Her parents state that she climbed into the bathtub alone. Which of the following is most important for the nurse to include in the documentation?**

   1. Treatment for the burns, parental visiting patterns and observations of the mother-child relationship.
   2. Parental visiting patterns, parents' comments to nurses and a description of the burns.
   3. Observation of the mother-child relationship, the types of toys the child has and whether the child is clean.
   4. Observation of relationship between parents and the client's siblings, treatment of the burns and the types of toys the child has.

   1. *No, this is only partially correct. The child has two parents, as stated in the stem, so the relationship with the father would also be observed.*

2. *Correct! This documentation provides information on the nurturing given by the parents to the child, care of the injury and response.*

3. *Not the best answer. The types of toys and the cleanliness of the child are more likely to be reflections of the family's socioeconomic status than their potential for further abusive patterns.*

4. *No, this is not the focus. Dysfunctional families may treat an abused child differently than other children in the family, but this is frequently not observable during the hospitalization.*

5. **Which of the following actions, if taken by a nurse to prepare a client for an electroencephalogram (EEG), is one that should be questioned?**

   1. The client is given a mild sedative the evening prior to the procedure.
   2. The client's intake of coffee and alcohol is restricted for 48 hours prior to the procedure.
   3. The client is told that the procedure is painless.
   4. The nurse washes and dries the client's hair prior to the procedure.

   1. *Yes, you have identified the inappropriate nursing action! Tranquilizers and stimulants should be withheld for 24 to 48 hours before an EEG because these medications can alter the EEG wave patterns or mask the abnormal wave patterns of a seizure disorder.*
   2. *No, this action is correct and should not be questioned. Stimulants and tranquilizers should be withheld because they can alter EEG wave patterns or mask abnormal wave patterns.*
   3. *No, this is a correct action. Electrodes are arranged on the scalp to record the electrical activity in various regions of the head. The procedure takes 45 to 60 minutes or longer if a sleep EEG is performed. The procedure does not cause an electric shock.*
   4. *No, this is a correct action. The hair should be clean and dry prior to the test. Remember that electrodes are going to be placed on the scalp.*

6. **A client was treated four weeks previously for a streptococcal pharyngitis and is seeking treatment for recurrent symptoms. The nurse understands that the most likely cause of the client's recurring symptoms is which of the following?**

   1. Enlarged cervical lymph node involvement.
   2. Failure to complete his oral antibiotic therapy.
   3. Contact with his co-workers.
   4. Failure to change his toothbrush.

   1. *Wrong. This is a clinical symptom of strep, not a cause, and it would not necessarily only occur now.*
   2. *Good choice! Strep usually resolves within five to seven days even without antibiotic therapy. This is the best answer since non-suppurative compli-*

cations, such as recurrence, result when the full course of antibiotic therapy is not completed.

3. *Incorrect, because the type of contact is not specified. Contact must be airborne. This distractor just says contact with co-workers.*

4. *This is recommended to all clients, but it is not the best answer. The client will still resolve his illness, even if he doesn't change his toothbrush.*

7. **The home health nurse knows to assess a client for what additional complications as a result of long-term morphine use?**

   1. Diuresis.
   2. Diarrhea.
   3. Constipation.
   4. Mydriasis.

   1. *No. Urinary retention is more likely to occur, due to an increase in tone of the bladder sphincter.*
   2. *Wrong. Diarrhea is highly unlikely with morphine use.*
   3. *Correct! Morphine decreases peristalsis and increases the tone of the anal sphincter.*
   4. *Wrong. In long-term use of morphine, miosis (pupil constriction) occurs and vision is impaired, leading to safety concerns. Mydriasis is pupil dilatation, the opposite of miosis.*

8. **A client complains of a throbbing headache after a lumbar puncture. Which action by the nurse would be most appropriate at this time?**

   1. Darken the client's room and close the door.
   2. Keep the client flat in bed for six to eight hours after the procedure.
   3. Encourage the client to limit fluid intake for eight hours after the procedure.
   4. Report the headache to the nurse in charge.

   1. *No, this action would not be the most appropriate as it doesn't address the cause of the headache. Although this action is helpful for any client in pain, there is another option that is more therapeutic in this case.*
   2. *Yes! The headache following a lumbar puncture is probably due to continuing cerebrospinal fluid (CSF) leakage through the opening in the dura made by the needle. The headache is usually relieved when the client lies down. Increasing fluids to 2,000-3,000 mL in 24 hours is also helpful in replacing fluid and CSF quickly, unless contraindicated.*
   3. *No! Just the opposite should be done. Fluid intake should be encouraged to replace the cerebrospinal fluid that was removed during the test. This will help to decrease the likelihood of post-spinal headaches.*

4. *Wrong action at this time. There are independent nursing actions that you can take to decrease the severity of post-spinal headaches, an uncomfortable but not life-threatening side effect of a lumbar puncture.*

9. **A discharged client will continue taking lithium and will be seen in the clinic on a regular basis after discharge. The nurse's discharge teaching would include information on which of the following behaviors, likely to lead to the occurrence of dose-related lithium toxicity?**

   1. Fasting.
   2. Mild exercise.
   3. Increasing sodium intake.
   4. Receiving Carbamazepine (Tegretol) therapy.

   1. **Correct. Crash dieting or fasting can lead to lithium toxicity because the sodium and electrolyte balance would be altered, causing the blood levels of lithium to rise.**
   2. *Mild exercise would not lead to lithium toxicity. Most clients are able to engage in exercise without difficulty, but they should take care to replace any sodium that has been lost through profuse sweating. This cannot be the correct answer.*
   3. *No. Increasing sodium intake will lead to excretion of lithium and a drop in the lithium level. If the lithium level should drop below the therapeutic range, the client may have a relapse of his bipolar disorder.*
   4. *Tegretol is an anticonvulsant that is used to treat acute mania and prevent future manic episodes. It is most often used alone in clients who cannot take lithium. When given with lithium, it has to be closely monitored because the combination can produce symptoms of neurotoxicity in the client. It is not associated with a dose-related lithium toxicity.*

10. **A client is to undergo various diagnostic tests and procedures for evaluation of neurologic function. When the client asks the nurse which test uses a gas as a contrast medium, the nurse responds that the appropriate test is the:**

    1. Pneumoencephalogram.
    2. Echoencephalogram.
    3. Brain scan.
    4. Electroencephalogram.

    1. **Correct. A pneumoencephalogram involves the instillation of air or a gas into the ventricular and subarachnoid system through a lumbar puncture. This air or gas serves as a contrast medium because air is less dense than fluid to x-rays. The CSF is partially replaced by the gas, and x-rays are taken.**
    2. *Incorrect. An echoencephalogram is the recording of sound waves reflected by the brain structures in response to ultrasound signals. There is no contrast medium used.*
    3. *Incorrect. A brain scan involves the use of a radioisotope which is absorbed easily by abnormal tissue, such as a tumor. After the isotope is injected, the client waits one to three hours for absorption. A scintillation scanner is then used to image the brain.*
    4. *No. An electroencephalogram (EEG) is a diagnostic test that evaluates the electrical activity of the brain. Electrodes are applied on the scalp surface and a reading is taken on graph paper. There is no contrast medium used.*

11. **The nurse learns a client is a college sophomore who recently transferred to the local university from another school in his home state. He reports he has been feeling depressed since he arrived and tells the nurse, "I can't seem to get with it...I don't know anyone here and can't get interested in my classes." The nurse diagnoses one of his nursing problems as which of the following?**

    1. Guilt related to failure to achieve his goals.
    2. Inability to cope related to loss or separation from loved ones.
    3. Feelings of hopelessness related to change of residence.
    4. Low self-esteem related to lack of trust.

    1. *This is not correct. Although many depressed and suicidal clients have feelings of guilt related to perceived failures on their part, there is no information in the case scenario that indicates this particular client is feeling guilty.*
    2. **Correct. This client has recently moved to a new college, is away from home, and stated that he does not know anyone. Separation from loved ones and social isolation are major risk factors for suicide.**
    3. *This is not correct. Feelings of hopelessness are highly correlated with suicidal behavior, but there is no information in the case scenario to indicate that this client is feeling hopeless.*
    4. *This is not correct. Low self-esteem and lack of trust are often associated with depression and suicidal behavior. There is a better response, however, based on the data that is contained in the case scenario.*

12. **Following spinal cord injury at or above T6, the nurse should watch the client closely for signs of autonomic dysreflexia. The nurse is aware that this potentially dangerous response could be triggered by:**

    1. Elevated blood pressure.
    2. Severe headache.
    3. Distended bladder.
    4. Edema of the spinal cord.

1. *Incorrect. A rapid rise in blood pressure, severe hypertension, is the most serious response seen in autonomic dysreflexia, due to vasoconstriction of the arterioles. It is not a triggering factor, but a result.*
2. *Incorrect. A severe headache is one of the results of autonomic dysreflexia. It is not a causative agent.*
3. **Excellent! There are many kinds of stimulation that can precipitate autonomic dysreflexia. Most are related to the bladder, bowel, and skin of the client, such as catheter changes, a distended bladder or bowel, enemas, or sudden position changes.**
4. *Incorrect. Edema of the spinal cord is a natural result of a spinal cord injury, not a causative factor of autonomic dysreflexia.*

13. **A client in the oliguric phase of acute renal failure has a serum potassium level of 5.5 mEq/L. If the client's potassium level continues to rise, the nurse will expect to observe which of the following on the EKG?**

    1. Depressed ST segments.
    2. Peaked tall T waves.
    3. Prolonged QT interval.
    4. Presence of U waves.

    1. *Wrong! This pattern may be seen in hypertrophy, or as a digitalis effect.*
    2. **Correct! Peaked T waves and ventricular dysrhythmias are frequently associated with hyperkalemia.**
    3. *Wrong. This is associated with hypocalcemia.*
    4. *Wrong. This is associated with hypokalemia.*

14. **A 12-year-old with a myelomeningocele at L2 is being seen at the clinic. Which statement by the child would indicate the need for more client teaching?**

    1. "I always drink three extra glasses of water every day."
    2. "My teacher says I need remedial reading."
    3. "I only need to catheterize myself twice a day, now."
    4. "I do wheelchair exercises while watching TV."

    1. *No! Extra fluids will help maintain fluid balance, and flush the body's urinary system. The client does not need more teaching based on this statement.*
    2. *Wrong choice! Remedial reading would be the responsibility of the school teacher, not the nurse. Normally myelomeningocele does not result in cognitive impairment.*
    3. **Excellent, this statement does indicate that the client needs more teaching! Infrequent emptying of the bladder can result in stasis and urinary tract infections. Catheterization should be performed every four hours.**

4. *Wrong choice! Wheel chair exercises maintain skin condition and upper body strength. These should be performed on a routine basis, so this statement does not indicate a need for more teaching.*

15. **A 76-year-old client was admitted to the hospital for surgery for a fractured hip. The client says to the nurse, "I guess I've lived long enough, and my number's up". Which of the following is the most therapeutic response by the nurse?**

    1. "You are in really good shape for your age."
    2. "This is just a minor setback. You will be on your feet in no time."
    3. "You feel that your life is ending?"
    4. "The doctors and nurses are going to take good care of you while you are here. There's nothing to worry about."

    1. *No. This response does not address the client's concerns. He has made a statement that implies that he is going to die. The nurse needs to explore these feelings further to be able to promote therapeutic communication. This response devalues the client's feelings and is an inhibitor to effective communication.*
    2. *This response devalues the client's feelings about himself dying. It uses a cliché and false reassurance, both of which inhibit communication. The nurse needs to address this client's feelings of doom.*
    3. **Excellent! This response uses restatement and clarification of the client's feelings to promote therapeutic communication. It addresses the client's immediate concerns.**
    4. *This response focuses on the doctors and the nurses and not on the client. This is inappropriate when promoting therapeutic communication. The feelings of the client concern death, and this response also devalues and puts off these feelings.*

16. **A client who had surgery 24 hours earlier is experiencing dyspnea and tachycardia, and has developed a fever. The nurse suspects atelectasis. If this complication is present, the nurse's auscultation of the client's lung sounds would reveal:**

    1. Diminished breath sounds.
    2. Rhonchi.
    3. A pleural friction rub.
    4. Absent breath sounds.

    1. **Correct. Assessment of atelectasis (collapse of lung tissue) would include increased pulse and temperature, and decreased breath sounds or fine crackles on auscultation.**
    2. *No, rhonchi are coarse, low-pitched, sonorous rattling sounds caused by secretions in the larger air passages. They are heard in clients with bronchitis, pulmonary edema, and resolving pneumonia.*

3. *Incorrect. A pleural friction rub, which is a grating or scratchy sound similar to creaking shoe leather, occurs when irritated visceral and parietal pleura rub against each other, as in pleurisy.*

4. *Wrong. Lung sounds would be absent in the case of a pneumothorax, which is the presence of air or gas within the pleural cavity.*

17. **When beginning ampicillin (Omnipen) 250 mg p.o. q six hours for a client's infection, the nurse should monitor which of the following?**

    1. Urine output.
    2. Urticaria or skin rash.
    3. Potassium level.
    4. Heart rate.

    1. *Wrong! Assessing for renal output would be necessary only when administering IV penicillins that contain sodium and potassium and could therefore impair renal function and urine output.*

    2. **Excellent! Allergic reactions such as urticaria or skin rash are a significant problem in the use of any of the penicillins. Assessing for allergies is a priority when administering penicillins.**

    3. *This is not correct. Potassium level is an indication of renal function and does not need to be assessed at this time.*

    4. *Ampicillin does not affect cardiac status.*

18. **The client's last menstrual period began on April 2nd. She is certain that she conceived on April 16th. According to Nagele's rule, which of the following would be her expected date of confinement?**

    1. *January 23rd.*
    2. *January 9th.*
    3. *July 9th.*
    4. *July 23rd.*

    1. *Incorrect. To calculate the expected date of confinement, you use the first day of the last menstrual period, count back three months and add seven days. The date of conception is not considered.*

    2. **Excellent work! You calculated the expected date of confinement using the correct formula: take the first day of the last menstrual period, count back three months and add seven days.**

    3. *Incorrect. To calculate the expected date of confinement, use the first day of the last menstrual period, count back three months and add seven days. The date of conception is not considered.*

    4. *Incorrect. To calculate the expected date of confinement, use the first day of the last menstrual period, count back three months and add seven days. The date of conception is not considered.*

19. **In planning care for a newborn with a surgical repair of a myelomeningocele, the nurse should**

be aware that this child is prone to developing which of the following?

1. Osteomyelitis.
2. Decubitus.
3. Otitis media.
4. Hydrocephalus.

1. *Wrong! Osteomyelitis results from an organism gaining access into the bone. This is unlikely in the surgical repair of a myelomeningocele.*

2. *Wrong! If the child suffers neurological impairment and motor loss, decubiti may be a concern. In the postoperative period, however, decubiti are unlikely.*

3. *Wrong choice! Otitis media results from dysfunctioning eustachian tubes. These are not related to neural tube defects.*

4. **Great choice! In the surgical repair of the myelomeningocele, the pathway for the cerebral spinal fluid has been altered. Therefore, the child is at risk for hydrocephalus.**

20. **Before giving preoperative medication to a client going to surgery, the nurse must make sure that:**

    1. The client has an empty bladder.
    2. Vital signs are documented on the preoperative check list.
    3. Dentures are removed.
    4. The consent form has been signed.

    1. *Incorrect. This assessment is desirable, but not critical prior to administering the preoperative medication. If a client expresses the need to urinate after the medication has been given, then the urinal or bedpan would be used. Remember that the client cannot get out of bed after the preoperative medication has been given (for safety reasons).*

    2. *No, this is important prior to the client's transport to the surgical suite, but it's not necessary that the data be documented prior to preoperative medication. What would be important is the fact that the vital signs were TAKEN prior to the administration of the preoperative medication.*

    3. *Incorrect. The client may wish to keep the dentures in place until called to the operating room. It is not critical that they be removed at this time.*

    4. **Correct. For legal reasons, the nurse must always check to see that a consent form has been signed before giving the preoperative medication. The client cannot be under the influence of narcotics or sedatives when signing, or the client's "mental competence" could be challenged.**

21. **A nurse working in an adolescent clinic should know which of the following about obesity?**

1. In teenagers, it is commonly due to hypothyroidism, hypopituitarism, or other endocrine problem.
2. Obesity is no more likely to be associated with emotional conflicts in teenagers who are not obese, than in teenagers who are obese.
3. During adolescence, obesity is highly correlated with significant psychopathology.
4. Obesity is often associated with poor recognition of either hunger or satiation.

1. *Not correct! Obesity in adolescence is rarely caused by an endocrine disturbance.*
2. *Wrong! Obese teenagers are more likely to experience emotional conflicts than their normal weight peers. The emotional conflict is often associated with the effects of being overweight rather than the cause of their obesity.*
3. *Obesity is not correlated with significant psychopathology.*
4. *Correct. Persons who become obese have poor recognition of feelings of hunger or satiation after eating. Normal-weight persons tend to eat when they feel hungry, but obese individuals tend to eat when they see food, whether they are hungry or not.*

22. **A client was told that her doctor found a lump in her breast and that a biopsy would have to be done. The client asks the nurse, "Do you think it is cancer?" Which of the following would be the best initial response by the nurse?**

1. "You seem to be worried about what the doctor may find."
2. "Do you have a family history of breast cancer?"
3. "We won't know anything until the biopsy is done."
4. "Most lumps are not cancerous, so you really shouldn't worry."

1. *Correct choice. Communication theory holds that the nurse should focus on the client's feelings. This answer focuses on the client's feelings of concern that she may have cancer. The response addresses the "here and now" and clarifies how the client is feeling.*
2. *This response focuses on the client's family history, not on the client's feelings. The stem of the question asks which response is "best initially." After the client's feelings are addressed the nurse may want to obtain this information but it is not the best initial response.*
3. *Wrong. This response does not answer the client's question or promote further expression of the client's feelings. This communication block puts the client's feelings of fear on hold.*
4. *Wrong choice. This response offers false reassurance and does not encourage the client to express her feelings concerning the fear of cancer. Saying "Don't worry" devalues the client's feelings.*

23. **A three-month-old client is being admitted with pyloric stenosis. She has an IV of D5 & 0.2 N/S at 22 mL/hour. She is NPO awaiting surgery. Which nursing assessment takes priority?**

1. Urine output of 30 mL in two hours.
2. IV site red.
3. Skin turgor elastic.
4. Baby acts slightly irritable.

1. *No. Hydration status is important with pyloric stenosis but a urine output of 30 mL in two hours time is normal for a three-month-old infant.*
2. *Excellent choice! Because the child is NPO, maintaining IV access is critical. These children often come into the hospital with fluid and electrolyte imbalances because of the vomiting. IV fluids are essential.*
3. *Wrong choice! Elastic skin turgor is a sign of normal hydration and would not be of concern.*
4. *Wrong choice! The infant is probably hungry or may be uncomfortable due to the new environment and the IV. Being slightly irritable may be normal. If the irritability increases considerably, then the nurse needs to become more concerned.*

24. **A client who is seven weeks pregnant is complaining of urinary frequency. She asks the nurse if this will continue throughout the pregnancy. Which of the following is the best response by the nurse?**

1. "Yes, it will, but if you decrease your fluid intake it won't be so bothersome."
2. "No, it should only last until 12 weeks of gestation, but it will return near the end of the pregnancy."
3. "No, it should only last until 28 weeks of gestation unless you have poor bladder tone."
4. "There is no way to predict how long it will last, we'll just have to wait and see."

1. *Incorrect. Urinary frequency usually disappears at about 12 weeks of gestation when the uterus rises out of the pelvis, thus reducing pressure on the bladder. Fluid intake should not be restricted because it is important for the expectant woman.*
2. *Correct. Urinary frequency usually disappears at about 12 weeks of gestation but returns at the end of the pregnancy following engagement, or the dropping of the fetal head into the pelvis.*
3. *Incorrect. The presence or absence of bladder tone has no bearing on urinary frequency in pregnancy; rather pressure on the bladder is the reason.*
4. *Incorrect. Since we know that most women report that urinary frequency disappears at about 12 weeks of gestation.*

25. **A client is hypertensive. The nurse is preparing to do client teaching. Which of the following goals is least appropriate?**

    1. The client eliminates sodium from the diet.
    2. The client exercises moderately each day.
    3. The client maintains weight appropriate for height.
    4. The client discontinues use of birth control pills.

    1. *Very good! Eliminating sodium from the diet is not a reasonable goal because sodium is present in so many foods. A diet appropriate for a hypertensive client will restrict intake of sodium, not eliminate it.*
    2. *Exercising moderately each day is an appropriate goal for a hypertensive client. This question has a false response stem, so the correct answer is a goal that is NOT appropriate for a hypertensive client.*
    3. *Maintaining weight appropriate for height is an appropriate goal for a hypertensive client. This question has a false response stem, so the correct answer is a goal that is NOT appropriate for a hypertensive client.*
    4. *Discontinuing use of birth control pills is an appropriate goal for a hypertensive client. This question has a false response stem, so the correct answer is a goal that is NOT appropriate for a hypertensive client.*

26. **A client's behavior becomes a problem on the unit because he talks incessantly with everyone he sees. He also tends to intrude on private conversations as well as constantly interrupt others when they are speaking. During a team conference, various ways of handling the client's behavior are discussed. Which of the following is the best course of action to follow?**

    1. Escort the client back to his room each time the staff observe him talking with other clients.
    2. Discuss this problem in a community meeting with all the clients on the unit present.
    3. Discuss the problem with the client and identify specific limits or consequences that the staff will apply if he is not able to control his behavior.
    4. Wait until his lithium levels are in the therapeutic range, when he will have better self-control.

    1. *Preventing the client from interacting with others on the unit will isolate him and tend to further lower his self-esteem. This cannot be the correct option.*
    2. *Using peer pressure to control undesirable behaviors is a principle of treatment in a therapeutic milieu. However, there is an important intervention that should be implemented prior to discussing the problem in a community meeting.*

3. *Excellent choice! The client needs to have clear limits set on his behavior by the staff members. This is best done by discussing the problem behaviors with the client and informing him of external controls that will be imposed by staff members if he is not able to exercise self-control.*
4. *Wrong choice! The client will be better able to control his behavior when his lithium levels are in the therapeutic range but his out-of-control behavior should not be ignored while waiting for his serum levels to rise.*

27. **A client is admitted to the hospital after complaining of chest pain. The client's history reveals congestive heart failure. He has been receiving digoxin (Lanoxin). The nurse understands that the purpose of giving the client digoxin is to:**
    1. Increase cardiac size.
    2. Decrease cardiac output.
    3. Increase the force of cardiac contraction.
    4. Slow the pulse rate.

    1. *Incorrect! The client has a history of congestive heart failure. His heart is not pumping effectively, so the blood is backing up in the pulmonary system and increasing his heart size. Digoxin helps reduce (not increase) the size of the poorly working heart.*
    2. *Incorrect! The client has a poorly functioning heart due to congestive heart failure. His heart is not pumping adequately. Digoxin increases (not decreases) cardiac output.*
    3. *Congratulations! Digoxin increases the strength of the heart's contractions, increases output, and slows the heart rate, which decreases the heart size, reduces edema, and increases urine output. This answer requires an analysis of digoxin.*
    4. *Incorrect choice! Digoxin slows the heart rate and increases cardiac output.*

28. **A client is an insulin dependent diabetic. He is scheduled for a gall bladder x-ray in the Outpatient Department. He was given medication to take as a prep for this test. Which of the following nursing actions is most important when preparing the client for this test?**

    1. Explain the procedure to the client, and ask if he has any questions.
    2. Give the client directions to the Outpatient Department and the parking lot.
    3. Explain to the client that he should not take his insulin before the x-ray.
    4. Tell the client to take his insulin and eat breakfast before leaving home.

1. *Wrong! Any client scheduled for a test should be given an explanation and an opportunity to ask questions but this is not the most important nursing action in preparing the client for the test.*
2. *No. The client should be given directions to the Outpatient Department and information about where to park but this is not the most important nursing action in preparing him for the test.*
3. ***You selected the correct answer! If the client takes his insulin before the test but remains NPO as required for the procedure, potentially life-threatening hypoglycemia may result. Maintaining the glucose level is a physiological need that should receive highest priority based on Maslow's Hierarchy of Needs.***
4. *This option is not correct! The client should not eat breakfast. The test for which he is scheduled requires that he remain NPO. It is also very important that the client not take his insulin, because taking his insulin without eating breakfast may cause a potentially life-threatening hypoglycemia.*

29. **When doing a physical assessment on a client with early common bile duct obstruction, the nurse would expect to see which clinical manifestation?**

    1. Dark yellow urine.
    2. Ascites.
    3. Clay-colored feces.
    4. Petechiae.

    1. *Incorrect. Dark yellow urine is a normal manifestation in clients with concentrated urine, possibly due to low fluid intake or dehydration. It is not symptomatic of a common bile duct obstruction.*
    2. *No, ascites is a complication of liver failure caused by portal hypertension. This accumulation of fluid in the abdominal cavity is not an early symptom of common bile duct obstruction.*
    3. ***Correct. Clay-colored feces indicates that bile has been obstructed from entering the intestinal tract, causing the absence of urobilin (which gives the characteristic brown color to feces).***
    4. *Wrong choice. Petechiae, small pinhead hemorrhages, are typically associated with bleeding disorders, not with bile duct obstruction.*

30. **The nurse is speaking to a group of young couples regarding the process of conception. Some of them are interested in preventing conception, and others are trying to achieve conception. Which of the following information should be related to these couples who wish to plan the timing of pregnancy?**
    1. The female ovum is only capable of fertilization for 48 hours after ovulation.
    2. The male sperm is capable of fertilization for up to three days after ejaculation.

3. Abstinence of intercourse for 48 hours after a rise in basal body temperature will prevent pregnancy.
4. The ideal time for fertilization to occur is day 12-16 of the menstrual cycle.

1. *Incorrect, the female ovum is only capable of fertilization for 24 hours following ovulation.*
2. ***Correct, the male sperm is capable of fertilization for up to 72 hours or three days after ejaculation.***
3. *Incorrect, a rise in basal body temperature occurs 24 to 36 hours after ovulation. Since the male sperm is capable of fertilization for 72 hours, abstinence of intercourse following a rise in BBT will not prevent conception.*
4. *Wrong, most women ovulate 14, plus or minus two days, prior to the onset of the next menses. In a normal 28-day menstrual cycle this would be days 12-16, but in a 40 day cycle, for example, it would be days 26-30.*

31. **The nursing assistant says to the nurse, "This client is incontinent of stool three or four times a day. I get angry when I think that he is doing it just to get attention. I think adult diapers should be used for him." Which of the following is the best initial nursing response?**

    1. "You are probably right. Soiling the bed is one way of getting attention from the nursing staff."
    2. "Changing his bed and cleaning him must be tiresome for you. Next time it happens, I'll help you."
    3. "It's upsetting to see an adult regress."
    4. "Why don't you spend more time with him if you think that he is behaving this way to get more attention?"

    1. *This response is not therapeutic because it does not address the nursing assistant's feelings. The response offers no encouragement of expression of feelings. The communication block of showing approval can be identified by the phrase, "you are right."*
    2. *This response shows empathy on the part of the nurse, but it does not encourage any further expression of feelings. The nurse needs to obtain more information about the nursing assistant's statement concerning the client's soiling the bed purposely, to provide therapeutic communication.*
    3. ***Excellent! This response encourages the nursing assistant to clarify her feelings that the client is soiling the bed for attention. The question asks which is the best "initial" response. Since this is the only option that addresses the feelings of the client, it is the best choice.***
    4. *This response does not address the feelings of the client. It offers advice instead of focusing on how the client feels. This action may be the solution to the problem but it isn't the best initial response.*

STRATEGY ALERT! *This communication question asks you to prioritize the nursing responses. The correct option also uses assessment to gather further information before taking action. The nursing process requires that assessment always takes priority over implementation.*

32. When transferring a client from a bed to a chair, the nurse should use which of the following techniques to avoid a back injury?

1. Bend at the waist while maintaining a wide stance, lift the client to a standing position, and then pivot the client toward the chair.
2. Have the client lock his or her hands around the nurse's neck, so that the client will feel more secure during the transfer.
3. Place the bed in an elevated position so that the client's hips are at the same level as the nurse's hip, resulting in the center of gravity being the same for both individuals.
4. Bend at the knees, while maintaining a wide stance and straight back, with the client's hands on the nurse's shoulders and the nurse's hands at the client's axillae.

1. *Wrong. Bending at the waist places strain on the small lower back muscles, which are prone to injury.*
2. *Wrong. If the client's hands are locked around the nurse's neck and then the client starts to fall, all of the client's weight is placed on the cervical vertebrae of the nurse, which can result in a serious injury. The client's hands should rest on the shoulders of the nurse.*
3. *Wrong. The bed should be in the low position, which provides a place for the client to sit if he is unable to stand. With the bed elevated, once the client attempts to stand, the client cannot sit back down on the bed if he becomes weak or faint, because the bed is too high.*
4. ***That's right! Bending at the knees results in the use of the large muscles of the legs. Keeping the back straight avoids using the small, easily injured back muscles. When the client's hands rest on the nurse's shoulders, this provides security for the client. Placing the hands under the axillae of the client avoids placing pressure on the chest, which can be uncomfortable for the client.***

33. A six-month-old infant is one day postoperative after receiving a colostomy. When the nurse positions him on his side, he stiffens and begins to cry. Which initial nursing action would the nurse take?

1. Leave the baby to rest, as infants' pain perception is not the same as older children.
2. Check when the last pain medication was given to see if able to give it now.

3. Check the abdominal dressing, as this may indicate an infection.
4. Call the mother in, as this is a sign of decreased attachment.

1. *Wrong! Thinking that infants do not feel pain is a myth that some hold to be true. Infants do feel pain and there is ample research to back this.*
2. ***Best choice! Stiffening and crying may be indicators of pain. This infant is only one day postoperative. Pain relief is essential for healing and recovery.***
3. *Wrong! Stiffening alone is not an indicator of infection. You would need to look at other assessment data such as redness, swelling, drainage, and perhaps increased body temperature.*
4. *False. A six-month-old would benefit from mother's presence, but there is not enough data here to indicate decreased attachment.*

34. The nurse administering digoxin (Lanoxin) to a client notices that his breakfast is untouched. He also is complaining of nausea. The nurse checks his vitals, which are BP 118/72, P 60, R 22. How would the nurse interpret the data?

1. The client is anxious and fearful.
2. The client needs a change in diet.
3. This is a normal reaction to the hospital.
4. He may be exhibiting a drug reaction.

1. *There is no information that would lead to the conclusion that the client is feeling anxious.*
2. *This is not the best choice! This might be true if the client were not taking digoxin.*
3. *Wrong! Nausea is not normal. The nurse needs to further assess what is causing the client's nausea.*
4. ***Good job! Digoxin toxicity includes nausea and vomiting, and bradycardia. In the assessment the nurse notes that the pulse rate is marginal. Bradycardia is usually defined as 60 or less. Therefore the client may be exhibiting a drug reaction.***

35. A physician has prescribed oral neomycin as well as a neomycin enema for a client with cirrhosis who is having central nervous system changes. The nurse would know that the neomycin has been effective if which of these laboratory values are decreased?

1. White blood cell count.
2. Ammonia.
3. Creatinine.
4. Serum albumin.

1. *Incorrect. A decreased white blood cell count would be evident after antibiotic therapy for an infection. Cirrhosis is not an infectious process.*

2. *Yes. The antibiotic neomycin is given to reduce the number of intestinal bacteria capable of converting urea to ammonia. As the serum ammonia level decreases, the central nervous system changes decrease. Keeping the serum ammonia level within normal limits will help to decrease the chances of hepatic encephalopathy.*

3. *No. Creatinine is a measure of kidney glomerular filtration, not liver function, and would not be affected by neomycin therapy.*

4. *Wrong. Serum albumin levels are not affected by neomycin, an antibiotic. In cirrhosis, the serum albumin level is already decreased due to altered protein metabolism.*

36. **A client has been incontinent of loose stool and is complaining of a painful perineum. The most appropriate nursing action initially is to:**

    1. Notify the physician to obtain an order for the loose stools.
    2. Check the client's perineum.
    3. Turn the client every two hours.
    4. Increase the client's fluid intake to prevent dehydration.

    1. *Informing the physician is a possibility but it does not address the client's concern, and the issue in the question, which is perineal pain. Also, note that this is an implementation action. The key word in this question is "initially." The nurse should always assess first!*

    2. **Excellent! This option addresses the client's concern, which is the painful perineum. This option is also the best because it is an assessment action. The nurse should always assess first!**

    3. *Turning an immobilized client every two hours will help prevent skin breakdown but it does not address the issue of the question, which is a perineal pain.*

    4. *Preventing dehydration is important for the client with loose stools. Although this is the client's medical diagnosis, it is not the issue this question. The issue is perineal pain, which is the subject of the client's complaint.*

37. **A client with advanced cirrhosis is admitted with bleeding esophageal varices. A Sengstaken-Blakemore tube has been inserted. In planning care for this client, the nurse knows that the primary purpose of the Sengstaken-Blakemore tube is to:**

    1. Coagulate the bleeding varices.
    2. Prevent the aspiration of blood into the lungs.
    3. Apply direct pressure to the bleeding varices.
    4. Provide a means for removing blood from the stomach.

1. *No, the Sengstaken-Blakemore tube does not have the capability to coagulate the bleeding varices; only a cautery can do this.*

2. *Wrong. Although the Sengstaken-Blakemore tube, when properly inflated, will prevent aspiration of blood into the lungs, that is not the primary purpose for the tube. The three openings in the tube are for specific purposes: gastric aspiration, inflation of the gastric balloon, and inflation of the esophageal balloon.*

3. **Correct. The Sengstaken-Blakemore tube compresses the bleeding vessels through inflation of the esophageal balloon, which applies direct pressure to the site. This is the primary purpose of the Sengstaken-Blakemore tube.**

4. *Incorrect. The Sengstaken-Blakemore tube does have one opening that is used for aspirating gastric contents, but that is not the primary function of the tube.*

38. **A pregnant client on iron supplements for iron-deficiency anemia calls and reports that her stools are black. She has no abdominal pain or cramping. What is the best response by the nurse?**

    1. "Come right in and we will check things out."
    2. "Go to the emergency room and your doctor will meet you there."
    3. "This is normal because of the way that iron is broken down during digestion."
    4. "What else have you been eating? This is unusual."

    1. *No, this would not be an appropriate response because coming to the office would not be necessary.*

    2. *Wrong choice! This would not be an appropriate response since the symptom is a normal side effect of high iron intake and not a medical emergency.*

    3. **Correct. Iron does turn the stools black. In the absence of cramping and abdominal pain, this is nothing to worry about. The client should have been instructed to watch for black stools.**

    4. *Incorrect. Black stools are expected from iron tablet therapy.*

39. **The nurse finds an elderly client with her IV pulled out, standing next to her bed with the side rails in the up position. The client is confused, does not have an identification bracelet on, and cannot remember her name. What should the nurse do first?**

    1. Help the client into bed, and remind her to call the nurse when she wants to get out of bed.
    2. Help the client into bed, and then restart the IV.
    3. Place a restraining vest on the client.
    4. Put an identification bracelet on the client and help her back to bed.

1. *Reminding a confused client to use a call light is not an appropriate nursing action. The case scenario tells you that the client cannot remember her name, so she will probably not remember to use a call light. Since a physiological need is not identified in this question, the safety of the client is the most important nursing consideration at this time. Which priority setting guideline will you use in this question?*

2. *The case scenario does not tell you whether the IV has life-saving medications or fluids infusing, so you cannot assume that the IV is a physiological need. Do not "read into" the question! Since a physiological need is not identified, the safety of the client is the most important nursing consideration at this time. Which priority setting guideline will you use in this question?*

3. ***Excellent! The case scenario tells you that the client got out of a bed that had the side rails up. This is an unsafe situation, since the client is at risk of falling. Such an injury can be life-threatening. Placing a restraining vest on the client will provide for her safety.***

4. *Wrong, although the client's lack of an identification bracelet is an important safety concern. The case scenario tells you that the client got out of a bed that had the side rails up. This is an unsafe situation, since the client is at risk for falling. Such an injury can be life-threatening. After the immediate physical safety of the client is assured, an identification bracelet can be obtained. Which priority setting guideline will you use in this question?*

40. **A client's husband asks to speak to the nurse about what effects he and his wife should expect after she is treated with electroconvulsive therapy. He says, "I know it will improve her depression but couldn't it also turn her into a vegetable?" After explaining that ECT will not cause any brain damage, what additional information can the nurse ethically give him?**

    1. "The main side effects, which are only temporary, are mild confusion, a slight headache, and short-term memory problems."
    2. "Most clients have no adverse effects to this treatment. In rare cases it has been known to cause fractures resulting from the induced seizure."
    3. "Some clients with cardiac problems have been known to have a heart attack, but we will monitor her closely to be certain this does not happen."
    4. "There are no permanent adverse effects associated with this treatment. The only common side effect is short-term memory problems, which can last for a few weeks."

    1. *Correct. The main side effects are mild disorientation and confusion immediately after the treatment, a slight headache, and short-term memory*

problems. Information about the treatment should be presented by the treating psychiatrist, but the nurse should reinforce this information and answer any questions the client and family may have.

2. *Wrong. There are several possible adverse effects to ECT but fractures are not one of them. Before receiving the treatment, the client is medicated with a muscle relaxant to prevent any muscle contractions, with resulting fractures, during the brain seizure.*

3. *This statement is not factually correct and would be inappropriate to present to a client or family member. Clients receive a complete medical history and physical exam before being scheduled for ECT. In addition, any client with heart disease should receive a cardiology consultation and clearance before receiving ECT. ECT is not done when a client has a history of recent myocardial infarction or aneurysm.*

4. *This statement, while technically correct, is not truthful. Whenever general anesthesia is used there is a small risk of death. Clients need to be accurately informed of both the risks and benefits so they can make an informed decision.*

41. **A 39-year-old client is having surgery on his bowel. The doctor orders a cleansing enema for the morning of surgery. Which of the following nursing interventions is most appropriate?**

    1. Wear gloves to insert the tubing.
    2. Use universal precautions and provide comfort measures to help the client relax during the procedure.
    3. Lubricate the tubing well prior to insertion.
    4. Position the client on his side and drape the client for warmth and privacy.

    1. *Gloves should be worn to prevent contamination. This is a possible answer but there is a better statement of the most appropriate nursing intervention.*

    2. ***Very good. This is a comprehensive statement of the best nursing intervention. Using universal precautions and providing comfort measures will prevent contamination and provide for the well-being of the client.***

    3. *Close. Lubricating the tube provides for the safety and comfort of the client by facilitating insertion. There is an even better statement of the most appropriate nursing intervention.*

    4. *Positioning and privacy are important aspects of administering an enema but there is a better statement of the most appropriate nursing intervention.*

42. **A client, admitted with ascites and an elevated serum ammonia level secondary to cirrhosis, is receiving dietary instructions. The nurse will know that the client has accurate understanding of his dietary needs if he selects a menu that is:**

1. High in protein, low in salt.
2. High in calories, moderate in protein.
3. Low in carbohydrates, high in fat.
4. Low in calcium, low in potassium.

1. *No, this diet is not therapeutic for this client. A high protein diet is only indicated when the client with cirrhosis has no ascites or edema and exhibits no signs of impending coma. Low salt would be appropriate for a client with ascites to reduce fluid retention.*
2. ***Correct choice. The client needs calories to promote liver tissue healing, but moderate to low protein intake to decrease ammonia production (a result of protein metabolism). Excessively high levels of ammonia in the blood are a primary cause of the neurologic changes that constitute hepatic encephalopathy, a dangerous complication of cirrhosis.***
3. *Incorrect. The client needs a therapeutic diet to promote healing of the liver and to prevent further ammonia production. A high fat diet is indicated when the goal is to delay gastric emptying, as in clients with "dumping syndrome" secondary to a gastric resection.*
4. *No, this type of diet is not indicated in clients with cirrhosis. Electrolyte disturbances are not indicated in the symptoms listed above.*

43. **A 14-month-old girl is admitted to the hospital with a fractured femur. Which of the following lunches would be most appropriate for the nurse to provide?**

    1. Infant formula.
    2. Chicken fingers and string beans.
    3. Strained chicken and strained beans.
    4. Hamburger and french fries.

    1. *Wrong. Solids would have been introduced to the child at around six months of age.*
    2. ***Best choice! These "finger foods" appeal to a 14-month-old and offer appropriate nutrition as well. A fractured femur does not require a special diet.***
    3. *Wrong. This may be a nutritious meal, but it offers little variety in texture, and the child cannot easily feed herself.*
    4. *Not the best choice! It is best to avoid fried foods when possible. Foods should be poached, broiled, or baked rather than fried.*

44. **An 82-year-old client is diagnosed with colon cancer. She asks the nurse several questions about what the doctor might be planning to do. The nurse does not know which options the physician may have decided to recommend to the client. The physician will be making rounds within the hour. Which of the following nursing actions is most appropriate?**

1. Help the client write down the questions to ask her physician, so that she doesn't forget when the doctor rounds in 30 minutes.
2. Assure the client that the doctor will tell her what has been planned.
3. Tell the client to have her daughter call the doctor to ask what options the doctor plans to recommend.
4. Provide the client with articles from several medical journals that discuss colon cancer.

1. ***Excellent! Forgetfulness is a part of the aging process. Since the nurse does not know the answers to the client's questions, and the physician will be making rounds soon, this action addresses the client's needs.***
2. *This response by the nurse blocks communication by putting the client's concern on hold and giving false reassurance. The nurse does not know what the doctor will tell the client. The nurse must always be in a therapeutic role and should address the client's needs. Which of the four options is the best response?*
3. *Having the client tell her daughter to call implies that the client's concerns can wait, and that her daughter is more important or more competent than she is. This option uses the communication blocks of putting the client's concerns on hold, and referring to inappropriate persons. The nurse must always be in a therapeutic role, and therapeutic communication must address the feelings and concerns of the client.*
4. *This option fails to address the client's concerns about what the doctor is going to prescribe for her, and it is also inappropriate because the client may not understand the information presented in the articles. This action does not promote therapeutic communication and is the wrong choice.*

45. **A 16-year-old, 5'4" high school student is admitted to an eating disorders program by her psychiatrist. She tells the admitting nurse she has lost 25 pounds over the past month and now weighs 85 pounds. The nursing assessment identifies several behaviors that are characteristic of clients in the beginning stages of anorexia nervosa, which could include:**

1. Appetite loss, amenorrhea, bradycardia, loss of 15% of pre-illness body weight.
2. Appetite loss, amenorrhea, tachycardia, hyperactivity.
3. Tachycardia, insomnia, fear of obesity, bulimia.
4. Amenorrhea, bradycardia, disturbed body image, loss of 15% of pre-illness body weight.

1. *This is not totally correct. Clients with anorexia usually experience amenorrhea, bradycardia, and*

loss of 15% of pre-illness body weight. Although they voluntarily refuse to eat, they do not typically experience appetite loss until they have been ill for a long time.

2. *This is not totally correct. Clients with anorexia do experience amenorrhea and hyperactivity, but do not experience tachycardia. Appetite loss does not occur until the late stages of the illness.*

3. *This is not totally correct. Clients with anorexia do experience amenorrhea, and fear of obesity. They do not experience insomnia. While many clients do have bulimia, many do not.*

4. ***Correct. Amenorrhea, bradycardia, disturbed body image, and loss of 15% of pre-illness body are among the most common symptoms experienced by anorexic clients.***

46. **The nurse is assisting a frail elderly client to eat. The client begins to choke and indicates to the nurse that she cannot talk. The first nursing action is to:**

    1. Perform the Heimlich maneuver to obtain a patent airway.
    2. Begin mouth to mouth resuscitation.
    3. Place an oxygen mask on the client.
    4. Go to the nurses' station to get some help.

    1. ***You are correct! The client is beginning to choke, which is a life-threatening situation. Performing the Heimlich maneuver on this client may alleviate the obstruction and provide the client with a patent airway.***
    2. *Because the client does not have a patent airway and is conscious, mouth to mouth resuscitation is an inappropriate first nursing action.*
    3. *Oxygenation correctly identifies a physiological need in this question but administering oxygen to a client who does not have a patent airway is inappropriate. There is no access for air exchange, so oxygen is of no value to this client.*
    4. *Leaving a client who is in distress is very inappropriate! If immediate nursing measures are ineffective, help can be summoned without leaving the client. The nurse can summon help by calling out, using the call system, or using the emergency call system.*

47. **A client is discharged from the hospital. She will continue taking lithium and will be seen in the clinic on a regular basis after discharge. The nurse knows that the client on long-term lithium therapy risks developing which condition?**

    1. Hyperthyroidism.
    2. Hypoglycemia.
    3. Impaired kidney function.
    4. Gall stones.

1. *Hypothyroidism, not hyperthyroidism, is a risk of long-term lithium therapy. This cannot be the correct answer.*
2. *This is not correct. Long-term lithium therapy is associated with diabetes insipidus but not diabetes mellitus or hypoglycemia. Read the options again to identify the correct answer.*
3. ***Excellent! A major risk of long-term lithium therapy is impairment of the kidney's ability to concentrate urine, which can progress to nephrogenic diabetes insipidus. Good work!***
4. *This is not correct. Long-term lithium therapy is not associated with gall bladder disease.*

48. **A client is gravida 5 para 4. During admission, the nurse assesses that contractions are occurring every two minutes and lasting approximately 45 seconds. The client says she has been in labor for approximately 10 hours. The priority assessment the nurse needs to make at this time is which of the following?**

    1. Time the client last ate.
    2. Cervical dilatation.
    3. Allergies to medications.
    4. Vital signs.

    1. *Incorrect! The time the client last ate is not the first priority for this client.*
    2. ***Great choice! Based upon your knowledge of the stages of labor, full dilatation usually takes approximately eight hours in a multi-gravida woman. Since this woman has already been in labor for 10 hours, the first priority is to assess cervical dilatation to best plan for a safe delivery.***
    3. *Wrong choice! This is not the priority assessment.*
    4. *Incorrect. While vital signs are important to assess in the mother and the fetus, if she delivers while the nurse is taking them, the conditions for delivery may not be safe.*

49. **The physician has ordered a client to be discharged on a 2000 calorie diabetic diet. What is the most important nursing action in developing a teaching plan for this client's diet?**

    1. Obtaining sample menus from the dietitian to give to the client.
    2. Asking the client to identify the types of foods that she usually eats and prefers.
    3. Telling the client that she will have to change all of her previous eating habits.
    4. Advising the client to buy only dietetic foods.

    1. *Sample menus may be helpful in providing the client with ideas for new foods or exchanges. It is not the most important nursing action. This question requires use of the nursing process, and this is an implementation action.*

2. *Excellent! Asking the client what types of foods she prefers provides an opportunity for the nurse to include these foods in the client's diet, which will promote compliance.*

3. *No! The client may have to change some of her eating habits, but not all of them! Telling the client what to do is inappropriate and this response does not give the client any information that the client can use in complying. Note that the absolute word "all" is a clue that this is probably a false statement.*

4. *This is not even good advice! Fresh fruits and vegetables and many other unprepared foods are permitted in a diabetic diet, and the diabetic may also use some prepared foods that are not labeled "dietetic." The statement is also incorrect because there are not enough dietetic foods available to meet all of the client's dietary requirements.*

50. **While changing a surgical dressing, the nurse notes green, foul-smelling drainage at the incision site. Another postoperative client is sharing the same room with this client. The most appropriate nursing action is to:**

    1. Place the client with the drainage in a private room.
    2. Institute drainage and secretion precautions.
    3. Move the other client to another room.
    4. Place the client in strict isolation until the organism has been cultured and identified.

    1. *This action is not necessary. A client with a wound infection does not need a private room. However, the integrity of the other client in the room needs to be taken into consideration. The nurse should institute measures that will meet the basic needs of both clients.*

    2. *Very good! Implementing drainage and secretion precautions protects not only the client with the wound infection, but other clients and the nurse as well. This option meets the physiological needs of all of the people mentioned in the case scenario by maintaining their physiological integrity in preventing the spread of infection.*

    3. *Moving the other client is not appropriate in the care of a client with a wound infection. Other, less drastic nursing measures can be instituted that will meet the basic needs of both clients.*

    4. *Placing the client in strict isolation is not an appropriate nursing action for a client with a wound infection. Strict isolation is used to prevent the transmission of highly communicable diseases. A wound infection is not considered to be highly communicable. Other nursing measures can be instituted to prevent possible spread of the infection.*

51. **The nurse walked into the room to assess a four-year-old admitted with croup. The mother says, "He never wets the bed at home, I am so embarrassed." The nurse helps the mother and then**

invites her into the hall. Which of the following statements is the nurse's most appropriate response to the mother's statement?

1. "I know this can really be embarrassing, but I have kids myself, so I understand and it doesn't bother me."
2. "It is not uncommon for children to regress during a hospitalization. His toileting skills will return when he is feeling better."
3. "It's probably due to the medication we are giving him for his infection."
4. "I plan to discuss your child's incontinency with the physician as this may require further investigation."

1. *No. Though you may have heard nurses say this, this is not therapeutic communication, since it offers no information about the source or treatment of the incontinence. It also inappropriately focuses on the nurse's feelings rather than the client's.*

2. *Good! This is correct. A recently gained skill such as toilet training is often temporarily lost due to the stress of hospitalization. It is appropriate to reassure the mother that this is an expected behavior in young children and the previous continence will be regained when his health is regained.*

3. *No. The medications most likely to be administered for croup would be antibiotics and acetaminophen; neither have side effects of incontinence.*

4. *Not likely, with the information given. Are you reading into the question? Symptoms such as hematuria, abdominal pain, or pain during urination would be necessary to warrant follow-up from this one.*

52. **The nurse would expect to make which of the following observations about a client to relate to a diagnosis of myocardial infarction rather than angina?**

    1. A feeling of an intermittent strangling sensation.
    2. Complaints of sudden substernal pain after an argument.
    3. Feelings of numbness or weakness in arms and wrists.
    4. Profuse perspiration with nausea and vomiting.

    1. *Wrong! A feeling of an intermittent strangling sensation is related to angina. Angina is characterized by pain or discomfort that is intermittent or acts at intervals.*

    2. *Wrong! Angina is caused by loss of blood flow or oxygen to the heart muscle. This discomfort or pain is temporary and is frequently caused by stress such as an argument.*

    3. *Wrong! Feelings of numbness or weakness are characteristics of angina. These feelings are associated with a decrease of oxygen to the heart muscle.*

4. *Excellent! This is the only option that is characteristic of a myocardial infarction. This is a priority assessment. Any client demonstrating extreme sweating, nausea and vomiting may be experiencing a heart attack. Immediate medical help is needed. In a myocardial infarction, a portion of the heart muscle is destroyed because of a blocked blood supply. This is an assessment question that focuses on identifying what the nurse needs to identify for a client who may be experiencing a myocardial infarction.*

53. **A 22-year-old client has had surgery on his foot and has just been returned to his room from the recovery room. The initial assessment indicates that he is stable. An hour later, his roommate turns on the call light and tells the nurse that the client has gotten up and hopped on one foot to the bathroom, using his IV pole for support. Which of the following actions would the nurse do first?**

1. Open the bathroom door to assess if the client is okay.
2. Help the client back to bed and get him a urinal.
3. Explain to the client that it is not safe for him to be hopping around on one foot.
4. Get a wheelchair and help the client back to bed when he is done in the bathroom.

1. *Incorrect choice! Even though the client should not have hopped to the bathroom, the nurse should respect his privacy and knock on the door to determine if he is okay.*
2. *Wrong choice! The client will have to hop back to bed with the nurse helping him, which is not a very stable method of ambulation. This is not safe.*
3. *This intervention is appropriate, but it is not the priority action. Getting the client safely back to bed is the priority issue for the nurse.*
4. *Good choice! Since the client is already in the bathroom, the nurse should allow him to void, and then return him to his bed safely in a wheel chair. This is an implementation question, and the stem asks you to prioritize the actions. This option meets the physiological and safety needs of the client.*

54. **A client who is incontinent of stool has been placed on a bowel training program. The nurse understands that the goal of bowel training is:**

1. To prevent soiling of the bed.
2. To prevent cancer of the colon.
3. To prevent loose stools.
4. To provide the client with control over his bowels.

1. *Bowel training will help the client to avoid soiling of the bed, but preventing soiling of the bed is not the goal of bowel training.*

2. *Bowel training does not prevent cancer.*
3. *Loose stools cannot be prevented by bowel training.*
4. *Very good. Bowel training provides the client with the ability to control bowel elimination.*

55. **A client is sitting by his food tray and pushing the food around on his plate. He says to the nurse, "I hate hospital food. Is this the only thing that I can get to eat?" Which of the following responses would be the best initial response by the nurse?**

1. "What is it about the food that you dislike?"
2. "Well, the other clients haven't complained about the food. Is something else bothering you?"
3. "I'll call the kitchen and order something else for you."
4. "Is there something special that you would like to eat?"

1. *Very good! This response promotes communication by addressing the feelings that the client has about the food. This response asks for clarification of the statement made by the client. Clarification is a tool that promotes therapeutic communication.*
2. *Wrong. This response focuses on the other clients and tells the client that his feelings about the food are not valid. It is also a defensive response that does not promote therapeutic communication. Asking the client if something else is bothering him may elicit an expression of feelings by the client, but the first part of the nurse's response makes this option incorrect.*
3. *Wrong. This response does not promote further communication by the client. Therapeutic communication is not developed when the nurse attempts to solve a problem without clarifying exactly what the problem is.*
4. *Wrong. The response doesn't focus on the client's feelings. He states that he hates "hospital food," not just this particular meal. This is a possible indicator of other problems. The nurse needs to explore the client's feelings before offering to get other food for him. This not the best "initial" response.*

56. **The alcoholic client tells the nurse he has not had anything to drink for 24 hours prior to admission. He complains of feeling anxious and shaky. Based on a knowledge of alcohol withdrawal, what other behaviors could the nurse expect him to display during the early phase of alcohol withdrawal?**

1. Coarse tremors, tachycardia, insomnia.
2. Confusion, visual hallucinations, delusions.
3. Disorientation, confabulation, memory deficits.
4. Incoordination, impaired thinking, irregular eye movements.

1. *Correct. The earliest signs of alcohol withdrawal are anxiety, anorexia, insomnia, and tremor. Tachycardia of 120-140 beats per minute persists throughout withdrawal. Pulse rates are closely monitored during the withdrawal process to assess the client's condition and need for medication.*

2. *This is not correct. The onset of confusion, visual hallucinations, and delusional activity indicates delirium tremens (DT's), a complication of untreated alcohol withdrawal. Delirium tremens, now called alcohol withdrawal delirium, is a potentially fatal complication of alcohol withdrawal that occurs when the withdrawal process has not been medically managed. It begins the second or third day after the client's last drink and lasts 48 to 72 hours.*

3. *This is not correct. Disorientation, confabulation and memory deficits are symptoms of alcohol amnestic disorder or Korsakoff's syndrome. Thiamine deficiency, a physical disorder associated with chronic alcoholism, is thought to cause this syndrome.*

4. *This is not correct. Incoordination, impaired thinking, and irregular eye movements are seen in Wernicke's syndrome, a rare disorder of central nervous system metabolism associated with thiamine deficiency and seen chiefly in chronic alcoholics.*

57. **A client diagnosed with schizophrenia says, "They lied about me and are trying to poison my food." Which of the following statements is the nurse's best response to the client?**

    1. "You are mistaken. Nobody has told lies about you or tried to poison you."
    2. "You're having very frightening thoughts."
    3. "Tell me more about your concerns about being poisoned."
    4. "Tell me who would do such things to you?"

    1. *This statement, if made by the nurse, is directly confronting the client's delusion, which could make the client feel more angry and misunderstood. There is a better option.*
    2. *Correct. Instead of responding literally to the words, the nurse is responding to the feelings that the client was attempting to communicate. By so doing, the nurse is shifting the focus from beliefs that are not real to the client's fear, which is real.*
    3. *Not correct. This statement supports the content of the delusion, so it is not a therapeutic response. Look again at the other options.*
    4. *Incorrect. This statement supports the client's delusional thinking.*

58. **A client delivers a six-pound 12-ounce male infant at 39 weeks of gestation. She experienced an** unremarkable labor and delivery. The nurse caring for the client 14 hours after delivery, assesses the following: Breasts soft; fundus firm, U +1, slightly deviated to the right; lochia moderate rubra; T 100° F, P 88, R 18. Which of the following nursing actions should be initiated?

    1. Ask her to empty her bladder.
    2. Report her temperature elevation.
    3. Suggest that she begin to nurse more frequently so her milk will come in.
    4. Nothing, these are normal assessments for 14 hours after delivery.

    1. *Excellent choice! Whenever the fundus is deviated from the midline a full bladder must be considered. A full bladder could result in complications such as uterine atony or infection.*
    2. *Wrong. A temperature up to 100.4° F following delivery is often the result of dehydration. Once the client is hydrated the temperature returns to normal.*
    3. *Wrong choice. The breasts would be expected to be soft 14 hours after delivery.*
    4. *Incorrect, since the fundus should be firm at the midline following delivery.*

59. **A client, age 63, is being discharged after insertion of a pacemaker for a persistent dysrhythmia. Which of the following statements made by the client indicates the need for further teaching?**

    1. "I know that I have to check my pulse every day, preferably in the morning."
    2. "I sure will miss being able to continue with my bowling league. I guess I'll take up walking as a sport!"
    3. "I'll stay away from my wife's microwave oven so that it doesn't interfere with my pacemaker."
    4. "If I start having any palpitations or dizziness, I'll call my doctor right away."

    1. *No, the client does understand the need to check the pacemaker's functioning every day. A pulse rate significantly above or below the programmed rate should be reported to the physician.*
    2. *Good for you! You recognized that the client does not have correct information regarding his participation in sports. He should avoid all contact sports, but should be able to resume bowling without problems.*
    3. *No, the client is correct in making this statement. He should avoid microwave ovens, arc welders, and electrical generators, as well as holding electrical equipment such as blow dryers next to his pacemaker. These activities may cause interfer-*

ence, place the pacemaker in a fixed mode or shut it off.

4. The client is correct when he knows to report any signs of decreased cardiac output, such as dizziness, fatigue, "palpitations", or dyspnea. Look for a statement that is incorrect.

60. **An ASO titer is drawn on an 11-year-old in the hospital with acute glomerulonephritis. The mother asks the nurse why the titer was drawn. Which response by the nurse is most justifiable?**

1. "This will tell us if he's ever had the measles."
2. "This will tell us if he's had a recent strep infection."
3. "This lab work is done routinely on all patients."
4. "This is done to determine the level of antibiotic is his blood."

1. *Incorrect. Titers are drawn to determine an antibody response to an infection. This titer will not tell if the child had measles. You may be thinking of a rubeola or a rubella titer.*
2. *You are correct! ASO (anti-streptolysin) titer indicates that the child has had a recent strep infection. In determining a definitive diagnosis for acute glomerulonephritis, this must be documented as it is usually the result of a recent strep infection.*
3. *Besides being a poor response to a mother who is concerned, this information is not correct. ASO titers are only drawn when a recent strep infection needs to be documented to determine the medical diagnosis.*
4. *Wrong! Blood work that is drawn to determine antibiotic levels in the blood falls under the category of therapeutic blood levels. ASO titers are drawn to determine whether the child has had a recent strep infection.*

61. **An 88-year-old client is admitted to the hospital with chest pain. His daughter tells the nurse that he has certain routines for his personal hygiene and for taking his medicine. She is concerned that he will be uncooperative while in the hospital. Which of the following would be the best initial response by the nurse?**

1. Assure the daughter that everything possible will be done to accommodate her father's needs.
2. Ask the daughter what routines and medicines her father uses at home.
3. Inform the daughter that the hospital has policies that have to be followed, and that the best care will be provided for her father.
4. Tell the daughter that she should inform the doctor about her father's routines so that orders can be written to meet the client's needs.

1. *Wrong choice. This option does not address the client's daughter's concerns. The correct answer has to address the daughter.*
2. *Excellent! This option encourages the daughter to tell the nurse about her concerns and promotes communication. This response also focuses on the nurse's responsibility to assess the client's needs.*
3. *This response devalues the daughter's concerns about her father. This is a block to therapeutic communication and therefore not an appropriate nursing response.*
4. *This response "passes the buck" to the doctor and puts the client's feelings and concerns on hold. This response inhibits communication.*

62. **The client is to receive a medication for control of tachycardia and an irregular heart rate. The nurse obtains the following vital signs prior to administering this medication: BP 98/54, P 48, R 30, T 98° F. The client's skin is cool, with cyanosis of the fingers and lips. Which of the following is the priority nursing action?**

1. Administer the medication as ordered by the physician.
2. Omit the medication for a day or two, depending on the client's response and symptoms.
3. Notify the physician concerning the client's status before administering the medication.
4. Give the client one half of the ordered dose.

1. *Administering a medication that decreases the heart rate of a client with a pulse of 48 is inappropriate, since the pulse rate may decrease even further. A pulse rate of 48 does not fall within the normal range, and results in a physiological need for oxygen for this client.*
2. *Withholding the medication is a possible nursing action, since the result of this action may be a increase in pulse rate. However, withholding the medication alone does not address all of the physiological needs identified in the case scenario.*
3. *Very good! The assessment data gathered by the nurse indicate that the client is exhibiting signs and symptoms that are not within the normal parameters. A pulse rate of 48 results in a physiological need for oxygen for this client. Withholding the medication until the physician has been notified addresses the immediate physiological need of the client. The information needs to be communicated to the physician, who will determine which medical interventions are necessary.*
4. *Changing or altering an ordered medication is a medical intervention, not a nursing action!*

63. **A client is receiving an intravenous infusion. The nurse observes the client for signs of infiltration of the IV solution. Which symptom, if noted by the**

nurse, is associated with a complication other than infiltration?

1. The infusion rate slows or stops while the tubing is not kinked.
2. The area around the injection site feels warm to the touch.
3. Swelling, hardness or pain located around the needle site.
4. Blood fails to return in the tubing when the bottle is lowered.

1. *Not the correct choice. One sign of infiltration is that the infusion rate slows or stops while the tubing is not kinked. Since this question has a negative response stem, you are looking for an exception — something that would not result from an infiltrated IV.*
2. ***Very good! The area around the injection site would not feel warm to the touch when the IV is infiltrated. The IV fluid is at room temperature, so the area around the injection site will feel cool to the touch when the IV is infiltrated. If the area around the injection site feels warm to the touch, it may indicate infection or phlebitis.***
3. *Incorrect choice. One sign of infiltration is swelling, hardness or pain located around the needle site. Since this question has a false response stem, you are looking for an exception — something that would NOT be a result of an IV being infiltrated.*
4. *Wrong choice! One sign of infiltration is that the blood fails to return in the tubing when the bottle is lowered. Since this question has a negative response stem, you are looking for an exception — something that would NOT be a result of an IV being infiltrated.*

64. **A client is admitted to the hospital with respiratory difficulty, wheezing on expiration, coughing, and diaphoresis. An intravenous infusion of aminophylline is ordered. The nurse knows that which of the following best describes the purpose of giving this medication?**

1. To relax the bronchial smooth muscles.
2. To increase the tone in the respiratory passages.
3. To cause bronchoconstriction.
4. To decrease the inflammatory reaction.

1. ***Good job! The primary purpose of aminophylline is to relax bronchial smooth muscles, which allows air to flow in and out more easily. This analysis question requires an understanding of the pathophysiological principles involved in the use of aminophylline.***
2. *No. Increasing tone in the respiratory passage is the same as bronchoconstriction. Options 2 and 3 are similar distractors. Bronchoconstriction blocks the flow in and out of the airway.*

3. *No. Bronchoconstriction and increasing the tone in the respiratory passages are similar distractors that can be eliminated. Constriction of the respiratory passages blocks the flow of air and causes respiratory distress.*
4. *Aminophylline is not an anti-inflammatory or antihistamine drug. Aminophylline is a xanthine, a spasmolytic, which relaxes the bronchial smooth muscles. The drug may be taken orally, rectally or IV.*

65. **The first, most important nursing action when a nurse discovers a fire in a client's room is which of the following?**

1. Pull the fire alarm and notify the hospital operator.
2. Close fire doors and client room doors.
3. Remove the client from the room.
4. Place moist towels or blankets at the threshold of the door of the room with the fire.

1. *This is an appropriate action but it is not the most important action. Pulling the fire alarm and alerting the hospital operator notifies the appropriate individuals who are needed to fight a fire but the immediate safety of the client in the room with the fire takes priority.*
2. *Closing fire doors helps prevent the spread of a fire to other areas of the hospital. Closing the clients' room doors helps prevent smoke and fumes from entering their rooms. While this is an important intervention to help protect the other hospitalized clients, there is another action that should be implemented first. The immediate safety of the client in the room with the fire takes priority.*
3. ***Excellent! The client in the room with the fire is at highest risk for injury. The smoke from a fire can deprive a client of adequate oxygenation, and the fire poses a direct threat to the safety of this client. Moving this client to safety receives first priority.***
4. *Placing moist towels or blankets at the threshold of the door where the smoke is coming from helps prevent the smoke and fumes from entering other areas. This is not an appropriate action to take at this time, however, because the client is at risk for injury and oxygen deprivation.*

66. **A 74-year-old client is admitted with respiratory acidosis as a complication of chronic COPD. Her blood gases reveal she is in primary respiratory acidosis. The nurse knows that this probably results from which of the following?**

1. Decreased exhalation of carbon dioxide.
2. Increased mucous secretion.
3. Long-term theophylline administration.
4. Recent vomiting and diarrhea.

1. *Good job! Clients with chronic lung disease have difficulty exhaling CO_2 due to loss of elastic recoil in the lungs. This results in respiratory acidosis.*
2. *No. Although increased mucous secretion is a symptom of COPD, it does not contribute to respiratory acidosis.*
3. *Incorrect choice. An increased respiratory rate is the only respiratory system side effect of theophylline administration.*
4. *Wrong. Recent vomiting and diarrhea would lead to metabolic alkalosis.*

67.   A client is readmitted to the hospital. After two weeks, her lithium level is within the therapeutic range and she no longer has manic symptoms. Before discharge, what information should the nurse give to the client about diet when taking lithium?

1. Sodium intake should be restricted.
2. Fluid intake should be restricted to 1000 mL per day.
3. An adequate daily intake of sodium and fluids should be maintained.
4. Sodium and fluid intake should be increased.

1. *This information would be incorrect! Restricting sodium intake would cause the lithium level to rise, leading to a state of toxicity. A loss of sodium through profuse sweating, vomiting, or diarrhea would also lead to toxicity.*
2. *No. Clients on lithium should drink six to eight glasses of water a day to maintain a normal state of hydration. This cannot be the correct answer.*
3. ***Correct! Clients should be cautioned to maintain a consistent intake of sodium and fluids to avoid developing lithium toxicity. If they should become physically ill, they should notify their psychiatrist at once.***
4. *Wrong advice! Increasing sodium or fluid intake would tend to lower the client's lithium level. If the level should drop below the therapeutic range, the client might relapse.*

68.   In providing care to a client who is hyperventilating, the nurse knows that which of the following conditions is most likely to be associated with hyperventilation?

1. Fatigue.
2. Opiate withdrawal.
3. Anxiety.
4. Petit mal epilepsy.

1. *Incorrect. Hyperventilation is not a sign of fatigue.*
2. *Incorrect. Opiate withdrawal is associated with*

yawning but not hyperventilation.
3. ***Correct. Hyperventilation frequently is a sign of severe to panic levels of anxiety.***
4. *Not correct. Hyperventilation is not associated with petit mal epilepsy.*

69.   A client asks the nurse how much weight is safe for her to gain during her pregnancy. The nurse appropriately teaches the client, that in relation to gaining weight during pregnancy, which of the following is recommended?

1. A maximum weight gain of about 15 pounds (6.8 kg).
2. A weight gain of about 12 pounds (5.5 kg) each trimester.
3. As long as the client does not feel hungry, the actual amount of weight gain has little significance.
4. A range of about 20 to 30 pounds (9 to 14.5 kg).

1. *No. This little weight gain is associated with poor fetal outcome.*
2. *No, this would result in a total gain of 36 pounds, which is excessive. A gain of four pounds in the first trimester and 12 pounds each for the 2nd and 3rd trimester is recommended.*
3. *Incorrect. The amount of weight gain is important.*
4. ***Correct, a weight gain of 20-30 pounds is associated with good fetal outcome.***

70.   The nurse is caring for a client who had abdominal surgery two days ago. Which of the following assessment data requires immediate action by the nurse?

1. A urinary drainage bag with 100 cc's of straw colored urine.
2. A wound dressing with thick light green drainage.
3. A blood pressure reading of 98/66.
4. Shallow respirations, with a rate of 30.

1. *Wrong! The amount of urine in the drainage bag does not provide any useful data, since the clinical situation does not include a time frame for measuring the client's output. More information is needed.*
2. ***Good choice! Thick light green drainage is indicative of an infection and should be reported to the physician immediately. The stem of the question requires analysis of the data by the nurse. This option also addresses a client safety issue, which requires an immediate response by the nurse.***
3. *Wrong! Since baseline data is not provided in the question, the nurse cannot determine whether or not the blood pressure reading is normal for this*

client. Further assessment is needed.

4. *Shallow respirations are not unusual for the client who has undergone abdominal surgery. Although the nurse needs to address this issue by having the client deep breathe and cough, it is not the priority action.*

71. **A nine-year-old is admitted for surgery for slipped capital femoral epiphysis. Aware of the main concerns of a child of this age, the nurse would want to plan to do which of the following?**

    1. Arrange for his parents to be with him continuously.
    2. Obtain a telephone to be at his bedside.
    3. Plan with the physician to obtain Patient Controlled Analgesia postoperatively.
    4. Provide special hospital pajamas.

    1. *Wrong! The presence of parents is important in helping the child cope with hospitalization. This is especially true of a young child such as an infant, toddler, or preschooler because separation from their parents is one of this age's major stressors. At the age of nine, however, fear of procedures and needles are more stressful than separation. Also, the nurse cannot force parents to stay with their children.*

    2. *No, he's too young to be helped much by this. A telephone would be very important to assist this child with his hospitalization if he were an adolescent. This would help him connect with his peer group.*

    3. ***Great choice! School age children have an extreme fear of needles. They will endure large amounts of pain just to avoid an injection. Obtaining Patient Controlled Analgesia will help avoid some injections, while obtaining pain relief for this child.***

    4. *Wrong! Normalizing the hospital experience is one of the goals in pediatrics. Giving children a choice of what they wear gives them more control in this stressful experience and can help them to cope better. In this case, the child may prefer to wear his own clothes or pajamas. This would be something that the nurse would do for all children, not specifically for this nine-year-old.*

72. **Two weeks after a client started taking amitriptyline (Elavil) she reported that she was sleeping better and her appetite had improved. She said, however, that she still felt hopeless and sad. In response to this, the best action for the nurse to take is to:**

    1. Notify her physician so that she can be switched to another drug.
    2. Ask her physician to increase her dose of Elavil.
    3. Explain that antidepressants often take three to

four weeks to be fully effective.
    4. Chart her complaints in the nursing notes.

    1. *This would not be a correct action. The client's physician will want to know how she is responding to her medication, but this is not the best option. Her antidepressant most likely will not be changed if she is experiencing some improvement in her target symptoms. Read the other options to identify the best nursing action.*

    2. *This is a possibility, but it is not the best nursing action because it does not deal with client education, which is issue this question is addressing. Look at the other options for a better choice.*

    3. ***Correct. The lag time for tricyclic antidepressants is three to four weeks before the client will experience significant improvement. The client has only taken her medication for two weeks, so she still has symptoms of a depressed mood, even though her sleep patterns and appetite have improved.***

    4. *This is an appropriate action, but it is not the best action for the nurse to take. Try again.*

73. **In the middle of making morning rounds, a client says to the nurse, "I almost died last night." Which of the following is the most therapeutic nursing response?**

    1. "You made it through the night."
    2. "Patients do have dreams that they die when they are hospitalized."
    3. "Are you feeling okay now?"
    4. "That must have been frightening for you. Tell me more about it."

    1. *This response is flippant and does not place any value on the client's concerns or feelings. Therapeutic responses focus on the client's feelings and promote further expression of feelings. This option makes light of what might have been a serious situation.*

    2. *This response focuses on other clients, and not on the feelings of the client at hand. It is a generalization that offers false reassurance. The nurse needs to validate and clarify the client's concerns.*

    3. *This response does not address the client's concern about "almost dying." It implies that his concern about dying is not valid if the client is "okay" now. Although the client should be assessed for his present status, his conversation indicates that he is concerned most about "almost dying".*

    4. ***Excellent choice! This response directly addresses the concern of the client. The nurse uses the communication tool of empathy in responding to this client's concerns and clarifies the client's feelings. This is the best response.***

74. **A client returns from surgery with two penrose**

drains in place. In anticipation of frequent dressing changes, what should the nurse use to most effectively reduce skin irritation around the incision area?

1. Montgomery straps.
2. Silicone spray.
3. Hypoallergenic tape.
4. Large, bulky absorbent pads.

1. Correct. Montgomery straps are adhesive strips applied to the skin on either side of the surgical wound. The strips have holes for the use of gauze to "tie" the dressing secure. When the dressing needs changing, the ties are released, the dressing changed, and the ties then secured again without removing the adhesive strips. This taping technique will decrease irritation to the skin around the wound edges.

2. Incorrect choice -- silicone spray is appropriate, but its purpose is not to reduce skin irritation. Silicone spray is used OVER the adhesive to hold the dressing in place. The silicone waterproofs the dressing so that the client can bathe. It also isolates the area from contamination.

3. Incorrect choice -- hypoallergenic tape is used when a client is sensitive to adhesive material, but it still has to be removed with each dressing change. This could increase the risk of skin irritation.

4. Wrong. The large, bulky absorbent pads would certainly absorb more wound drainage, but would not prevent skin irritation around the incisional area.

75. A client has congestive heart failure and is on digoxin (Lanoxin). In response to this client's question, the nurse explains that digoxin affects cardiac function through which of the following mechanisms?

1. Decreasing the strength of cardiac contractions and increasing the heart rate and conduction time.
2. Increasing the strength of cardiac contractions, the heart rate and conduction time.
3. Increasing the strength of contractions while decreasing the conduction time and heart rate.
4. Decreasing the strength of cardiac contractions, the heart rate and conduction time.

1. Not correct! Digoxin increases the strength of contractions and decreases heart rate and conduction time.

2. No! Digoxin does increase the strength of contractions, but does not increase the heart rate and conduction time.

3. Correct! Digoxin makes contractions stronger and slows the heart rate and conduction time. In other words, digitalis drugs have a positive inotropic action and a negative chronotropic and dromo-

tropic action. This improves cardiac output.

4. Wrong! Cardiac contractions are strengthened. Conduction time and heart rate are decreased.

76. During administration of medications to a client, the priority nursing assessment is which of the following?

1. Help the client swallow medications without aspirating by keeping the head in a neutral position.
2. Identify the client by checking the client's identification bracelet and asking for his name.
3. Keep all prepared medications in sight.
4. Check the client for desired or undesired drug effects within an hour after administration of the medication.

1. Maintaining the head in a neutral or slightly flexed position is an appropriate nursing action that facilitates the movement of tablets or capsules down the esophagus and into the stomach. This question requires use of the nursing process to prioritize. This option is an implementation action. What is the first step in the nursing process?

2. Very good! Identification of the client helps to ensure that the medication will be given to the right client. This is one of the "five rights" of administering medications: the right client, the right drug, the right dose, the right route, and the right time.

3. Keeping prepared medications in sight is important in assuring that the right medication will be administered in the right dose. The nurse can ensure that the medications will not be disturbed and will not be taken by others. This nursing action is part of the implementation phase of the nursing process. Can you identify the priority assessment action?

4. Evaluating the client's response to a medication is important for identifying undesired signs of toxicity or side effects. For example, after administering a narcotic pain medication, the nurse might observe signs of respiratory depression. The nurse may also evaluate whether the medications are helpful, which can be seen in relief of pain. Evaluation is the last phase of the nursing process. Can you identify the priority assessment action?

77. A 78-year-old diabetic who is blind was admitted to the hospital for an infected leg ulcer. The nurse would avoid which nursing intervention in caring for this client?

1. Place her food tray directly in front of her on the overbed table and remind her that the tea is hot.
2. Speak to the client when entering her room, and identify oneself.
3. Show her where everything is in the room.

4. Place her belongings within easy reach.

1. *Very good! You have identified the inappropriate action. The issue in this question is blindness. It is not a sufficient safety measure to simply place the tray directly in front of the client and remind her that the tea is hot. To prevent the client from getting burned by spilling the tea, the nurse should also show or tell the client where the tea and other items on the tray are located.*

2. *This is an appropriate action in caring for a blind client. The nurse should speak on entering (and leaving) as well as ensure that the client knows the nurse's name, so that she will not become startled and will know who is entering (or leaving) the room. This question has a false response stem. Look for the option that is INAPPROPRIATE.*

3. *Showing the blind client where objects in the room are located is an appropriate action that provides for the client's safety and makes the client more comfortable in the hospital environment. This question has a false response stem. Look for the action that is INAPPROPRIATE.*

4. *Placing belongings within easy reach provides for the client's safety. If objects are not within easy reach, the client may become injured when getting out of bed unnecessarily to locate them, or may fall out of bed trying to reach them. This is an appropriate nursing action in caring for a blind client. This question has a false response stem. Look for the option that is INAPPROPRIATE.*

78. **A four-year-old is brought into the emergency room with burns to her neck and face. Which of the following has the highest nursing priority for this child at this time?**

1. Potential for infection.
2. Ineffective individual coping.
3. Fluid volume deficit.
4. Potential for ineffective airway clearance.

1. *Wrong. Infection is always a very important risk factor in burns but, in this case, it is not the immediate priority.*

2. *Wrong. Coping may be a concern because of the severity of the burns but it is not the immediate priority initially.*

3. *Wrong! Burns may cause fluid shifting in the body and fluid volume deficit can result. This is important, but not the immediate and most life-threatening priority initially.*

4. *Correct! An ineffective airway is the immediate and most life-threatening possible complication for this child. The location of the burns around the head and neck make this even more of a risk factor due to potential swelling in this area. Children's airways are also considerably smaller than an adults until approximately seven years of age, which increases this risk also.*

79. **When administering ear drops with a dropper, which of the following actions taken by the nurse best prevents contamination of the bottle of medication?**

1. Washing hands prior to preparing the medication.
2. Holding the dropper with the tip above the ear canal.
3. Washing the client's ear prior to instilling the medication.
4. Filling the dropper with only the prescribed number of drops.

1. *Good try. Hands should be washed before preparing any medication but ear drops should not come in contact with the hands, so this action will not prevent contamination of the solution.*

2. *Yes! Holding the dropper above the ear canal prevents the tip of the dropper from touching the ear. Touching the dropper tip to the skin would contaminate the end of the dropper, which will contaminate the solution when the dropper is placed in the bottle.*

3. *Wrong! The ear may be cleansed if dried secretions or drainage will interfere with absorption of the medication. This action, however, will not protect the bottle of solution from contamination.*

4. *This is not a correct action. The dropper should be filled with sufficient medication to assure that enough drops are available for use at the time of instillation, since it is difficult to determine how many drops are available in every size of dropper.*

80. **The primary nurse learns that an obsessive-compulsive client has a full set of dentures because he eroded all his tooth enamel with his brushing rituals. He also brushes his tongue several times a day, and has developed several ulcerations on it. His nursing care plan should set the highest initial priority for which of the following?**

1. Eliminating his brushing and mouth care rituals.
2. Verbalizing the underlying cause of his behavior.
3. Seeking out the nurse when he is feeling anxious.
4. Reestablishing healthy tissue in his mouth and tongue.

1. *This option is the goal of his treatment and not the highest initial priority.*

2. *This may or may not be appropriate, as behavioral methods will most likely be used to treat the client's problems. This is not the correct response as it would not be the highest initial priority.*

3. *This is an appropriate goal but is not the highest initial priority for his care.*

4. *Correct. Restoring physiological integrity is the highest initial priority for this client. This will be done while working on the long-term goal of decreasing the mouth care rituals.*

81. **The nurse caring for a client with a history of congestive heart failure is aware that which condition is likely to contribute to digoxin (Lanoxin) toxicity?**

    1. Hypokalemia.
    2. Hypocalcemia.
    3. Obesity.
    4. Hyponatremia.

    1. *Correct! Potassium actually inhibits the excitability of the heart. A depletion of potassium, therefore, will increase excitability. Potassium loss increases the likelihood of digitalis cardiotoxicity.*
    2. *No. Hypocalcemia may interfere with the effectiveness of digoxin therapy, but it is not associated with digoxin toxicity.*
    3. *Wrong! Digoxin is not affected by obesity.*
    4. *No. Digoxin toxicity is unlikely to result from hyponatremia.*

82. **A 77-year-old client was hospitalized for observation after a fall that he experienced when he was walking for exercise. He is to ambulate for the first time since his fall. He tells the nurse that he is afraid to get up. Which of the following statements would be the best response by the nurse?**

    1. "There is nothing to be afraid of. Your doctor wouldn't have written the order if the doctor didn't think that you were ready."
    2. "Tell me what concerns you about getting up today?"
    3. "I will have another person here to help you when you get up."
    4. "Are you afraid of falling again?"

    1. *Wrong choice. This response does not facilitate a response from the client. It devalues his concerns by making the doctor's orders seem more important. It also focuses on the doctor and not on the client. A therapeutic response focuses on the client's feelings.*
    2. *Excellent! This nursing response focuses on the client's feelings. It gives value to the client's statement by directly addressing it and clarifying what the client is feeling concerning ambulating.*
    3. *This response may not address the client's concerns, since the nurse does not know why the client is afraid. Clarification is necessary before the nurse can plan to meet the client's needs. This response focuses on the nurse's action and not on the client's feelings.*
    4. *Wrong. The question may lead the nurse to assume that the client is afraid of falling, but the nurse cannot be sure of that assumption. Communication theory states that clarification is an important aspect of effective communication. The response*

also inhibits communication since the client can answer the question with just a "yes" or "no".

83. **After six months, the physician determines that the client is no longer responding well to lithium. After discontinuing the lithium, the physician prescribes valproic acid (Myproic Acid), an anticonvulsant that is also effective in bipolar disorders. What special instructions should the nurse give the client about valproic acid?**

    1. A pretreatment EEG must be done and repeated in six months.
    2. Liver function and hematology levels must be monitored.
    3. Thyroid function tests must be done every six months.
    4. The white blood count must be monitored regularly.

    1. *EEGs would be done on clients who are being treated for a seizure disorder. They are not indicated for clients who are being treated for a bipolar disorder. This is not the correct answer.*
    2. *Correct. Pancreatitis and severe hepatic dysfunction are two adverse effects associated with this medication. Even though they are relatively rare, blood testing should be done every three to six months.*
    3. *Hypothyroidism is a long-term risk for clients on lithium, not valproic acid. This is not the correct answer.*
    4. *Agranulocytosis is an adverse effect associated with carbamazepine (Tegretol) and clozapine (Clozaril), not valproic acid. This is not the correct answer.*

84. **The nurse would instruct an antepartum client to call the physician if she experiences which of the following symptoms in her pregnancy?**

    1. Facial edema.
    2. Urinary frequency.
    3. Nausea and vomiting.
    4. Breast leakage.

    1. *Good choice! Facial edema is an indication of pregnancy induced hypertension and needs to be reported immediately to the health care provider.*
    2. *Wrong choice! Urinary frequency is a normal symptom of pregnancy caused by pressure on the bladder.*
    3. *Incorrect. Nausea and vomiting are often a response to high hormone levels in pregnancy. Only if they continue for long periods of time would they be a cause for concern.*
    4. *Incorrect. Breast leakage is often seen during the second and third trimesters and is related to the woman's prolactin level.*

85. A client is to be transferred from her bed to a stretcher, in order to be transported to surgery for a fractured hip. The first most important nursing action is to:

   1. Provide for the client's privacy with a blanket.
   2. Lock the wheels on the stretcher and the bed.
   3. Have four people available for lifting the client.
   4. Provide a lifting device to assist with moving the client.

   1. Covering the client with a blanket for privacy provides for the client's comfort and self-esteem. Maslow's Hierarchy of Needs identifies self-esteem as a high level need. Look for an option that addresses a more basic need.
   2. Excellent! Locking the wheels on the bed and the stretcher stops their movement and helps prevent client falls between the bed and the stretcher. Safety is the priority concern in this question.
   3. If the nurse requires help with a transfer, the number of assistants required will depend upon the situation. More or fewer people may be needed to assist the nurse. This action might be appropriate, but this cannot be the best option. Look for an accurate statement that identifies a priority action.
   4. A transfer device can assist with transferring a client from a bed to a stretcher by decreasing the amount of strength and energy required by the nurses or persons who are performing the transfer. This action might be appropriate, but this cannot be the best option. Look for an accurate statement that identifies a priority action.

86. After a bronchoscopy, which assessment, if made by the nurse, would require immediate action by the nurse?

   1. Blood-tinged mucous.
   2. Complaints of hoarseness when speaking.
   3. Irritation and discomfort when swallowing.
   4. Difficulty breathing.

   1. Blood-tinged mucous and sputum is normal after this procedure. The bronchoscope when inserted may cause trauma to the tissue of the larynx, trachea or bronchi.
   2. The client may complain of hoarseness after the bronchoscopy because of the trauma to tissue of the larynx and the trachea.
   3. This is another normal symptom after a bronchoscopy. The swallowing reflex is usually blocked for about six hours after the procedure. Initially the client may have some discomfort and difficulty when the swallowing reflex is restored.
   4. Good choice! This is a priority assessment that needs immediate medical treatment. The difficulty in breathing may be caused by edema in the larynx or trachea and is a serious complication.

87. A 38-year-old client is admitted with PIH (pregnancy induced hypertension). The physician orders a urinalysis. When the nurse collects the urine specimen, which of the following measures taken by the nurse is the most important?

   1. Labeling the container with the client's room number.
   2. Checking the identification of the client.
   3. Using sterile gloves when handling a urine specimen.
   4. Instructing the client to put the specimen on the counter at the nurses' station for pick-up.

   1. This is not the most important measure, and it is not sufficient for identifying the specimen.
   2. Yes, you are correct! In order to avoid errors, the most important thing to do is to identify the client. After the client is identified, the next action is to make sure the specimen label has the client's name and identification number.
   3. No. Gloves should be worn when handling any specimen, for the protection of the nurse. Sterile gloves are not necessary, however, since the nurse should not be touching any sterile surfaces.
   4. This is not proper technique. The nurse should take the specimen container in the dirty utility room.

88. A client is hospitalized for a closed reduction of a fractured femur and application of a cast. A vital nursing action in the care of this client is to:

   1. Perform neurovascular checks of the extremities.
   2. Use the palms of the hands when moving an extremity with a wet cast.
   3. Provide an instrument for the client to scratch the itching areas of skin under the cast.
   4. Petal the edges of the cast to provide smooth edges.

   1. Excellent! This is an important aspect of care for the client with a fracture. Circulation can become compromised and cause nerve and tissue damage. This action is more "vital" than the other three options.
   2. Using fingertips on a wet cast can cause indentations in the cast, resulting in pressure areas inside the cast. Using palms only when moving the still wet cast is an appropriate nursing action, but it is not the most important or "vital" action.
   3. This is not an appropriate nursing action! Scratching under the cast can cause injury to the skin and potential infection.
   4. Petaling the edges of the cast should be done to prevent injury to the skin caused by uneven edges of the cast. This answer is similar to another choice in that it concerns care of the cast, but it is not the most important or "vital" action.

89. In planning preoperative care for a client, the nurse is aware that obtaining legal, informed consent to perform surgery is the responsibility of:

    1. The nurse.
    2. The surgeon.
    3. The client's family physician.
    4. The client.

    1. *Incorrect. The nurse's responsibility is to ensure that an informed consent has been obtained voluntarily from an informed and comprehending person. The nurse may present a form for the client to sign, and the nurse may sign the form as a witness to the signature. However, this does not transfer legal liability for informed consent for medical care to the nurse.*
    2. ***Yes. To attain the right to operate, it is necessary for the surgeon to obtain a voluntary and informed consent from the client. Before the client signs the consent form, the surgeon should inform the client in clear and simple terms what a reasonable person would want to be told, including an explanation of what the surgery will entail, as well as the possible risks and complications of the surgical procedure.***
    3. *No. The client's family physician does not have responsibility for obtaining the informed consent. The family physician's role is purely advisory in this situation.*
    4. *No. The client's family physician does not have responsibility for obtaining the informed consent. His role is purely advisory in this situation.*

90. A 21-year-old client is admitted to the hospital because of extreme weight loss. It is noted on the admission assessment that the client believes that she is overweight at 88 pounds. What aspect of care should the nurse consider the patient's first priority?

    1. Assessing the client's nutritional status.
    2. Obtaining a psychiatric consult.
    3. Planning a therapeutic diet for the client.
    4. Talking to the family members to find out more about the client's self- concept.

    1. ***Excellent! The client's nutritional status should receive first priority, because nutrition is a basic physiological need. If the client's nutritional needs are not met, the situation may be life-threatening.***
    2. *Obtaining a psychiatric consult may be an appropriate intervention, but with only the information given in this case scenario, it would not take priority at this time.*
    3. *Close. You are correct in identifying nutrition as a basic physiological need and a high priority. Planning a nursing intervention, however, should come after one of the other options in this question.*

    4. *Obtaining further information from the family may be appropriate, but it is not the priority action in this situation.*

91. A client has an intravenous fluid infusing per gravity at 125 mL/hour. Which of the following assessment findings indicates to the nurse that the IV site needs to be changed?

    1. The IV is infusing at 75 mL/hour regardless of the height of the IV bag.
    2. The area around the IV site is reddened but not tender.
    3. There is fluid leaking at the connecting site.
    4. There is blood backing up in the IV tubing.

    1. *Although the height of the bag has an impact on the flow of the IV fluids to the client, height alone does not control flow rate. There is not enough information, about the drip control or roller valve for instance, with which to make a determination that the IV site should be changed.*
    2. ***Good choice! Redness noted at the IV site is an indication of possible phlebitis or infection, and the IV site should be changed. The stem of this question requires the nurse to analyze the assessment data.***
    3. *Wrong. Fluid leaking at the connecting site may be an indication that the connection is loose and in need of tightening.*
    4. *Wrong. Blood backing up in the tubing is an indication that there is not enough pressure from the IV bag to push the fluid into the client. This could be caused by an empty IV bag or a bag that is too low.*

92. A post-mastectomy client returns to the surgical unit with a closed-wound suction device (Hemovac) in place. Which action by the nurse will ensure proper operation of the device?

    1. Irrigate the tubing with sterile normal saline once each shift.
    2. Empty the device when it's full.
    3. Keep the tubing above the level of the surgical incision.
    4. Recollapse the device whenever it's one-half to two-thirds full of air.

    1. *No! The Hemovac has a drainage catheter connected to a spring-loaded drum. It is not possible to irrigate the tubing. Patency is accomplished through another option.*
    2. *No! The device should be emptied when it STARTS to fill, to prevent the weight of the collected drainage from pulling on the insertion site. There is no suction if the collecting device is full of drainage.*
    3. *No! This action would defeat the purpose of a portable suction device. The tubing should always be below the level of the incision to enhance drainage.*

4. *Yes, you understand the functioning of the Hemovac! The Hemovac, which has a drainage catheter connected to a spring-loaded drum, must be collapsed periodically to create the desired suction, which pulls fluid into the collection area of the device. As drainage or air accumulates, it is emptied and the Hemovac recompressed.*

93. **An antepartum client's lab work reveals that she has a negative rubella titer. The nurse knows that the result of the test:**

    1. Means that the client does not have rubella at this time.
    2. Means that the client is immune to rubella and need not worry about exposure in this pregnancy. She does not need to be immunized.
    3. Means that the client is not immune to rubella and needs to be immunized as soon as possible.
    4. Means the client is not immune to rubella and will need an immunization following delivery.

    1. *Incorrect. A negative rubella titer means that the client has never had rubella. Although she may not have rubella at this time, this is not how it is verified.*
    2. *Incorrect. A negative rubella titer means that the client has never had rubella and has no protection against the rubella virus.*
    3. *Wrong. The first part of this answer is correct, but immunization during pregnancy is contraindicated because of possible damage to the developing fetus.*
    4. *Correct! This negative rubella titer means that the client is susceptible to the rubella virus and needs vaccination after delivery. Further teaching not to conceive for three months after immunization is indicated.*

94. **A two-year-old boy is brought to the emergency room with nausea and diarrhea. Which statement by the parents would cause the nurse to be most concerned?**

    1. "His last wet diaper smelled very strong."
    2. "He is very quiet when he is playing."
    3. "His lips are dry and crusty."
    4. "He cries whenever I put him down."

    1. *Wrong option! Strong smelling urine may indicate concentrated urine but the child is still voiding.*
    2. *Wrong choice! A lethargic child may be cause for alarm. This child, however, is still playing and the parents give no indication of decreased alertness.*
    3. *Excellent choice! A dry and crusty mouth are classic signs of dehydration, which would be a cause for immediate concern.*
    4. *Sorry, wrong choice! A sick child, or a child in a new situation may feel fearful and irritable and cry to be held. This in itself is an expected finding.*

95. **A four-year-old who had hydrocephalus as an infant is admitted with a malfunctioning ventriculo-peritoneal shunt. Following new shunt placement, the nurse conducts a postoperative check. Which assessment would demand an immediate response from the nurse?**

    1. Sleepy, very difficult to arouse.
    2. Pupils equal and reactive to light.
    3. BP 100/60, apical pulse of 90.
    4. Urine output 33 mL in two hours.

    1. *You are correct! The child may be sleepy following surgery, but should be easily aroused. Lethargy could indicate increased intracranial pressure.*
    2. *Wrong! The nurse should expect to find pupils equal and reactive to light. This indicates normal neurological function.*
    3. *Wrong! These vital signs are well within normal range for a four-year-old. They do not indicate any need for action.*
    4. *Incorrect! A urine output of 30 mL in two hours indicates adequate renal function. It does not necessitate immediate action.*

96. **A client is admitted to the hospital for cataract surgery of the left eye. The physician has ordered eye drops to be administered to both eyes at frequent intervals prior to surgery. Which of the following nursing actions is most appropriate?**

    1. Use aseptic technique and avoid dropping the medication onto the cornea.
    2. Gently wash away any crust along the eyelid margin with warm water.
    3. Have the client look up toward the ceiling prior to instillation of drops.
    4. Drop prescribed number of drops into the conjunctival sac.

    1. *Excellent! Aseptic technique is always used when administering medications. The cornea is very sensitive to anything applied to it and should be avoided.*
    2. *Cleansing the eyelid provides a clean area for instillation of the drops. This is an appropriate nursing action but there is another, more global option that is better. Read the other options and try to identify the best option.*
    3. *Having the client look up protects the cornea from the drops landing on it. The cornea is very sensitive to anything applied to it and should be avoided. This is an appropriate nursing action but not the best answer. Read the other options and try to identify the best option.*
    4. *The drops should be instilled into the conjunctival sac to avoid placement on the cornea, which is very sensitive. This is an appropriate nursing action. Read the other options and try to identify the best option.*

97. **The nurse can evaluate the agoraphobic client's progress as improving when the client is able to attend which of the following activities?**

1. Daily community/milieu meetings.
2. Occupational therapy on the unit.
3. The hospital gift shop.
4. A unit picnic in a local park.

1. *This is not correct, since the community meetings are held on the hospital unit. The client's phobia does not concern exposure to other people.*
2. *This is not correct. Occupational therapy sessions are held on the unit.*
3. *This is not correct. The gift shop is within the hospital building. This client will show improvement when she is able to leave the building.*
4. ***Correct. The park is outside of the hospital building, so the client would be demonstrating some improvement if she were able to leave the hospital to attend a picnic.***

98. **A client is seen in the emergency room for abdominal pain, and is scheduled for emergency surgery. Which of the following is most important for the nurse to include in preoperative teaching for the client?**

1. An explanation of the hospital billing process for clients receiving surgery.
2. Instruction about deep breathing and coughing, with abdominal splinting.
3. Having the client sign the surgical consent.
4. An explanation of where the incision will be and how much drainage to expect on the dressing after surgery.

1. *Explaining this process to the client is informative, but is not appropriate prior to emergency surgery. This option does not address the issue of the question, which is preoperative teaching.*
2. ***Excellent! Any client having abdominal surgery should be taught deep breathing and coughing.***
3. *Obtaining the surgical consent is not a part of preoperative teaching, which is the issue in this question.*
4. *There is not enough information to permit the nurse to explain the location of the incision and amount of drainage. There is another option that is more important in preoperative teaching.*

99. **A 75-year-old man is a psychiatric client who is taking lithium for a bipolar mood disorder. The nurse knows that elderly clients:**

1. Cannot be safely treated with lithium.
2. Take the same dosage of lithium as younger adults.
3. Treated with lithium have a therapeutic range of 0.6-0.8 mEq/L.
4. Treated with lithium have a therapeutic range of 0.6-1.4 mEq/L.

1. *Incorrect. Elderly clients who do not have cardiovascular problems or other medical problems that would be contraindications, can be treated safely with lithium.*
2. *This would tend to be an incorrect statement. In general, elderly clients are treated with lower doses of lithium. The dose is determined by the serum levels, so some elders may take the same dosage as younger adults.*
3. ***Correct. The therapeutic range for elderly clients is narrower with 0.8 mEq/L as the upper level. This is because elderly clients, or clients with medical illness, may develop symptoms of neurotoxicity such as confusion and disorientation.***
4. *This is not the correct therapeutic range for elderly adults. Read the other options.*

100. **The nurse enters a client's room. The client's son tells the nurse, "You people can't do anything right. Ever since my father was admitted to this hospital, it has been one mistake after another. I am taking him out of here before you kill him." The most therapeutic response by the nurse is which of the following?**

1. "You feel that your father is not being well taken care of?"
2. "We have the best intentions for the clients."
3. "I'll get the supervisor for you."
4. "Your father hasn't complained about the care. What specifically is the problem?"

1. ***Excellent! This response uses the communication tool of restatement and focuses on the issue. This response encourages the son to express his concerns to the nurse. The nurse needs more information from the client before problem-solving can occur. This response also focuses on the "here and now".***
2. *Incorrect. This response is a defensive remark by the nurse, which is a communication block. This response implies that whatever is bothering the son cannot be valid, and this response may escalate the situation. A therapeutic response would encourage the son to tell the nurse why he feels upset concerning his father's care.*
3. *This response puts the feelings of the son on hold by asking him to wait until the supervisor arrives. Therapeutic communication addresses the "here and now," and does not "pass the buck" to another person. Indeed, the supervisor may become involved, but the best response by the nurse is to address the client's immediate needs.*
4. *This response focuses on the father, but the son is the one with the concerns. It implies that the son's feelings cannot be valid since his father has not voiced any complaints. This is not a therapeutic nursing response and contains the communication blocks of not addressing the client and devaluing his feelings.*

NOTES

NCLEX-RN

Test 3

NCLEX-RN TEST 3

1. **A client diagnosed with urolithiasis is advised to follow a low calcium diet after his pathology report reveals calcium oxalate stones. Which of the following menu selections indicates to the nurse the need for further teaching?**

   1. Hamburger, baked potato, squash.
   2. Shrimp, scalloped potatoes, broccoli.
   3. Chicken, wild rice, green beans.
   4. Roast pork, whipped potatoes, carrots.

2. **A teenager informs the nurse at the women's health clinic that she had sexual intercourse with a man who she "heard" is HIV positive. She asks what she should do. The nurse's best response is:**

   1. "Did you use protection such as a condom?"
   2. "Have you confirmed that the man is HIV positive?"
   3. "Would you like to have an AIDS test done?"
   4. "You shouldn't worry. You don't even know if he is positive."

3. **The nurse is working in a busy pediatric emergency room. In which of the following cases would the nurse maintain a high index of suspicion of physical abuse?**

   1. A three-year-old female with 15% burns in a splash pattern over the face and chest reportedly sustained when she pulled on the tablecloth and a teapot fell, spilling over her.
   2. A 14-month-old male with many bruises on bony prominences, in various stages of healing. The child is reportedly clumsy.
   3. A six-year-old with a spiral fracture of the tibia and fibula, which reportedly occurred while riding his bicycle.
   4. A nine-month-old near drowning, who reportedly climbed into the tub and turned on the water.

4. **A 56-year-old client has been treated for angina pectoris, which has become unstable in the past two months. The client is scheduled for a cardiac catheterization. The nurse's first priority when caring for the client post-catheterization is which of the following?**

   1. Check that the call light is readily accessible.
   2. Maintain immobility in the affected extremity.
   3. Monitor urinary output.
   4. Ask open-ended questions about the procedure to promote further effective communication with the client.

5. **It is usually best to avoid taking any medications during pregnancy. Some psychiatric drugs are particularly harmful, especially during the first trimester. The nurse should know that all but which one of the following drugs should never be taken by pregnant women?**

   1. Lithium.
   2. Imipramine (Tofranil).
   3. Diazepam (Valium).
   4. Haloperidol (Haldol).

6. **The nurse is planning care for a group of clients who visit the Hypertension Clinic weekly. Which of the following clients should the nurse recognize as being at the greatest risk for a potentially life-threatening complication when nadolol (Corgard) is used to manage the blood pressure?**

   1. A 34-year-old pregnant woman.
   2. A 52-year-old female diabetic.
   3. A 65-year-old male with congestive heart failure (CHF).
   4. A 72-year-old male with impaired renal function.

7. **A client, age 56, diagnosed with pneumonia, is being treated with penicillin G sodium 3 million units IV every four hours. When completing the drug history, it is especially important for the nurse to assess a client for allergies to which of the following medications?**

   1. Antituberculars.
   2. Calcium channel blockers.
   3. Aminoglycosides.
   4. Cephalosporins.

8. **The physician orders labetalol (Trandate) for a client to treat severe hypertension secondary to a pheochromocytoma. The nurse recognizes that this drug is a potent antihypertensive because of its action as:**

   1. An ACE inhibitor.
   2. A calcium channel blocker.
   3. An alpha- and beta-adrenergic blocker.
   4. A selective beta-adrenergic blocker.

9. **Upon assessing a baby, the nurse determines that he is 40 weeks gestational age. Which of the following characteristics are most likely to be found in this baby?**

1. Lanugo abundant over shoulders and lower coccyx.
2. Pinna of ear springs back slowly when folded.
3. Vernix well distributed over entire body.
4. Creases covering the entire bottom of both feet.

10. **A nurse working in a mental health clinic should know predisposing factors for suicide would include all of the following except:**

    1. Alcoholism and substance abuse.
    2. Age younger than 40 years of age.
    3. Male.
    4. Unmarried.

11. **A client has been told by the doctor that he has cancer and that it has advanced so far that treatment will not help. When the nurse enters the room to set up his bath equipment, he says to the nurse, "I'm not an invalid, you know. I can take care of myself. Get out and leave me alone". Which of the following is the best nursing response?**

    1. "I know that you are not an invalid. I was only trying to help you."
    2. "It sounds to me like you are angry about something. Did somebody do something wrong?"
    3. "You are pretty upset. Let's talk about it."
    4. "I'll just set up this equipment for you to bathe and come back later when you're not so angry."

12. **A complete blood count is ordered on a two-month-old child with cyanotic heart disease. The results are a hemoglobin of 18 g/dL and a hematocrit of 51%. Which of the following statements by the nurse reflects the most appropriate interpretation of this information?**

    1. The body is compensating for tissue hypoxia by increasing RBC production.
    2. The child may be anemic. This is a low hemoglobin for a two-month-old child and the hematocrit is within normal limits.
    3. The child is severely dehydrated, and the loss of vascular fluid has elevated the hematocrit. The hemoglobin is within normal limits.
    4. This laboratory data would be considered within normal limits for a two-month-old child.

13. **While making an initial home visit, the community health nurse notes several suspicious bruises and old burns on the 10-month-old child. Which is the nurse's priority action?**

    1. Call the child protection hotline and report possible abuse.
    2. Discuss the family with the physician and social worker at the next team meeting.

3. Tell the mother that child protection will be notified if injuries are noted on the next visit.
4. Carefully record the visit for follow-up.

14. **The nurse is informed during report that a postoperative client has not voided for eight hours. The initial nursing action would be to:**

    1. Assist the client to the bathroom.
    2. Place the client on a bed pan and pour warm water over her perineum.
    3. Palpate and percuss the client's bladder.
    4. Catheterize the client.

15. **A two-year-old is admitted to the hospital with vomiting and possible dehydration. Which of the following findings would most concern the nurse?**

    1. Potassium 2.5 mEq/L.
    2. Blood glucose 150 mg/dL.
    3. Weight loss of 10 grams.
    4. Urine specific gravity 1.020.

16. **When presented with a group of clients, the nurse should recognize which client as the best candidate for a low forceps delivery?**

    1. A client, gravida 1, who has been pushing for one hour with repeated early decelerations and good variability.
    2. A client, gravida 1, who is fully dilated, and has caput in view, and an FH monitor strip showing severe late decelerations with every contraction.
    3. A client, gravida 1, who says she can't push anymore, and has a FH monitor strip with good variability.
    4. A client, gravida 2, who is fully dilated with her baby remaining at minus one station in a LOP position for the past hour.

17. **A pregnant diabetic arrives in the emergency room at 30 weeks of gestation with symptoms of hyperglycemia. Her blood sugar is 348 mg/dL. The resident orders 30 units of NPH insulin, to be given subcutaneously, stat. The nurse should do which of the following?**

    1. Give the dosage immediately.
    2. Start the dextrose IV the resident also ordered before giving the insulin.
    3. Question the large dosage.
    4. Question the type of insulin.

18. **Which of the following statements made by a client indicates to the nurse the need for further teaching regarding a scheduled arthroscopy of the knee?**

    1. "I know the doctor will be looking at my joint to check for cartilage damage."

2. "I'll have to limit my exercising for a few weeks after this procedure."

3. "I hope the incision heals quickly with those staples in place."

4. "I know that I'll have to keep my knee straight and elevated to reduce the swelling after the surgery."

19. **A 12-year-old girl had a ventriculo-peritoneal shunt placed to treat hydrocephalus in infancy. In counseling the child about health management of the shunt, the nurse would consider the teaching effective if the child states:**

1. "I should drink plenty of fluids and stay rested."

2. "I may need to wear glasses as a teenager"

3. "I can take prochlorperazine (Compazine) for vomiting."

4. "If I get a really bad headache, I should call the doctor."

20. **A client, age 73, is receiving IV carbenicillin (Geocillin) for pharyngitis. Which of the following signs/symptoms manifested by the client would be of immediate concern to the nurse?**

1. Anorexia and nausea.

2. Abdominal cramping with diarrhea.

3. Macular rash on lower extremities.

4. Decreased visual acuity and tinnitus.

21. **The nurse would expect that psychological factors, such as anxiety, could be responsible for which of the following?**

1. Contributing to the development and progress of coronary artery disease.

2. Causing coronary artery disease.

3. Affecting the prognosis, only, for a client with coronary artery disease.

4. Affecting a client's ability to adjust to a diagnosis of coronary artery disease, while having little direct effect on treatment outcomes.

22. **A physician prescribes tocainide (Tonocard) PO for a client who has occasional to frequent premature ventricular contractions (PVCs). The nurse should teach the client to report which of the following side effects when taking Tonocard?**

1. Double vision.

2. Dry mouth.

3. Petechiae.

4. Photosensitivity.

23. **The nurse asks a suicidal client to make a safety contract whereby he promises that if he has thoughts of harming himself he will not act on them, but will discuss them with either her or another staff member. The client tells the nurse**
that he cannot make this safety contract because he cannot promise that he will not harm himself. In the nurse's plan of care, which initial action would best ensure this client's safety?

1. Provide a relaxed and accepting environment to develop trust.

2. Sterilize the environment by removing belts, glass objects, or sharp instruments that could be used for self-harm.

3. Lock the doors to the unit and secure all windows so they cannot be opened.

4. Assign a staff member to stay with the client at all times.

24. **A 72-year-old client is admitted to the hospital with congestive heart failure and will be started on digoxin (Lanoxin). Vitals on admission are BP 110/60, pulse 100, respirations 22. What is the expected outcome of digitalization?**

1. Respiratory rate of 26.

2. Heart rate greater than 100.

3. Urine output of 50 mL per hour.

4. Increased thirst.

25. **Which of the following foods should the nurse teach the client to include in a daily diet to minimize the most critical electrolyte loss when taking furosemide (Lasix)?**

1. Grains.

2. Milk.

3. Red meats.

4. Dried fruits.

26. **An antepartum client tells the nurse she has been vomiting her breakfast nearly every morning. Which of the following measures is most likely to help the client overcome early morning nausea and vomiting?**

1. Sipping whole milk with breakfast.

2. Drinking only liquids for breakfast.

3. Eating some crackers before arising from bed in the morning.

4. Drinking a carbonated beverage before arising from bed in the morning.

27. **A client who was diagnosed with cancer of the testes is being discharged from the hospital with an intravenous catheter in place for administration of chemotherapy. The nurse is to teach the client how to flush the catheter at home. Which information about the client's actions during the teaching session would indicate that the nurse's teaching is successful?**

1. The client looks at the ceiling during the teaching session.
2. The client asks the nurse to show his wife how to flush the catheter.
3. The client asks the nurse if it is all right to flush the catheter before going to work in the morning.
4. The client tells the nurse that he will have the nurses at the clinic flush the catheter when he receives his chemotherapy.

28. **The nurse realizes that typical characteristics of girls with anorexia nervosa include which of the following?**

    1. They fail to comply with their parents' wishes or societal expectations.
    2. They exercise relentlessly.
    3. They are truthful in reporting their eating habits.
    4. They have problems with self-control.

29. **A client is in a nursing home and is confined to bed. What is the most important nursing intervention that will lessen the possibility of skin breakdown and decubitus ulcers?**

    1. Massage all bony prominences with lotion to increase circulation.
    2. Keep the skin clean and dry.
    3. Turn the client at least every two hours.
    4. Place an egg crate mattress on the bed.

30. **A client, admitted with hypertension, is taking furosemide (Lasix) 40 mg p.o. twice a day. Which of the following interventions, if included in the plan of care by the nurse, would require further clarification?**

    1. Daily weights before breakfast.
    2. Monitor intake and output.
    3. Orthostatic blood pressure checks every eight hours.
    4. Limit fluid intake to 1000 mL in 24 hours.

31. **A mother brings her 18-month-old to the pediatric emergency room. The child has sustained a fractured left femur. Which statement by the mother might make the nurse suspect a problem of child abuse?**

    1. "She is so active and gets into everything."
    2. "She was riding her bicycle and her foot got caught in the spokes."
    3. "My daughter slipped out of her high chair because the strap was too loose."
    4. "My daughter climbed up on a chair and fell down."

32. **The nurse tells a client that the doctor has ordered an intravenous to be started. The client appears to be upset but says nothing to the nurse.**

Which of the following is the best nursing response?

1. "Do you have any questions about the procedure?"
2. "The doctor wants you to have antibiotics, and this method eliminates getting frequent injections."
3. "What is there about this procedure that concerns you?"
4. "It only hurts a little bit. It'll be over before you know it."

33. **A client has active herpes type 2. Which of the following describes the best plan for delivery, assuming the lesions remain active?**

    1. The mother should be induced close to term so that the nursery can be prepared for an infected infant.
    2. The mother should be instructed to call the doctor when her contractions become regular and increase in intensity. She may or may not need a C-section.
    3. The client should be delivered by C-section prior to the onset of labor.
    4. The client should be delivered by C-section as soon after rupture of membranes as possible.

34. **At a boy scout camp the nurse encounters a child who exhibits a high-pitched inspiratory sound, and cyanosis. Describe the procedure that the nurse should institute.**

    1. Stand behind the child and apply an upward thrust below the xiphoid.
    2. Monitor the child; if respirations cease, use the Heimlich maneuver.
    3. Bend the child forward and deliver back blows to dislodge the object.
    4. Begin cardiopulmonary resuscitation.

35. **An 18-month-old is being admitted with a diagnosis of Wilm's tumor. Which nursing intervention takes priority?**

    1. Checking vital signs every eight hours for incidence of hypertension.
    2. Placing a sign over the bed that says "Do Not Palpate the Abdomen."
    3. Raising the head of the bed to ease breathing.
    4. Monitoring the urinary output every two hours.

36. **A client, diagnosed with hypertension, is started on chlorothiazide (Diuril). The nurse is aware that this thiazide is often one of the preferred Step I diuretics in the management of hypertension because:**

    1. The drug is more potent than that of loop diuretics.
    2. The client only has to take the medication once each day.

3. Side effects from the drug are relatively less extensive.

4. Loss of electrolytes, especially potassium, is minimal.

37. **A client who has been diagnosed with CHF two days earlier begins to exhibit symptoms of left-sided heart failure. Which of the following would the nurse observe?**

1. Peripheral edema.
2. Dyspnea.
3. Abdominal distention.
4. Fatigue.

38. **A 75-year-old client is taking lithium for a bipolar mood disorder. He asks the nurse whether psychiatric problems run in the family, because his alcoholic 45-year-old son and bulimic 20-year-old granddaughter are also taking lithium. In considering how to respond to the client, the nurse knows that lithium, while useful for certain other disorders, in addition to bipolar disorders, is least useful in treating which of the following?**

1. Unipolar depressions.
2. Aggressive conduct disorder.
3. Bulimia.
4. Alcoholism.

39. **A client is taking propranolol (Inderal) as an anti-anginic. Inderal relieves angina because of which of the following actions?**

1. Increase in cardiac output.
2. Increase in heart rate.
3. Inhibition of vasodilatation in coronary vessels.
4. Decrease in myocardial oxygen requirements.

40. **A postoperative client is to ambulate for the first time after surgery. Which action to ensure safety is least appropriate for the nurse to use in preparing the client to ambulate?**

1. Have the client get up and sit in the chair next to the bed.
2. Have the client sit on the edge of the bed with his feet down for a few minutes before he starts to ambulate.
3. Have the client stand at the side of the bed for a few minutes before taking his first steps.
4. Encourage the client to try to walk straight ahead while assisting him with his walking.

41. **The nurse assigned to care for a child with cerebral palsy should obtain information concerning his abilities, limitations, interests, and habits, because the aim of therapy is to:**

1. Assess the child's assets and potentialities and capitalize on these in the habilitative process, while ignoring limitations.
2. Reverse abnormal functioning and restore brain damage through rehabilitation.
3. Provide a therapeutic program that avoids subjecting the child to frustrating experiences that decrease his achievement.
4. Develop an individualized therapeutic program that utilizes the child's assets and abilities and provides experiences that permit him to achieve success as well as help to cope with frustration and failure.

42. **An 18-year-old client is hospitalized for treatment of depression. The client was married at a young age, but is now separated from her husband. Because of the client's condition, which of the following approaches should be included in her plan of care?**

1. Giving the client choices.
2. Spending time with the client.
3. Providing a chess game.
4. Encouraging decision-making.

43. **During an office visit early in her pregnancy, a primigravida confides to the nurse that even though she and her husband planned this pregnancy she is experiencing many ambivalent feelings about the pregnancy. What response by the nurse would be most appropriate?**

1. "Perhaps you should see a counselor to discuss these feelings."
2. "Have you told your husband about these feelings?"
3. "These feelings are quite normal at the beginning of pregnancy; there is no reason for you to feel guilty."
4. "I am quite concerned about these feelings, could you explain more about them."

44. **A client is re-hospitalized because she discontinued her medication on her own accord. The client's discharge plans include living with her parents and attending a job training program during the day. What is the most important goal for her remaining sessions with the nurse?**

1. Reinforce the importance of taking her medications as prescribed.
2. Anticipate future problems and how she might handle them.
3. Terminate the nurse-client relationship.
4. Promote the client's self-confidence.

45. **During a well-child visit, the mother of a five-year-old expresses concern that her son will not**

wear his helmet while riding his bicycle. What is the most appropriate response?

1. "Tell him the bike doesn't leave the garage without the helmet."
2. "It isn't that important, since he won't be riding in the road."
3. "Gradually encourage the wearing of the helmet with small rewards."
4. "I'll explain the potential for injury without a helmet."

46. A 16-year-old adolescent sustained an open fracture of his left femur after being thrown from his motorcycle. A Steinmann pin is inserted and he is placed in ninety-ninety traction. In performing the initial assessment, the nurse finds the traction weight resting on the floor. Which of the following is the initial nursing action?

1. Help the client use the trapeze to pull himself up in bed.
2. Check the pedal pulse and capillary refill of the right foot.
3. Notify the attending orthopedic physician.
4. Remove the weight and move the client to correct alignment in bed.

47. During open heart surgery, a 59-year-old client is placed on cardiopulmonary bypass in order to accomplish which of the following?

1. Maintain systemic circulation.
2. Provide a bloodless field.
3. Eliminate ectopic rhythms.
4. Restore blood supply to the myocardium.

48. A 45-year-old man is admitted to the emergency room complaining of chest pain and dyspnea. He is also flushed and perspiring profusely. He says, "I feel like I am going to die. Am I having a heart attack?" The medical exam and lab work are negative. He is diagnosed with anxiety. The nurse assesses his level of anxiety as:

1. Mild.
2. Moderate.
3. Severe.
4. Panic.

49. An eight-year-old is in the hospital for second and third degree burns to his left arm. He was playing with matches with his friends. The others were not injured. While acutely ill in the hospital, the nursing diagnosis with the highest priority for the child at this time is:

1. Potential for infection.
2. Potential altered parenting.

3. Knowledge deficit regarding injury prevention.
4. Ineffective airway clearance.

50. A client is taking triamterene (Dyrenium) in addition to hydrochlorothiazide (Hydrodiuril) to control hypertension. The nurse is aware that the rationale for this combination medication therapy is to prevent or treat:

1. Mild hypokalemia.
2. Dehydration.
3. Moderate hyponatremia.
4. Hypotension.

51. A client who has just been diagnosed with cancer tells the nurse that he would rather be dead than go through the treatment for cancer. The most appropriate nursing response is:

1. "What is it about the cancer treatment that concerns you?"
2. "If you don't receive the treatment, you will get your wish."
3. "Why don't you talk to your doctor about your feelings?"
4. "That wouldn't be fair to your family, would it?"

52. A confused elderly client is on strict bed rest, secondary to left-sided heart failure. Which of the following interventions would provide for this client's safety?

1. Place the client in a room away from the noise and confusion of the nurses' station.
2. Avoid the use of nightlights, since they tend to distort images and confuse clients.
3. Discuss with the client the need for restraints if she continues to get out of bed.
4. Provide opportunities for regular toileting, and include this information in the client's care plan.

53. An elderly, confused client is on bed rest. A nursing action that is least likely to help prevent a fall for this client is:

1. Providing regular toileting.
2. Explaining to the client that she should use the call light if she needs to get up.
3. Placing the side rails in the up position and checking on the client often.
4. Proper use of restraints.

54. In caring for a client taking digoxin (Lanoxin), the nurse would give immediate attention to which of the following statements?

1. "I have a headache and backache."
2. "I feel nauseated and have no appetite."
3. "I've gained a half-pound in the last two days."

4. "I'm having muscle cramps in my legs."

55. **A six-month-old was admitted to the hospital after he had been in a car accident. He was placed on phenytoin (Dilantin) after he had a seizure. He had no further seizures, and will be going home on this medication. Which of the following is inaccurate information that the nurse would avoid giving to the parents?**

   1. Watch for signs of gingival hyperplasia.
   2. Note any increase in seizure activity.
   3. Have therapeutic blood levels drawn after one year on dapitalize Dilantin.
   4. Drowsiness may occur when therapy is initially begun.

56. **Before administering lithium, the nurse checks the client's latest lab report for her serum lithium level and notes a level of 1.2 mEq/L. What is the best action for the nurse to take next?**

   1. Administer the next prescribed dose of lithium.
   2. Suggest the blood test be repeated.
   3. Withhold the next dose of lithium and notify the psychiatrist of the lab results.
   4. Ask the client how she is feeling, to identify any untoward effects.

57. **A client has an indwelling Foley catheter. The nurse would avoid including which nursing actions in the plan for irrigation of the catheter?**

   1. Instill sterile distilled water in the catheter.
   2. Use minimal pressure to clear the catheter of clots or mucous plugs.
   3. Use sterile equipment for irrigation.
   4. Use gravity to achieve a return flow of the irrigant.

58. **The nurse would expect which pattern of contractions when the client reports that they are four minutes apart?**

   1. A contraction that lasts for four minutes followed by a period of relaxation.
   2. Contractions that last for 60 seconds with a four-minute rest between contractions.
   3. Contractions that last for 60 seconds with a three-minute rest between contractions.
   4. Contractions that last for 45 seconds with a three-minute rest between contractions.

59. **An elderly client is admitted to the hospital with pneumonia. His daughter, who takes care of him at home, says to the nurse, "I'm so glad he is here. You can take much better care of him than I can." The best nursing response to the daughter's statement is which of the following?**

   1. "We do have the equipment and people to take care of sick clients."
   2. "It is not easy to care for the elderly. How do you manage?"
   3. "Sir, your daughter takes good care of you at home, doesn't she?"
   4. "Are you feeling guilty because your father has pneumonia?"

60. **The nurse knows that the two basic types of arrhythmias, listed in order of those that make the heart go faster, and those that make the heart go slower are:**

   1. Bradyarrhythmias and tachyarrhythmias.
   2. Tachyarrhythmias and bradyarrhythmias.
   3. Supraventricular and ventricular.
   4. Ventricular and supraventricular.

61. **A client comes to the clinic to be tested for tuberculosis. Which is the most valuable diagnostic tool currently used to screen for TB?**

   1. Chest x-ray.
   2. Sputum culture.
   3. Bronchial washings.
   4. Mantoux skin test.

62. **The charge nurse is preparing the staffing assignment. A six-month-old on the unit has AIDS and cytomegalovirus (CMV). Which staff person should be assigned as the primary care giver for this child?**

   1. An experienced nurse who is six months pregnant.
   2. A male graduate nurse, recently oriented to pediatrics.
   3. An experienced nurse's aide who is healthy.
   4. A licensed practical nurse with eczema.

63. **A cholecystectomy client is three days postoperative. A postoperative wound infection is suspected because the nurse notes that the drainage from his dressing is yellow and thick. This describes which type of drainage?**

   1. Serous.
   2. Purulent.
   3. Serosanguineous.
   4. Sanguineous.

64. **A client with hypertension is being treated with chlorothiazide (Diuril) 500 mg p.o. twice a day. In taking the client's medication history, the nurse notes that the client is a diabetic and has been taking chlorpropamide (Diabinese) 250 mg p.o. daily. The nurse is aware that the potential interaction of Diabinese with Diuril may result in:**

   1. Hypocalcemia.

2. Hyperglycemia.
3. Aplastic anemia.
4. Hypoglycemia.

65. **The nurse is preparing to do client teaching for a hypertensive client. Which of the following goals is least appropriate?**

    1. The client eliminates sodium from her diet.
    2. The client exercises moderately each day.
    3. The client maintains weight appropriate for height.
    4. The client discontinues use of birth control pills.

66. **A client is admitted to a nursing home. She has difficulty seeing and hearing. Which of the following nursing actions is least important for this client?**

    1. Showing the client where all of the furniture and personal items are in the room.
    2. Talking loudly when entering the client's room.
    3. Telling the client that because of her increased risk of falling and injuring herself, she is not allowed out of her room.
    4. Assisting the client to identify the placement of food items during meals.

67. **The physician orders peripheral pulse checks every eight hours on a client who was admitted to the hospital with decreased circulation to his left leg. The nurse performing the peripheral pulse checks should include documentation of which of the following?**

    1. Strength and rate.
    2. Amplitude, rhythm and symmetrical comparison of both extremities.
    3. Temperature of the skin.
    4. Color of the extremity.

68. **While providing care for a client, the nurse should avoid which action in order to prevent muscle strain?**

    1. Move muscles quickly, using short tugs in order to avoid muscle fatigue.
    2. Use the longest and strongest muscles of the body whenever possible.
    3. Lean toward objects being pushed, such as a stretcher.
    4. Carry objects close to the body without touching your clothing.

69. **The nurse knows that quinidine sulfate (Quinidex) is used to treat atrial and ventricular arrhythmias because of which of the following effects?**

    1. Increase of automaticity and excitability.
    2. Increase of vagal action in the SA and AV nodes.
    3. Shortening the refractory period of atrial and ven-

tricular fibers.
    4. Cell membrane stabilization through the prevention of movement of sodium and potassium.

70. **A 56-year-old female client is started on hydrochlorothiazide (Hydrodiuril) and spironolactone (Aldactone) for treatment of hypertension. The nurse's discharge instructions should include an admonition to the client that she should:**
    1. Contact her physician if blood pressure control is not achieved in two to three days.
    2. Take the Aldactone between meals to increase absorption.
    3. Watch for signs of hypokalemia and include potassium-rich foods in her diet.
    4. Report any muscle twitching or numbness in extremities to the physician.

71. **While caring for the client with an IV, it is most important for the nurse to:**

    1. Report any signs of infection to the physician.
    2. Record the condition of the IV site and the rate of infusion, and report any unusual findings.
    3. Record intravenous intake.
    4. Ask the client if the IV site is painful or tender.

72. **A vaginal exam reveals the following information on a laboring woman and her fetus: two centimeters, 50%, +1, ROA. Based on this information which of the following is the presentation of the fetus?**

    1. ROA.
    2. Two centimeters.
    3. Vertex.
    4. +1.

73. **A 78-year-old client has been in the hospital for a week on bed rest. She complains of elbow pain. The best nursing action is to:**

    1. Place elbow pads on the client.
    2. Examine the elbow.
    3. Call the physician for an order for pain medication.
    4. Reposition the client so that she is more comfortable.

74. **A client is to have a nasogastric tube inserted because of an obstruction in his bowel. The nurse explains the procedure to him and is about to begin the insertion, when the client says, "No way! You are not putting that hose down my throat. Get away from me." Which of the following statements is the best nursing response?**

    1. "You have the right to refuse treatment. Why don't you talk to your doctor about it?"
    2. "Something is upsetting you. Can you tell me

what it is:"

3. "What do you feel about this hose?"
4. "I would just get it over with, because you won't get better without this tube."

75. A nine-year-old is admitted to the hospital with acute glomerulonephritis. Which nursing action should be included in the plan of care for this child?

1. Elevating the HOB to decrease edema of face and eyes.
2. Monitoring blood pressure every four hours.
3. Administering prednisone as ordered to facilitate diuresis.
4. Reporting any hematuria to the physician immediately.

76. A 49-year-old client has been diagnosed with iron deficiency anemia. The nurse should recommend an increased intake of which of the following foods when teaching the client about her diet.

1. Fresh fruits.
2. Milk and cheese.
3. Organ meats.
4. Whole grain breads.

77. A client is hospitalized for a surgical procedure. The most important nursing intervention when administering the preoperative medication is which of the following?

1. Have the client void before going to the operating room.
2. Put the side rails up, and instruct the client to remain in bed.
3. Ask the client if she has signed all of the admission forms for the surgery.
4. Have the family leave, since the medication will decrease the client's inhibitions and she may say or do something that is out of character for her.

78. A 50-year-old client is being discharged following bilateral vein ligation and stripping. While doing discharge planning, the nurse instructs the client that it is important to do which of the following when she goes home?

1. Wear slacks and opaque hose regularly for cosmetic reasons.
2. Purchase and wear above-the-knee support hose only.
3. Join a local diet center to facilitate weight loss.
4. Elevate her legs above the heart level four times a day for 15-20 minutes.

79. A client is to be up in a chair three times a day. He is paralyzed from the waist down. What is the best nursing approach when transferring this client from a bed into a wheelchair?

1. Place the wheelchair close to the foot of the bed.
2. Utilize the principles of body mechanics while providing a safe transfer for the client.
3. Slide the client to the edge of the bed, keeping the nurse's back straight and using a rocking motion to pull the client.
4. Place the nurse's arms under the client's axillae from the back of the client.

80. A client, 35 years old, was admitted to the hospital for possible gall bladder surgery. Following a gall bladder x-ray, the doctor decided that a cholecystectomy was necessary. The nurse should include which of the following in preoperative teaching for the client?

1. After this type of surgery, many clients are admitted to the intensive care unit.
2. Minor discomfort is expected in the operative site during the first few postoperative days.
3. Moving as little as possible will decrease the discomfort following this procedure.
4. A demonstration and return demonstration of coughing and deep breathing.

81. The nurse knows that lidocaine hydrochloride (Xylocaine) exerts its most important cardiac effect by which of the following?

1. Depressing excessive automaticity of ectopic pacemakers in the His-Purkinje fibers.
2. Suppressing conduction velocity in the AV node and purkinje fibers.
3. Depressing myocardial contractility.
4. Suppressing the SA node impulses.

82. Of the following information, which should be recorded first in the client's record by the nurse admitting the client?

1. The client's vital signs.
2. The plan that was developed for the care of the client while in the hospital.
3. Nursing actions performed for the client.
4. Assessment of the client.

83. A client is on the telemetry unit, and the monitor shows he is in ventricular fibrillation ("V-Fib"). Which of the following actions should be given priority by the nurse?

1. Prepare the client for cardioversion.
2. Assess the client's responsiveness and begin CPR.
3. Administer Lidocaine IV push.
4. Obtain a permit for insertion of a permanent pacemaker.

84. A 21-year-old client has sustained a basal skull fracture. The nurse notices drainage from his right nostril. The priority nursing action is which of the following?

1. Notify his physician.
2. Suction his nostril.
3. Test the drainage for glucose.
4. Ask the client to blow his nose.

✓ 85. **A confused elderly client continually grabs at the nurses from her wheelchair. Which of the following is the most appropriate nursing action?**

1. Move the wheelchair to a location where she cannot grab people.
2. Apply a chest restraint for her own safety.
3. Use wrist restraints and move her to the visitor's room.
4. Remove her hands and firmly tell her not to grab.

86. **After several days of furosemide (Lasix) therapy, a client begins to complain of muscle weakness, drowsiness, abdominal cramping, and nausea. The nurse is aware that the most likely explanation for these symptoms is:**

1. Hyponatremia.
2. Hypokalemia.
3. Metabolic alkalosis.
4. Uremia.

87. **On vaginal examination the presenting part was at station plus two. Which of the following is the proper interpretation by the nurse?**

1. Presenting part is two centimeters above the level of the ischial spines.
2. Biparietal diameter is at the level of the ischial spines.
3. Presenting part is two centimeters below the level of the ischial spines.
4. Biparietal diameter is two centimeters above the ischial spines.

88. **A client is very suspicious of the nursing staff and other clients. Her primary nurse would like to establish a therapeutic relationship with her. Which plan of care is the best for doing this:**

1. Avoid pressuring the client by waiting for her to initiate interactions with the nurse.
2. Approach the client frequently during the day for brief interactions.
3. Set aside a specific time each day to spend with the client.
4. Approach the client in a friendly manner offering to disclose some personal information so she will feel she knows the nurse better.

89. **The initial plan of care for a 10-year-old child admitted for orthopedic surgery who has a history of cerebral palsy should include strategies for which of the following?**

1. Keeping a calm, quiet environment to prevent seizures.
2. Explaining all information to the child's parents, as the child is not able to understand.
3. Facilitating communication with the child by his/her usual means.
4. Obtaining IV access immediately, as children with cerebral palsy have difficulty drinking.

90. **A client with a history of previous cesarean section asks the nurse whether she might be able to deliver vaginally this time. The nurse, in framing an answer, knows that a trial of labor for vaginal delivery after cesarean is more likely if the client's experience was:**

1. First cesarean through a classic incision as a result of severe fetal distress.
2. First low transverse cesarean for breech position; this pregnancy fetus is in a vertex presentation.
3. First and second caesareans were for cephalopelvic disproportion.
4. First low transverse cesarean was for active herpes, type 2 infection; vaginal culture at 39 weeks this pregnancy was positive.

91. **Which of the following electrolyte levels must be monitored most closely by the nurse while the client is taking chlorothiazide (Diuril)?**

1. Calcium.
2. Magnesium.
3. Potassium.
4. Sodium.

92. **What should the nurse emphasize in developing the initial nursing care plan for a client with an acute schizophrenia?**

1. Establishing a daily routine to promote orientation to the unit.
2. Providing a variety of activities to keep the client focused on reality-based topics.
3. Encouraging the client to enter into simple group activities.
4. Assigning the same members of the nursing staff to work with the client each day.

93. **After complaining of severe chest pain for the last hour, a client is admitted to MICU with acute myocardial infarction. The admitting nurse reviews the client's chart and notes that cardiac enzyme studies were done on admission. The nurse knows that the purpose of the studies were to evaluate which of the following?**

1. The degree of damage to the myocardium.
2. The location of the myocardial infarction.

3. The size of the myocardial infarction.
4. The coexistence of pulmonary congestion.

94. **Which nursing assessment would be a priority for postoperative care of a four-year-old following an appendectomy?**

1. Vital signs every eight hours.
2. Measure intake and output every eight hours.
3. Auscultate the lungs every four hours.
4. Check the extremities for phlebitis every four hours.

95. **A client is being discharged following major abdominal surgery. Which of the following is most important for the nurse to include in the teaching plan since the client will be doing her own dressing changes at home?**

1. Appropriate opening of bandages to maintain their sterility.
2. Discussion of proper aseptic technique.
3. Proper gloving technique.
4. Discussion of good handwashing technique.

96. **An 82-year-old widower is admitted to the psychiatric unit. His diagnosis is depression with agitation. A behavior the nurse would least likely expect to be associated with this diagnosis would be:**

1. Difficulty concentrating and memory loss.
2. Irritability and extreme annoyance with other people.
3. Jitteriness and hand wringing.
4. Sleeping 10 to 12 hours a day.

97. **A 48-year-old woman is accompanied by her 24-year-old daughter to the psychiatric hospital for an evaluation. The client explains that she has been unable to leave her house for the past 10 years without her husband or daughter. If she tries to go out alone, she becomes very anxious and must quickly return inside. The nurse interviewing her identifies the problem as most likely due to which of the following disorders?**

1. Conversion disorder.
2. Agoraphobia.
3. Panic disorder.
4. Obsessive-compulsive disorder.

98. **The nurse observes a 72-year-old client trying to climb over the side rails of the bed. The nurse obtains a vest restraint and is placing it on the client when the daughter arrives and says to the nurse, "My mother does not need to be tied down in bed. I've been caring for her for years, and she hasn't fallen out of bed yet." The best initial response by the nurse is which of the following statements?**

1. "I just saw your mother trying to climb over the side rails. Since I am concerned about her falling and hurting herself, I think this is best for her safety."
2. "Tell me how you managed to care for her at home."
3. "Hospital policy requires restraint vests on clients who are at risk for falling. I just saw your mother trying to climb over the rails. You don't want her to get hurt, do you?"
4. "The elderly may become confused in an unfamiliar place and do things they wouldn't do at home. It is difficult to see her restrained. While you are with her, the restraints can be off. Let me know when you are ready to leave."

99. **A mother arrives at the emergency room with her child, who is wet, and the color of his skin is blue. She shouts to the nurse, "I think that I have killed my son. I wasn't watching him like I should have and he fell in the pool." While the doctor and other nursing staff are providing care for the child, a nurse stays with the mother to obtain information. What is the most therapeutic response by the nurse?**

1. "These things happen. Don't blame yourself."
2. "You are right. A child should always be watched when he is playing near a pool."
3. "You didn't kill him. He is still alive. It is going to be all right."
4. "It must feel terrible to have something like this happen to your child."

100. **A client asks the nurse how the relaxation techniques will help his gastric pain. "Can't I just take the cimetidine (Tagamet) that my physician has prescribed?" In responding to his question, the nurse is guided by the knowledge that:**

1. Gastric ulcer is a stress-related illness, and his stress levels and emotional issues are contributing to the exacerbation of his symptoms.
2. He is in denial because he is refusing to acknowledge that stress is playing a role in the progress of his illness.
3. Gastric ulcer, and other psychosomatic illnesses, are caused by stress and can't be cured with only medical or surgical treatments.
4. The client is displaying the "typical ulcer personality" of a competitive, aggressive person who is defending against unresolved dependency needs.

NOTES

NCLEX-RN

Test 3

Questions with Rationales

NCLEX-RN TEST 3 WITH RATIONALES

1.   **A client diagnosed with urolithiasis is advised to follow a low calcium diet after his pathology report reveals calcium oxalate stones. Which of the following menu selections indicates to the nurse the need for further teaching?**

   1.   Hamburger, baked potato, squash.
   2.   Shrimp, scalloped potatoes, broccoli.
   3.   Chicken, wild rice, green beans.
   4.   Roast pork, whipped potatoes, carrots.

   1.   *No, this menu selection is low in calcium. The client would be correct in choosing this menu.*
   2.   ***Absolutely! Shellfish, broccoli, and the milk and cheese used to make the scalloped potatoes are all high in calcium. The client would need further teaching if he chose these menu items.***
   3.   *No, this menu is low in calcium and would be acceptable. You are to select an option that has food high in calcium.*
   4.   *Incorrect. These food items are acceptable on a low calcium diet. The client would not need further teaching with this menu selection.*

2.   **A teenager informs the nurse at the women's health clinic that she had sexual intercourse with a man who she "heard" is HIV positive. She asks what she should do. The nurse's best response is:**

   1.   "Did you use protection such as a condom?"
   2.   "Have you confirmed that the man is HIV positive?"
   3.   "Would you like to have an AIDS test done?"
   4.   "You shouldn't worry. You don't even know if he is positive."

   1.   ***Good choice! Obtaining this information by clarification will prevent a misunderstanding and allow for the appropriate direction.***
   2.   *Incorrect. This response does not answer her question, but offers advice. Offering advice is a communication block.*
   3.   *Incorrect. Assuming that she most likely is HIV positive takes the decision-making away from the client.*
   4.   *Incorrect. This offers false reassurance, which may discourage open communication.*

3.   **The nurse is working in a busy pediatric emergency room. In which of the following cases would the nurse maintain a high index of suspicion of physical abuse?**

   1.   A three-year-old female with 15% burns in a splash pattern over the face and chest reportedly sustained when she pulled on the tablecloth and a teapot fell, spilling over her.
   2.   A 14-month-old male with many bruises on bony prominences, in various stages of healing. The child is reportedly clumsy.
   3.   A six-year-old with a spiral fracture of the tibia and fibula, which reportedly occurred while riding his bicycle.
   4.   A nine-month-old near drowning, who reportedly climbed into the tub and turned on the water.

   1.   *No. The history is consistent with the injury. Toddlers frequently help pull themselves up by pulling on objects that may be unstable. The splash of burns would occur from head downward.*
   2.   *No. Toddlers have recently mastered walking and do have many falls and collisions. Since the bruises are in various stages of healing and over bony prominences, this indicates falling on several occasions.*
   3.   *Incorrect. Spiral fractures can be caused by physical abuse, but this six-year-old child is just mastering the riding of a bicycle and this injury is consistent with having a foot caught in the spokes of the bike, which would cause the twisting and fracture.*
   4.   ***Yes! Maybe a nine-month-old could climb into the tub, but turn the water on? This should definitely be followed up. The reported cause of the accident seems inconsistent with the developmental abilities of most nine-month-olds.***

4.   **A 56-year-old client has been treated for angina pectoris, which has become unstable in the past two months. The client is scheduled for a cardiac catheterization. The nurse's first priority when caring for the client post-catheterization is which of the following?**

   1.   Check that the call light is readily accessible.
   2.   Maintain immobility in the affected extremity.
   3.   Monitor urinary output.
   4.   Ask open-ended questions about the procedure to promote further effective communication with the client.

   1.   *No. This is important, yet it is not the first priority.*
   2.   ***Correct. This must be done to prevent breaking the seal over the entry site to the artery, which can result in hemorrhage.***
   3.   *No. Although contrast medium acts as an osmotic diuretic, and monitoring diuresis is important, it is not the first priority.*

4. No. Even though this stressful procedure can produce a high degree of anxiety, a psychological need should not take priority over immobility, which addresses a physiological concern.

5. **It is usually best to avoid taking any medications during pregnancy. Some psychiatric drugs are particularly harmful, especially during the first trimester. The nurse should know that all but which one of the following drugs should never be taken by pregnant women?**

    1. Lithium.
    2. Imipramine (Tofranil).
    3. Diazepam (Valium).
    4. Haloperidol (Haldol).

    1. This is not correct. Lithium crosses the placental barrier and has been associated with babies born with congenital anomalies. Look again at the options to select the drug that is least harmful.

    2. This is not correct. Tofranil is a tricyclic antidepressant. These drugs can cause congenital anomalies or toxic effects to the fetus, so they are contraindicated in pregnant or lactating women. Look again at the options to select the drug that is least harmful.

    3. This is not correct. Valium is a benzodiazepine anti-anxiety drug. Use of these drugs during pregnancy has been associated with infant cleft lip/cleft palate, multiple congenital anomalies, and intrauterine growth retardation. When used late in pregnancy or during lactation, these drugs have been associated with "floppy infant," neonatal withdrawal symptoms, poor sucking, and hypotonia. Look again at the options to select the drug that is least harmful.

    4. ***Correct. There is no conclusive evidence that Haldol, or some other antipsychotics, are harmful to the pregnant woman or the baby. These drugs are less likely to cause harm than the other types of psychotropic medication.***

6. **The nurse is planning care for a group of clients who visit the Hypertension Clinic weekly. Which of the following clients should the nurse recognize as being at the greatest risk for a potentially life-threatening complication when nadolol (Corgard) is used to manage the blood pressure?**

    1. A 34-year-old pregnant woman.
    2. A 52-year-old female diabetic.
    3. A 65-year-old male with congestive heart failure (CHF).
    4. A 72-year-old male with impaired renal function.

    1. Wrong choice. Corgard should be used cautiously during pregnancy because of potential problems in the newborn, but is not contraindicated.

    2. Incorrect. Corgard is not contraindicated. Diabetic clients should monitor serum glucose closely, especially if weakness, fatigue, or irritability occur. Corgard may mask increased blood pressure and tachycardia as signs of hypoglycemia, but dizziness and sweating may still occur. When Corgard is used with insulin, prolonged hypoglycemia may occur.

    3. ***Yes! Nadolol, a beta-adrenergic blocker, decreases the excitability of the heart, decreasing cardiac output and oxygen consumption, and lowering blood pressure. Nadolol is contraindicated in clients with CHF because the drug's action can worsen existing CHF and lead to pulmonary edema. Both conditions can be life-threatening to the client.***

    4. No. Corgard should be used cautiously in clients with renal impairment (the dosage interval should be increased if the creatinine clearance is less than 50 mL/min), but renal failure is not a complication of this drug.

7. **A client, age 56, diagnosed with pneumonia, is being treated with penicillin G sodium 3 million units IV every four hours. When completing the drug history, it is especially important for the nurse to assess a client for allergies to which of the following medications?**

    1. Antituberculars.
    2. Calcium channel blockers.
    3. Aminoglycosides.
    4. Cephalosporins.

    1. Incorrect. There is no known cross-sensitivity between penicillin and antitubercular medications.

    2. Wrong choice. There is no evidence of any significant drug interaction when a client is concurrently taking penicillin and calcium channel blockers.

    3. Incorrect choice. There is no known cross-sensitivity between penicillin and aminoglycosides, which is another group of antibiotics.

    4. ***Good choice! Many clients who are allergic to penicillins are also allergic to cephalosporins, and vice versa. A definite cross-sensitivity may exist.***

8. **The physician orders labetalol (Trandate) for a client to treat severe hypertension secondary to a pheochromocytoma. The nurse recognizes that this drug is a potent antihypertensive because of its action as:**

    1. An ACE inhibitor.
    2. A calcium channel blocker.
    3. An alpha- and beta-adrenergic blocker.
    4. A selective beta-adrenergic blocker.

    1. Incorrect. ACE inhibitors work to lower vascular resistance and lower blood volume. Examples are captopril (Capoten), enalapril (Vasotec), and lisinopril (Zestril).

2. Wrong choice. Calcium channel blockers limit the movement of calcium ions across the cell membrane, decreasing conductivity from the SA node to the AV node as well as contractility. Examples are nifedipine (Procardia), verapamil (Calan), and diltiazem (Cardizem).

3. **Excellent! Labetalol is a nonselective beta-adrenergic blocker, blocking stimulation of beta-1 and beta-2 receptor sites as well as alpha-adrenergic receptors. This drug is an extremely potent antihypertensive agent.**

4. No. Labetalol is not a selective beta-adrenergic blocker like atenolol (Tenormin) and metoprolol (Lopressor).

9. **Upon assessing a baby, the nurse determines that he is 40 weeks gestational age. Which of the following characteristics are most likely to be found in this baby?**

1. Lanugo abundant over shoulders and lower coccyx.
2. Pinna of ear springs back slowly when folded.
3. Vernix well distributed over entire body.
4. Creases covering the entire bottom of both feet.

1. No, abundant lanugo in a newborn is indicative of prematurity.
2. Incorrect. The lack of cartilage in the ear is seen in premature infants.
3. No, abundant vernix on the body is seen in preterm infants.
4. **Correct. The full-term infant should have creases on the soles of his feet.**

10. **A nurse working in a mental health clinic should know predisposing factors for suicide would include all of the following except:**

1. Alcoholism and substance abuse.
2. Age younger than 40 years of age.
3. Male.
4. Unmarried.

1. These are risk factors for suicide so this is not the correct option.
2. **Correct. The majority of completed suicides occur after the age of 40. Elderly white males have the highest suicides rates, although the suicide rate among adolescents is growing rapidly.**
3. Wrong choice. Although women attempt suicide more often, about 70% of completed suicides are men.
4. Wrong choice. Divorced, widowed or separated persons are at higher risk of suicide than are those who are married.

11. **A client has been told by the doctor that he has cancer and that it has advanced so far that treatment will not help. When the nurse enters the room to set up his bath equipment, he says to the nurse, "I'm not an invalid, you know. I can take care of myself. Get out and leave me alone". Which of the following is the best nursing response?**

1. "I know that you are not an invalid. I was only trying to help you."
2. "It sounds to me like you are angry about something. Did somebody do something wrong?"
3. "You are pretty upset. Let's talk about it."
4. "I'll just set up this equipment for you to bathe and come back later when you're not so angry."

1. This is an incorrect option because this response focuses on the nurse and not on the client.
2. This option assumes that the client is angry. By asking if "somebody" did something wrong, it focuses on "somebody" else instead of focusing on the client's feelings.
3. **Good choice! This option addresses the emotional state of the client by stating that he is upset. The communication tool of clarification is used to promote therapeutic communication, which focuses on the client's feelings.**
4. This option does not promote any communication with the client. It implies that his behavior is inappropriate and that the nurse is not willing to deal with it.

12. **A complete blood count is ordered on a two-month-old child with cyanotic heart disease. The results are a hemoglobin of 18 g/dL and a hematocrit of 51%. Which of the following statements by the nurse reflects the most appropriate interpretation of this information?**

1. The body is compensating for tissue hypoxia by increasing RBC production.
2. The child may be anemic. This is a low hemoglobin for a two-month-old child and the hematocrit is within normal limits.
3. The child is severely dehydrated, and the loss of vascular fluid has elevated the hematocrit. The hemoglobin is within normal limits.
4. This laboratory data would be considered within normal limits for a two-month-old child.

1. **Correct! The body is attempting to compensate. Both values are elevated to increase the oxygen-carrying capacity to the tissues.**
2. No. These values are elevated for a two-month-old.
3. Half right, but no credit! Both values are elevated, so the rationale offered doesn't correctly interpret both laboratory results.
4. Incorrect. The normal hemoglobin for a two-month-old is 9-14 g/dL and normal hematocrit is 28-42%.

13. While making an initial home visit, the community health nurse notes several suspicious bruises and old burns on the 10-month-old child. Which is the nurse's priority action?

   1. Call the child protection hotline and report possible abuse.
   2. Discuss the family with the physician and social worker at the next team meeting.
   3. Tell the mother that child protection will be notified if injuries are noted on the next visit.
   4. Carefully record the visit for follow-up.

1. Absolutely correct! As a mandated reporter the nurse is obligated to report any cases of suspected abuse. The nurse does not need to prove the case, just report the facts as known. This is the law.
2. No. The nurse could be considered negligent. This is too long a delay before possible action that could protect the child.
3. No. This is destined to drive the family underground and will not help the nurse develop a therapeutic relationship with the mother. She is likely not to be at home the next time the nurse visits. Choose again.
4. No, the nurse didn't do anything that will either stop the abuse or provide immediate investigation. Hint—what does "mandated reporter" mean?

14. The nurse is informed during report that a postoperative client has not voided for eight hours. The initial nursing action would be to:

   1. Assist the client to the bathroom.
   2. Place the client on a bed pan and pour warm water over her perineum.
   3. Palpate and percuss the client's bladder.
   4. Catheterize the client.

1. Assisting the client to the bathroom may be helpful if the client needs to urinate. This information needs to be obtained before action is taken.
2. Placing the client on a bed pan is not always conducive to urinating. If the client is allowed out of bed, sitting on the toilet while pouring warm water over the perineum can facilitate the client to void. This is not the priority action. The client should have the need and an urge to void before this intervention is implemented.
3. Very good! Assessing the client's bladder provides information concerning the need to void. This is the priority action and the only option that provides for assessment of the client.
4. Catheterizing the client should only be done after it has been determined that the client has a full bladder and is unable to void. The nurse must assess first.

15. A two-year-old is admitted to the hospital with vomiting and possible dehydration. Which of the following findings would most concern the nurse?

   1. Potassium 2.5 mEq/L.
   2. Blood glucose 150 mg/dL.
   3. Weight loss of 10 grams.
   4. Urine specific gravity 1.020.

1. Congratulations, you are correct! The normal potassium level is 3.5-5.0 mEq/L. This level indicates hypokalemia, which could cause arrhythmias or even cardiac arrest.
2. Incorrect! The normal blood glucose level is 80-120 mg/dL. This level is slightly elevated. It would need to monitored, but will not cause life-threatening complications unless it were to go much higher. A low glucose level, on the other hand, could be more serious. Hypoglycemia can progress more rapidly and can easily lead to unconsciousness if intervention is not initiated.
3. Wrong. Ten grams of weight loss is not significant for a two-year-old child. Yes, children should always be growing and gaining weight. Under these circumstances, since the child is vomiting, a small weight loss would not be significant. Larger weight loss could indicate the severity of the dehydration and must be monitored.
4. No. The normal urine specific gravity is between 1.010-1.020. This measurement is on the upper limits of urine concentration and bears watching; however, it is not the main concern. It's the body's natural mechanism to conserve urine when fluids are being lost in other places.

16. When presented with a group of clients, the nurse should recognize which client as the best candidate for a low forceps delivery?

   1. A client, gravida 1, who has been pushing for one hour with repeated early decelerations and good variability.
   2. A client, gravida 1, who is fully dilated, and has caput in view, and an FH monitor strip showing severe late decelerations with every contraction.
   3. A client, gravida 1, who says she can't push anymore, and has a FH monitor strip with good variability.
   4. A client, gravida 2, who is fully dilated with her baby remaining at minus one station in a LOP position for the past hour.

1. Incorrect! There is no reason to interfere with this delivery. The fetus is not in danger and the primigravida mother has only been pushing for one hour.
2. Good choice. The fetal head is visible and the fetal heart reflects a problem with fetal oxygenation. A low forceps delivery is indicated in this situation.

3. *Incorrect, because there is no clinical indication to interfere with this delivery process. Most clients complain of being tired at this point in their labor.*

4. *Incorrect. This fetal head is one cm above the ischial spines in a posterior position. A forceps delivery in this situation would be difficult. If the condition does not correct itself, a cesarean section is indicated.*

17. **A pregnant diabetic arrives in the emergency room at 30 weeks of gestation with symptoms of hyperglycemia. Her blood sugar is 348 mg/dL. The resident orders 30 units of NPH insulin, to be given subcutaneously, stat. The nurse should do which of the following?**

    1. Give the dosage immediately.
    2. Start the dextrose IV the resident also ordered before giving the insulin.
    3. Question the large dosage.
    4. Question the type of insulin.

    1. *Incorrect. This client needs a quick acting insulin. NPH is an intermediate acting insulin.*
    2. *Wrong. This client already has a blood sugar of 348, and an IV with dextrose will only cause it to go higher.*
    3. *No, the dose of the insulin is not wrong, the type of insulin is.*
    4. **Correct. When a the client's blood sugar is 348, she needs a quick acting insulin, not an intermediate acting such as NPH.**

18. **Which of the following statements made by a client indicates to the nurse the need for further teaching regarding a scheduled arthroscopy of the knee?**

    1. "I know the doctor will be looking at my joint to check for cartilage damage."
    2. "I'll have to limit my exercising for a few weeks after this procedure."
    3. "I hope the incision heals quickly with those staples in place."
    4. "I know that I'll have to keep my knee straight and elevated to reduce the swelling after the surgery."

    1. *No, the client is correct. The arthroscopy is done to visualize the joint, including the synovium, articular surfaces, and joint structures. Look for an incorrect fact.*
    2. *The client is well-advised to limit activity following the procedure. Look for a statement that would indicate lack of knowledge about this procedure.*
    3. **You're right! An arthroscopy only involves puncture wounds with no need for staples following completion of this procedure. On occasion, a suture may be needed after insertion of the large-bore needle, but it's not standard procedure.**

4. *No, this is a correct understanding of post-procedure activity. These measures will help to reduce the swelling after the arthroscopy. Ice is also used for 24 hours afterwards. Choose an option that reflects the client's lack of knowledge.*

19. **A 12-year-old girl had a ventriculo-peritoneal shunt placed to treat hydrocephalus in infancy. In counseling the child about health management of the shunt, the nurse would consider the teaching effective if the child states:**

    1. "I should drink plenty of fluids and stay rested."
    2. "I may need to wear glasses as a teenager"
    3. "I can take prochlorperazine (Compazine) for vomiting."
    4. "If I get a really bad headache, I should call the doctor."

    1. *Wrong! Fluids and rest are good general health rules; however, they do not indicate knowledge of shunt management.*
    2. *Wrong! Controlled hydrocephalus is unlikely to cause changes in visual acuity. It is possible that the child may need glasses, but that would be unrelated to the shunt.*
    3. *Wrong! Effective teaching would result in the child's understanding of the need to notify the physician for vomiting, since vomiting is an early sign of increased intracranial pressure.*
    4. **Great choice! A headache is a sign of increased intracranial pressure. The child correctly identifies this as an indication to notify the physician.**

20. **A client, age 73, is receiving IV carbenicillin (Geocillin) for pharyngitis. Which of the following signs/symptoms manifested by the client would be of immediate concern to the nurse?**

    1. Anorexia and nausea.
    2. Abdominal cramping with diarrhea.
    3. Macular rash on lower extremities.
    4. Decreased visual acuity and tinnitus.

    1. *Incorrect. Anorexia and nausea are common side effects of antibiotics experienced by clients of all ages. Look for an option that addresses a potentially life-threatening complication for an elderly client.*
    2. **Good choice. Reducing or eliminating normal bowel flora with antibiotics provides an environment conducive to the growth of undesirable bacteria; in this case, a toxin produced by Clostridium difficile. These two symptoms may suggest the severe, life-threatening superinfection known as pseudomembranous colitis, which is characterized by diarrhea and abdominal cramping.**
    3. *Not the best option. Skin rashes should be monitored in all clients and may indicate hypersensitiv-*

ity. The question asks for a symptom seen more in the elderly that would be of immediate concern to the nurse. Try again.

4. *Wrong choice! Visual changes and tinnitus are not adverse effects associated with penicillins.*

21. **The nurse would expect that psychological factors, such as anxiety, could be responsible for which of the following?**

    1. Contributing to the development and progress of coronary artery disease.
    2. Causing coronary artery disease.
    3. Affecting the prognosis, only, for a client with coronary artery disease.
    4. Affecting a client's ability to adjust to a diagnosis of coronary artery disease, while having little direct effect on treatment outcomes.

    1. *Correct. Although theories that individuals with certain personality types (such as "Type A" persons) are more prone to develop cardiac disease have been disputed, anxiety and other psychological factors are still believed to play a significant role in the development and progress of cardiac disorders.*
    2. *Psychological factors are only one of the risk factors involved in the development of coronary artery disease. Psychological factors, alone, do not cause cardiac problems.*
    3. *This statement is only partially true, so it cannot be the correct option. Anxiety and other psychological factors are believed to play a significant role in the development and progress of cardiac disorders.*
    4. *This statement is inaccurate because psychological factors can have a profound effect on treatment outcomes.*

22. **A physician prescribes tocainide (Tonocard) PO for a client who has occasional to frequent premature ventricular contractions (PVCs). The nurse should teach the client to report which of the following side effects when taking Tonocard?**

    1. Double vision.
    2. Dry mouth.
    3. Petechiae.
    4. Photosensitivity.

    1. *Incorrect. Tocainide may cause blurred vision — not double vision. Make another selection.*
    2. *No, this is not a side effect of tocainide therapy. Dry mouth is typically seen in clients who take medications that contain atropine.*
    3. *Yes! Potential life-threatening side effects of tocainide therapy are leukopenia, neutropenia, and thrombocytopenia. The client should be instructed to notify the physician if unusual bleeding or bruising occurs, e.g., petechiae, hematuria, melena, or epistaxis.*

    4. *Wrong choice. Photosensitivity is a side effect of tetracycline therapy, not tocainide. The dermatologic side effects of tocainide are rashes, sweating, and flushing. Choose again.*

23. **The nurse asks a suicidal client to make a safety contract whereby he promises that if he has thoughts of harming himself he will not act on them, but will discuss them with either her or another staff member. The client tells the nurse that he cannot make this safety contract because he cannot promise that he will not harm himself. In the nurse's plan of care, which initial action would best ensure this client's safety?**

    1. Provide a relaxed and accepting environment to develop trust.
    2. Sterilize the environment by removing belts, glass objects, or sharp instruments that could be used for self-harm.
    3. Lock the doors to the unit and secure all windows so they cannot be opened.
    4. Assign a staff member to stay with the client at all times.

    1. *Wrong. These are important components of the nursing care plan, but this is not the best option for this question because it does not guarantee the client's safety.*
    2. *Removing sharp objects and other potentially dangerous items is important, but this is not the best option for ensuring the client's safety.*
    3. *The doors and windows could be secured so the client cannot leave the unit or jump from the window. However, this is not the best option for ensuring this client's safety.*
    4. *Correct. The client who is at high risk for suicidal behavior requires constant supervision at all times to ensure his safety. The nurse has both a legal and professional responsibility to provide a safe environment for the suicidal client.*

24. **A 72-year-old client is admitted to the hospital with congestive heart failure and will be started on digoxin (Lanoxin). Vitals on admission are BP 110/60, pulse 100, respirations 22. What is the expected outcome of digitalization?**

    1. Respiratory rate of 26.
    2. Heart rate greater than 100.
    3. Urine output of 50 mL per hour.
    4. Increased thirst.

    1. *No. Digoxin does not speed up the respiratory rate.*
    2. *No. Digoxin does not speed up the heart rate. Choose again.*
    3. *Excellent work! As the cardiac output improves, the kidney perfusion will improve, and urine output will increase.*

4. No. Increased thirst is not related to digitalization, but it may be indicative of diabetes.

25. **Which of the following foods should the nurse teach the client to include in a daily diet to minimize the most critical electrolyte loss when taking furosemide (Lasix)?**

1. Grains.
2. Milk.
3. Red meats.
4. Dried fruits.

1. Incorrect. Grains, which are high in fiber and iron, would not be indicated to prevent electrolyte loss.
2. Wrong choice. Milk, high in calcium and Vitamin D, would not correct the major electrolyte lost by the administration of Lasix.
3. Absolutely not. Red meats are high in fat and cholesterol (lean meats are iron-rich). This protein product would not affect the electrolyte loss caused by Lasix.
*4. **Yes! Dried fruits, avocadoes, broccoli, cantaloupe, grapefruit, lima and navy beans, oranges, nuts, bananas, peaches, potatoes, prunes, spinach, and tomatoes are potassium-rich foods. You remembered that Lasix causes the loss of potassium, along with the loss of sodium, chloride, magnesium, and calcium.***

26. **An antepartum client tells the nurse she has been vomiting her breakfast nearly every morning. Which of the following measures is most likely to help the client overcome early morning nausea and vomiting?**

1. Sipping whole milk with breakfast.
2. Drinking only liquids for breakfast.
3. Eating some crackers before arising from bed in the morning.
4. Drinking a carbonated beverage before arising from bed in the morning.

1. No. Clients are taught to decrease their fluid intake with meals to prevent overdistension of the stomach, thus reducing the risk of nausea and vomiting.
2. No, because large amounts of fluids tend to increase the nausea associated with pregnancy.
*3. **Good choice! Dry foods eaten before rising in the morning tend to reduce the risk of nausea in the pregnant woman.***
4. No. Fluids seem to increase the risk of nausea.

27. **A client who was diagnosed with cancer of the testes is being discharged from the hospital with an intravenous catheter in place for administration of chemotherapy. The nurse is to teach the client how to flush the catheter at home. Which**

information about the client's actions during the teaching session would indicate that the nurse's teaching is successful?

1. The client looks at the ceiling during the teaching session.
2. The client asks the nurse to show his wife how to flush the catheter.
3. The client asks the nurse if it is all right to flush the catheter before going to work in the morning.
4. The client tells the nurse that he will have the nurses at the clinic flush the catheter when he receives his chemotherapy.

1. Successful teaching is dependent on the client's willingness and readiness to learn. A client who looks at the ceiling during a teaching session is not ready or motivated to learn this skill. The client is blocking out the information being provided by the nurse. Which priority setting guideline will you use in this question?
2. Asking the nurse to show his wife how to perform the flushes indicates that the client is not motivated to perform this skill himself, and is not ready to learn the skill. Which priority setting guideline will you use in this question?
*3. **Excellent! When a client asks a question about how to implement the skills that are being taught, he is indicating that he has adopted the goal of providing for his own health care needs. This question by the client indicates that the teaching program will probably be successful.***
4. Saying that he will have the nurses at the clinic perform the flushes indicates that the client is not motivated to perform the task himself. This lack of motivation is an indication that the client is not ready to learn and that the discharge teaching will most likely not be successful.

28. **The nurse realizes that typical characteristics of girls with anorexia nervosa include which of the following?**

1. They fail to comply with their parents' wishes or societal expectations.
2. They exercise relentlessly.
3. They are truthful in reporting their eating habits.
4. They have problems with self-control.

1. This is not correct. Girls with anorexia nervosa are often described as thoughtful, obedient at home, and excellent students.
*2. **Great choice! Many girls with anorexia nervosa participate in sports and other athletic activities. They also tend to exercise relentlessly in their efforts to lose more weight.***
3. This is not correct. Clients with anorexia nervosa will often do whatever is necessary to continue losing weight, including lying to their parents and physicians about their eating patterns.

4. *Wrong. Clients with anorexia nervosa do not have problems with self-control. They are most often preoccupied with compulsive over-control.*

29. **A client is in a nursing home and is confined to bed. What is the most important nursing intervention that will lessen the possibility of skin breakdown and decubitus ulcers?**

    1. Massage all bony prominences with lotion to increase circulation.
    2. Keep the skin clean and dry.
    3. Turn the client at least every two hours.
    4. Place an egg crate mattress on the bed.

    1. *This is not the best choice. Massage of the bony prominences helps in preventing skin breakdown, but massage alone will not eliminate breakdown if the client is left in one position for long periods of time.*
    2. *Clean, dry skin is helpful in the prevention of skin breakdown. However, if the client has clean dry skin and is not moved frequently, skin breakdown will still occur.*
    3. ***This is the best choice! Turning the client frequently is the most important nursing intervention, since this measure alternates the pressure of the mattress against the skin, which decreases circulation and causes skin breakdown. This question reflects the planning phase of the nursing process.***
    4. *An egg crate mattress will help alleviate some of the pressure on the skin, but the client must be turned in order to eliminate pressure at a particular site.*

30. **A client, admitted with hypertension, is taking furosemide (Lasix) 40 mg p.o. twice a day. Which of the following interventions, if included in the plan of care by the nurse, would require further clarification?**

    1. Daily weights before breakfast.
    2. Monitor intake and output.
    3. Orthostatic blood pressure checks every eight hours.
    4. Limit fluid intake to 1000 mL in 24 hours.

    1. *Wrong. This intervention would be appropriate for the client's plan of care because of the need to monitor for fluid volume deficits that can be caused by Lasix. Remember that daily weights are the best indicators of fluid balance (a gain or loss of 1 kg is equal to a gain or loss of 1 liter of fluid).*
    2. *Incorrect. Monitoring intake and output would be important for the client on furosemide therapy. Recall that this drug is a very potent diuretic that can easily cause dehydration.*
    3. *No. It would be wise to make this assessment because Lasix can cause orthostatic hypotension. The*

client is cautioned to make position changes slowly to minimize the incidence of orthostatic hypotension, which can result from hypovolemia.
4. ***Correct option. This intervention would need to be discussed further. Lasix, a potent diuretic, can frequently cause dehydration. Limiting a client's fluid intake may contribute to this problem. This would not be a safe nursing measure.***

31. **A mother brings her 18-month-old to the pediatric emergency room. The child has sustained a fractured left femur. Which statement by the mother might make the nurse suspect a problem of child abuse?**

    1. "She is so active and gets into everything."
    2. "She was riding her bicycle and her foot got caught in the spokes."
    3. "My daughter slipped out of her high chair because the strap was too loose."
    4. "My daughter climbed up on a chair and fell down."

    1. *No, 18-month-old children are normally very active. This statement seems reasonable.*
    2. ***Correct! This statement does not seem reasonable because 18-month-old children are not developmentally ready to be riding bikes. This should make the nurse suspicious that the mother may be trying to hide something.***
    3. *Wrong! Even though the mother should have tied the strap on the high chair to prevent a fall, the statement seems reasonable. After the crisis is over, safety teaching could be given.*
    4. *No, 18-month-old children are very active and will climb on anything available. This statement seems reasonable. Perhaps some safety strategies could be discussed with the mother after the initial crisis is over.*

32. **The nurse tells a client that the doctor has ordered an intravenous to be started. The client appears to be upset but says nothing to the nurse. Which of the following is the best nursing response?**

    1. "Do you have any questions about the procedure?"
    2. "The doctor wants you to have antibiotics, and this method eliminates getting frequent injections."
    3. "What is there about this procedure that concerns you?"
    4. "It only hurts a little bit. It'll be over before you know it."

    1. *Wrong. This response focuses on the procedure, not on the client's feelings. This communication block places the client's feelings on hold instead of focusing on the procedure.*
    2. *Wrong. This response focuses on an inappropriate person (the doctor) and on an inappropriate issue (antibiotics by injection). This is a block to*

communication, since the client's feelings aren't addressed.

3. *Excellent choice! This response uses the communication tools of clarification and offering self. The nurse inquires about the client's concerns in the statement. The nurse offers self by offering to talk to the client about both the procedure and the client's feelings.*

4. *This option is incorrect. An intravenous puncture hurts more than a little bit. This communication block is identified as false assurance.*

33. **A client has active herpes type 2. Which of the following describes the best plan for delivery, assuming the lesions remain active?**

1. The mother should be induced close to term so that the nursery can be prepared for an infected infant.

2. The mother should be instructed to call the doctor when her contractions become regular and increase in intensity. She may or may not need a C-section.

3. The client should be delivered by C-section prior to the onset of labor.

4. The client should be delivered by C-section as soon after rupture of membranes as possible.

1. *Incorrect. The client who has a diagnosis of active herpes simplex type 2 needs to be delivered by C-section to prevent neonatal herpes.*

2. *Wrong. The active herpes type 2 client is instructed to call the physician as soon as she experiences any contractions so she can be admitted for an emergency cesarean section.*

3. *Correct. Whenever possible, the cesarean section should be scheduled prior to the onset of labor or rupture of membranes to reduce the risk of neonatal transmission of herpes.*

4. *Incorrect. The cesarean section should be planned prior to the rupture of membranes. If rupture of membranes does occur, an emergency cesarean section should be done as soon as possible, but every attempt should be made to prevent this situation.*

34. **At a boy scout camp the nurse encounters a child who exhibits a high-pitched inspiratory sound, and cyanosis. Describe the procedure that the nurse should institute.**

1. Stand behind the child and apply an upward thrust below the xiphoid.

2. Monitor the child; if respirations cease, use the Heimlich maneuver.

3. Bend the child forward and deliver back blows to dislodge the object.

4. Begin cardiopulmonary resuscitation.

1. *Yes, you have correctly evaluated the data as a child with an inadequate gas exchange, and then*

selected the correct procedure for the Heimlich maneuver on a child.

2. *No, do not delay treatment. The cyanosis and high-pitched inspiratory sound indicate an inadequate gas exchange. This child needs assistance now.*

3. *No, this is the treatment for an infant with an airway obstruction.*

4. *Why? There is no indication in the assessment that a cardiac arrest has occurred. Most children are primary respiratory arrests.*

35. **An 18-month-old is being admitted with a diagnosis of Wilm's tumor. Which nursing intervention takes priority?**

1. Checking vital signs every eight hours for incidence of hypertension.

2. Placing a sign over the bed that says "Do Not Palpate the Abdomen."

3. Raising the head of the bed to ease breathing.

4. Monitoring the urinary output every two hours.

1. *Wrong. Hypertension is not commonly found with Wilm's tumor, although you would want to check for stable vital signs as you would for any other client.*

2. *This is very important. These tumors are usually encapsulated. It is very important to protect this encapsulation and help contain the tumor. Decreasing palpation of the abdomen may protect this encapsulation.*

3. *The tumors vary in size, but unless the tumor is very large, it should not affect the child's breathing in most instances.*

4. *Wrong choice! I&O should be monitored as with any child. Usually urine output is not commonly affected, so that monitoring it every two hours may not be necessary.*

36. **A client, diagnosed with hypertension, is started on chlorothiazide (Diuril). The nurse is aware that this thiazide is often one of the preferred Step I diuretics in the management of hypertension because:**

1. The drug is more potent than that of loop diuretics.

2. The client only has to take the medication once each day.

3. Side effects from the drug are relatively less extensive.

4. Loss of electrolytes, especially potassium, is minimal.

1. *Incorrect. Thiazides act to slightly inhibit sodium and water loss. Their therapeutic effects are less potent than those of the loop diuretics.*

2. *Wrong. Depending on the type of thiazide diuretic used, the client may need to take the medication more than once a day.*

3. *Correct choice. The side effects of thiazide diuretics are less extensive than those of the loop diuretics, such as furosemide. Electrolyte losses (except for potassium) are seen infrequently with thiazides.*

4. *No. Potassium loss (hypokalemia) is a frequently occurring side effect of thiazide therapy—just as with loop diuretics.*

37. **A client who has been diagnosed with CHF two days earlier begins to exhibit symptoms of left-sided heart failure. Which of the following would the nurse observe?**

    1. Peripheral edema.
    2. Dyspnea.
    3. Abdominal distention.
    4. Fatigue.

    1. *No, this is seen in right-sided failure, due to the elevated venous pressure associated with right-sided failure.*

    2. *Excellent! A classic symptom of left-sided heart failure is that the left atrium cannot effectively empty its contents into the ventricle and left atrial pressure rises, causing increased pulmonary hydrostatic pressure. Fluid moves from circulation into interstitial spaces and into alveoli.*

    3. *No, this is seen in right-sided failure, due to the elevated venous pressure associated with right-sided failure.*

    4. *No, this is seen in right-sided failure, due to the elevated venous pressure associated with right-sided failure.*

38. **A 75-year-old client is taking lithium for a bipolar mood disorder. He asks the nurse whether psychiatric problems run in the family, because his alcoholic 45-year-old son and bulimic 20-year-old granddaughter are also taking lithium. In considering how to respond to the client, the nurse knows that lithium, while useful for certain other disorders, in addition to bipolar disorders, is least useful in treating which of the following?**

    1. Unipolar depressions.
    2. Aggressive conduct disorder.
    3. Bulimia.
    4. Alcoholism.

    1. *A low dose of lithium is sometimes given with an antidepressant when the antidepressant alone has not been effective. Lithium, alone, is also used on occasion to treat depression. This cannot be the correct answer.*

    2. *Some clients with aggressive conduct disorder respond well to treatment with lithium and its mood stabilizing properties. Read the options to identify the disorder that is not treated with lithium.*

    3. *Correct. Although lithium is sometimes used to*

treat eating disorders, it would not be the drug of choice for a client with bulimia because of the risks associated with an unstable fluid and electrolyte balance.

4. *In the past, lithium was used more widely to treat alcoholism than it is currently. It is still used in some settings. This is not the correct answer.*

39. **A client is taking propranolol (Inderal) as an anti-anginic. Inderal relieves angina because of which of the following actions?**

    1. Increase in cardiac output.
    2. Increase in heart rate.
    3. Inhibition of vasodilatation in coronary vessels.
    4. Decrease in myocardial oxygen requirements.

    1. *No! The effect of Inderal is to lower cardiac output, heart rate, conduction velocity, and myocardial contractility.*

    2. *Incorrect! Inderal lowers heart rate.*

    3. *Wrong choice! Inderal inhibits vasodilatation and arterial spasms, so it can be used for vascular headaches.*

    4. *Excellent! Inderal lowers the heart rate and contractility, which causes the heart to use less oxygen. It prevents angina.*

40. **A postoperative client is to ambulate for the first time after surgery. Which action to ensure safety is least appropriate for the nurse to use in preparing the client to ambulate?**

    1. Have the client get up and sit in the chair next to the bed.
    2. Have the client sit on the edge of the bed with his feet down for a few minutes before he starts to ambulate.
    3. Have the client stand at the side of the bed for a few minutes before taking his first steps.
    4. Encourage the client to try to walk straight ahead while assisting him with his walking.

    1. *This is the correct response since you are looking for an inappropriate action. If a client is to ambulate, placing him in a chair next to the bed does not meet the requirements for preparing for ambulation.*

    2. *Wrong choice! It is appropriate to have the client sit at the edge of the bed with his feet dangling. The action allows assessment of the client for weakness and dizziness, which may place the client at increased risk of falling.*

    3. *Wrong choice! Having the client stand at the edge of the bed is appropriate because it allows for assessment of the client's tolerance of this activity. He is still close to the bed, so if he becomes faint or weak he can easily be assisted back to bed.*

    4. *No. It is appropriate to assist a client during the*

initial ambulation following surgery, so assessment can be made of the client's tolerance to this activity.

41. **The nurse assigned to care for a child with cerebral palsy should obtain information concerning his abilities, limitations, interests, and habits, because the aim of therapy is to:**

    1. Assess the child's assets and potentialities and capitalize on these in the habilitative process, while ignoring limitations.
    2. Reverse abnormal functioning and restore brain damage through rehabilitation.
    3. Provide a therapeutic program that avoids subjecting the child to frustrating experiences that decrease his achievement.
    4. Develop an individualized therapeutic program that utilizes the child's assets and abilities and provides experiences that permit him to achieve success as well as help to cope with frustration and failure.

    1. *Although this goal is stated in general terms, the last part of the statement is not true—ignoring any aspect of the client is never the aim of therapy! An option that is partially true and partially false is always incorrect.*
    2. *Incorrect. Brain damage cannot be reversed or restored. This is a false statement, and this option should be eliminated.*
    3. *Wrong. It cannot be an aim of therapy to avoid frustrating experiences; this would be unrealistic. Although this option might appear to be a possibility and is stated in general terms, it is a false statement.*
    4. ***You chose the correct answer! This goal statement includes recognizing the client's assets and helping him cope with frustrations and failures due to his limitations. This option is a global response. It states appropriate goals of therapy in general terms, and it also includes the true part of Option 1.***

42. **An 18-year-old client is hospitalized for treatment of depression. The client was married at a young age, but is now separated from her husband. Because of the client's condition, which of the following approaches should be included in her plan of care?**

    1. Giving the client choices.
    2. Spending time with the client.
    3. Providing a chess game.
    4. Encouraging decision-making.

    1. *Wrong! Making choices is difficult for a depressed client. Note that this option is similar to Option 4, and these similar options should be eliminated.*
    2. ***Yes! You made the right selection! Because depressed clients frequently have suicidal tendencies, the best nursing action for the client is to***

spend time with her.
    3. *Wrong! An intellectual game such as chess would not be a good activity for a depressed client. Non-intellectual activities such as latch hook or needle work would be a better choice. Read all of the other options and then try to select the best one.*
    4. *Wrong! Decision-making is difficult for a depressed client. Note that this option is similar to Option 1, and these similar options can be eliminated.*

43. **During an office visit early in her pregnancy, a primigravida confides to the nurse that even though she and her husband planned this pregnancy she is experiencing many ambivalent feelings about the pregnancy. What response by the nurse would be most appropriate?**

    1. "Perhaps you should see a counselor to discuss these feelings."
    2. "Have you told your husband about these feelings?"
    3. "These feelings are quite normal at the beginning of pregnancy; there is no reason for you to feel guilty."
    4. "I am quite concerned about these feelings, could you explain more about them."

    1. *Incorrect, since this insinuates that she needs a counselor when in fact ambivalence is considered normal in most pregnancies.*
    2. *Wrong. This response insinuates that there is a problem that needs to be resolved.*
    3. ***Excellent choice! This client needs reassurance that these feelings are normal in pregnant women and there is no reason for concern.***
    4. *Incorrect. This is an inappropriate response because these feelings are normal in pregnant women and there is no reason for concern.*

44. **A client is re-hospitalized because she discontinued her medication on her own accord. The client's discharge plans include living with her parents and attending a job training program during the day. What is the most important goal for her remaining sessions with the nurse?**

    1. Reinforce the importance of taking her medications as prescribed.
    2. Anticipate future problems and how she might handle them.
    3. Terminate the nurse-client relationship.
    4. Promote the client's self-confidence.

    1. *Wrong! Reinforcing her medication regime is important for this client who had to be re-hospitalized because she had stopped taking her medications. However, it is not the most important goal at this time. There is a better option.*
    2. *This is an important component of discharge plan-*

ning, but it is not the most important goal at this time.

3. *Correct. The nurse should focus on ending their relationship by exploring the client's responses to the separation and dealing with any feelings of rejection that the client may have. This is the most important goal because it greatly affects the client's ability to establish positive relationships with health care providers in the future.*

4. *Promoting self-confidence is usually a component of the nursing care plan, but it is not the most important goal at this time.*

45. **During a well-child visit, the mother of a five-year-old expresses concern that her son will not wear his helmet while riding his bicycle. What is the most appropriate response?**

1. "Tell him the bike doesn't leave the garage without the helmet."
2. "It isn't that important, since he won't be riding in the road."
3. "Gradually encourage the wearing of the helmet with small rewards."
4. "I'll explain the potential for injury without a helmet."

1. *Even though this may sound very tough, it is direct, and is an appropriate method of obtaining compliance. The parent must believe that the helmet is necessary and apply the rule consistently.*
2. *No, any fall anywhere can potentially cause a head injury.*
3. *No, this response implies inconsistency. Children respond more favorably to consistency. A reward system should not be necessary, since this is expected rather that an optional behavior.*
4. *Not likely to be effective.*

46. **A 16-year-old adolescent sustained an open fracture of his left femur after being thrown from his motorcycle. A Steinmann pin is inserted and he is placed in ninety-ninety traction. In performing the initial assessment, the nurse finds the traction weight resting on the floor. Which of the following is the initial nursing action?**

1. Help the client use the trapeze to pull himself up in bed.
2. Check the pedal pulse and capillary refill of the right foot.
3. Notify the attending orthopedic physician.
4. Remove the weight and move the client to correct alignment in bed.

1. *Correct! When the traction weight is resting on the floor, the traction is no longer effective. Provided that nothing is out of alignment, the nurse should help the client resume his normal position in bed, making the system work again.*

2. *Wrong! Checking the pedal pulse and capillary refill is a way of measuring circulation. The leg of most concern is the left one, which is in traction because of the fracture.*
3. *Wrong! Helping the client slide up in bed should alleviate the problem and restore the function of the traction. There is no need to notify the orthopedic physician unless the traction is out of alignment or other assessments are not within the normal range.*
4. *Wrong! Never remove the traction weight! Besides possibly causing pain, this could interfere with the ends of the fracture being aligned. Always leave the traction set up as it is. If it does not look correct, notify the physician.*

47. **During open heart surgery, a 59-year-old client is placed on cardiopulmonary bypass in order to accomplish which of the following?**

1. Maintain systemic circulation.
2. Provide a bloodless field.
3. Eliminate ectopic rhythms.
4. Restore blood supply to the myocardium.

1. *Correct! After determining that the vein graft is functioning adequately, the client is slowly weaned from extracorporeal circulation.*
2. *Wrong. This is not the rationale for placement on cardiopulmonary bypass.*
3. *Wrong. Ectopic rhythms are a cause of arrhythmias, not a result of open heart surgery or a reason for cardiopulmonary bypass.*
4. *Wrong choice! This is a goal of surgery, but, nevertheless, systemic circulation must be maintained.*

48. **A 45-year-old man is admitted to the emergency room complaining of chest pain and dyspnea. He is also flushed and perspiring profusely. He says, "I feel like I am going to die. Am I having a heart attack?" The medical exam and lab work are negative. He is diagnosed with anxiety. The nurse assesses his level of anxiety as:**

1. Mild.
2. Moderate.
3. Severe.
4. Panic.

1. *The severity of this client's symptoms indicate that he has more than a mild level of anxiety. This is not the correct option.*
2. *In moderate anxiety, the person's perceptual field narrows but he is able to cope with some assistance. This client's symptoms indicate a higher level of anxiety.*
3. *In severe anxiety, the person's perceptual field is scattered and he is not able to focus on anything except relieving his anxiety. This does not describe this client because he is currently immobilized.*

4. Correct. This client's symptoms indicate he is experiencing the panic level of anxiety. His symptoms are also classic symptoms of a panic disorder.

49. An eight-year-old is in the hospital for second and third degree burns to his left arm. He was playing with matches with his friends. The others were not injured. While acutely ill in the hospital, the nursing diagnosis with the highest priority for the child at this time is:

1. Potential for infection.
2. Potential altered parenting.
3. Knowledge deficit regarding injury prevention.
4. Ineffective airway clearance.

1. Great work! Infection is the main concern in this case because skin is the body's first line of defense against infection. Much of this client's skin has been burned away so the client is now very susceptible to microorganisms.
2. Potential altered parenting is a diagnosis that makes reference to potential abuse or neglect. Although there are grave concerns here regarding the availability of parental supervision, there is not enough data at this time. The nurse would want to collect more data about this to determine the actual events surrounding the incident.
3. Teaching about injury prevention would be very important to consider in the long range plan for this client. In dealing with acute priorities, however, infection is the greatest concern. This also is not the most appropriate time to teach parents and child, when they're in this crisis state.
4. Wrong. Ineffective airway clearance is always a potential problem with an extensive burn or one that involves the head and neck area but, due to the location of this burn, infection is more of a priority.

50. A client is taking triamterene (Dyrenium) in addition to hydrochlorothiazide (Hydrodiuril) to control hypertension. The nurse is aware that the rationale for this combination medication therapy is to prevent or treat:

1. Mild hypokalemia.
2. Dehydration.
3. Moderate hyponatremia.
4. Hypotension.

1. Correct! Potassium-sparing diuretics, such as Dyrenium, are used to prevent or treat mild hypokalemia due to the concurrent use of drugs that are potassium-wasting, such as Hydrodiuril.
2. No. Dyrenium and Hydrodiuril both cause excretion of sodium, which can lead to dehydration. These drugs cannot be used to prevent a problem they might cause!

3. Incorrect. These drugs can cause hyponatremia because both are diuretics.
4. Wrong choice. Dyrenium and Hydrodiuril can cause hypotension due to their diuretic effect.

51. A client who has just been diagnosed with cancer tells the nurse that he would rather be dead than go through the treatment for cancer. The most appropriate nursing response is:

1. "What is it about the cancer treatment that concerns you?"
2. "If you don't receive the treatment, you will get your wish."
3. "Why don't you talk to your doctor about your feelings?"
4. "That wouldn't be fair to your family, would it?"

1. Excellent! This response is therapeutic because it focuses on the client's feelings and concerns. This response encourages the client to further express his feelings about cancer treatments. The nurse may also be able to clarify any misinformation that the client may have concerning the treatments.
2. This response is inappropriate and unprofessional. It fails to respect the client's feelings and does not address the client's immediate concerns. This response blocks further communication, instead of encouraging the client to express his feelings concerning the treatments.
3. With this response, the nurse avoids the discussion with the communication block of putting the client's concern on hold. This response is not appropriate, because it tells the client that the nurse does not want to hear about the client's feelings.
4. This response uses the communication block of referring to an inappropriate person. By addressing the needs of the family instead of the needs of the client, the nurse indicates that the needs of the family are more important. This statement also expresses disapproval by the nurse.

52. A confused elderly client is on strict bed rest, secondary to left-sided heart failure. Which of the following interventions would provide for this client's safety?

1. Place the client in a room away from the noise and confusion of the nurses' station.
2. Avoid the use of nightlights, since they tend to distort images and confuse clients.
3. Discuss with the client the need for restraints if she continues to get out of bed.
4. Provide opportunities for regular toileting, and include this information in the client's care plan.

1. This is an inappropriate nursing action. Any client who is confused should be placed in a room near the nursing station—not away from it.

2. *This is incorrect. A nightlight is generally used for confused clients, because it decreases image distortion and enhances reality. Also, the use of a nightlight helps orient clients to the hospital environment.*

3. *This option is a good distractor, because it implies that by talking to the client, the nurse may be able to lessen her confusion. Wrong! If the client is confused, then the issue of safety requires that the nurse should focus on how to adapt the client's environment to decrease the risk of accidents.*

4. ***Very good! This client is confused, which means there is a high safety risk due to decreased ability to perceive danger. Providing opportunities for regular toileting helps ensure that the client's basic needs for elimination will be met, and will greatly reduce the risk of the client's falling while trying to get up and go to the bathroom without the assistance of the nurse. This nursing action provides for the comfort and safety of the client, and it should be recorded in the plan of care.***

53. **An elderly, confused client is on bed rest. A nursing action that is least likely to help prevent a fall for this client is:**

    1. Providing regular toileting.
    2. Explaining to the client that she should use the call light if she needs to get up.
    3. Placing the side rails in the up position and checking on the client often.
    4. Proper use of restraints.

    1. *No. This is an important and necessary nursing action. When a confused, elderly client has the physiological need to void or have a bowel movement, an attempt is usually made to find a bathroom. This attempt may result in a fall for the confused client.*

    > **TEST-TAKING TIP:** Since this question has a false response stem, the correct answer is something that will NOT help prevent a fall.

    2. ***Excellent! If the client is confused, as identified in the case scenario, she is not likely to remember instructions concerning the use of the call light. This action is not likely to prevent a fall, and does not provide for the client's safety. Since this question has a false response stem, the answer is something that will NOT prevent a fall.***

    > **SAFETY ALERT!** This client is confused, and thus may not be able to perceive danger.

    3. *Wrong. The side rails should be in the up position to prevent the client from falling out of bed, and to serve as a reminder to the client to remain in bed.*

    > **TEST-TAKING TIP:** Since this question has a false response stem, the correct answer is something that will NOT help prevent a fall.

4. *Wrong. If the client is assessed and it is determined that she needs to be restrained in order to avoid injury, then restraints may be applied, and the physician notified of the situation.*

> **TEST-TAKING TIP:** Since this question has a false response stem, the correct answer is something that will NOT help prevent a fall.

54. **In caring for a client taking digoxin (Lanoxin), the nurse would give immediate attention to which of the following statements?**

    1. "I have a headache and backache."
    2. "I feel nauseated and have no appetite."
    3. "I've gained a half-pound in the last two days."
    4. "I'm having muscle cramps in my legs."

    1. *Wrong choice! Headaches and backaches are not related to the use of digoxin.*
    2. ***Excellent! Anorexia, nausea, vomiting and abdominal discomforts are early signs of digoxin toxicity.***
    3. *Not the best choice! A weight gain of half a pound is not significant. Diuresis is likely to occur, with some weight loss.*
    4. *No. This usually indicates other electrolyte abnormalities like hypokalemia, but is not a direct symptom of digoxin toxicity.*

55. **A six-month-old was admitted to the hospital after he had been in a car accident. He was placed on phenytoin (Dilantin) after he had a seizure. He had no further seizures, and will be going home on this medication. Which of the following is inaccurate information that the nurse would avoid giving to the parents?**

    1. Watch for signs of gingival hyperplasia.
    2. Note any increase in seizure activity.
    3. Have therapeutic blood levels drawn after one year on dapitalize Dilantin.
    4. Drowsiness may occur when therapy is initially begun.

    1. *This statement is accurate and refers to a common side effect of Dilantin. Parents need to be aware of this so they don't become alarmed and so that the proper dental precautions can be taken to prevent mouth infections.*
    2. *This is accurate and important for the parents to know. While on this medication no seizure activity should occur. If a seizure does occur, the physician needs to be aware so that medication adjustments can occur.*
    3. ***You chose the correct answer! Therapeutic blood levels need to be drawn to make sure the medication is at a high enough level to control the seizures, but not a toxic level to cause harm. Chil-***

dren also grow and their weight changes may create the need for a higher dose for the drug to still be effective. These blood levels should be drawn soon after the therapy has begun and periodically thereafter. One year is too long to wait to draw the first level.

4. *Incorrect! Drowsiness is a common side effect when the Dilantin is first begun. Parents need to be prepared for this so that they don't think something is wrong.*

56. Before administering lithium, the nurse checks the client's latest lab report for her serum lithium level and notes a level of 1.2 mEq/L. What is the best action for the nurse to take next?

1. Administer the next prescribed dose of lithium.
2. Suggest the blood test be repeated.
3. Withhold the next dose of lithium and notify the psychiatrist of the lab results.
4. Ask the client how she is feeling, to identify any untoward effects.

1. *Although the lithium level is still within the therapeutic range, it is at the very top of the range. This action is a possibility but it could be unsafe. Read the other options to see if there is a better choice.*
2. *This action could be appropriate, but it is not the best action for the nurse to take next. Read the other options.*
3. *This is not correct. The lithium level is still within the normal range, so withholding the lithium is not an appropriate nursing action.*
4. *Correct! A lithium level of 1.2 mEq/L is at the top of the therapeutic range. Before the next dose can be safely given, the nurse must assess the client for any signs of lithium toxicity. If the client has none, the nurse can give the medication as prescribed.*

57. A client has an indwelling Foley catheter. The nurse would avoid including which nursing actions in the plan for irrigation of the catheter?

1. Instill sterile distilled water in the catheter.
2. Use minimal pressure to clear the catheter of clots or mucous plugs.
3. Use sterile equipment for irrigation.
4. Use gravity to achieve a return flow of the irrigant.

1. *Great job! Sterile solution is necessary but distilled water is hypotonic and may be absorbed by body tissues. Sterile normal saline is the solution of choice, since it is the most similar to normal body tissue fluid.*

STRATEGY ALERT! *This option is different from the other three and is a false statement. Note that this planning question has a negative response stem.*

2. *Wrong choice! Minimal pressure is used to avoid trauma to the bladder tissue. This appropriate action is not correct because this question has a negative response stem.*
3. *Wrong choice! The bladder is a sterile cavity, and any procedure that introduces foreign substances into it should utilize surgical asepsis. This is a proper action so it is not the correct choice because this question has a false response stem.*
4. *The irrigant should be allowed to return by gravity. Negative pressure or suction can cause injury to bladder tissue. This appropriate action is not the correct answer to this question with a false response stem.*

58. The nurse would expect which pattern of contractions when the client reports that they are four minutes apart?

1. A contraction that lasts for four minutes followed by a period of relaxation.
2. Contractions that last for 60 seconds with a four-minute rest between contractions.
3. Contractions that last for 60 seconds with a three-minute rest between contractions.
4. Contractions that last for 45 seconds with a three-minute rest between contractions.

1. *Wrong! When timing the interval of contractions, count from the beginning of one contraction to the beginning of the next. The total time will include the contraction plus the relaxation period. This pattern is longer than four minutes.*
2. *Wrong! This contraction interval is five minutes apart.*
3. *Correct. A 60-second contraction with a relaxation period of three minutes is equivalent to contractions every four minutes.*
4. *Wrong! This contraction pattern is less than four minutes apart.*

59. An elderly client is admitted to the hospital with pneumonia. His daughter, who takes care of him at home, says to the nurse, "I'm so glad he is here. You can take much better care of him than I can." The best nursing response to the daughter's statement is which of the following?

1. "We do have the equipment and people to take care of sick clients."
2. "It is not easy to care for the elderly. How do you manage?"
3. "Sir, your daughter takes good care of you at home, doesn't she?"
4. "Are you feeling guilty because your father has pneumonia?"

1. *This response does not focus on the appropriate person (the daughter). This response also focuses*

on inappropriate issues concerning other people and hospital equipment. To be therapeutic, the nurse's response should focus on the daughter's feelings and concerns.

2. ***Very good! This response uses the communication tool of showing empathy, and asks for clarification of the statement made to the nurse.***

> **STRATEGY ALERT!** *Be sure to correctly identify the client in communication questions! The daughter is the client in this question, and the nurse's response should address her concerns. Note that Options 1 & 3 focus on inappropriate issues, and Option 4 implies to the client that she may be to blame for her father's pneumonia.*

3. *This response is not directed towards the appropriate person (the daughter). The father is the person with the medical problem, but his daughter is the client in this test question. The nurse's response should be addressed to the daughter.*

4. *This response indirectly places blame on the daughter for her father's pneumonia. This type of response can put the client on the defensive, which is not therapeutic.*

60. **The nurse knows that the two basic types of arrhythmias, listed in order of those that make the heart go faster, and those that make the heart go slower are:**

    1. Bradyarrhythmias and tachyarrhythmias.
    2. Tachyarrhythmias and bradyarrhythmias.
    3. Supraventricular and ventricular.
    4. Ventricular and supraventricular.

    1. *No. You chose the correct terminology, but in the wrong order. Remember, arrhythmias that make the heart go faster are called tachyarrhythmias, and arrhythmias that make the heart go slower are called bradyarrhythmias.*

    2. ***You are right! Arrhythmias that make the heart go faster are called tachyarrhythmias, and arrhythmias that make the heart go slower are called bradyarrhythmias.***

    3. *Wrong! In addition to two types of arrhythmias that make the heart go faster and slower, arrhythmias can arise from different areas in the heart as well. These areas are usually divided into supraventricular (from above the ventricles), and ventricular (from within the ventricle) arrhythmias.*

    4. *Wrong! In addition to two types of arrhythmias that make the heart go faster and slower, arrhythmias can arise from different areas in the heart as well. These areas are usually divided into ventricular (from within the ventricle) arrhythmias, and supraventricular (from above the ventricles).*

61. **A client comes to the clinic to be tested for tuberculosis. Which is the most valuable diagnostic tool currently used to screen for TB?**

    1. Chest x-ray.
    2. Sputum culture.
    3. Bronchial washings.
    4. Mantoux skin test.

    1. *Wrong. A chest x-ray is sometimes used for diagnosis and is always used as a follow-up for changes.*
    2. *Wrong! It is necessary to obtain a good deep cough to get adequate sputum. Clients with TB are unable to cough deep enough.*
    3. *Wrong choice! It is sometimes used but often requires multiple specimens.*
    4. ***Good choice! It is designated as the most accurate and valuable tool.***

62. **The charge nurse is preparing the staffing assignment. A six-month-old on the unit has AIDS and cytomegalovirus (CMV). Which staff person should be assigned as the primary care giver for this child?**

    1. An experienced nurse who is six months pregnant.
    2. A male graduate nurse, recently oriented to pediatrics.
    3. An experienced nurse's aide who is healthy.
    4. A licensed practical nurse with eczema.

    1. *No. You probably selected this nurse due to her status and experience. However, this assignment would place the nurse's fetus at undue risk, since pregnant women should avoid exposure to CMV.*
    2. ***Yes! A graduate nurse should be able to carry out the care, maintaining appropriate technique based on the principles of communicable disease transmission.***
    3. *No. Although the aide is "healthy" and experienced, this client should have a licensed caregiver. The implied level of care is above that of the aide.*
    4. *No, this nurse is at risk for injury from this assignment. She has open areas on her skin, which is the body's first line of defense from communicable disease.*

63. **A cholecystectomy client is three days postoperative. A postoperative wound infection is suspected because the nurse notes that the drainage from his dressing is yellow and thick. This describes which type of drainage?**

    1. Serous.
    2. Purulent.
    3. Serosanguineous.
    4. Sanguineous.

1. *No, this describes clear, watery plasma.*
2. ***Correct, purulent describes thick yellow, green, or brown drainage.***
3. *No, this describes pale, very watery drainage.*
4. *No, this indicates fresh bleeding.*

64. **A client with hypertension is being treated with chlorothiazide (Diuril) 500 mg p.o. twice a day. In taking the client's medication history, the nurse notes that the client is a diabetic and has been taking chlorpropamide (Diabinese) 250 mg p.o. daily. The nurse is aware that the potential interaction of Diabinese with Diuril may result in:**

    1. Hypocalcemia.
    2. Hyperglycemia.
    3. Aplastic anemia.
    4. Hypoglycemia.

    1. *Wrong choice. Hypocalcemia does not result from the combined use of Diuril and Diabinese.*
    2. ***Correct! Thiazides, such as Diuril, may decrease the effectiveness of Diabinese, resulting in hyperglycemia. Diabetic clients require close monitoring and may require increased antidiabetic medication.***
    3. *No. Aplastic anemia is a life-threatening side effect of Diabinese therapy (and all oral hypoglycemic agents). It is not a result of an interaction between Diuril and Diabinese.*
    4. *Incorrect. Hypoglycemia is the most common side effect of Diabinese therapy and does not result from an interaction between Diuril and Diabinese.*

65. **The nurse is preparing to do client teaching for a hypertensive client. Which of the following goals is least appropriate?**

    1. The client eliminates sodium from her diet.
    2. The client exercises moderately each day.
    3. The client maintains weight appropriate for height.
    4. The client discontinues use of birth control pills.

    1. ***Very good! Eliminating sodium from the client's diet is not a reasonable goal because sodium is present in so many foods. A diet appropriate for a hypertensive client will restrict intake of sodium, not eliminate it.***
    2. *True, but not correct! Exercising moderately each day is an appropriate goal for a hypertensive client. This question has a false response stem, so the correct answer is a goal that is NOT appropriate for a hypertensive client.*
    3. *Not the correct choice! Maintaining weight appropriate for height is an appropriate goal for a hypertensive client. This question has a false response stem, so the correct answer is a goal that is NOT appropriate for a hypertensive client.*

4. *Discontinuing use of birth control pills is an appropriate goal for a hypertensive client. This question has a false response stem, so the correct answer is a goal that is NOT appropriate for a hypertensive client.*

66. **A client is admitted to a nursing home. She has difficulty seeing and hearing. Which of the following nursing actions is least important for this client?**

    1. Showing the client where all of the furniture and personal items are in the room.
    2. Talking loudly when entering the client's room.
    3. Telling the client that because of her increased risk of falling and injuring herself, she is not allowed out of her room.
    4. Assisting the client to identify the placement of food items during meals.

    1. *Wrong choice. Since the client has difficulty seeing, the nursing staff should familiarize her with the location of pertinent items in her room.*

    > **TEST-TAKING TIP:** *This question has a false response stem, so the correct answer to the question is an option that is LEAST appropriate.*

    2. *Wrong choice. A client who is sight and hearing impaired needs to be alerted to the presence of another individual entering the room. This can be done by speaking loudly enough for the client to hear.*
    3. ***Correct answer. Confining the client to her room is least appropriate. She has sensory deprivation and is at risk for falling, but she should not be isolated from others. She can be assisted by staff when attending other activities. This inappropriate action is the correct answer to the question, however, because the question has a false response stem.***

    > **SAFETY ALERT!** *A client with sensory deprivation is at risk, because of impaired ability to perceive danger.*

    4. *Wrong choice! It is important that the client know where food items are located to prevent potential burns, spills, and injuries.*

67. **The physician orders peripheral pulse checks every eight hours on a client who was admitted to the hospital with decreased circulation to his left leg. The nurse performing the peripheral pulse checks should include documentation of which of the following?**

1. Strength and rate.
2. Amplitude, rhythm and symmetrical comparison of both extremities.
3. Temperature of the skin.
4. Color of the extremity.

1. Although strength and rate are important aspects of a peripheral pulse, this option does not indicate that a comparison is to be made with the other leg.

2. Good job! The amplitude gives information concerning the strength, and the rhythm provides information concerning the rate and regularity of the pulse. An important aspect of this option is the fact that symmetry is assessed, which is most important for comparison of extremities. This question reflects the assessment phase of the nursing process.

3. The temperature of the skin is important for this client, but it is not a part of the peripheral pulse check.

4. Color of the extremity is very important and should be assessed, but it is not part of the procedure for performing peripheral pulse checks.

68. **While providing care for a client, the nurse should avoid which action in order to prevent muscle strain?**

1. Move muscles quickly, using short tugs in order to avoid muscle fatigue.
2. Use the longest and strongest muscles of the body whenever possible.
3. Lean toward objects being pushed, such as a stretcher.
4. Carry objects close to the body without touching your clothing.

1. This is the correct answer, because the question is asking you to select an action that the nurse should avoid. Jerky movements produce increased strain on muscles and are usually uncomfortable for the client.

2. Wrong choice! The longest, strongest muscles are less likely to become injured than the small muscles. This is not an action the nurse should AVOID.

3. Body weight adds force to muscle action when pushing any object. This is a correct action, but the question is asking you to select an option that the nurse should AVOID.

4. When objects are close to the body, the line of gravity is within the body's base of support, which improves balance and reduces strain on the arm muscles. This is a correct action, but the question is asking you to select an option that the nurse should AVOID.

69. **The nurse knows that quinidine sulfate (Quinidex) is used to treat atrial and ventricular arrhythmias because of which of the following effects?**

1. Increase of automaticity and excitability.
2. Increase of vagal action in the SA and AV nodes.
3. Shortening the refractory period of atrial and ventricular fibers.
4. Cell membrane stabilization through the prevention of movement of sodium and potassium.

1. Incorrect! Quinidine and Group I-A drugs like Pronestyl and Norpace decrease automaticity and excitability.

2. Incorrect! The indirect anticholinergic effect of quinidine inhibits vagal action on the SA and AV nodes.

3. No. The main reason quinidine is used is to prolong the effective refractory period of atrial and ventricular muscles. It can therefore be used for both atrial and ventricular arrhythmias.

4. Correct! By stabilizing the cell membrane and preventing sodium and potassium from moving, cardiac impulses are suppressed. Quinidine works in various areas of the heart — ectopic areas in the atria and ventricles, and the AV node.

70. **A 56-year-old female client is started on hydrochlorothiazide (Hydrodiuril) and spironolactone (Aldactone) for treatment of hypertension. The nurse's discharge instructions should include an admonition to the client that she should:**

1. Contact her physician if blood pressure control is not achieved in two to three days.
2. Take the Aldactone between meals to increase absorption.
3. Watch for signs of hypokalemia and include potassium-rich foods in her diet.
4. Report any muscle twitching or numbness in extremities to the physician.

1. Incorrect. It will take one to two weeks for the client's blood pressure to be controlled. The client should be taught the correct technique for monitoring the blood pressure weekly.

2. Wrong choice. Aldactone commonly causes nausea/vomiting, anorexia, and diarrhea. The drug should be given with food or milk to minimize GI irritation and to increase bioavailability.

3. Not necessary. Remember that Aldactone is a potassium-sparing diuretic; therefore, hypokalemia is not a major concern.

4. Yes! Aldactone is often combined with other diuretic agents because of its potassium-sparing effect. With increased retention of potassium, hyperkalemia may develop if the client's intake of potassium is high.

71. **While caring for the client with an IV, it is most important for the nurse to:**

1. Report any signs of infection to the physician.
2. Record the condition of the IV site and the rate of infusion, and report any unusual findings.
3. Record intravenous intake.
4. Ask the client if the IV site is painful or tender.

1. *This is an appropriate nursing action, since the physician may need to provide orders to alleviate the problem. However, this is not the best option.*
2. **Observing the site and infusion rate is part of providing safe care to the client receiving intravenous therapy. This option is the most comprehensive and includes the ideas in the other options.**
3. *This action is standard care for the client receiving intravenous therapy and is a possible choice. However, this is not the best option.*
4. *This action is part of assessing the site for possible infiltration or phlebitis. This is an appropriate action, but there is a better choice.*

72. **A vaginal exam reveals the following information on a laboring woman and her fetus: two centimeters, 50%, +1, ROA. Based on this information which of the following is the presentation of the fetus?**

1. ROA.
2. Two centimeters.
3. Vertex.
4. +1.

1. *Wrong! ROA (Right, Occipital Anterior) is the position of the fetus. This describes the relationship of the presenting part of the fetus to the mother's pelvis. In this case the occipital bone is located anteriorly in the mother's right side.*
2. *Incorrect. Two centimeters describes the dilation of the cervix.*
3. **Good job! Based upon the position of the fetus (ROA) the presenting part (the part of the fetus lowermost in the pelvis) must be the head or vertex.**
4. *No, this describes the degree of descent of the fetus into the pelvis, called the fetal station.*

73. **A 78-year-old client has been in the hospital for a week on bed rest. She complains of elbow pain. The best nursing action is to:**

1. Place elbow pads on the client.
2. Examine the elbow.
3. Call the physician for an order for pain medication.
4. Reposition the client so that she is more comfortable.

1. *Since the case scenario does not relate what is causing the elbow pain, you cannot assume that it is*

related to pressure or skin breakdown. More information must be obtained by the nurse before implementing any actions.
2. **Very good! Examining the elbow is an assessment of the client's complaint. The nurse does not know enough about the elbow pain or its probable cause. The elbows can be assessed for redness, swelling, or joint pain. Then, after assessing, the nurse can analyze the situation and develop a plan of care and implement the appropriate nursing interventions.**
3. *Calling the physician at this time is not appropriate! The nurse does not know enough about the elbow pain or what is causing it. After obtaining further information, the nurse may not need to notify the physician if nursing interventions will alleviate the problem. If the physician must be notified, the nurse will need to give the physician the information needed to analyze the problem and order appropriate medical treatment.*
4. *Repositioning the client may provide for the client's comfort, however, the nurse still does not know what is causing the pain. Repositioning the client should not precede the nurse's investigation of the client's complaint of pain. The nursing process requires that assessment be performed before planning or implementing any other nursing action, because these actions must be based on information obtained during the assessment. Choose another option!*

74. **A client is to have a nasogastric tube inserted because of an obstruction in his bowel. The nurse explains the procedure to him and is about to begin the insertion, when the client says, "No way! You are not putting that hose down my throat. Get away from me." Which of the following statements is the best nursing response?**

1. "You have the right to refuse treatment. Why don't you talk to your doctor about it?"
2. "Something is upsetting you. Can you tell me what it is:"
3. "What do you feel about this hose?"
4. "I would just get it over with, because you won't get better without this tube."

1. *Incorrect choice. The client certainly has this right, but it is not the best response by the nurse. This response puts the client's feelings on hold, referring them to another person at a later time. This response blocks communication.*
2. **Very good. This response addresses the client's feelings. It is more global than Option 3, which focuses only on the client's feelings about the nasogastric tube. This option uses the communication tool of clarification, which helps the nurse assess the situation.**

3. *Wrong choice. This option asks for a response from the client concerning the hose. The nurse does not need information concerning the hose. The nurse needs information concerning the client's feelings about the whole situation.*

4. *Incorrect choice! In this response, the nurse is blocking communication by giving advice.*

75. **A nine-year-old is admitted to the hospital with acute glomerulonephritis. Which nursing action should be included in the plan of care for this child?**

1. Elevating the HOB to decrease edema of face and eyes.
2. Monitoring blood pressure every four hours.
3. Administering prednisone as ordered to facilitate diuresis.
4. Reporting any hematuria to the physician immediately.

1. *Wrong. Glomerulonephritis does sometimes cause mild edema. Usually this is not one of the major concerns. This symptom may be confused with nephrotic syndrome, which causes marked edema. This intervention is most appropriate for marked edema.*

2. **Correct. One of the associated problems that must be monitored during an episode of acute glomerulonephritis is hypertension. The nurse needs to be aware of this and make frequent assessments of blood pressure as necessary.**

3. *Wrong. Prednisone is not given for acute glomerulonephritis, but for nephrotic syndrome. Treatment for acute glomerulonephritis is primarily symptomatic.*

4. *Wrong. Hematuria is expected during the initial stages of acute glomerulonephritis. It must be monitored, however, as the child must remain on bedrest until it clears. Frank blood in the urine may need to be reported.*

76. **A 49-year-old client has been diagnosed with iron deficiency anemia. The nurse should recommend an increased intake of which of the following foods when teaching the client about her diet.**

1. Fresh fruits.
2. Milk and cheese.
3. Organ meats.
4. Whole grain breads.

1. *Wrong! Fruits provide the body with a rich source of Vitamins A and C; this client is deficient in iron.*

2. *Wrong. Dairy products are good sources of high quality complete protein, not iron.*

3. **Right choice! A diet rich in organ meats provides iron, which is what the client needs to improve her anemia.**

4. *Wrong. Whole grain breads are rich in carbohydrates and dietary fiber, not iron.*

77. **A client is hospitalized for a surgical procedure. The most important nursing intervention when administering the preoperative medication is which of the following?**

1. Have the client void before going to the operating room.
2. Put the side rails up, and instruct the client to remain in bed.
3. Ask the client if she has signed all of the admission forms for the surgery.
4. Have the family leave, since the medication will decrease the client's inhibitions and she may say or do something that is out of character for her.

1. *Incorrect. It is standard preoperative care to have clients void prior to surgery but the nurse should have the client void before administering the pre-operative medication.*

> **TEST-TAKING TIP:** The stem of the question asks about administering the preoperative medication — not about preoperative preparation of the client. This option does not address the issue in the question.

2. *Yes! Preoperative medications may cause the client to become disoriented, drowsy, and unsteady when walking. It is very important that the side rails are up and the client remain in bed in order to protect the client from an injury caused by a fall.*

> **SAFETY ALERT!** Preoperative medications are identified as a priority risk factor, because they impair the client's ability to perceive and respond to danger.

3. *No. The necessary forms should be signed prior to surgery; however, the client does not know what forms are required by the hospital. It is the nursing staff's responsibility to check the forms for completion. This is not an appropriate nursing action and cannot be the correct answer.*

4. *No. Although preoperative medications can alter a person's behavior, educating the family about the possible side effects is more appropriate than separating the family at this time, when support for the client is important.*

78. **A 50-year-old client is being discharged following bilateral vein ligation and stripping. While doing discharge planning, the nurse instructs the client that it is important to do which of the following when she goes home?**

1. Wear slacks and opaque hose regularly for cosmetic reasons.
2. Purchase and wear above-the-knee support hose only.

3. Join a local diet center to facilitate weight loss.
4. Elevate her legs above the heart level four times a day for 15-20 minutes.

1. *Incorrect. This certainly can be suggested, but is not necessary.*
2. *Incorrect, because above-the-knee support hose will cause pressure in the popliteal area. Below-the-knee hose are recommended.*
3. *Incorrect. The client must be ready to lose weight. The nurse's responsibility is to teach proper nutrition, not to suggest the client join a diet center to learn proper nutrition.*
4. *Yes! This position is necessary to decrease venous hydrostatic pressure, reduce stasis, and relieve symptoms.*

79. **A client is to be up in a chair three times a day. He is paralyzed from the waist down. What is the best nursing approach when transferring this client from a bed into a wheelchair?**

1. Place the wheelchair close to the foot of the bed.
2. Utilize the principles of body mechanics while providing a safe transfer for the client.
3. Slide the client to the edge of the bed, keeping the nurse's back straight and using a rocking motion to pull the client.
4. Place the nurse's arms under the client's axillae from the back of the client.

1. *This is not correct. The wheelchair should be placed as close to the position of the client's buttocks as possible for a safe and easy transfer. The wheelchair should not be placed at the foot of the bed.*
2. *Very good! The nurse is in control of the nurse's own body and the client's movement during the transfer. Providing for the safety of the client, and utilizing the principles of body mechanics to provide safety for the nurse and the client, is the best nursing approach. Maslow's Hierarchy of Needs assigns top priority to safety needs when no physiological need is identified.*
3. *This is an appropriate nursing action that addresses the safety of the nurse and client. Positioning the client near the edge of the bed will reduce the energy required to move the client to the wheelchair, and will protect the nurse's back by using leg and arm muscles to move the client to the edge of the bed. However, there is another option that better describes the best nursing approach when transferring this client. Read all the options before you select the best one!*
4. *This is a correct action that helps provide for the nurse's and the client's safety. Supporting the upper portion of the client's body helps to place the weight of the client over the nurse's center of gravity. However, there is another option that better describes the best nursing approach in transferring this client. Read all the options before you select the best one!*

80. **A client, 35 years old, was admitted to the hospital for possible gall bladder surgery. Following a gall bladder x-ray, the doctor decided that a cholecystectomy was necessary. The nurse should include which of the following in preoperative teaching for the client?**

1. After this type of surgery, many clients are admitted to the intensive care unit.
2. Minor discomfort is expected in the operative site during the first few postoperative days.
3. Moving as little as possible will decrease the discomfort following this procedure.
4. A demonstration and return demonstration of coughing and deep breathing.

1. *Incorrect. Following cholecystectomy, clients usually return to the general nursing unit from the post anesthesia recovery room.*
2. *Incorrect. Following cholecystectomy, clients usually experience acute pain in the operative site for several days.*
3. *Moving as little as possible is contraindicated following surgery because it contributes to the complications associated with immobility. Clients are encouraged to turn, cough, deep breathe, and ambulate postoperatively to decrease the possibility of complications. Acute postoperative discomfort can be managed by giving medications as ordered.*
4. *Good choice! A demonstration and return demonstration of coughing and deep breathing will facilitate the client's ability to participate in her care postoperatively. Coughing and deep breathing helps prevent postoperative respiratory complications.*

81. **The nurse knows that lidocaine hydrochloride (Xylocaine) exerts its most important cardiac effect by which of the following?**

1. Depressing excessive automaticity of ectopic pacemakers in the His-Purkinje fibers.
2. Suppressing conduction velocity in the AV node and purkinje fibers.
3. Depressing myocardial contractility.
4. Suppressing the SA node impulses.

1. *Excellent! Lidocaine works directly in the bundle and in the Purkinje fibers, so it is used to treat ventricular arrhythmias.*
2. *No! Lidocaine is different from quinidine in that it has little effect on conduction time or refractory period in AV or Purkinje fibers. It suppresses automaticity, not velocity, in ventricular fibers.*
3. *No. Lidocaine does not depress contractility; it suppresses automaticity.*
4. *Incorrect! Lidocaine does not suppress the SA node and is not used to treat atrial arrhythmias.*

82. **Of the following information, which should be recorded first in the client's record by the nurse admitting the client?**

    1. The client's vital signs.
    2. The plan that was developed for the care of the client while in the hospital.
    3. Nursing actions performed for the client.
    4. Assessment of the client.

    1. *The client's vital signs should be recorded in the client's record in order to document that the nurse assessed the client's condition on admission. This is an appropriate nursing action and a possible answer, but not the best option. Read all the options before you select your answer!*
    2. *The plan of care should be documented but a plan cannot be developed until the nurse finds out more about the client. What should be recorded first?*
    3. *Nursing actions are documented as the plan of care is implemented. Since the case scenario tells you that the client is being admitted, the nursing process requires that the nurse gather data and develop a plan before implementing actions.*
    4. ***Excellent! The nurse should document assessment findings in order to provide information concerning the status of the client on admission.***

83. **A client is on the telemetry unit, and the monitor shows he is in ventricular fibrillation ("V-Fib"). Which of the following actions should be given priority by the nurse?**

    1. Prepare the client for cardioversion.
    2. Assess the client's responsiveness and begin CPR.
    3. Administer Lidocaine IV push.
    4. Obtain a permit for insertion of a permanent pacemaker.

    1. *Wrong! Cardioversion is used in atrial fibrillation to convert the client to normal sinus rhythm. Cardioversion is similar to defibrillation but uses less wattage, and is not an emergency procedure.*
    2. ***Good choice! Yes, the treatment protocol for V-Fib is to begin CPR until defibrillation is available.***
    3. *Not the best choice! This is done, but not until an IV line is established.*
    4. *This is not an emergency treatment for V-Fib, although it may be necessary if defibrillation does not convert the client to normal sinus rhythm.*

84. **A 21-year-old client has sustained a basal skull fracture. The nurse notices drainage from his right nostril. The priority nursing action is which of the following?**

    1. Notify his physician.
    2. Suction his nostril.
    3. Test the drainage for glucose.
    4. Ask the client to blow his nose.

    1. *Incorrect. The nurse must determine the source of drainage. The next action is to then notify the physician.*
    2. *Wrong. This is contraindicated if the drainage is cerebral spinal fluid, due to complications of meningitis.*
    3. ***Good choice! Positive glucose on a reagent strip signifies that the drainage is cerebrospinal fluid. This must then be reported to the physician.***
    4. *Incorrect. This is contraindicated because it may prolong closure of a dural tear and increase the risk of infection.*

85. **A confused elderly client continually grabs at the nurses from her wheelchair. Which of the following is the most appropriate nursing action?**

    1. Move the wheelchair to a location where she cannot grab people.
    2. Apply a chest restraint for her own safety.
    3. Use wrist restraints and move her to the visitor's room.
    4. Remove her hands and firmly tell her not to grab.

    1. *Incorrect choice! Moving her to another location away from people does not really deal with the problem of her grabbing at people. Isolating the client will increase agitation.*
    2. *Wrong choice! Applying a chest restraint increases a client's restlessness and agitation.*
    3. *Incorrect choice! The use of wrist restraints increases a confused irritated client's feelings of agitation.*
    4. ***Right choice! Setting limits by removing her hand and telling her not to grab at people is the most effective way of dealing with the behavior problem. This question requires the ability to plan nursing care for a elderly client with a specific problem.***

    STRATEGY ALERT! *Options 2 and 3 both use restraints. Similar options tend to be incorrect!*

86. **After several days of furosemide (Lasix) therapy, a client begins to complain of muscle weakness, drowsiness, abdominal cramping, and nausea. The nurse is aware that the most likely explanation for these symptoms is:**

    1. Hyponatremia.
    2. Hypokalemia.
    3. Metabolic alkalosis.
    4. Uremia.

    1. *Incorrect. Signs and symptoms of hyponatremia are muscle weakness and twitching, progressing to convulsions if unrelieved; alterations in level of consciousness; mental confusion; and anxiety.*
    2. ***Correct. Furosemide causes increased excretion***

of potassium in the urine. The symptoms that the client describes are typical of hypokalemia: muscle weakness, drowsiness, abdominal cramping, and nausea.

3. *No. Signs and symptoms of metabolic alkalosis include muscle weakness, irritability, confusion, muscle twitching, and shallow, slow respirations.*

4. *Wrong. Signs and symptoms of uremia are those of end-stage renal disease: hyperkalemia, hypertension, nausea/vomiting, pruritus, anemia.*

87.   On vaginal examination the presenting part was at station plus two. Which of the following is the proper interpretation by the nurse?

1. Presenting part is two centimeters above the level of the ischial spines.
2. Biparietal diameter is at the level of the ischial spines.
3. Presenting part is two centimeters below the level of the ischial spines.
4. Biparietal diameter is two centimeters above the ischial spines.

1. *No, station describes the level of the top of the presenting part to an imaginary line between the ischial spines. At the spines is documented as O station, a plus number indicates the number of centimeters below the spines, and a negative number the number of centimeters above the spines. This fetus is at plus two station.*

2. *Incorrect. The biparietal diameter (a diameter on the fetal head) is not used when determining fetal station.*

3. *Good job, this fetus is at plus two station or two centimeters below the ischial spines.*

4. *Incorrect. Biparietal diameter is not used to assess fetal station.*

88.   A client is very suspicious of the nursing staff and other clients. Her primary nurse would like to establish a therapeutic relationship with her. Which plan of care is the best for doing this:

1. Avoid pressuring the client by waiting for her to initiate interactions with the nurse.
2. Approach the client frequently during the day for brief interactions.
3. Set aside a specific time each day to spend with the client.
4. Approach the client in a friendly manner offering to disclose some personal information so she will feel she knows the nurse better.

1. *The nurse is not demonstrating trustworthiness by waiting for the client to initiate the interaction. This is not correct.*

2. *This approach might be effective, however, there is a better option.*

3. *To promote a therapeutic relationship, it is best to set aside a specific time for the nurse and client to meet together. It is also important that the nurse be consistent in order to earn the client's trust.*

4. *This approach is promoting a social relationship and is not appropriate if the nurse's goal is to form a therapeutic relationship.*

89.   The initial plan of care for a 10-year-old child admitted for orthopedic surgery who has a history of cerebral palsy should include strategies for which of the following?

1. Keeping a calm, quiet environment to prevent seizures.
2. Explaining all information to the child's parents, as the child is not able to understand.
3. Facilitating communication with the child by his/her usual means.
4. Obtaining IV access immediately, as children with cerebral palsy have difficulty drinking.

1. *Incorrect! Children with cerebral palsy often have associated seizure disorder and are treated with anti-seizure medications. Keeping a quiet environment is important in cases of meningitis in order to prevent seizures, but not in the case of cerebral palsy.*

2. *Incorrect! Children with cerebral palsy may have difficulty communicating because the muscles needed for speech are often affected. However, these children may have normal or even superior intelligence. They need to be properly prepared and treated as any other child in the hospital.*

3. **Correct! Children with cerebral palsy may have speech and communication difficulties because the muscles that control speech are often affected, as are the muscles needed for writing. However, they can understand what is going on and are fearful of the hospital experience, as are normal children, and need to be prepared for what is happening. They also need to be able to express their needs and fears in some way. A communication board or use of sign language may be helpful, depending on what the child uses at home.**

4. *Wrong choice! Children with cerebral palsy may have difficulty drinking because the oral muscles are often affected. The nurse needs to find out what best facilitates drinking for that particular child and employ those measures while in the hospital. No extra invasive measures need to be employed for this child than for any other child.*

90.   A client with a history of previous cesarean section asks the nurse whether she might be able to deliver vaginally this time. The nurse, in framing an answer, knows that a trial of labor for vaginal delivery after cesarean is more likely if the client's experience was:

1. First cesarean through a classic incision as a result of severe fetal distress.
2. First low transverse cesarean for breech position; this pregnancy fetus is in a vertex presentation.
3. First and second caesareans were for cephalopelvic disproportion.
4. First low transverse cesarean was for active herpes, type 2 infection; vaginal culture at 39 weeks this pregnancy was positive.

1. *No, because clients who have a classical (vertical) uterine incision into the uterus are at high risk for a uterine rupture and must be delivered by cesarean section in all future pregnancies.*
2. ***Correct! This type of client has no obstetrical indication for a cesarean section as she did with her first cesarean delivery.***
3. *No, because when the first two C-sections are done for cephalopelvic disproportion (CPD) the risk is very high that this fetus is also too big for safe vaginal delivery. A careful assessment of fetal weight may indicate a much smaller fetus, but this option does not give that information.*
4. *Incorrect. Whenever a client has active herpes type 2, a cesarean section is indicated to prevent transmission of herpes to the infant.*

91. **Which of the following electrolyte levels must be monitored most closely by the nurse while the client is taking chlorothiazide (Diuril)?**

    1. Calcium.
    2. Magnesium.
    3. Potassium.
    4. Sodium.

    1. *Wrong choice. Hypochloremia is seen in clients who are taking loop diuretics such as furosemide.*
    2. *Incorrect. Hypomagnesemia is a concern when the client is taking furosemide, a loop diuretic.*
    3. ***Yes! You remembered that the thiazide diuretics can cause potassium loss. Signs and symptoms of hypokalemia are fatigue, muscle weakness, leg cramps, restlessness, and confusion.***
    4. *No. Thiazides act to slightly inhibit sodium and water resorption; therefore, hyponatremia is not the major concern.*

92. **What should the nurse emphasize in developing the initial nursing care plan for a client with an acute schizophrenia?**

    1. Establishing a daily routine to promote orientation to the unit.
    2. Providing a variety of activities to keep the client focused on reality-based topics.
    3. Encouraging the client to enter into simple group activities.
    4. Assigning the same members of the nursing staff to work with the client each day.

1. *A daily routine is important to help the client become adjusted to the unit, but this is not the best option for the client with an acute schizophrenic illness.*
2. *Initially, too much activity would overwhelm the acutely ill client. This is not the correct option.*
3. *This is not correct because the acutely ill client will become too anxious in group situations to cope with the demands of the activity.*
4. ***Correct. Establishing trust is the primary initial goal for clients who are acutely ill with a schizophrenic disorder. This can best be achieved by assigning the same nursing staff members to work with the client each day.***

93. **After complaining of severe chest pain for the last hour, a client is admitted to MICU with acute myocardial infarction. The admitting nurse reviews the client's chart and notes that cardiac enzyme studies were done on admission. The nurse knows that the purpose of the studies were to evaluate which of the following?**

    1. The degree of damage to the myocardium.
    2. The location of the myocardial infarction.
    3. The size of the myocardial infarction.
    4. The coexistence of pulmonary congestion.

    1. ***Good choice! Cardiac enzyme studies are checked on admission, and then daily for several days, because their degree of elevation can reflect the degree of damage to the myocardium.***
    2. *Wrong. The location of the MI is determined by ECG findings.*
    3. *Incorrect, because the size of the infarct can be determined through a PET scan, a noninvasive method of assessment of the size of the infarct.*
    4. *Incorrect. This can be a complication of MI, however, enzyme studies do not reflect coexistence of pulmonary congestion.*

94. **Which nursing assessment would be a priority for postoperative care of a four-year-old following an appendectomy?**

    1. Vital signs every eight hours.
    2. Measure intake and output every eight hours.
    3. Auscultate the lungs every four hours.
    4. Check the extremities for phlebitis every four hours.

    1. *Incorrect! Postoperatively, vital signs should be checked every four hours, not every eight hours.*
    2. *Incorrect! Intake and output should be monitored, but it will not indicate the major complication following surgery, which is pneumonia.*
    3. ***Correct! Because of the child's anesthesia, decreased cough, and immature lungs, pneumonia***

is a major complication of an appendectomy. Auscultating the lungs will indicate adventitious breath sounds, which signify fluid collection in the lungs.

4. *Wrong choice! Phlebitis is an uncommon postoperative complication. Pneumonia is a more likely complication.*

95. **A client is being discharged following major abdominal surgery. Which of the following is most important for the nurse to include in the teaching plan since the client will be doing her own dressing changes at home?**

1. Appropriate opening of bandages to maintain their sterility.
2. Discussion of proper aseptic technique.
3. Proper gloving technique.
4. Discussion of good handwashing technique.

1. *Incorrect choice. The client is at risk for the transmission of microorganisms that may cause an infection. Very often the home environment does not lend itself to the practice of aseptic technique, and the nurse must help the client improvise with the resources available.*
2. *Incorrect. The client is at risk for the transmission of microorganisms that may cause an infection. Very often the home environment does not lend itself to the practice of aseptic technique, and the nurse must help the client improvise with the resources available.*
3. *Incorrect. The client is at risk for the transmission of microorganisms that may cause an infection. Very often the home environment does not lend itself to the practice of aseptic technique, and the nurse must help the client improvise with the resources available.*
4. *Correct! This is the most important and most basic technique in preventing and controlling the transmission of pathogens.*

96. **An 82-year-old widower is admitted to the psychiatric unit. His diagnosis is depression with agitation. A behavior the nurse would least likely expect to be associated with this diagnosis would be:**

1. Difficulty concentrating and memory loss.
2. Irritability and extreme annoyance with other people.
3. Jitteriness and hand wringing.
4. Sleeping 10 to 12 hours a day.

1. *Wrong. Difficulty concentrating and memory loss are common behaviors seen in a client who has an agitated depression. Many times these symptoms in an elderly client are mistaken for a beginning dementia. When the depression is treated, these cognitive problems return to normal.*

2. *Wrong choice! Extreme annoyance with others and irritability are common behaviors displayed by clients with agitated depressions.*
3. *Wrong. Jitteriness and hand wringing are common behaviors displayed by clients with agitated depressions. This cannot be the correct option.*
4. *Right! Clients with an agitated depression usually have great difficulty sleeping and suffer from insomnia. Excessive sleeping is a symptom of depression with psychomotor retardation but not psychomotor agitation.*

97. **A 48-year-old woman is accompanied by her 24-year-old daughter to the psychiatric hospital for an evaluation. The client explains that she has been unable to leave her house for the past 10 years without her husband or daughter. If she tries to go out alone, she becomes very anxious and must quickly return inside. The nurse interviewing her identifies the problem as most likely due to which of the following disorders?**

1. Conversion disorder.
2. Agoraphobia.
3. Panic disorder.
4. Obsessive-compulsive disorder.

1. *This is not correct. Conversion disorder is an anxiety disorder where the client has the physical symptoms suggesting a medical problem (such as blindness or paralysis) for which no organic pathology can be diagnosed.*
2. *Correct. Agoraphobia is the fear and subsequent avoidance of places or situations from which escape might be difficult. The most common form of this disorder is avoiding open public places, such as shopping malls, and fear of leaving one's home.*
3. *This is not correct. Panic disorder is characterized by recurrent panic attacks that are not associated with any specific stimulus or situation, but seem to occur spontaneously.*
4. *This is not correct. Obsessive-compulsive disorders are characterized by recurrent obsessional thoughts and/or ritual behaviors.*

98. **The nurse observes a 72-year-old client trying to climb over the side rails of the bed. The nurse obtains a vest restraint and is placing it on the client when the daughter arrives and says to the nurse, "My mother does not need to be tied down in bed. I've been caring for her for years, and she hasn't fallen out of bed yet." The best initial response by the nurse is which of the following statements?**

1. "I just saw your mother trying to climb over the side rails. Since I am concerned about her falling and hurting herself, I think this is best for her safety."
2. "Tell me how you managed to care for her at home."
3. "Hospital policy requires restraint vests on clients who are at risk for falling. I just saw your mother trying to climb over the rails. You don't want her to get hurt, do you?"
4. "The elderly may become confused in an unfamiliar place and do things they wouldn't do at home. It is difficult to see her restrained. While you are with her, the restraints can be off. Let me know when you are ready to leave."

1. *Wrong. The client's safety is the issue in this question. Since the daughter and nurse are with her, she is not in immediate danger. It is important to note that the client in this test question is the daughter, and the nurse should address the daughter's statement. This response focuses on safety and restraints, and not on the client's (the daughter's) concerns about her mother being tied down.*
2. *Wrong. This response does not focus on the issue in the question, which concerns the client's feelings about restraints being placed on her mother. This option may be appropriate later in the conversation, but is not the best initial response.*
3. *Wrong. This response implies that the daughter is not interested in her mother's safety and makes her defensive. It focuses on hospital policy and not the daughter's concerns.*
4. ***Excellent! This option focuses on the daughter's concerns and provides information and rationale for the restraints. It also provides for safety and offers a compromise to the daughter that addresses her concerns and gives her some control.***

99. **A mother arrives at the emergency room with her child, who is wet, and the color of his skin is blue. She shouts to the nurse, "I think that I have killed my son. I wasn't watching him like I should have and he fell in the pool." While the doctor and other nursing staff are providing care for the child, a nurse stays with the mother to obtain information. What is the most therapeutic response by the nurse?**

1. "These things happen. Don't blame yourself."
2. "You are right. A child should always be watched when he is playing near a pool."
3. "You didn't kill him. He is still alive. It is going to be all right."
4. "It must feel terrible to have something like this happen to your child."

1. *This response uses a communication block by utilizing a cliché when talking to the mother. It does not promote further effective communication from the client.*
2. *Wrong. This option implies that the mother was at fault by not supervising her child. It passes judgment and expresses the nurse's opinion about the situation. This is not a therapeutic response.*
3. *Not the best choice! The part of this option that makes it incorrect is the statement, "It is going to be all right." This statement offers false reassurance, which is never appropriate when fostering therapeutic communication.*
4. ***Very good. This option is an example of the nurse using empathy when responding to the client. This response lets the client know that the nurse is not blaming her for the accident and promotes further effective communication.***

100. **A client asks the nurse how the relaxation techniques will help his gastric pain. "Can't I just take the cimetidine (Tagamet) that my physician has prescribed?" In responding to his question, the nurse is guided by the knowledge that:**

1. Gastric ulcer is a stress-related illness, and his stress levels and emotional issues are contributing to the exacerbation of his symptoms.
2. He is in denial because he is refusing to acknowledge that stress is playing a role in the progress of his illness.
3. Gastric ulcer, and other psychosomatic illnesses, are caused by stress and can't be cured with only medical or surgical treatments.
4. The client is displaying the "typical ulcer personality" of a competitive, aggressive person who is defending against unresolved dependency needs.

1. ***Correct. The client's question indicates that he does not readily perceive the relationship between stress and the exacerbation of his ulcer. The nurse, guided by this knowledge, can formulate a response to help him better understand his illness.***
2. *This is not correct. The client's question does not necessarily indicate denial. The nurse could not know that he is refusing to acknowledge the role of stress in his illness without additional assessment data.*
3. *Wrong. Stress alone does not cause a psychosomatic illness. There are physiological factors that are more directly involved.*
4. *Wrong. Current research indicates that a "typical ulcer personality" does not exist. Therefore, this cannot be the correct option.*

NCLEX-RN

Test 4

|————————————————————————————|

0.1 mg/Kg/dose   0.2 mg/Kg/dose

NCLEX-RN TEST 4

1. **The nurse assists an asthmatic client with a face mask delivering humidified oxygen at 35%. The nurse knows that the effectiveness of this therapy is best demonstrated by:**

    1. Absence of adventitious breath sounds.
    2. PaO_2 of 92.
    3. Heart rate increase of 25 beats/min.
    4. Bicarbonate level of 25 mEq/liter.

2. **The nurse admitting a newly diagnosed obsessive-compulsive client understands that he is using which defense mechanism when he performs his rituals?**

    1. Introjection and fixation.
    2. Repression and projection.
    3. Displacement and undoing.
    4. Suppression and sublimation.

3. **A pale five-year-old with leukemia has been receiving chemotherapy. He is receiving total parenteral nutrition via a central line. Which nursing diagnosis has the highest priority for this child?**

    1. Activity intolerance.
    2. Potential for infection.
    3. Potential fluid volume deficit.
    4. Altered nutrition, less than body requirements.

4. **A six-month-old child is recovering from surgery. The child is crying and appears to be in pain. Morphine 1.9 mg, sc, every four hours p.r.n. is ordered. The child weighs seven kilograms. The medication manual states that morphine can be given 0.1 mg/kg/dose - 0.2 mg/kg/dose, up to a maximum of 15 mg/dose. The nurse's best response would be which of the following?**

    1. Discuss the dose with the physician because the dose is too high.
    2. Question giving morphine to a six-month-old infant.
    3. Give the morphine as ordered because the dose is within the safe range.
    4. Discuss the dose with the physician because the dose is too low.

5. **A client asks the nurse if he will feel a lot of pain during the a sigmoidoscopy. The best nursing response is:**

    1. "No, you should only feel a small amount of pain, since the area is anesthetized."
    2. "No, the test does not cause pain."
    3. "You will feel slightly uncomfortable and will have the urge to defecate when the instrument is inserted."
    4. "You will most likely experience little discomfort except for lying on the hard examination table."

6. **A client is in the hospital and he is dying. He is very weak, tired, and short of breath. The plan of care for the client and his family should include which of the following?**

    1. Limiting visiting hours to help conserve his energy.
    2. Have the client do as much as he can for himself to increase his self-esteem and independence.
    3. Encourage the family to spend as much time as possible with him and do whatever they feel comfortable with in caring for him.
    4. Plan all of his care to be done at one time so he can rest for long intervals.

7. **An elderly client is constantly putting her call light on. When the nurse answers the light, the client does not appear to need anything. The nurse would consider many interventions, but the least appropriate solution would be to:**

    1. Ask the members of the family if they can spend more time with the client.
    2. Remove the call light from easy reach of the client.
    3. Make frequent visits to the client's room.
    4. Spend more time in the client's room while charting.

8. **A 48-year-old man is hospitalized for an obsessive-compulsive disorder. He has recurring thoughts that he has mouth odors that are offensive to others. He also has mouth care rituals that occupy a good deal of his waking hours and caused him to be fired from his last job. The nurse understands that these symptoms most likely represent:**

    1. A method of reducing anxiety.
    2. A form of manipulation to avoid work.
    3. An attention-getting strategy.
    4. A rationalization for avoiding social contact.

9. **The nurse caring for a child with Tetralogy of Fallot notes that he is easily fatigued. The nurse**

understands that the etiology of the fatigue is:

1. Inadequate intake of high calorie foods and vitamins.
2. Poor muscular tone and development.
3. Oxygenation of tissues is inadequate to support energy metabolism.
4. Restricted blood flow leaving the heart.

10. A three-year-old girl is admitted for a myringotomy after being diagnosed with chronic otitis media. Following the surgery, the nurse prepares discharge teaching. Which statement by the parents indicates effective client teaching?

1. "Now my daughter will not have ear infections."
2. "I must keep her away from other children with colds."
3. "I will only call the doctor if she gets a fever."
4. "I will keep water out of her ears."

11. A client is admitted with a possible ectopic pregnancy. Which of the following best describes the clinical picture of a client experiencing a ruptured ectopic pregnancy?

1. Large amount of vaginal bleeding, tender abdomen, drop in BP at three to four weeks gestation.
2. Moderate to large amount of vaginal bleeding, abdominal pain and fainting spells at 10 to 12 weeks gestation.
3. Vague complaints of abdominal pain and severe nausea and vomiting at eight to 10 weeks gestation.
4. Small amounts of vaginal spotting, severe abdominal pain, signs and symptoms of shock at eight to 10 weeks gestation.

12. A client started methyldopa (Aldomet) to lower his blood pressure. The nurse must emphasize to the client the importance of keeping appointments for which of the following lab studies?

1. Renal function studies.
2. Blood cell counts and hepatic function studies.
3. Aldomet blood levels.
4. Cardiac enzymes.

13. A client is very upset about the loss of her baby. She is discharged and will be seen at regular intervals by the visiting nurse. At which of the following times would it be most appropriate for the nurse to begin teaching about future pregnancies?

1. The nurse should begin teaching during the first home visit.
2. When the client begins to ask questions about having another baby.
3. As soon as the nurse has developed a good relationship with the client.
4. Teaching should not begin for about six months.

14. A client is admitted to the hospital with congestive heart failure. He has been on bed rest at home and has been incontinent of urine. His wife has been caring for him, and there is a strong odor of urine when he is placed in the bed on the nursing unit. She tells the nurse that she is sorry and embarrassed about the unpleasant smell. The best nursing response is:

1. "It must be difficult to care for someone who is confined to bed. How have you been able to manage?"
2. "Don't worry about it. He will get a bath, and that will take care of the odor."
3. "A lot of clients that are cared for at home have the same problem."
4. "When was the last time that he had a bath?"

15. Which of the following would the nurse expect to be commonly used to manage alcohol withdrawal?

1. Antipsychotic drugs.
2. Barbiturates.
3. Anti-anxiety agents.
4. Anticonvulsants.

16. A client is taking acetaminophen (Tylenol) for muscular aches and pains. She reports to the nurse that she is lonely and has been drinking heavily in the evenings. What drug interaction should the nurse discuss with the client?

1. Alcohol and Tylenol may result in a diuretic effect, depleting fluid volume and electrolytes.
2. Sodium and fluid retention may result from this combination.
3. Alcoholic beverages increase the risk of liver toxicity when taken with Tylenol, so the combination should be avoided.
4. This combination has an increased potential for causing palpitations.

17. CPR has been initiated on a client in the emergency room. The nurse understands that which of the following would indicate effective cardiac compressions?

1. An EKG pattern with each compression.
2. Compression depth of one and one-half to two inches.
3. A palpable femoral pulse during each compression.
4. Pupils changing from pinpoint to dilated.

18. Upon returning from the recovery room, the fluid in the chest tube bottle has stopped fluctuating. The nurse most appropriately interprets this assessment to indicate which of the following?

    1. All the fluid and air has been removed.
    2. The tubing may be kinked.
    3. The lungs have re-expanded.
    4. The suction is set too low.

19. An 18-year-old client admitted with ulcerative colitis is being treated with sulfasalazine (Azulfidine). The nurse explains to the client that the major action of Azulfidine is to:

    1. Suppress inflammation of the bowel wall.
    2. Reduce peristaltic activity.
    3. Neutralize gastrointestinal tract acidity.
    4. Prevent a secondary infection.

20. A client takes ibuprofen (Motrin) for her arthritis. How should the nurse advise her to take the medication to reduce the complication of esophageal irritation?

    1. Don't take with meals.
    2. Take with a full glass of water and remain upright for 15-30 minutes afterwards.
    3. Take before meals with a snack.
    4. Take after meals; then lie down for an hour.

21. A client is admitted with acute leukemia. The nurse can anticipate that the client will report which of the following clusters of symptoms?

    1. Nausea/vomiting, diarrhea.
    2. Fatigue, weakness.
    3. Fever, chills.
    4. Nosebleed, headache.

22. An anorexic client tells the nurse that she thinks too much fuss is being made about what she eats. "I have plenty of energy and get all A's in school. I do not think I am too thin. Look, my hips are fat." What is the most appropriate nursing response to her statement?

    1. "You say your hips look fat to you, but you seem very thin to me."
    2. "Let's go over to the mirror so you can see how thin you really are."
    3. "You are such a bright girl. I don't understand how you can do this to yourself."
    4. "You would be much more attractive if you were not so skinny."

23. A client's blood pressure rises to 200/120, which is considered a hypertensive emergency. Diazoxide (Hyperstat) is administered. When should the expected response be noticeable to the nurse?

    1. Between one and five minutes of administration.
    2. Within one hour of administration.
    3. After the second dose.
    4. After the first few doses.

24. The nurse is interviewing the mother of a four-year-old at a well child clinic. Which finding would concern the nurse the most?

    1. His speech is intelligible 80% of the time.
    2. He is fearful about being examined.
    3. He occasionally stutters when he speaks.
    4. He has an imaginary playmate named "Red."

25. A client diagnosed with AIDS is placed on zidovudine (formerly AZT). The nurse monitors the client for which life-threatening side effect of this drug?

    1. Fever.
    2. Aplastic anemia.
    3. Renal failure.
    4. Cardiac dysrhythmia.

26. While caring for a client during treatment of pregnancy induced hypertension, which of the following parameters would most concern the nurse?

    1. Respiratory rate of 22.
    2. Complaint of a mild headache.
    3. Urine output of 80 mL in four hours.
    4. Deep tendon reflexes of plus two.

27. The client tells the nurse that he does not know how he is ever going to stay on the low cholesterol diet that his doctor ordered after his heart attack. The best response by the nurse is:

    1. "If you don't follow the diet, you will probably have another heart attack, which could kill you."
    2. "What is it about the low cholesterol diet that seems to be a problem for you?"
    3. "I've been on that same diet for the last five years, and I'm sure you will learn how to change your eating habits after a while."
    4. "I will have the dietitian talk to you before you are discharged. She's the expert, and she can be really helpful."

28. A client is 85 years old. Which of the following assessment findings by the nurse should be re-

ported to the physician?

1. The client is unable to discriminate between hot and cold sensations below the knee of his left extremity.
2. The client walks into the furniture that is in his room.
3. The client does not respond with appropriate answers to the questions asked by the nurse.
4. The client refuses to remove his clothing.

29. **A client, age 26, has been diagnosed with AIDS and is currently hospitalized for treatment of Pneumocystis carinii pneumonia. Which of the following symptoms would the nurse least expect to observe in a client with this type of pneumonia?**

1. Hemoptysis
2. Fever
3. General malaise
4. Dyspnea

30. **A client is admitted to the hospital with congestive heart failure and the physician orders stat blood work. The laboratory technician says to the nurse, "I can't do the stat blood work because the client doesn't have an identification bracelet on." The best nursing action would be which of the following?**

1. Since the nurse knows the client, draw the blood for the laboratory technician.
2. Assure the laboratory technician that the nurse can verify that he has the correct client.
3. Obtain an identification bracelet for the client as quickly as possible.
4. Ask the client to identify himself to the laboratory technician.

31. **The nurse working in a community health clinic knows which of the following statements about suicide is most accurate?**

1. Suicide rates increase dramatically during natural catastrophes such as earthquakes or floods, or in times of natural uprisings such as strikes or riots.
2. Suicide is the leading cause of death in the 15- to 19-year-old age group.
3. Suicide attempts are preceded by a visit to a physician or primary care provider in a significant number of cases.
4. The majority of people who commit suicide are psychotic.

32. **A client who has right-sided paralysis following a stroke is not able to talk, but can make gestures to make himself understood. To effectively**

communicate with the client, the nurse should do which of the following?

1. Speak very loudly to the client.
2. Speak quickly to the client, since his attention span may be short.
3. Use gestures while speaking slowly.
4. Wait until the family comes in, so they can interpret his behavior.

33. **The nurse is talking with the mother of a six-year-old child. Which statement by the mother would concern the nurse most?**

1. "His teacher says he's been squinting to see the blackboard."
2. "He has lost both of his top teeth."
3. "He cheats when we play Candyland."
4. "He acts bossy sometimes."

34. **A client is diagnosed as hypertensive and prescribed hydralazine (Apresoline). What statement would indicate to the nurse that the client understands the action of his medication?**

1. "I will eat plenty of foods high in sodium to keep my fluid level up."
2. "I will limit my fluid intake."
3. "I realize that I need to get up more slowly than before."
4. "I will always remember to take this medication on an empty stomach."

35. **In assessing postoperative clients for signs and symptoms of early hypovolemic shock, the nurse notes that an initial observation would most likely be:**

1. Thirst.
2. Warm, flushed skin.
3. Irritability.
4. Bradycardia.

36. **An unconscious client is to have an electroencephalogram (EEG). The first nursing action is which of the following?**

1. Notify the EEG Department that the client is ready for the scan.
2. Check to see that the client is wearing an identification bracelet.
3. Shampoo the client's hair.
4. Prepare a sedative in case the client becomes conscious prior to the procedure.

37. **A trauma client, admitted through the Emergency Room, has a urinary catheter inserted to monitor kidney function and assess for early signs**

of shock. The nurse would report which urinary output measurements as suggestive of cardiac failure or hypovolemia?

1. 20 mL/hour.
2. 35 mL/hour.
3. 40 mL/hour.
4. 50 mL/hour.

38. A client is scheduled for abdominal surgery, and the nurse is demonstrating deep breathing and coughing exercises. Which of the following information about the client indicates to the nurse that the client may not be ready to learn?

1. The client gives a return demonstration of deep breathing to the nurse.
2. The client is experiencing severe pain.
3. The client asks the nurse how often deep breathing is done after surgery.
4. The client tells the nurse that this exercise will probably be painful after surgery.

39. During the administration of a medication, a nineteen-year-old client tells the nurse that he has never had that particular pill before. The best nursing action is which of the following?

1. Check the client's identification bracelet again.
2. Check the physician's orders to see if this is a new medication.
3. Assure the client that the medication package has his name on it.
4. Ask the client to take the medication, since the identification bracelet and medication administration record indicate the client is to receive the medication.

40. A client is six days post-craniotomy for removal of an intracerebral aneurysm and has been transferred from the ICU to the surgical unit. The nurse suspects he may be developing increased intracranial pressure when the client says which of the following?

1. He would like to go home.
2. He feels nauseated.
3. He has a slight headache.
4. He is extremely sleepy.

41. A high school student speaks to the school nurse about a friend who is abusing cocaine. He wants to know what is the best way to influence his friend to stop. The best nursing response is based on what knowledge about cocaine?

1. Cocaine use rarely interferes with academic or career activities.
2. Cocaine abuse is difficult to treat because of its

abstinence syndrome.
3. Cocaine does more psychological harm than physical damage.
4. Cocaine use is highly reinforcing.

42. The emergency room nurse is concerned that an 18-month-old child's home situation may include child abuse. Which action by the nurse is most appropriate?

1. Notify the physician.
2. Admit the child to the pediatric unit.
3. Remove the mother from the child's room.
4. Report the suspected abuse.

43. A four-year-old client is seen at the clinic and is to receive an injection. When preparing to administer a medication for injection from an ampule, the nurse should avoid performing which action?

1. Score the neck of the ampule with a file.
2. Protect the thumb and fingers with a gauze square or alcohol wipe.
3. Snap the neck of the ampule toward the body when breaking the top free from the ampule.
4. Insert the needle into the ampule without touching the needle to the edges of the ampule.

44. A gravid client is admitted to the hospital at 38 weeks with a large amount of bright red vaginal bleeding. A diagnosis of partial abruptio placenta is made. She is on the fetal monitor and the nurse assesses her as follows: FH 138 regular, BP 98/52, pulse 118, respirations 24, temperature 97.6° F. Assuming all of the following are ordered by the physician, which should be the nurse's first priority?

1. Abdominal prep.
2. Insert a Foley catheter.
3. Sign informed consent for surgery.
4. Start an IV.

45. A client returns from surgery for a lung resection due to cancer. Of the following postoperative orders, which should receive highest priority?

1. Oxygen per mask at six liters per minute.
2. Change dressings as needed.
3. Vital signs every hour.
4. Cough and deep breathe every two hours.

46. The nurse administering aspirin knows that it is prescribed to reduce the risk of TIA's and strokes, because of its ability to inhibit which of the following?

1. Prostaglandins.
2. Platelet aggregation.
3. Leukocyte migration.
4. Lysosomal enzymes.

47. The nurse requests to be assigned to stay with an elderly client when she returns to the unit after her surgery. Preoperatively, the client had been disoriented to time and place. What is the most likely rationale for this request?

    1. The elderly client requires close postoperative supervision because of her unpredictable preoperative behavior.
    2. The elderly client will most likely be agitated when she regains consciousness after surgery.
    3. The many stresses associated with surgery could lead to further cognitive impairment in this elderly client.
    4. Elderly clients are particularly vulnerable to the development of postoperative complications.

48. A 54-year-old client is hospitalized with congestive heart failure and is to receive an x-ray. The nurse enters the client's room and asks the client if she is ready to go to x-ray. The client nods her head "yes." The initial nursing action is which of the following?

    1. Explain the x-ray procedure to the client.
    2. Help the client into a wheelchair, so that she will be ready when the transporter arrives to take her to x-ray.
    3. Ask the client if she has any questions.
    4. Look at the client's identification bracelet.

49. A client scheduled for surgery asks the nurse if she can put on some makeup before going to surgery. Which of the following would be the best response by the nurse?

    1. "Only a light application of makeup is allowed."
    2. "Hospital policy states that all makeup must be removed before surgery."
    3. "I will check with the charge nurse to find out the regulations."
    4. "Makeup will interfere with the ability to see your skin color during surgery."

50. While performing a vaginal exam, the nurse notes a glistening white cord hanging from the vagina. Which of the following would be the first nursing action?
    1. Return to the nurses' station to place an emergency call to the physician.
    2. Start oxygen at 6 to ten liters, and assess the client's vital signs.
    3. Cover the cord with a sterile moist saline dressing.
    4. Apply manual pressure on the presenting part and have the mother get into a knee-chest position.

51. An elderly client with Alzheimer's disease is admitted to the hospital. His daughter says to the nurse, "I really feel guilty about leaving my father, but I need to go home." Which of the following is the most therapeutic response by the nurse?

    1. "Your father is well cared for here."
    2. "Your worried feelings are normal."
    3. "When you are getting ready to leave, tell me. I will sit with your father."
    4. "Can I call another family member to stay with him?"

52. A client is admitted to the hospital with a compound fracture. While making the client's bed, the nurse finds a capsule of medication in the sheets. It would be least appropriate for the nurse to:

    1. Administer the medication to the client.
    2. Notify the physician of the missed dose.
    3. Determine what medication the capsule contains.
    4. Document the incident in the nurse's notes.

53. A client is in the hospital and has weakness on her left side because of a stroke. She becomes upset when eating because liquids drool out of her mouth on her weak side. What nursing intervention would be most appropriate?

    1. Provide only pureed and solid foods to prevent drooling and to prevent the client from becoming upset.
    2. Have a member of the family assist with the client's feedings.
    3. Teach the client how to drink fluids on the unaffected side to prevent drooling.
    4. Have the client use a syringe to squirt liquids into the back of her mouth.

54. A client is instructed by the nurse to recognize beginning signs of lithium toxicity. Which of the following signs of lithium toxicity does the nurse include in this teaching?

    1. Nystagmus, irregular tremor, decreased urine output.
    2. Tinnitus, blurred vision, slurred speech.
    3. Incoordination, muscle twitching, severe diarrhea.
    4. Mild ataxia, coarse hand tremors, difficulty concentrating.

55. A 14-year-old with muscular dystrophy is noted to spend a lot of time in his room by himself. He sleeps late and has been noted to give his personal belongings away. The best intervention by the nurse would be to say:

1. "You still have a lot to live for!"
2. "You seem rather sad lately."
3. "Come play Nintendo with another client in the activities room."
4. "Perhaps I should leave you alone for a while."

56. **An elderly client is on strict bed rest. While making an occupied bed for this client, which of the following actions should be taken by the nurse to maintain proper body mechanics?**

    1. Place the bed in semi-Fowler's position.
    2. Place the bed in a low horizontal position.
    3. Ask the client to move to the foot of the bed.
    4. Place the bed in a high horizontal position.

57. **A 72-year-old man has gouty arthritis. His physician prescribes naproxen (Naprosyn). The nurse understands that the geriatric implications for this drug include:**

    1. A higher incidence of agranulocytosis and aplastic anemia.
    2. A higher incidence of perforated peptic ulcers and/or bleeding.
    3. A higher incidence of central nervous system side effects.
    4. None, as all NSAIDs are relatively safe medications for any age group.

58. **A client is visually impaired from a childhood injury. When ambulating this visually impaired client, the most important nursing action is which of the following?**

    1. The nurse does not leave the client alone in an unfamiliar area.
    2. The nurse should stand on the client's non-dominant side.
    3. The nurse has the client use his dominant hand to reach out for barriers or landmarks.
    4. The nurse describes the route to be taken and removes any obstacles.

59. **A client is admitted to the ER for an acute asthmatic attack. Which of the following should be the initial intervention by the nurse?**

    1. Assist the client to a high Fowler's position.
    2. Offer oral fluids to loosen secretions.
    3. Monitor respiratory rate for changes.
    4. Reduce all unnecessary environmental stimuli.

60. **In planning postpartum nursing care for a client with cardiac disease, which of the following statements is inaccurate?**

    1. The client needs to be on strict intake and output to assess for a fluid overload.
    2. The client needs to be on a high residue diet to decrease the risk of constipation.
    3. The client needs to force fluids to prevent dehydration, which could result in cardiac irregularities.
    4. The client needs her vital signs taken more frequently than the standard routine.

61. **A client says to the nurse, "I am so frustrated with having five kids. My husband won't do anything to help keep me from getting pregnant." Which of the following should be the initial nursing action?**

    1. Refer the client and spouse to family planning services.
    2. Find out if she could use a contraceptive that would not involve her husband.
    3. Assess what the client means by "being frustrated."
    4. Ask the client if her husband is interested in birth control.

62. **A client has pneumonia and is being treated with erythromycin ethylsuccinate (E.E.S.) 400 mg p.o. every six hours. The nurse should observe the client for side effects of this drug, which include which of the following?**

    1. Hearing loss.
    2. Jaundice.
    3. Hypotension.
    4. Diarrhea.

63. **A postoperative client's knee dressing becomes completely saturated with blood one hour after returning to the clinical unit. Initially, the nurse should:**

    1. Reinforce the knee dressing.
    2. Apply a tourniquet around the closest artery.
    3. Apply direct pressure to the knee.
    4. Apply ice to the knee.

64. **The best approach for the nurse to take initially with a client who has severe anxiety is:**

    1. Move the person to a calm, non-stimulating environment.
    2. Encourage expression of feelings without attempting to modify defensive behavior.
    3. Lower the client's level of anxiety by offering medication.
    4. Suggest the client engage in some automatic behavior, such as pacing, to reduce his anxiety level.

65. **A client diagnosed with a frontal lobe mass is admitted following an MRI and is scheduled for a supratentorial craniotomy. Postoperatively, the nurse would correctly position the client in which**

of the following positions?

1. Dorsal recumbent.
2. Trendelenburg.
3. Semi-Fowler's.
4. Prone.

66. A 70-year-old man with a severe systemic infection is being treated with a 10-day course of gentamicin sulfate (Garamycin). What important assessments should the nurse make during this treatment?

    1. Assess for visual disturbances and seizures.
    2. Check IV site after three days.
    3. There are few complications with Garamycin and relatively minor assessments for the nurse to make.
    4. Monitor for dizziness or buzzing in ears.

67. Which of the following interventions would be most important for the nurse to include in the plan of care for a client with hepatitis B?

    1. Bedrest with bathroom privileges.
    2. High calorie, high protein diet.
    3. Force fluids to 3,000 mL in 24 hours.
    4. Medicate for pain every three to four hours as needed.

68. During a client's postoperative recovery from an ileostomy, the nurse begins teaching her stoma care. She refuses to look at her ostomy and states "I'd rather be dead than have to live with this all my life." The most therapeutic nursing response is to say?

    1. "I can't imagine what you must be feeling like; it must be awful."
    2. "I'll call your physician and see if something can be ordered to help you to relax."
    3. "There's no reason to feel like that, things will get better."
    4. "You appear upset, would you like to talk?"

69. A client is awake at 1:00 a.m. He is irritable and tells the nurse that the staff is making too much noise and that he hasn't had a decent night's sleep since his wife died a year ago. He asks the nurse to get him a cup of hot tea to help him relax and quench his thirst. Which of the following is the best nursing intervention?

    1. Get the client the cup of hot tea that he requested.
    2. Close the door to eliminate noise from the hallway.
    3. Use techniques that promote relaxation and suggest a warm glass of milk for the client.
    4. Tell the client that he should try to get some exercise so that he will be tired enough to sleep at night.

70. The most important nursing goal for a client who is admitted with an acute exacerbation of ulcerative colitis is which of the following?

    1. To provide emotional support.
    2. To prevent skin breakdown.
    3. To maintain fluid and electrolyte balance.
    4. To promote physical rest.

71. A 34-year-old client who weighs 288 pounds says to the nurse, "I'm going to have surgery and have my stomach stapled in order to lose weight. I've tried everything else, and nothing seems to work." Which of the following is the most therapeutic response by the nurse?

    1. "That's a pretty drastic measure. Are you sure that is what you want to do?"
    2. "I hear that the surgery is only a temporary measure, and if you have the staples removed you will only gain the weight back again."
    3. "It must be difficult to be overweight and not able to lose weight. What does your husband think about the surgery?"
    4. "Can you tell me about the possible consequences and side effects of this type of surgery?"

72. When orienting a severely depressed client to the unit, which of the following approaches by the nurse would be best?

    1. Introduce the client to the others on the unit and staff members.
    2. Tour the unit and introduce her to everyone they meet on the way.
    3. Explain the unit policies and answer any questions she may have.
    4. Accompany the client to her room and stay with her while she unpacks, offering only minimal information.

73. A 30-month-old male is being admitted with asthma. The nurse will discuss with the parents the emotional impact of hospitalization for their child. Which of the following actions will best minimize the stress of hospitalization for this client?

    1. Explain procedures and routines.
    2. Encourage contact with children of the same age.
    3. Provide for privacy.
    4. Encourage rooming-in.

74. When inserting a nasogastric tube in a comatose client for tube feedings, the nurse needs to avoid:

    1. Measuring the amount of the tube to be inserted.
    2. Lubricating the distal portion of the tube.
    3. Tilting the client's head back when inserting the

tube.
4. Checking placement of the tube.

75. **A 26-year-old man is seen in the clinic for a dermatological problem. The nurse is to apply topical ointment to the client's skin. Which of the following actions should be avoided?**

1. Massaging the ointment into the skin.
2. Removing excess ointment.
3. Applying ointment with ungloved fingertips.
4. Documenting a description of the skin prior to application of the ointment.

76. **Prior to a paracentesis for a client with cirrhosis and ascites, the nurse should encourage the client to do which of the following?**

1. Drink two liters of water.
2. Empty his bladder.
3. Cleanse the abdominal area thoroughly.
4. Eat a meal high in sodium.

77. **A child is born with a Simian crease and other characteristics of Down's syndrome. The diagnosis of Down's syndrome is confirmed. Which nursing intervention may be most beneficial to the family at this time?**

1. Seeking information from the family about prenatal care received.
2. Discussing positive aspects of foster care for the baby.
3. Assessing the baby's developmental level.
4. Encouraging family members to express concerns about the baby.

78. **A client is admitted with esophageal varices. The most appropriate intervention that will decrease the risk of esophageal bleeding is which of the following?**

1. Apply an ice collar.
2. Maintain semi-Fowler's position.
3. Administer stool softeners.
4. Provide a diet high in Vitamin D.

79. **The nurse is concerned about a depressed client's weight loss and continued refusal to eat. Which one of the following approaches to this problem by the nurse would be least appropriate?**

1. Encourage small, frequent meals to help increase caloric intake.
2. Offer highly nutritious foods that are easy to chew and nutritional supplements that require little effort to eat.
3. Determine what foods the client likes and make

them available at meals or for snacks.
4. Remind her she will become ill if she does not eat.

80. **In evaluating a mother's adaptation to motherhood, which of the following behaviors would the nurse expect to see in the "taking in" phase?**

1. Anxiety because the baby is not nursing well.
2. Eager to return the bath demonstration you gave to her yesterday.
3. Upset because her lunch is late.
4. Confident in her ability to nurse the baby without difficulty.

81. **When attempting to obtain information from a hearing impaired client, the nurse should do which of the following?**

1. Face the client and speak slowly.
2. Speak frequently and exaggerate lip movements.
3. Speak loudly.
4. Speak directly into the impaired ear.

82. **A 22-year-old client sustained a T4 spinal cord injury. While doing morning assessments four weeks post-injury, the nurse discovers his BP is 280/140 and he is complaining of nasal stuffiness and a severe, pounding headache. The first nursing action is which of the following?**

1. Sit the client upright.
2. Call the physician.
3. Check the client's bladder for distension.
4. Administer the prescribed antihypertensive.

83. **A client has been taking her iron for two weeks but is still complaining of fatigue from her anemia. What is the best response by the nurse, assuming that the client is taking her medication properly?**

1. "Perhaps you should go to bed earlier."
2. "This is really unusual, I'll tell your doctor."
3. "I guess your anemia must be really bad."
4. "It will take one to two months for your hemoglobin level to get back to normal, so keep taking your iron tablets."

84. **A client awaits surgery to remove an obstruction in his small intestine. The nurse notices his vomitus contains fecal material. Which of the following actions should the nurse do immediately?**

1. Provide frequent mouth cleansing.
2. Notify the physician.
3. Check his bowel sounds.
4. Administer a prescribed antiemetic.

85. When obtaining a urine specimen for a culture and sensitivity from an indwelling catheter, the nurse should:

    1. Empty the drainage bag from the urometer port.
    2. Wear sterile gloves.
    3. Cleanse the entry site prior to inserting the needle.
    4. Drain the bag and wait for a fresh urine sample to send from the drainage bag.

86. When assessing a client in the oliguric-anuric stage of acute renal failure, the nurse notices a respiratory rate of 28, and the client complains of nausea, a dull headache, and general malaise. The priority nursing action should be?

    1. Notify the physician.
    2. Check the chart for her latest electrolyte values.
    3. Administer an analgesic and an antiemetic.
    4. Provide O_2 at two liters, by nasal cannula.

87. A three-year-old is being admitted with nephrotic syndrome. The best roommate for this client is:

    1. A 16-year-old postoperative from removal of a ruptured appendix.
    2. An eight-year-old with leukemia.
    3. Another toddler with rheumatic fever.
    4. No roommate, isolation is required.

88. Second and third degree burns of the head, neck and chest place the client initially at greatest risk for which of the following?

    1. Infection.
    2. Airway obstruction.
    3. Fluid imbalance.
    4. Paralytic ileus.

89. A client, admitted with salicylate intoxication, has arterial blood gases drawn with the following results: pH 7.50, $PaCO_2$ 32, HCO_3 24. This client's blood gas values indicate which of the following acid-base disturbances?

    1. Metabolic alkalosis
    2. Respiratory alkalosis
    3. Metabolic acidosis
    4. Respiratory acidosis

90. On the day of delivery a client is assisted out of bed for the first time. She becomes frightened when she passes a blood clot and notices an increase in her lochia. Which of the following should the nurse include in her explanation?

    1. The lochia pools in the vagina when lying in bed.
    2. Placental fragments have probably been retained in the uterus.
    3. She probably has a uterine or urinary tract infection.
    4. The amount of lochia will increase during the postpartum period.

91. A four-year-old child is admitted to the hospital with periorbital cellulitis. The child weighs 15 kg and the physician orders cefazolin (Kefzol) 600 mg IV every eight hours. The medication manual states that Kefzol can be given 50-100 mg/kg/24 hours. The nurse's best response would be which of the following statements?

    1. Discuss the dose with the physician because the dose is too high.
    2. Question giving Kefzol to treat periorbital cellulitis.
    3. Give the Kefzol as ordered because the dose is in the safe range.
    4. Discuss the dose with the physician because it is too low.

92. A client, age 36, is diagnosed with active tuberculosis. He and his family have many questions for the nurse. They ask, "How did this happen? What can we do to prevent this? What will happen next?" Which of the following statements would be the best response by the nurse?

    1. "The tuberculosis was probably contracted from someone else with TB."
    2. "You need not be concerned, TB is very curable."
    3. "Tuberculosis can be treated at home with medications."
    4. "You seem very worried about tuberculosis. What concerns you most?"

93. The nurse understands that clients who are diagnosed with agoraphobia display which of the following defense mechanisms?

    1. Denial.
    2. Isolation.
    3. Displacement.
    4. Undoing.

94. A client is referred to a high risk prenatal clinic by a midwife. She thinks she is about three months pregnant but is to be examined for the presence of hydatidiform mole. The nurse expects which of the following symptoms to be present if she has a hydatidiform mole?

    1. Seizure activity.
    2. Periods of amnesia.
    3. Rapidly enlarging uterus.
    4. Painful uterine contractions.

95. An eight-year-old child complains of a stomachache while visiting the school nurse. Which statement by the child would concern the nurse most?

    1. "My stomachache goes away if I rest for a few minutes."
    2. "My friends are picking on me and calling me fatso."
    3. "My brother just had his appendix out."
    4. "My friends won't let me play kickball with them the way I want to."

96. A client, 42 years old, is admitted to the psychiatric hospital for the third time with a diagnosis of schizophrenic disorder, paranoid type. During her admission interview, she tells the nurse, "I'm in the hospital because they told lies about me. They are trying to poison my food." This comment is an example of which of the following?

    1. A grandiose delusion.
    2. An illusion.
    3. An auditory hallucination.
    4. A persecutory delusion.

97. A nursing mother asks the nurse how she will know if the baby is getting enough milk. The nurse tells the client that the best way to evaluate adequate intake for the newborn is by which of the following methods?

    1. Fit of his clothes.
    2. Amount of crying he does.

    3. Number of wet diapers.
    4. Number of hours he sleeps after each feeding.

98. A client, age 25, comes to the health clinic for the results of her HIV testing. When the nurse tells her that the results are negative, the client states, "Thank God that I don't have AIDS!" What would be the nurse's most appropriate response?

    1. "Yes, that is good news. You have not been infected with the virus this time. Please be careful in the future."
    2. "You are fortunate that you have immunity to the AIDS virus—some people are not so lucky."
    3. "The results mean that antibodies to the virus are not present at this time. Use the safe sex guidelines and consider retesting in three months."
    4. "This test result indicates that you don't have AIDS now, but the disease may be dormant and become active up to 10 years from now."

99. A nurse working with a client with agoraphobia recognizes that the most effective technique for treatment of agoraphobia is:

    1. Continual exposure to situations that she fears.
    2. Distraction each time she brings up her problem.
    3. Teaching relaxation techniques.
    4. Gradual desensitization by controlled exposure to the situation she fears.

100. Which of the following interventions would the nurse anticipate using, following a Shirodkar procedure at 14 weeks of gestation?

    1. Administration of betamethasone.
    2. Nonstress testing.
    3. Administration of tocolytic drugs.
    4. Administration of oxytocic drugs.

NOTES

NCLEX-RN

Test 4

Questions with Rationales

NCLEX-RN TEST 4 WITH RATIONALES

1. **The nurse assists an asthmatic client with a face mask delivering humidified oxygen at 35%. The nurse knows that the effectiveness of this therapy is best demonstrated by:**

    1. Absence of adventitious breath sounds.
    2. PaO$_2$ of 92.
    3. Heart rate increase of 25 beats/min.
    4. Bicarbonate level of 25 mEq/liter.

    1. *Not the best indicator of oxygen therapy treatment. The absence of adventitious sounds means that crackles and wheezing are not audible, but does not tell you if there is adequate gas exchange.*
    2. ***Tremendous, you selected correctly. The goal of oxygen therapy is achievement of a PaO$_2$ above 80 and no signs or symptoms of oxygen toxicity.***
    3. *No, the opposite should occur if the oxygen is effective. The myocardial workload should be decreased, allowing for a slowing of the heart rate.*
    4. *Incorrect. The value given is a normal bicarbonate, but is not an indicator of the client's response to oxygen therapy. This value is used to detect acid-base deviations.*

2. **The nurse admitting a newly diagnosed obsessive-compulsive client understands that he is using which defense mechanism when he performs his rituals?**

    1. Introjection and fixation.
    2. Repression and projection.
    3. Displacement and undoing.
    4. Suppression and sublimation.

    1. *Wrong! Fixation is becoming arrested at a particular stage of emotional development, while introjection is internalizing another's qualities or values.*
    2. *Wrong! Repression is involuntarily forgetting an unacceptable or painful thought or impulse, and projection is attributing one's own unacceptable thoughts or feelings to another.*
    3. ***Great job! The rituals are a form of undoing to reverse or negate unacceptable impulses that have been displaced onto the behavior.***
    4. *This is not correct. Suppression is consciously excluding thoughts from one's awareness, and sublimation is diverting unacceptable impulses into socially acceptable channels.*

3. **A pale five-year-old with leukemia has been receiving chemotherapy. He is receiving total parenteral nutrition via a central line. Which nursing diagnosis has the highest priority for this child?**

    1. Activity intolerance.
    2. Potential for infection.
    3. Potential fluid volume deficit.
    4. Altered nutrition, less than body requirements.

    1. *Try again. Chemotherapy does cause bone marrow suppression, so these children are usually anemic. They would naturally be tired. This is definitely a concern, but not the priority at this time.*
    2. ***Yes. This is the main concern. Children with leukemia are often leukopenic, and receiving chemotherapy increases this risk because of the bone marrow suppression. Receiving total parenteral nutrition, which has a high sugar content, via a central line doubles the risk for infection.***
    3. *No. Having IV access cuts down the risk for fluid volume deficit considerably, because there is a way to maintain hydration even if the child refuses to drink.*
    4. *No. Nutrition is a major concern with cancer clients, especially those receiving chemotherapy. The total parenteral nutrition should help with this problem. It is an important concern, but not as important as the risk of infection.*

4. **A six-month-old child is recovering from surgery. The child is crying and appears to be in pain. Morphine 1.9 mg, sc, every four hours p.r.n. is ordered. The child weighs seven kilograms. The medication manual states that morphine can be given 0.1 mg/kg/dose - 0.2 mg/kg/dose, up to a maximum of 15 mg/dose. The nurse's best response would be which of the following?**

    1. Discuss the dose with the physician because the dose is too high.
    2. Question giving morphine to a six-month-old infant.
    3. Give the morphine as ordered because the dose is within the safe range.
    4. Discuss the dose with the physician because the dose is too low.

    1. ***This is correct. In order to see if the dose falls within the safe range, multiply each end of the range by the child's weight to see the safe range for that child.***
    7 kg x 0.1 mg/kg/dose = 0.7 mg/dose.
    7 kg x 0.2 mg/kg/dose = 1.4 mg/dose.
    The ordered dose is 1.9 mg, which is higher than the safe range and must be questioned.
    2. *No. Infants need pain relief like other children and adults. Morphine that is given presents no greater risk than for other children and adults, if given in the safe range.*

3. *No. The nurse should not give this dose because it is too high and could cause respiratory depression, among other side effects.*

4. *Wrong! The dose is too high, not too low. Try the math again.*

5. **A client asks the nurse if he will feel a lot of pain during the a sigmoidoscopy. The best nursing response is:**

    1. "No, you should only feel a small amount of pain, since the area is anesthetized."
    2. "No, the test does not cause pain."
    3. "You will feel slightly uncomfortable and will have the urge to defecate when the instrument is inserted."
    4. "You will most likely experience little discomfort except for lying on the hard examination table."

    1. *This is an incorrect response because the area is not anesthetized and the pain felt during a sigmoidoscopy is not accurately described.*
    2. *This is incorrect. A sigmoidoscopy does cause pain.*
    3. ***Correct! This accurately describes the sensations the client will experience during the procedure.***
    4. *Incorrect. This describes what a client would experience during an upper GI series.*

6. **A client is in the hospital and he is dying. He is very weak, tired, and short of breath. The plan of care for the client and his family should include which of the following?**

    1. Limiting visiting hours to help conserve his energy.
    2. Have the client do as much as he can for himself to increase his self-esteem and independence.
    3. Encourage the family to spend as much time as possible with him and do whatever they feel comfortable with in caring for him.
    4. Plan all of his care to be done at one time so he can rest for long intervals.

    1. *Wrong! The question tells you that the client is dying. Limiting visiting hours serves no purpose and denies the client, family and friends time together that cannot be given at a later time.*
    2. *Wrong choice! The client is weak and short of breath. Self-care activities will increase oxygen needs and cause more physiological distress for the client.*
    3. ***Correct choice! This plan provides support systems for the client and allows the family to spend as much time as possible with the client before his death, which is important when working through the grieving process.***
    4. *Wrong! The question tells you that the client is short of breath and weak. Therefore, providing frequent rest periods is more important than getting all of the care done at one time, since this will further*

exhaust the client and increase oxygen consumption.

7. **An elderly client is constantly putting her call light on. When the nurse answers the light, the client does not appear to need anything. The nurse would consider many interventions, but the least appropriate solution would be to:**

    1. Ask the members of the family if they can spend more time with the client.
    2. Remove the call light from easy reach of the client.
    3. Make frequent visits to the client's room.
    4. Spend more time in the client's room while charting.

    1. *Wrong choice! Family members are often willing to help in caring for a client if they are asked, or given some direction. Look for an INAPPROPRIATE action.*
    2. ***Correct answer! The call light should never be taken from a client. The client may try to reach for the call light and sustain a fall, or attempt to get out of bed in order to get someone's attention.***
    3. *Wrong choice! Frequently stopping by the client's room is appropriate because it reassures the client that someone is available to assist if needed. Many times clients feel alone and isolated, and use the call bell to get attention.*
    4. *Wrong choice! To help alleviate the client's feelings of isolation, the caregiver can perform tasks such as charting while sitting in a chair in the client's room, rather than at the nurses' station. This would be appropriate. Since this question has a negative response stem, the correct answer is an action that would be INAPPROPRIATE.*

8. **A 48-year-old man is hospitalized for an obsessive-compulsive disorder. He has recurring thoughts that he has mouth odors that are offensive to others. He also has mouth care rituals that occupy a good deal of his waking hours and caused him to be fired from his last job. The nurse understands that these symptoms most likely represent:**

    1. A method of reducing anxiety.
    2. A form of manipulation to avoid work.
    3. An attention-getting strategy.
    4. A rationalization for avoiding social contact.

    1. ***Correct. The ritualized behaviors of a person with an obsessive-compulsive disorder are an attempt to control anxiety.***
    2. *This is not correct. The behavioral rituals performed by a person with an obsessive-compulsive disorder cannot be controlled, so they cannot be considered attempts to manipulate the environment.*
    3. *This is not correct. Obsessive-compulsive behav-*

iors may draw attention to the individual, but the individual is most often embarrassed about them and will go to great lengths to conceal the rituals from others.

4. *No. Persons with obsessive-compulsive behaviors are compelled to perform their rituals and usually derive no pleasure from carrying them out.*

9. **The nurse caring for a child with Tetralogy of Fallot notes that he is easily fatigued. The nurse understands that the etiology of the fatigue is:**

1. Inadequate intake of high calorie foods and vitamins.
2. Poor muscular tone and development.
3. Oxygenation of tissues is inadequate to support energy metabolism.
4. Restricted blood flow leaving the heart.

1. *No, this is the result, not the etiology, of the fatigue. The child tires too easily to take in adequate nutrition.*
2. *No. Poor muscle tone and development is a symptom of the fatigue.*
3. *Right! Fatigue is a direct result of the child circulating poorly oxygenated blood. The defects of Tetralogy of Fallot cause left to right shunting of blood.*
4. *No. This is the pathophysiology of aortic stenosis.*

10. **A three-year-old girl is admitted for a myringotomy after being diagnosed with chronic otitis media. Following the surgery, the nurse prepares discharge teaching. Which statement by the parents indicates effective client teaching?**

1. "Now my daughter will not have ear infections."
2. "I must keep her away from other children with colds."
3. "I will only call the doctor if she gets a fever."
4. "I will keep water out of her ears."

1. *Wrong. Myringotomies will decrease the possibility of otitis media; it does not guarantee that the child will not get any ear infections.*
2. *Wrong choice! Keeping the child away from children with colds is a good general health practice, but is not specific to myringotomy surgery.*
3. *Wrong. Fever is not the only indicator of illness. Irritability and loss of appetite may also indicate an ear infection.*
4. *Congratulations! After placement of tympanostomy tubes, water, and especially soapy water, may enter the middle ear if the ears are not protected from water.*

11. **A client is admitted with a possible ectopic pregnancy. Which of the following best describes the clinical picture of a client experiencing a ruptured ectopic pregnancy?**

1. Large amount of vaginal bleeding, tender abdomen, drop in BP at three to four weeks gestation.
2. Moderate to large amount of vaginal bleeding, abdominal pain and fainting spells at 10 to 12 weeks gestation.
3. Vague complaints of abdominal pain and severe nausea and vomiting at eight to 10 weeks gestation.
4. Small amounts of vaginal spotting, severe abdominal pain, signs and symptoms of shock at eight to 10 weeks gestation.

1. *Incorrect. Rarely is an ectopic pregnancy associated with a large amount of vaginal bleeding, and symptoms are rarely seen prior to eight weeks gestation.*
2. *Wrong! A ruptured ectopic pregnancy is rarely associated with the described blood loss.*
3. *Wrong! The pain associated with an ectopic pregnancy is sudden, severe and associated with syncope. The presence of nausea and vomiting is not related to a ruptured ectopic pregnancy.*
4. *Correct! The client with a ruptured ectopic pregnancy has sudden, severe abdominal pain associated with symptoms of shock.*

12. **A client started methyldopa (Aldomet) to lower his blood pressure. The nurse must emphasize to the client the importance of keeping appointments for which of the following lab studies?**

1. Renal function studies.
2. Blood cell counts and hepatic function studies.
3. Aldomet blood levels.
4. Cardiac enzymes.

1. *No! Liver toxicity is of prime importance with this medication, not kidney function.*
2. *Correct! Aldomet may cause hepatotoxicity within two to four weeks of beginning the drug. Hemolytic anemia occurs in four percent of clients.*
3. *This is incorrect. Blood levels are not drawn for Aldomet.*
4. *Wrong! Cardiac enzymes are not indicated for this drug.*

13. **A client is very upset about the loss of her baby. She is discharged and will be seen at regular intervals by the visiting nurse. At which of the following times would it be most appropriate for the nurse to begin teaching about future pregnancies?**

1. The nurse should begin teaching during the first home visit.
2. When the client begins to ask questions about having another baby.
3. As soon as the nurse has developed a good relationship with the client.

4. Teaching should not begin for about six months.

1. *Wrong! Teaching is best done when the client is ready to learn. The client may not be ready on the first home visit because she continues to be very upset.*
2. ***Congratulations! When the client begins to ask questions about having another baby, she is indicating that she is motivated to learn. Teaching/ Learning theory indicates that motivation should receive priority.***
3. *Good try. A good relationship between the nurse and the client is essential to allow the nurse to be therapeutic. However, the nurse should first help the client deal with her feelings before beginning to teach the client about future pregnancies. After the client has dealt with her feelings, she will be more motivated to learn.*
4. While it may be best for the client to wait for several months prior to becoming pregnant, teaching can begin before that time has passed. Teaching should begin when the client is motivated to learn.

14. **A client is admitted to the hospital with congestive heart failure. He has been on bed rest at home and has been incontinent of urine. His wife has been caring for him, and there is a strong odor of urine when he is placed in the bed on the nursing unit. She tells the nurse that she is sorry and embarrassed about the unpleasant smell. The best nursing response is:**

1. "It must be difficult to care for someone who is confined to bed. How have you been able to manage?"
2. "Don't worry about it. He will get a bath, and that will take care of the odor."
3. "A lot of clients that are cared for at home have the same problem."
4. "When was the last time that he had a bath?"

1. ***Excellent! The wife is the client in this question. The nurse's response must be therapeutic for the client. This response addresses the feelings of the client by using the communication tool of showing empathy. It also facilitates therapeutic communication because it is nonjudgmental and encourages the client to express her feelings.***
2. *Telling the client not to worry blocks communication by devaluing her feelings and her concern about the odor. This is a communication question, and the nurse's response must be therapeutic for the client. Look for a response by the nurse that addresses the feelings of the client and uses a therapeutic communication tool.*
3. *This response implies that caregivers in the home are not able to keep the client odor free. It is a judgmental statement that is not therapeutic. Look for a response by the nurse that addresses the feel-*

ings of the client and uses a therapeutic communication tool.
4. *Asking about the last bath implies to the client that the odor of urine indicates that her husband has not been bathed for some time. This is a communication question, and the nurse's response must be therapeutic for the client. Who is the client in this question? Look for a response by the nurse that addresses the feelings of the client and uses a therapeutic communication tool.*

15. **Which of the following would the nurse expect to be commonly used to manage alcohol withdrawal?**

1. Antipsychotic drugs.
2. Barbiturates.
3. Anti-anxiety agents.
4. Anticonvulsants.

1. *This is not correct. Antipsychotics are used to treat psychotic symptoms. They are not used to manage alcohol withdrawal.*
2. *This is not correct. Barbiturates are potent central nervous system depressants. They are not used during alcohol withdrawal.*
3. ***Correct. Anti-anxiety agents, such as Librium and Valium, are long acting central nervous system depressants that are used to treat alcohol withdrawal. They are substituted for alcohol during the withdrawal process to prevent the occurrence of delirium tremens and to minimize withdrawal symptoms.***
4. *This is not correct. Magnesium sulfate or other anticonvulsants may be used to prevent seizures during detoxification in clients with a history of seizures. Anticonvulsants are not commonly used in alcohol withdrawal for clients who do not have a history of seizures.*

16. **A client is taking acetaminophen (Tylenol) for muscular aches and pains. She reports to the nurse that she is lonely and has been drinking heavily in the evenings. What drug interaction should the nurse discuss with the client?**

1. Alcohol and Tylenol may result in a diuretic effect, depleting fluid volume and electrolytes.
2. Sodium and fluid retention may result from this combination.
3. Alcoholic beverages increase the risk of liver toxicity when taken with Tylenol, so the combination should be avoided.
4. This combination has an increased potential for causing palpitations.

1. This is incorrect. The diuretic effect occurs when alcohol is taken with ibuprofen.
2. This is incorrect. Sodium and fluid retention occurs when NSAIDs are given with steroids.

3. Good! Liver toxicity is likely to occur, as alcohol potentiates the hepatic effects of Tylenol.
4. This is incorrect. Alcohol and Tylenol taken together will cause hepatic changes, not cardiac changes.

17. CPR has been initiated on a client in the emergency room. The nurse understands that which of the following would indicate effective cardiac compressions?

1. An EKG pattern with each compression.
2. Compression depth of one and one-half to two inches.
3. A palpable femoral pulse during each compression.
4. Pupils changing from pinpoint to dilated.

1. *No. The EKG only indicates an electrical impulse and does not guarantee that there is contraction of the myocardium. There will be an electrical pattern generated by any movement of the chest wall by the compressor.*
2. *Incorrect. This is the correct technique, but it is not an evaluation of effective compression.*
3. ***Absolutely! The nurse should place several fingers on the femoral pulse during artificial compressions. If a pulse is generated with the compression it is considered effective in circulating blood.***
4. *No, this is backwards! If the pupils change from pinpoint to dilated, this would indicate that the brain is not receiving adequate oxygen, due to inadequate ventilations or compressions.*

18. Upon returning from the recovery room, the fluid in the chest tube bottle has stopped fluctuating. The nurse most appropriately interprets this assessment to indicate which of the following?

1. All the fluid and air has been removed.
2. The tubing may be kinked.
3. The lungs have re-expanded.
4. The suction is set too low.

1. *Highly unlikely. This would be expected to take several days.*
2. ***Correct. The nurse should first investigate the entire length of tubing from the collection bottle to the client for patency. It is expected in this early postoperative period that a fluctuation would occur with each respiration.***
3. *No, the lungs will not fully re-expand this quickly.*
4. *No. Fluctuation should occur within the system even if it is only to gravity drainage.*

19. An 18-year-old client admitted with ulcerative colitis is being treated with sulfasalazine (Azulfidine). The nurse explains to the client that the major action of Azulfidine is to:

1. Suppress inflammation of the bowel wall.
2. Reduce peristaltic activity.
3. Neutralize gastrointestinal tract acidity.
4. Prevent a secondary infection.

1. ***Correct. Azulfidine, an antibiotic, exhibits some antibacterial activity but also serves as an anti-inflammatory agent to decrease irritation within the colon.***
2. *Incorrect. Azulfidine will not reduce peristaltic activity. In fact, some of the common side effects of the drug are nausea, vomiting, and diarrhea.*
3. *Incorrect. Azulfidine does not act to reduce GI tract acidity. This would be the action of an antacid.*
4. *Incorrect. Azulfidine, although classified as an antibiotic, is not used to prevent a secondary infection. Recall that the client with ulcerative colitis already has an infection and treatment is aimed at correcting this problem first.*

20. A client takes ibuprofen (Motrin) for her arthritis. How should the nurse advise her to take the medication to reduce the complication of esophageal irritation?

1. Don't take with meals.
2. Take with a full glass of water and remain upright for 15-30 minutes afterwards.
3. Take before meals with a snack.
4. Take after meals; then lie down for an hour.

1. *This is incorrect. Ibuprofen can be taken with a meal to prevent gastric irritation.*
2. ***Excellent choice! To reduce the serious risk of esophageal irritation caused by tablets lodging against the esophageal lining, the client should take water and remain upright.***
3. *Wrong choice! Taking ibuprofen with food helps reduce esophageal irritation, but there is an even better method.*
4. *This is incorrect. Lying down may cause gastric reflux into the esophagus.*

21. A client is admitted with acute leukemia. The nurse can anticipate that the client will report which of the following clusters of symptoms?

1. Nausea/vomiting, diarrhea.
2. Fatigue, weakness.
3. Fever, chills.
4. Nosebleed, headache.

1. *Incorrect. These symptoms may result from the treatment of leukemia chemotherapy, but they are not characteristics of the disease process.*
2. ***Good choice! Fatigue and weakness secondary to anemia are the most common presenting symptoms.***
3. *No. Fever and chills may result from an infection secondary to granulocytopenia, but they are not presenting symptoms of leukemia.*

4. No. Bleeding tendencies, such as nosebleeds, may occur due to thrombocytopenia, but the headache is seen when the client has meningeal leukemia and is not a common presenting symptom.

22. **An anorexic client tells the nurse that she thinks too much fuss is being made about what she eats. "I have plenty of energy and get all A's in school. I do not think I am too thin. Look, my hips are fat." What is the most appropriate nursing response to her statement?**

1. "You say your hips look fat to you, but you seem very thin to me."
2. "Let's go over to the mirror so you can see how thin you really are."
3. "You are such a bright girl. I don't understand how you can do this to yourself."
4. "You would be much more attractive if you were not so skinny."

1. Correct. The client's perception of her body is distorted. The nurse can be most therapeutic by responding to her statement in a factual, nonjudgmental way, that does not support her distorted body image.
2. This is not correct. The client's perception of her body image is distorted. Looking in the mirror will not change her problem with body image. There is a better option.
3. This is not correct. This statement by the nurse is demeaning and shows that she lacks an understanding of the client's problem.
4. This is not correct. This statement by the nurse is not therapeutic because it is harmful to the client's self-esteem.

23. **A client's blood pressure rises to 200/120, which is considered a hypertensive emergency. Diazoxide (Hyperstat) is administered. When should the expected response be noticeable to the nurse?**

1. Between one and five minutes of administration.
2. Within one hour of administration.
3. After the second dose.
4. After the first few doses.

1. Excellent! Results occur within one minute and peak action is within two to five minutes. The duration of the effect is from two to twelve hours.
2. No! Results occur more quickly.
3. This is incorrect. Results occur more quickly.
4. This is incorrect. Results occur more quickly.

24. **The nurse is interviewing the mother of a four-year-old at a well child clinic. Which finding would concern the nurse the most?**

1. His speech is intelligible 80% of the time.
2. He is fearful about being examined.

3. He occasionally stutters when he speaks.
4. He has an imaginary playmate named "Red."

1. Best option! By four years of age, a child's speech should be 100% intelligible. This is cause for concern and should be referred to check out hearing and/or developmental delays that can be treated to help the child learn better in school.
2. Wrong! Being fearful of the examination is completely normal for this age.
3. Wrong! Stuttering is normal for a child in the pre-school years.
4. False! Having an imaginary playmate is normal during the pre-school years.

25. **A client diagnosed with AIDS is placed on zidovudine (formerly AZT). The nurse monitors the client for which life-threatening side effect of this drug?**

1. Fever.
2. Aplastic anemia.
3. Renal failure.
4. Cardiac dysrhythmia.

1. Incorrect. Fever is not a side effect of AZT therapy.
2. Good! Severe bone marrow depression, resulting in anemia, is the most common life-threatening adverse reaction of AZT therapy.
3. No, AZT is not known as a nephrotoxic agent. It is rapidly metabolized to an inactive compound and excreted by the kidneys.
4. No, AZT has no known effects upon the heart.

26. **While caring for a client during treatment of pregnancy induced hypertension, which of the following parameters would most concern the nurse?**

1. Respiratory rate of 22.
2. Complaint of a mild headache.
3. Urine output of 80 mL in four hours.
4. Deep tendon reflexes of plus two.

1. Wrong! Respiratory rate of 22 is within normal limits. The nurse should continue to monitor vital signs regularly, but should not consider this finding cause for concern.
2. Wrong! A mild headache is not unusual in a client with pregnancy induced hypertension. The symptom should be treated with an analgesic, but the nurse should not consider this finding cause for concern.
3. Excellent! A urine output of 80 mL in four hours is too low. The kidneys should produce a minimum of 30 mL per hour. Renal damage is a further complication of pregnancy induced hypertension. The nurse should be alert for oliguria. This is the finding that would most concern the

nurse.

4. *Incorrect. Deep tendon reflexes of plus two is within normal limits. This finding would not be a cause of concern for the nurse.*

27. The client tells the nurse that he does not know how he is ever going to stay on the low cholesterol diet that his doctor ordered after his heart attack. The best response by the nurse is:

1. "If you don't follow the diet, you will probably have another heart attack, which could kill you."
2. "What is it about the low cholesterol diet that seems to be a problem for you?"
3. "I've been on that same diet for the last five years, and I'm sure you will learn how to change your eating habits after a while."
4. "I will have the dietitian talk to you before you are discharged. She's the expert, and she can be really helpful."

1. *Wrong. A low cholesterol diet decreases the amount of fat in the diet. High fat content in the diet causes placque to be deposited in the blood vessels, which results in narrowed blood vessels that can cause a heart attack. Telling the client that he may die if he doesn't follow this diet is perceived as a threat and blocks therapeutic communication.*
2. *Excellent! This response uses the therapeutic communication tool of clarification. It lets the client know that his concerns are important to the nurse, and encourages him to tell the nurse more about his concerns. When you cannot identify a therapeutic response focusing on the client's feelings, look for a response that addresses the client's concerns and uses a therapeutic communication tool.*
3. *The fact that the nurse has personal experience with this diet may be beneficial when teaching the client about the diet but, as a response to the client's comment in the case scenario, this response is not therapeutic. It blocks communication by focusing on an inappropriate person — the nurse — instead of on the client's feelings and concerns. The nurse must always be in a therapeutic role.*
4. *This response blocks communication by putting the client's concern on hold. The nurse should address the client's concern and should obtain more information from the client about the problem before deciding to ask the dietitian to talk with the client.*

28. A client is 85 years old. Which of the following assessment findings by the nurse should be reported to the physician?

1. The client is unable to discriminate between hot and cold sensations below the knee of his left extremity.
2. The client walks into the furniture that is in his

room.
3. The client does not respond with appropriate answers to the questions asked by the nurse.
4. The client refuses to remove his clothing.

1. *Best choice! Lack of feeling or sensation below the knee of the left leg can be a symptom of poor circulation to that extremity. The physician should be made aware of this assessment finding. It is not unusual for the elderly to have decreased sensation, but it should be symmetrical.*
2. *Wrong! The nurse should further assess this client for poor vision, which is not unusual for this age group.*
3. *Wrong! A decrease in the ability to hear clearly is a common developmental problem for the elderly. Further assessments needed to determine if the client is hard of hearing or is confused.*
4. *Fear of loss is a common developmental problem of the elderly. They lose friends, respect, independence, self-esteem and many other attributes that they possessed when they were younger. Fear of loss of personal belongings is not uncommon.*

29. A client, age 26, has been diagnosed with AIDS and is currently hospitalized for treatment of Pneumocystis carinii pneumonia. Which of the following symptoms would the nurse least expect to observe in a client with this type of pneumonia?

1. Hemoptysis
2. Fever
3. General malaise
4. Dyspnea

1. *Correct! Clients with pneumocystis pneumonia have a nonproductive cough. Hemoptysis is a late sign of lung cancer.*
2. *No, fever is a usual symptom of this opportunistic infection.*
3. *Incorrect. Clients with pneumocystis pneumonia have general malaise. You were asked to choose a symptom that is NOT expected.*
4. *Incorrect. Clients with this pneumonia do have dyspnea—as is true of all clients with pneumonia.*

30. A client is admitted to the hospital with congestive heart failure and the physician orders stat blood work. The laboratory technician says to the nurse, "I can't do the stat blood work because the client doesn't have an identification bracelet on." The best nursing action would be which of the following?

1. Since the nurse knows the client, draw the blood for the laboratory technician.
2. Assure the laboratory technician that the nurse can verify that he has the correct client.
3. Obtain an identification bracelet for the client as

quickly as possible.

4. Ask the client to identify himself to the laboratory technician.

1. *This is incorrect. Although the nurse may know the client, the client must have an identification band to ensure that the name and hospital numbers match the laboratory requisitions. This is necessary to prevent errors in reporting results.*

2. *In order to prevent erroneous reporting of lab results, the laboratory technician needs to match the client's name and number from the identification bracelet with those on the laboratory requisition.*

3. *Correct! The client needs an identification bracelet to provide for his safety in all aspects of hospitalization.*

4. *The client's name alone is not sufficient identification to ensure the safety of the client. Clients with the same name can be hospitalized in the same health care facility.*

31. **The nurse working in a community health clinic knows which of the following statements about suicide is most accurate?**

1. Suicide rates increase dramatically during natural catastrophes such as earthquakes or floods, or in times of natural uprisings such as strikes or riots.

2. Suicide is the leading cause of death in the 15- to 19-year-old age group.

3. Suicide attempts are preceded by a visit to a physician or primary care provider in a significant number of cases.

4. The majority of people who commit suicide are psychotic.

1. *No. Suicide rates fall dramatically during wars, mass strikes, and natural catastrophes.*

2. *No. Suicide is the second leading cause of death during adolescence. Suicide attempts in adolescence are most often precipitated by the loss of, or lack of, a meaningful relationship.*

3. *Correct. Research indicates that significantly more than half of the persons who attempt suicide have been seen by a primary care provider within a month of their suicide attempt. It is imperative that all physicians and nurses be familiar with the evaluation of and treatment of depression and suicidal risk as they are likely to encounter suicidal clients in their practice.*

4. *No. The majority of people who commit suicide are not psychotic, but many of them are depressed. Psychotic individuals who have "command" hallucinations telling them to harm themselves, however, are at high risk.*

32. **A client who has right-sided paralysis following a stroke is not able to talk, but can make gestures to make himself understood. To effectively communicate with the client, the nurse should do which of the following?**

1. Speak very loudly to the client.

2. Speak quickly to the client, since his attention span may be short.

3. Use gestures while speaking slowly.

4. Wait until the family comes in, so they can interpret his behavior.

1. *This option is incorrect, since the client is not hard of hearing.*

2. *This is incorrect because fast speech is difficult to understand. Also, there is no information that the client has a short attention span.*

3. *Right choice! This client is at a high safety risk, due to both impaired mobility and impaired ability to communicate. The nurse must use all appropriate means to be sure that the client understands what the nurse is saying, and to enable the client to express his needs.*

4. *No. The client may have needs that cannot wait for the family. This option does not respect the client's needs, or assure his comfort and safety.*

33. **The nurse is talking with the mother of a six-year-old child. Which statement by the mother would concern the nurse most?**

1. "His teacher says he's been squinting to see the blackboard."

2. "He has lost both of his top teeth."

3. "He cheats when we play Candyland."

4. "He acts bossy sometimes."

1. *Correct! Squinting to see the board may indicate a vision problem. It's essential to assess children for hearing and vision problems. If not caught early, they lead to frustration and decreased ability to learn. This can lead to decreased self-esteem.*

2. *Wrong! This is the age when children begin to lose their deciduous teeth and replace them with their permanent teeth. This would be an expected response.*

3. *Wrong. Children of five to seven years often cheat to win at games because they feel winning is most important. The nurse can help the mother understand this normal response. This would not, however, be a major concern.*

4. *Children of this age are often "bossy" and are learning how to interact with peers. They have to learn to appreciate how others feel, but this is a gradual process as they are still somewhat egocentric.*

34. **A client is diagnosed as hypertensive and prescribed hydralazine (Apresoline). What statement would indicate to the nurse that the client understands the action of his medication?**

1. "I will eat plenty of foods high in sodium to keep

my fluid level up."
2. "I will limit my fluid intake."
3. "I realize that I need to get up more slowly than before."
4. "I will always remember to take this medication on an empty stomach."

1. *Not right! Sodium intake should be reduced, as it causes water retention, which in turn raises blood pressure.*
2. *This is not correct. An adequate fluid volume is needed. As vasodilatation occurs, urine output will increase.*
3. ***Correct! Orthostatic hypotension occurs due to vasodilatation and the lowering of diastolic pressure.***
4. *Not correct! Taking this medication with food would minimize the first pass metabolism and enhance bioavailability.*

35. **In assessing postoperative clients for signs and symptoms of early hypovolemic shock, the nurse notes that an initial observation would most likely be:**

1. Thirst.
2. Warm, flushed skin.
3. Irritability.
4. Bradycardia.

1. *Incorrect. Thirst is not an early sign of hypovolemic shock. True thirst is caused by fluid volume deficits, but comes after other diagnostic signs and symptoms.*
2. *Incorrect. Warm, flushed skin is seen in early septic shock, which is usually caused by gram-negative bacteria. It is not an early sign of hypovolemic shock.*
3. ***Good work! Early in hypovolemic shock, hyperactivity of the sympathetic nervous system with increased secretion of epinephrine usually causes the client to feel anxious, nervous, and irritable.***
4. *Incorrect. Bradycardia is not seen in shock conditions. The pulse is rapid and becomes weaker, thready and irregular as shock progresses.*

36. **An unconscious client is to have an electroencephalogram (EEG). The first nursing action is which of the following?**

1. Notify the EEG Department that the client is ready for the scan.
2. Check to see that the client is wearing an identification bracelet.
3. Shampoo the client's hair.
4. Prepare a sedative in case the client becomes conscious prior to the procedure.

1. *Wrong. Although the department performing the procedure should be notified, this is not the first*

nursing action.
2. ***Right! Since the client is unconscious and cannot provide information, it is of utmost importance that an identification bracelet be in place.***
3. *No. Although the client's hair will need a shampoo prior to the test, one of the other options should be chosen prior to this intervention.*
4. *No. Sedatives may be ordered by the physicians prior to giving EEGs to help the client relax. However, because this client is unconscious, he does not need a sedative.*

37. **A trauma client, admitted through the Emergency Room, has a urinary catheter inserted to monitor kidney function and assess for early signs of shock. The nurse would report which urinary output measurements as suggestive of cardiac failure or hypovolemia?**

1. 20 mL/hour.
2. 35 mL/hour.
3. 40 mL/hour.
4. 50 mL/hour.

1. ***Correct. Normal urine flow is 50 mL/hour. A urinary output of 30 mL/hour or less is suggestive of cardiac failure or inadequate volume replacement.***
2. *Incorrect. This output would be in the safe parameters, but the client should be monitored closely to watch for further changes.*
3. *Incorrect. This urinary output amount is within safe limits. The client will need continued monitoring to evaluate further changes in urinary output.*
4. *Incorrect. Normal urine flow is 50 mL/hour. This output would suggest normal kidney function.*

38. **A client is scheduled for abdominal surgery, and the nurse is demonstrating deep breathing and coughing exercises. Which of the following information about the client indicates to the nurse that the client may not be ready to learn?**

1. The client gives a return demonstration of deep breathing to the nurse.
2. The client is experiencing severe pain.
3. The client asks the nurse how often deep breathing is done after surgery.
4. The client tells the nurse that this exercise will probably be painful after surgery.

1. *Incorrect choice. Deep breathing and coughing exercises help prevent respiratory complications following surgery. Return demonstration indicates to the nurse that the client understands and is able to perform the activity taught by the nurse. This question has a false response stem and is asking for a negative indication of the client's readiness to learn.*
2. ***Excellent! A client who is experiencing severe pain is not able to concentrate and therefore not***

ready to learn a new activity.

3. *Incorrect choice. Deep breathing and coughing help prevent postoperative respiratory complications. The client is motivated to perform the activity and wants to know how often. This question about the frequency of the activity indicates to the nurse that learning has taken place. This question has a false response stem and is asking for a negative indication of the client's readiness to learn.*

4. *Deep breathing and coughing can be uncomfortable after surgery. This statement indicates to the nurse that the client is motivated to learn, since it tells the nurse that the client knows the possible effects of this activity when an abdominal incision is present. This question has a false response stem, so the correct answer is a negative indication of the client's readiness to learn.*

39. **During the administration of a medication, a nineteen-year-old client tells the nurse that he has never had that particular pill before. The best nursing action is which of the following?**

    1. Check the client's identification bracelet again.
    2. Check the physician's orders to see if this is a new medication.
    3. Assure the client that the medication package has his name on it.
    4. Ask the client to take the medication, since the identification bracelet and medication administration record indicate the client is to receive the medication.

    1. *No. Rechecking the client's identification band does not resolve the question of a "new pill" for the client.*
    2. ***Right! Checking the physician's orders will confirm if this is a new medication ordered for the client, and addresses the client's concern.***
    3. *No. The client's name on the medication label does not address the client's concern about a "new pill." Mistakes can be made with medications. The situation needs to be clarified further in order to provide for the client's safety and to reassure him that he is supposed to receive this pill.*
    4. *No. The person responsible for transcribing the physician's orders onto the medication administration record could have made an error; therefore, the situation needs further clarification.*

40. **A client is six days post-craniotomy for removal of an intracerebral aneurysm and has been transferred from the ICU to the surgical unit. The nurse suspects he may be developing increased intracranial pressure when the client says which of the following?**

    1. He would like to go home.
    2. He feels nauseated.
    3. He has a slight headache.
    4. He is extremely sleepy.

1. *Incorrect. This is a normal response for anyone recovering from surgery.*
2. *Incorrect. Vomiting may occur infrequently with increased intracranial pressure, but it is not accompanied by nausea.*
3. *Incorrect. This is considered normal post-craniotomy. If a headache becomes intense, it may be indicative of increased intracranial pressure.*
4. ***Good choice! Deterioration in the LOC will occur because of reduced oxygen supply, and is the first symptom observed.***

41. **A high school student speaks to the school nurse about a friend who is abusing cocaine. He wants to know what is the best way to influence his friend to stop. The best nursing response is based on what knowledge about cocaine?**

    1. Cocaine use rarely interferes with academic or career activities.
    2. Cocaine abuse is difficult to treat because of its abstinence syndrome.
    3. Cocaine does more psychological harm than physical damage.
    4. Cocaine use is highly reinforcing.

    1. *This is not correct. Cocaine use is frequently associated with family, financial, academic, and career disruptions.*
    2. *This is not the best option. Cocaine abuse results in a powerful psychological dependence. Repeated abuse is associated with an abstinence syndrome of fatigue, depression, prolonged sleep and increased appetite with overeating. This abstinence syndrome is unpleasant but not life-threatening unless the depression becomes suicidal.*
    3. *This is not correct. Medical complications of cocaine include severe weight loss, hepatitis, cerebrovascular stroke, and cardiac arrest.*
    4. ***Correct. Because of cocaine's effects on the neurotransmitters that regulate mood and other psychological processes, it is highly reinforcing of self-administration. Cocaine abuse is very difficult to treat. Some abusers are treated successfully as outpatients, but many require inpatient treatment programs.***

42. **The emergency room nurse is concerned that an 18-month-old child's home situation may include child abuse. Which action by the nurse is most appropriate?**

    1. Notify the physician.
    2. Admit the child to the pediatric unit.
    3. Remove the mother from the child's room.
    4. Report the suspected abuse.

    1. *This response is appropriate, but not the best answer. The nurse needs to share this information*

with other members of the health care team, but the nurse's responsibilities do not necessarily end there. Read all the options and select again.

2. *Wrong. Nurses are not able to admit children to the hospital, but they can discuss their concerns with those able to do so.*

3. *Sorry, unless the nurse feels that the mother may be hurting the child by being in the room, this may not be the most appropriate intervention at this time. It would be appropriate to remove the mother for a short time to talk to the child alone. The mother may be a source of support for the child, and not the abuser. There is not enough data here to warrant removing the mother.*

4. ***Best answer! The nurse wants to discuss the concern about potential abuse with members of the health care team. But if all members of the health care team cannot agree about reporting, and the nurse feels the situation could be an abusive one, the nurse must report.***

43. **A four-year-old client is seen at the clinic and is to receive an injection. When preparing to administer a medication for injection from an ampule, the nurse should avoid performing which action?**

    1. Score the neck of the ampule with a file.
    2. Protect the thumb and fingers with a gauze square or alcohol wipe.
    3. Snap the neck of the ampule toward the body when breaking the top free from the ampule.
    4. Insert the needle into the ampule without touching the needle to the edges of the ampule.

    1. *No. This works well. Scoring the neck of the ampule provides a place for the ampule to break easily without jagged edges.*
    2. *No. Using a gauze or alcohol wipe protects the thumb and finger from being cut if contact is made with the hand and edges of the broken ampule.*
    3. ***The neck of the ampule should be broken away from the body, to prevent shattering of glass toward the hand or face.***
    4. *No. This action is correct. The rim of the ampule is considered contaminated. Touching the edges with the needle will contaminate the needle.*

44. **A gravid client is admitted to the hospital at 38 weeks with a large amount of bright red vaginal bleeding. A diagnosis of partial abruptio placenta is made. She is on the fetal monitor and the nurse assesses her as follows: FH 138 regular, BP 98/52, pulse 118, respirations 24, temperature 97.6° F. Assuming all of the following are ordered by the physician, which should be the nurse's first priority?**

    1. Abdominal prep.
    2. Insert a Foley catheter.
    3. Sign informed consent for surgery.
    4. Start an IV.

    1. *Incorrect. An abdominal prep can be delayed until just prior to the cesarean delivery, if it is done.*
    2. *Wrong. The Foley catheter can be inserted in the delivery room just prior to the delivery, if it is needed.*
    3. *Wrong. The consent form, if not signed immediately by the client can be signed by a family member, if the situation warrants.*
    4. ***Correct! Insertion of the IV line into this client is the first priority. She is at high risk for shock, and if that occurs it will be very difficult to insert an IV catheter. Inserting it now is the first priority for safe care.***

45. **A client returns from surgery for a lung resection due to cancer. Of the following postoperative orders, which should receive highest priority?**

    1. Oxygen per mask at six liters per minute.
    2. Change dressings as needed.
    3. Vital signs every hour.
    4. Cough and deep breathe every two hours.

    1. ***Very good. The postoperative surgical client may need supplemental oxygen in order to maintain normal blood oxygen levels as a result of the surgery and anesthesia.***
    2. *Changing the dressings provides the nurse with information concerning the amount and type of drainage that the client is having. However, this is not the priority postoperative action.*
    3. *Assessing vital signs provides information related to the present status of the client. In specifying the "hourly" assessment of vital signs, this order is an implementation order. This question does not use the nursing process as the priority setting guideline! Notice that one of the options identifies a basic physiological need.*
    4. *Coughing and deep breathing helps prevent postoperative respiratory complications. This nursing action is an appropriate intervention to prevent a potential problem. However, it is not the first priority in this question. Can you identify an option that identifies a basic physiological need?*

46. **The nurse administering aspirin knows that it is prescribed to reduce the risk of TIA's and strokes, because of its ability to inhibit which of the following?**

    1. Prostaglandins.
    2. Platelet aggregation.
    3. Leukocyte migration.
    4. Lysosomal enzymes.

    1. *This is incorrect. Prostaglandin inhibition blocks pain, rather than reducing risk of TIAs and strokes.*
    2. ***Correct! Platelets are inhibited by an enzyme, which then will prevent a thrombus from form-***

ing. A thrombus may block blood flow or develop into an embolus and travel to the brain.

3.   *Wrong! This is an anti-inflammatory response. It is not useful in preventing strokes.*

4.   *No. This is an anti-inflammatory response. It is not useful for preventing strokes.*

47.   The nurse requests to be assigned to stay with an elderly client when she returns to the unit after her surgery. Preoperatively, the client had been disoriented to time and place. What is the most likely rationale for this request?

1.   The elderly client requires close postoperative supervision because of her unpredictable preoperative behavior.

2.   The elderly client will most likely be agitated when she regains consciousness after surgery.

3.   The many stresses associated with surgery could lead to further cognitive impairment in this elderly client.

4.   Elderly clients are particularly vulnerable to the development of postoperative complications.

1.   *This is not the best option for this question. The client had disorientation to time and place preoperatively, but she was not described as unpredictable.*

2.   *This is not the best option. This client is at risk for many problems, including agitation, postoperatively.*

3.   **Correct. Many stresses, both physiological and psychological, associated with surgery, place this client at risk for further cognitive impairment postoperatively. Her postoperative behavior requires ongoing nursing assessment and intervention. This can be best provided by a nurse in constant attendance.**

4.   *This is an accurate statement but it is not the best answer for this question.*

48.   A 54-year-old client is hospitalized with congestive heart failure and is to receive an x-ray. The nurse enters the client's room and asks the client if she is ready to go to x-ray. The client nods her head "yes." The initial nursing action is which of the following?

1.   Explain the x-ray procedure to the client.

2.   Help the client into a wheelchair, so that she will be ready when the transporter arrives to take her to x-ray.

3.   Ask the client if she has any questions.

4.   Look at the client's identification bracelet.

1.   *No. Although the x-ray procedure should be explained to the client, this would not be the initial nursing action.*

2.   *No. Having the client ready for the transporter is very considerate; however, another option takes*

priority over this.

3.   *No! Answering any questions is an appropriate nursing action; however, this is not the initial action.*

4.   **Excellent! Once the client's identity is determined, the nurse can then proceed with the other options.**

49.   A client scheduled for surgery asks the nurse if she can put on some makeup before going to surgery. Which of the following would be the best response by the nurse?

1.   "Only a light application of makeup is allowed."

2.   "Hospital policy states that all makeup must be removed before surgery."

3.   "I will check with the charge nurse to find out the regulations."

4.   "Makeup will interfere with the ability to see your skin color during surgery."

1.   *Incorrect! Makeup of any kind masks the color of the skin or nails. Assessment of the circulatory system is monitored by observing the color of the skin, nails and mucosa.*

2.   *Wrong. Using hospital policy as an explanation is not very helpful. Clients deserve a better explanation. Using hospital policy for an answer is "passing the buck." It does not answer the question being asked.*

3.   *The nurse should know this information. With this response, the nurse is "passing the buck".*

4.   **Congratulations! Makeup colors the skin and masks the ability to assess the circulatory status. Before surgery, all makeup must be removed, including any colored nail polish.**

50.   While performing a vaginal exam, the nurse notes a glistening white cord hanging from the vagina. Which of the following would be the first nursing action?

1.   Return to the nurses' station to place an emergency call to the physician.

2.   Start oxygen at 6 to ten liters, and assess the client's vital signs.

3.   Cover the cord with a sterile moist saline dressing.

4.   Apply manual pressure on the presenting part and have the mother get into a knee-chest position.

1.   *Not the best choice. The physician needs to be called, but the health of the fetus is the first priority.*

2.   *Wrong choice! All the oxygen in the world is not going to help this fetus if it cannot get through the umbilical cord. The mother's vital signs are not a concern with a prolapsed cord, the viability of the fetus is of vital concern.*

3.   *Not the best choice! Covering the cord with a moist sterile dressing will keep the cord moist and sterile*

but it will not oxygenate the fetus.

4. *Best choice! It is essential to get any pressure off the umbilical cord to allow oxygen to get to this fetus. Manual pressure on the presenting part and a knee-chest position are two ways to relieve umbilical cord compression.*

51. An elderly client with Alzheimer's disease is admitted to the hospital. His daughter says to the nurse, "I really feel guilty about leaving my father, but I need to go home." Which of the following is the most therapeutic response by the nurse?

    1. "Your father is well cared for here."
    2. "Your worried feelings are normal."
    3. "When you are getting ready to leave, tell me. I will sit with your father."
    4. "Can I call another family member to stay with him?"

    1. *This may sound good, but it is not correct. This response blocks therapeutic communication by falsely reassuring the client. Remember, the client in this test question is the daughter!*
    2. *Wrong choice! This is an example of the communication block of false reassurance. Also, this response does not address the client's concern about leaving her father.*
    3. *Good choice! In this response the nurse offers to help the daughter by sitting with the father. In this response, the nurse is using the therapeutic communication tool of offering self.*
    4. *Wrong! By suggesting getting someone else to sit with the father, the nurse makes the daughter feel all the more guilty about leaving.*

52. A client is admitted to the hospital with a compound fracture. While making the client's bed, the nurse finds a capsule of medication in the sheets. It would be least appropriate for the nurse to:

    1. Administer the medication to the client.
    2. Notify the physician of the missed dose.
    3. Determine what medication the capsule contains.
    4. Document the incident in the nurse's notes.

    1. *Excellent choice! Since the nurse does not know which dose of the medication was not taken by the client, giving the client the capsule may result in an overdose if a capsule of the same medication has recently been given.*
    2. *Wrong choice! The physician should be notified to determine if the medication should be repeated or if omitting the dose will not be harmful to the client.*
    3. *Wrong choice! Determining what the capsule contains is necessary to determine if the client is at risk for injury if a dose was missed. Some medications*

are very critical for a client's well-being.

4. *Wrong choice! All incidents which can affect the client should be charted in the nurse's notes, in order to clarify any changes that may occur as a result of the incident.*

53. A client is in the hospital and has weakness on her left side because of a stroke. She becomes upset when eating because liquids drool out of her mouth on her weak side. What nursing intervention would be most appropriate?

    1. Provide only pureed and solid foods to prevent drooling and to prevent the client from becoming upset.
    2. Have a member of the family assist with the client's feedings.
    3. Teach the client how to drink fluids on the unaffected side to prevent drooling.
    4. Have the client use a syringe to squirt liquids into the back of her mouth.

    1. *Wrong! Eliminating liquids from the client's diet is inappropriate, since fluids are a basic physiological need.*
    2. *Wrong! This option does not solve the problem of the drooling fluids and does not promote independence in this client.*
    3. *Correct! This promotes independence and addresses the problem of drooling. The client still has control over swallowing and tongue motion on the unaffected side, which will address her concerns. This question reflects the implementation phase of the nursing process.*
    4. *Although this may help eliminate some drooling, it does not promote normalcy during eating, which can result in a decrease in self-esteem.*

54. A client is instructed by the nurse to recognize beginning signs of lithium toxicity. Which of the following signs of lithium toxicity does the nurse include in this teaching?

    1. Nystagmus, irregular tremor, decreased urine output.
    2. Tinnitus, blurred vision, slurred speech.
    3. Incoordination, muscle twitching, severe diarrhea.
    4. Mild ataxia, coarse hand tremors, difficulty concentrating.

    1. *These are signs of severe lithium intoxication. Read all the options to identify the signs of beginning intoxication.*
    2. *These are signs of moderate lithium intoxication. This cannot be the correct answer.*
    3. *These are signs of moderate lithium intoxication. Read the other options to identify the signs of beginning intoxication.*
    4. *Correct. These are beginning signs of lithium toxicity.*

55. A 14-year-old with muscular dystrophy is noted to spend a lot of time in his room by himself. He sleeps late and has been noted to give his personal belongings away. The best intervention by the nurse would be to say:

1. "You still have a lot to live for!"
2. "You seem rather sad lately."
3. "Come play Nintendo with another client in the activities room."
4. "Perhaps I should leave you alone for a while."

1. *Wrong response. The child is showing signs of depression which would normally accompany a progressive illness such as muscular dystrophy. This statement would not encourage expression of feelings, but could cause the adolescent to feel guilty about the feelings of sadness he is experiencing.*
2. *Correct response. This statement may open up communication and expression of feelings because it asks the person to validate it or deny it. It also conveys interest.*
3. *Wrong. While this may be a good idea to get the adolescent out of the room, it ignores any feelings of sadness that he may have and blocks the opportunity to talk about them.*
4. *No. This statement is no intervention at all. Children who are exhibiting signs of depression need to be encouraged to express feelings, not to be left alone.*

56. An elderly client is on strict bed rest. While making an occupied bed for this client, which of the following actions should be taken by the nurse to maintain proper body mechanics?

1. Place the bed in semi-Fowler's position.
2. Place the bed in a low horizontal position.
3. Ask the client to move to the foot of the bed.
4. Place the bed in a high horizontal position.

1. *Incorrect! The bed cannot be made correctly while in the semi-Fowler's position. Making the bed while it is in semi-Fowler's position will cause the nurse to reach while making the head of the bed, which places strain on the musculoskeletal system. It will also cause the linen to pull out when the bed is placed in the horizontal position.*
2. *This is incorrect. Bending over to reach a bed in low position causes more stress on the small muscles of the back.*
3. *This is not an appropriate nursing action. The client should be kept in good body alignment.*
4. *Great choice! In order to use good body mechanics, the bed should be in a high horizontal position. This prevents bending and excess stretching by the nurse.*

57. A 72-year-old man has gouty arthritis. His physician prescribes naproxen (Naprosyn). The nurse understands that the geriatric implications for this drug include:

1. A higher incidence of agranulocytosis and aplastic anemia.
2. A higher incidence of perforated peptic ulcers and/or bleeding.
3. A higher incidence of central nervous system side effects.
4. None, as all NSAIDs are relatively safe medications for any age group.

1. *Wrong! These side effects are more likely to occur with the drug phenylbutazone (Butazolidin), not with naproxen.*
2. *Good choice! Ulcers and bleeding are more common because administration results in a higher proportion (up to twice that in a younger person) of unbound (free) naproxen, which causes more side effects.*
3. *Incorrect. It's indomethacin (Indocin) that is responsible for causing confusion in the elderly.*
4. *Incorrect! Indocin, Naprosyn, and other NSAIDs have many side effects.*

58. A client is visually impaired from a childhood injury. When ambulating this visually impaired client, the most important nursing action is which of the following?

1. The nurse does not leave the client alone in an unfamiliar area.
2. The nurse should stand on the client's non-dominant side.
3. The nurse has the client use his dominant hand to reach out for barriers or landmarks.
4. The nurse describes the route to be taken and removes any obstacles.

1. *Correct! A client with a visual impairment should not be left alone in an unfamiliar environment because of the increased risk of injury.*
2. *The client can use the non-dominant hand to hold on to the nurse's arm during ambulation since the dominant hand should be utilized for feeling objects. Although this is a correct nursing action, it is not the most important action for the nurse to take.*
3. *The dominant hand should be utilized for feeling objects or barriers since it is stronger and more developed than the non-dominant hand. It is not, however, the most important action for the nurse to take in this situation.*
4. *Describing the route helps familiarize the client with surroundings and decreases the sense of social isolation. Removing obstacles provides for the client's safety. It is not, however, the most important nursing action in this situation.*

59. A client is admitted to the ER for an acute asthmatic attack. Which of the following should be the initial intervention by the nurse?

1. Assist the client to a high Fowler's position.
2. Offer oral fluids to loosen secretions.
3. Monitor respiratory rate for changes.
4. Reduce all unnecessary environmental stimuli.

1. Correct. This position is necessary and should be initiated first in order to lower abdominal organs to facilitate breathing.
2. Wrong! A client in an acute attack is unable to take oral fluids. Parenteral fluids are necessary to route medications and liquify secretions.
3. Incorrect. Tachypnea can indicate hypoxemia, yet changing her position is more important initially to promote adequate ventilation.
4. Wrong choice! The initial goal is to promote oxygenation, then allay fears.

60. In planning postpartum nursing care for a client with cardiac disease, which of the following statements is inaccurate?

1. The client needs to be on strict intake and output to assess for a fluid overload.
2. The client needs to be on a high residue diet to decrease the risk of constipation.
3. The client needs to force fluids to prevent dehydration, which could result in cardiac irregularities.
4. The client needs her vital signs taken more frequently than the standard routine.

1. Wrong choice. It is accurate to state that the postpartum woman with cardiac disease is at high risk for a fluid overload and must be on strict intake and output.
2. Wrong choice. Prevention of constipation in the postpartum cardiac woman is important to decrease the amount of straining needed to evacuate the bowel. Look for a statement that is INACCURATE.
3. Good job! The postpartum woman with cardiac disease is already at risk for a fluid overload due to the extra accumulation of fluids during pregnancy. An excessive fluid intake in this client would increase the already present risk.
4. Wrong choice. The postpartum woman does need more frequent vitals, look for a statement that is INACCURATE.

61. A client says to the nurse, "I am so frustrated with having five kids. My husband won't do anything to help keep me from getting pregnant." Which of the following should be the initial nursing action?

1. Refer the client and spouse to family planning services.
2. Find out if she could use a contraceptive that would not involve her husband.
3. Assess what the client means by "being frustrated."
4. Ask the client if her husband is interested in birth control.

1. Not the best choice. Referring both of them to family planning services may be an option. However, the key word in the stem of the question is "first." This option is not the best choice for the first action the nurse should take.
2. Good job! Before you can plan, the nurse needs to get more information. Assessment is the first step of the nursing process.
3. This might appear to be a good choice, but it is not correct. The nurse is assessing the wrong part of the problem. The client already stated that her frustration is due to the number of children. The nurse does not need to assess any more about the client's feelings of frustration.
4. This is incorrect because the client stated that her husband is not interested in birth control measures that directly involve him.

62. A client has pneumonia and is being treated with erythromycin ethylsuccinate (E.E.S.) 400 mg p.o. every six hours. The nurse should observe the client for side effects of this drug, which include which of the following?

1. Hearing loss.
2. Jaundice.
3. Hypotension.
4. Diarrhea.

1. Incorrect. Hearing loss is a possible adverse reaction when clients are taking high doses of IV Erythrocin, especially in the presence of renal impairment. It rarely occurs with oral use of E.E.S.
2. No. Jaundice, a sign of liver impairment, is more frequently seen in clients who are taking Erythromycin estolate (Ilosone). If the client has a prior history of liver disease, erythromycin should be used with caution and periodic hepatic function studies are monitored.
3. Wrong choice. There is no data to suggest a correlation between changes in blood pressure and erythromycin therapy.
4. Good choice! Diarrhea, abdominal cramping, nausea/vomiting are common adverse reactions to erythromycin therapy. Supportive care may include an order for an antiemetic or antidiarrheal agent and asking the physician about enteric-coated forms of erythromycin, which are associated with a lower incidence of GI distress.

63. A postoperative client's knee dressing becomes completely saturated with blood one hour after returning to the clinical unit. Initially, the nurse should:

1. Reinforce the knee dressing.
2. Apply a tourniquet around the closest artery.
3. Apply direct pressure to the knee.
4. Apply ice to the knee.

1. *No, this would not be effective. This action is more for cosmetic purposes and does not reflect the seriousness of the client's condition. Something must be done to stop or slow the bleeding.*
2. *No, this is not appropriate at this time. This action is somewhat drastic and should only be used as a last resort when the hemorrhage cannot be controlled by any other method.*
3. **Correct! Almost all bleeding can be stopped by direct pressure, except when a major artery has been severed. The charge nurse should then be notified, so that appropriate action can be taken by the surgeon. The client usually has to return to surgery for ligation of the bleeder(s).**
4. *No, this is inappropriate in this situation -- even though ice is a vasoconstrictor and will help decrease edema and hematoma formation.*

64. **The best approach for the nurse to take initially with a client who has severe anxiety is:**

1. Move the person to a calm, non-stimulating environment.
2. Encourage expression of feelings without attempting to modify defensive behavior.
3. Lower the client's level of anxiety by offering medication.
4. Suggest the client engage in some automatic behavior, such as pacing, to reduce his anxiety level.

1. *This might be a good intervention, but this is not the best initial action for the nurse to take.*
2. **Correct. The nurse should encourage the client to communicate by offering self and listening in a nonjudgmental manner. The initial goal is to support the client's defenses to help him gain more control over his anxiety.**
3. *Wrong! Medication is indicated for panic levels of anxiety. Clients with a severe level of anxiety can be helped without medication.*
4. *This might be a good intervention, but this is not the best initial action for the nurse. There is a better option.*

65. **A client diagnosed with a frontal lobe mass is admitted following an MRI and is scheduled for a supratentorial craniotomy. Postoperatively, the nurse would correctly position the client in which of the following positions?**

1. Dorsal recumbent.
2. Trendelenburg.
3. Semi-Fowler's.
4. Prone.

1. *No. This position is recommended following infratentorial surgery, since it prevents pressure on the brain stem.*
2. *No. This position is contraindicated following any cranial surgery, due to increased intracranial pressure.*
3. **Excellent choice! This position is recommended, since it approximates normal increased intracranial pressure.**
4. *No. The prone position very often is confining and suffocating because chest expansion is inhibited during respirations, thereby potentiating respiratory complications.*

66. **A 70-year-old man with a severe systemic infection is being treated with a 10-day course of gentamicin sulfate (Garamycin). What important assessments should the nurse make during this treatment?**

1. Assess for visual disturbances and seizures.
2. Check IV site after three days.
3. There are few complications with Garamycin and relatively minor assessments for the nurse to make.
4. Monitor for dizziness or buzzing in ears.

1. *Wrong. Garamycin will not cause changes in vision or seizures, it is toxic to the kidneys, ears, and nerves.*
2. *No. It is recommended that the IV site be checked after three days when administering cephalosporins.*
3. *Garamycin has many side effects and adverse reactions, therefore, this answer is not correct.*
4. **Great choice! Dizziness and buzzing in the ears would be complications of ototoxicity and should be monitored closely. Audiograms and vestibular studies may need to be done before and during administration of high doses.**

67. **Which of the following interventions would be most important for the nurse to include in the plan of care for a client with hepatitis B?**

1. Bed rest with bathroom privileges.
2. High calorie, high protein diet.
3. Force fluids to 3,000 mL in 24 hours.
4. Medicate for pain every three to four hours as needed.

1. **Yes, this is very important. Bed rest is usually recommended until the symptoms of hepatitis have subsided. Bed rest will "rest" the liver and decrease energy demands.**
2. *Wrong. Adequate nutrition should be maintained, but proteins are restricted when the liver's ability to metabolize protein by-products is impaired. Because the client tends to be anorexic, meals should be small, high-calorie, and provide only moderate*

protein.

3. *Incorrect. Clients with hepatitis B are anorexic and often experience nausea/vomiting. If emesis is a problem, the client is treated with intravenous therapy. It is not realistic to expect the client to drink 3,000 mL in 24 hours.*

4. *Wrong. Clients with hepatitis B may be anorexic and experience dyspepsia, generalized aching, malaise, and weakness. Non-pharmacological pain relief measures may be indicated but medications are avoided, if at all possible, in order to "rest" the liver.*

68. During a client's postoperative recovery from an ileostomy, the nurse begins teaching her stoma care. She refuses to look at her ostomy and states "I'd rather be dead than have to live with this all my life." The most therapeutic nursing response is to say?

1. "I can't imagine what you must be feeling like; it must be awful."
2. "I'll call your physician and see if something can be ordered to help you to relax."
3. "There's no reason to feel like that, things will get better."
4. "You appear upset, would you like to talk?"

1. *No. Expressing excessive approval can be as harmful to the nurse/client relationship as stating disapproval.*

2. *No, this ignores the client's statement and changes the subject, which conveys a lack of empathy.*

3. *No, this offers false reassurance to the client, which is a block to therapeutic communication.*

4. *Good choice. This conveys to client a caring attitude, and willingness to listen. This is the therapeutic communication tool of offering self.*

69. A client is awake at 1:00 a.m. He is irritable and tells the nurse that the staff is making too much noise and that he hasn't had a decent night's sleep since his wife died a year ago. He asks the nurse to get him a cup of hot tea to help him relax and quench his thirst. Which of the following is the best nursing intervention?

1. Get the client the cup of hot tea that he requested.
2. Close the door to eliminate noise from the hallway.
3. Use techniques that promote relaxation and suggest a warm glass of milk for the client.
4. Tell the client that he should try to get some exercise so that he will be tired enough to sleep at night.

1. *Although the case scenario refers to psychological needs as a result of his wife's death, sleep is a basic physiological need. Tea contains caffeine, a stimulant, which interferes with sleep. Getting him the hot tea is not the best nursing intervention.*

2. *Eliminating noise is helpful in promoting sleep, however, this action leaves the client alone and ignores his request for something to drink. The client's physiological needs of sleep and thirst must be addressed.*

3. *Very good! Relaxation is a preliminary step to sleep. Using these techniques not only helps the client relax but also promotes a therapeutic relationship with the nurse. The nurse offers self by spending time with the client. Milk will quench the client's thirst and contains an ingredient that promotes sleep.*

4. *Exercise promotes a feeling of well-being and may be a factor for this client, but the case scenario does not tell you whether the client does or does not exercise during the day. More importantly, however, this response by the nurse does not meet the client's present physiological needs. It doesn't address thirst or help the client get to sleep.*

70. The most important nursing goal for a client who is admitted with an acute exacerbation of ulcerative colitis is which of the following?

1. To provide emotional support.
2. To prevent skin breakdown.
3. To maintain fluid and electrolyte balance.
4. To promote physical rest.

1. *No. Emotional support is necessary, but physiological needs must be the priority in the acute stage.*

2. *Incorrect, because skin breakdown will be prevented if the client's fluid and electrolyte balance is maintained.*

3. *Correct! Problems related to fluid and electrolyte balance can affect all systems. The goal would be to treat imbalances.*

4. *Incorrect. Rest promotes a decreased metabolic rate, yet is not sufficient to counteract problems resulting from fluid and electrolyte imbalances.*

71. A 34-year-old client who weighs 288 pounds says to the nurse, "I'm going to have surgery and have my stomach stapled in order to lose weight. I've tried everything else, and nothing seems to work." Which of the following is the most therapeutic response by the nurse?

1. "That's a pretty drastic measure. Are you sure that is what you want to do?"
2. "I hear that the surgery is only a temporary measure, and if you have the staples removed you will only gain the weight back again."
3. "It must be difficult to be overweight and not able to lose weight. What does your husband think about the surgery?"
4. "Can you tell me about the possible consequences and side effects of this type of surgery?"

1. *Wrong! This response by the nurse is judgmental and questions the decision made by the client. There is no encouragement from the nurse that promotes further communication from the client. This is not a therapeutic response or intervention by the nurse.*

2. *This may or may not be a true statement, but it does not promote communication from the client. The client is frustrated about her weight and needs to express her feelings. This response indicates to the client that her situation is hopeless.*

3. *This response is only half correct. Asking about the husband's feelings focuses on someone other than the client, resulting in a block to further communication about the client's feelings, which is the issue in this question.*

4. ***Congratulations! This response asks for clarification of the client's understanding of the surgery and promotes further communication. This implementation question asks for an appropriate response by the nurse.***

72. **When orienting a severely depressed client to the unit, which of the following approaches by the nurse would be best?**

    1. Introduce the client to the others on the unit and staff members.
    2. Tour the unit and introduce her to everyone they meet on the way.
    3. Explain the unit policies and answer any questions she may have.
    4. Accompany the client to her room and stay with her while she unpacks, offering only minimal information.

    1. *This approach would be overwhelming for the client at this time.*
    2. *This is a possibility, but there is a better option.*
    3. *This is a possibility, but there is a better option.*
    4. ***Correct. Severely depressed persons have problems with concentration and easily become confused. A nursing approach that focuses on giving simple information, slowly and directly, is best. Also, the presence of the nurse will help her adjust to her new surroundings.***

73. **A 30-month-old male is being admitted with asthma. The nurse will discuss with the parents the emotional impact of hospitalization for their child. Which of the following actions will best minimize the stress of hospitalization for this client?**

    1. Explain procedures and routines.
    2. Encourage contact with children of the same age.
    3. Provide for privacy.
    4. Encourage rooming-in.

    1. *No. You can explain procedures, but given a choice,*

this is not the best answer. This becomes a more appropriate stress reducing technique as the child matures into school age and adolescence.

2. *No. The peer group is not the major support for the toddler. This would be a more successful plan with the school age or adolescent client.*

3. *Incorrect. Adolescence is the age in which stress may be reduced by providing privacy in order for them to cope more effectively.*

4. ***Right! Rooming-in is the most effective means of providing emotional support for the toddler. The family's presence provides a sense of security that will increase the child's ability to cope in an unfamiliar environment. This is well supported by nursing research.***

74. **When inserting a nasogastric tube in a comatose client for tube feedings, the nurse needs to avoid:**

    1. Measuring the amount of the tube to be inserted.
    2. Lubricating the distal portion of the tube.
    3. Tilting the client's head back when inserting the tube.
    4. Checking placement of the tube.

    1. *The nurse would not want to avoid this. Measurement from the tip of the client's nose to the ear lobe to the xiphoid process is the measurement considered to be approximately equal to the distance necessary for stomach placement. This question is asking for something that is NOT appropriate to do.*

    2. *Wrong choice. Remember, this question has a negative response stem and is looking for something NOT to do when inserting a nasogastric tube. Lubricating the tube allows it to pass through the nostril more easily.*

    3. ***Good work! This statement is incorrect. This is avoided, since it makes it difficult to swallow, and the likelihood of introducing the tube into the trachea is increased.***

    4. *Wrong choice. The nurse would not want to avoid this, because placement needs to be verified to assure that the tube is not in the trachea or lungs. Remember, this question has a negative response stem.*

75. **A 26-year-old man is seen in the clinic for a dermatological problem. The nurse is to apply topical ointment to the client's skin. Which of the following actions should be avoided?**

    1. Massaging the ointment into the skin.
    2. Removing excess ointment.
    3. Applying ointment with ungloved fingertips.
    4. Documenting a description of the skin prior to application of the ointment.

    1. *Massaging the ointment into the skin provides for penetration of the ointment into the skin. What*

action should be AVOIDED?

2. *Excess ointment should be removed, since it may stain clothing or come into contact with other areas of the body, or with other objects or people. What action should be AVOIDED?*

3. *Correct answer! Applying ointment with ungloved fingertips allows for absorption of the medication through the pores of the skin, which may cause some undesirable effects to the person applying the ointment.*

4. *Wrong choice! The skin should be described to determine if the ointment is having a positive effect.*

76. **Prior to a paracentesis for a client with cirrhosis and ascites, the nurse should encourage the client to do which of the following?**

1. Drink two liters of water.
2. Empty his bladder.
3. Cleanse the abdominal area thoroughly.
4. Eat a meal high in sodium.

1. *Incorrect, because fluids are restricted to 1-1.5 liters daily for clients with ascites.*

2. *Good choice! Voiding will help avoid puncture of the bladder when the trocar is inserted into the abdomen.*

3. *Incorrect. Cleansing of the skin with an antiseptic solution on the lower abdomen is done during the procedure by a physician or nurse.*

4. *Incorrect. Sodium is restricted to 800 mg in order to induce a negative sodium balance and permit diuresis.*

77. **A child is born with a Simian crease and other characteristics of Down's syndrome. The diagnosis of Down's syndrome is confirmed. Which nursing intervention may be most beneficial to the family at this time?**

1. Seeking information from the family about prenatal care received.
2. Discussing positive aspects of foster care for the baby.
3. Assessing the baby's developmental level.
4. Encouraging family members to express concerns about the baby.

1. *Wrong! Seeking information about prenatal care received may imply that something the parents did or did not do could have caused the Down's syndrome. This is added guilt for the parents.*

2. *Absolutely not! Down's children do not have to go into foster care. By letting the parents lead the discussion, the nurse can answer questions they have instead of implying that one method of care is better than another.*

3. *Wrong! While assessments made for all newborns*

should be done for this baby, no other specific developmental assessments need to be made at this time. During the newborn phase it is not possible to determine a lot about future development.

4. *This is the best answer because it will focus the nurse on the parents' concerns and open discussion of feelings and fears.*

78. **A client is admitted with esophageal varices. The most appropriate intervention that will decrease the risk of esophageal bleeding is which of the following?**

1. Apply an ice collar.
2. Maintain semi-Fowler's position.
3. Administer stool softeners.
4. Provide a diet high in Vitamin D.

1. *Incorrect. An ice collar cannot control portal hypertension.*

2. *Incorrect. This plays no role in decreasing the risk of bleeding for this client.*

3. *Good choice! Bleeding occurs as a result of straining when stooling; therefore, it is appropriate to decrease any possibility of straining, by administering stool softeners.*

4. *Incorrect. Foods high in Vitamin D help to stimulate the active transport of calcium and phosphorous, but play no role in controlling bleeding.*

79. **The nurse is concerned about a depressed client's weight loss and continued refusal to eat. Which one of the following approaches to this problem by the nurse would be least appropriate?**

1. Encourage small, frequent meals to help increase caloric intake.
2. Offer highly nutritious foods that are easy to chew and nutritional supplements that require little effort to eat.
3. Determine what foods the client likes and make them available at meals or for snacks.
4. Remind her she will become ill if she does not eat.

1. *This is an appropriate approach, but this negative response stem question is asking for an option that is NOT appropriate.*

2. *Wrong choice. This is a good way to encourage adequate nutrition in a client who has no appetite. This negative response stem is asking for an option that is NOT appropriate.*

3. *This is an appropriate approach, but this question is asking for an option that is NOT appropriate.*

4. *Correct option! This option is not appropriate because it would increase the guilt already felt by a depressed client.*

80. In evaluating a mother's adaptation to motherhood, which of the following behaviors would the nurse expect to see in the "taking in" phase?

    1. Anxiety because the baby is not nursing well.
    2. Eager to return the bath demonstration you gave to her yesterday.
    3. Upset because her lunch is late.
    4. Confident in her ability to nurse the baby without difficulty.

    1. *Wrong. While the mother is in the "taking in" phase, she is very self-centered.*
    2. *Wrong. This is a behavior seen in the "taking hold" phase, when the mother is more confident and in control.*
    3. ***Correct, the mother in this phase is very self-centered. Her needs are most important at this time.***
    4. *No, this behavior is not seen until the "taking hold" phase.*

81. When attempting to obtain information from a hearing impaired client, the nurse should do which of the following?

    1. Face the client and speak slowly.
    2. Speak frequently and exaggerate lip movements.
    3. Speak loudly.
    4. Speak directly into the impaired ear.

    1. ***Correct. You should always face the hearing impaired client and accentuate your words.***
    2. *Incorrect. Speaking frequently will not aid the client in hearing, and exaggerated lip movements are contraindicated.*
    3. *Incorrect. Shouting overemploys normal speaking movements, which may cause distortion and be too loud for the client.*
    4. *Incorrect. Speaking directly into the impaired ear is contraindicated. Moving closer and toward the better ear will facilitate communication.*

82. A 22-year-old client sustained a T4 spinal cord injury. While doing morning assessments four weeks post-injury, the nurse discovers his BP is 280/140 and he is complaining of nasal stuffiness and a severe, pounding headache. The first nursing action is which of the following?

    1. Sit the client upright.
    2. Call the physician.
    3. Check the client's bladder for distension.
    4. Administer the prescribed antihypertensive.

    1. ***Correct choice! Since autonomic hyperreflexia is a medical emergency, the first action is to lower the BP. By sitting the client upright, compensatory orthostatic hypotension is used to lower the***

BP.

2. *Incorrect. Calling the physician is important after nursing measures have been initiated to lower the BP.*
3. *Incorrect! This should be done to assess the cause of hyperreflexia, but the first goal is to lower the BP and, ultimately, to prevent stroke.*
4. *Incorrect, because causing orthostatic hypotension will provide the same results initially. Antihypertensives are used if non-pharmacologic methods are unsuccessful.*

83. A client has been taking her iron for two weeks but is still complaining of fatigue from her anemia. What is the best response by the nurse, assuming that the client is taking her medication properly?

    1. "Perhaps you should go to bed earlier."
    2. "This is really unusual, I'll tell your doctor."
    3. "I guess your anemia must be really bad."
    4. "It will take one to two months for your hemoglobin level to get back to normal, so keep taking your iron tablets."

    1. *Wrong. This would not be an appropriate response. It does not offer an explanation to the client.*
    2. *No, this is not appropriate, as it will take more than two weeks for her to see a response.*
    3. *No, this is not a professional response, and would worry the client unnecessarily. Reread the responses.*
    4. ***Correct. The hemoglobin level will take from one to two months to come up to normal. This response is correct and reassuring to the client.***

84. A client awaits surgery to remove an obstruction in his small intestine. The nurse notices his vomitus contains fecal material. Which of the following actions should the nurse do immediately?

    1. Provide frequent mouth cleansing.
    2. Notify the physician.
    3. Check his bowel sounds.
    4. Administer a prescribed antiemetic.

    1. *Incorrect. Although it is important to make the client comfortable and to prevent parotitis, this isn't the first priority.*
    2. ***Correct! Feculent vomitus requires immediate surgical intervention because this indicates complete obstruction, and the client is likely to develop septic shock.***
    3. *Incorrect. Checking bowel sounds will have no bearing on the client's vomitus; it only confirms his obstruction.*
    4. *Incorrect. Although antiemetics are valuable in controlling nausea, since this is an emergency situation, surgery is the treatment of choice.*

85. **When obtaining a urine specimen for a culture and sensitivity from an indwelling catheter, the nurse should:**

    1. Empty the drainage bag from the urometer port.
    2. Wear sterile gloves.
    3. Cleanse the entry site prior to inserting the needle.
    4. Drain the bag and wait for a fresh urine sample to send from the drainage bag.

    1. *Incorrect. The urometer port can only be used to obtain a non-sterile specimen; therefore, the nurse cannot obtain a urine culture and sensitivity from this port.*
    2. *Incorrect. Sterile gloves are unnecessary when obtaining culture and sensitivity, since the nurse does not disrupt the closed system except with a sterile needle.*
    3. ***Excellent choice! Disinfecting the needle insertion site removes or destroys any microorganisms on the surface of the catheter, thereby avoiding contamination of the needle and the entrance of microorganisms into the catheter.***
    4. *Incorrect choice, because if the urine is obtained from the drainage bag it is unsterile since the bag contains microorganisms.*

86. **When assessing a client in the oliguric-anuric stage of acute renal failure, the nurse notices a respiratory rate of 28, and the client complains of nausea, a dull headache, and general malaise. The priority nursing action should be?**

    1. Notify the physician.
    2. Check the chart for her latest electrolyte values.
    3. Administer an analgesic and an antiemetic.
    4. Provide O_2 at two liters, by nasal cannula.

    1. *Incorrect. The physician will want a complete assessment before being notified, and will require the nurse to relate the potassium level.*
    2. ***Correct, the nurse should look for the client's latest potassium level, since these symptoms indicate hyperkalemia, which can lead to death.***
    3. *This is not a priority since the client is exhibiting symptoms of an increased potassium level, which can lead to death.*
    4. *Incorrect. The client is not in respiratory distress, nor is he experiencing labored breathing.*

87. **A three-year-old is being admitted with nephrotic syndrome. The best roommate for this client is:**

    1. A 16-year-old postoperative from removal of a ruptured appendix.
    2. An eight-year-old with leukemia.
    3. Another toddler with rheumatic fever.
    4. No roommate, isolation is required.

    1. *Wrong, the child with nephrotic syndrome is at risk for infection.*
    2. ***Right. This child is not infectious; that's what you are looking for as a roommate for a child with nephrotic syndrome. The roommates may have nothing in common, but the potential for infection is a high priority nursing diagnosis for this admission.***
    3. *No, this isn't the best choice, since the child with rheumatic fever may still be infectious from the original causative organism.*
    4. *No, it is not necessary to place this child on isolation.*

88. **Second and third degree burns of the head, neck and chest place the client initially at greatest risk for which of the following?**

    1. Infection.
    2. Airway obstruction.
    3. Fluid imbalance.
    4. Paralytic ileus.

    1. *Incorrect. Although infection is necessary to prevent throughout burn treatment, a patent airway is the priority.*
    2. ***Good choice! Burns in this area may involve damage to the pulmonary tree, resulting in severe respiratory difficulty.***
    3. *Incorrect. Although adequate fluid replacement is necessary for cellular and organ function, initially, a patent airway is the priority.*
    4. *Incorrect. During the acute phase, paralytic ileus may occur, requiring nasogastric suction. However, it does not take precedence over a patent airway.*

89. **A client, admitted with salicylate intoxication, has arterial blood gases drawn with the following results: pH 7.50, $PaCO_2$ 32, HCO_3 24. This client's blood gas values indicate which of the following acid-base disturbances?**

    1. Metabolic alkalosis
    2. Respiratory alkalosis
    3. Metabolic acidosis
    4. Respiratory acidosis

    1. *Incorrect. Metabolic alkalosis is characterized by a high plasma bicarbonate concentration. The bicarbonate level for this client is within normal limits.*
    2. ***Excellent! You understand blood gases!! Respiratory alkalosis is recognized by the high pH (decreased hydrogen ion concentration and a $PaCO_2$ less than 35 mm Hg). It is always due to hyperventilation, which causes excessive "blowing off" of carbon dioxide and hence a decrease in plasma***

carbonic acid content.

3. *No, metabolic acidosis would initially be characterized by an increased hydrogen concentration. Recall what effect this would have on the blood pH.*

4. *Incorrect. You need to review your normal blood gas values and the parameters for identifying respiratory and metabolic imbalances. Remember to always look at the blood pH first, to determine if the imbalance is acidosis (low pH) or alkalosis (high pH).*

90. **On the day of delivery a client is assisted out of bed for the first time. She becomes frightened when she passes a blood clot and notices an increase in her lochia. Which of the following should the nurse include in her explanation?**

1. The lochia pools in the vagina when lying in bed.
2. Placental fragments have probably been retained in the uterus.
3. She probably has a uterine or urinary tract infection.
4. The amount of lochia will increase during the postpartum period.

1. *Congratulations! The client needs to be reassured that this is a normal occurrence following a period of time in bed.*

2. *No, this occurrence is the result of pooling of lochia rather than a complication such as retained placenta fragments.*

3. *No, this clinical picture is not indicative of a postpartum infection.*

4. *Incorrect. The amount of lochia is greatest immediately following delivery and should decrease as the uterus contracts.*

91. **A four-year-old child is admitted to the hospital with periorbital cellulitis. The child weighs 15 kg and the physician orders cefazolin (Kefzol) 600 mg IV every eight hours. The medication manual states that Kefzol can be given 50-100 mg/kg/24 hours. The nurse's best response would be which of the following statements?**

1. Discuss the dose with the physician because the dose is too high.
2. Question giving Kefzol to treat periorbital cellulitis.
3. Give the Kefzol as ordered because the dose is in the safe range.
4. Discuss the dose with the physician because it is too low.

1. *Right. Three doses of Kefzol are given per 24 hours. 600 mg x 3 doses/24 hours = 1800 mg/24 hours. Multiply the weight times each end of the range to give the amount for a child of this weight.*

15 kg x 50 mg/kg/24 hours = 750 mg/24 hours. 15 kg x 100 mg/kg/24 hours = 1500 mg/24 hours. Therefore, the dose is higher than the acceptable range. The nurse should question the order with the physician.

2. *Wrong. Periorbital cellulitis is an infection that can be treated with a cephalosporin such as Kefzol.*

3. *No. The dose is not within the safe range. The order must be questioned.*

4. *No. The dose is too high, not too low.*

92. **A client, age 36, is diagnosed with active tuberculosis. He and his family have many questions for the nurse. They ask, "How did this happen? What can we do to prevent this? What will happen next?" Which of the following statements would be the best response by the nurse?**

1. "The tuberculosis was probably contracted from someone else with TB."
2. "You need not be concerned, TB is very curable."
3. "Tuberculosis can be treated at home with medications."
4. "You seem very worried about tuberculosis. What concerns you most?"

1. *Not a good choice. This only answers one question and not very helpfully at that.*

2. *Incorrect. This pat response does not answer their questions or allay their fears.*

3. *Incorrect choice! This response only addresses one question.*

4. *Good choice. This is appropriate. It invites the family to ask questions and obtain answers to all that concerns them.*

93. **The nurse understands that clients who are diagnosed with agoraphobia display which of the following defense mechanisms?**

1. Denial.
2. Isolation.
3. Displacement.
4. Undoing.

1. *This is not correct. Denial is the avoidance of disagreeable realities by ignoring or refusing to recognize them.*

2. *This is not correct. Isolation is separating or blocking the feelings associated with a memory of a situation or person.*

3. *Great choice! Displacement is redirecting an emotion from the original object to a more acceptable substitute. In phobic disorders the anxiety is displaced from the original source to another object or situation, resulting in the phobia.*

4. *This is not correct. Undoing is an act or communication that reverses or negates a previous act that was unacceptable.*

94. A client is referred to a high risk prenatal clinic by a midwife. She thinks she is about three months pregnant but is to be examined for the presence of hydatidiform mole. The nurse expects which of the following symptoms to be present if she has a hydatidiform mole?

1. Seizure activity.
2. Periods of amnesia.
3. Rapidly enlarging uterus.
4. Painful uterine contractions.

1. *No. Seizure activity is not related to the presence of a hydatidiform mole.*
2. *Wrong. Amnesia is not a clinical finding in the client with a hydatidiform mole.*
3. ***Yes! A rapidly enlarging uterus along with severe nausea and vomiting is associated with the presence of a hydatidiform mole and would warrant ultrasound examination of the uterus.***
4. *No. Uterine contractions are not related to hydatidiform mole at three months gestation. An abortion needs to be considered as the cause.*

95. An eight-year-old child complains of a stomachache while visiting the school nurse. Which statement by the child would concern the nurse most?

1. "My stomachache goes away if I rest for a few minutes."
2. "My friends are picking on me and calling me fatso."
3. "My brother just had his appendix out."
4. "My friends won't let me play kickball with them the way I want to."

1. *Wrong choice! The nurse would want to make sure the child is afebrile and not in acute pain. Otherwise, this could be part of a viral illness. The nurse would want to monitor this, but it is not the most pressing issue of the choices.*
2. ***Right! Children rely heavily on what other children say to them and take things said literally. Being ridiculed can lead to problems with self-esteem. It's critical for the nurse to look into this statement further and try to intervene.***
3. *Wrong. Appendicitis is not contagious. However, the child may need reassurance or to talk about what has recently happened with the sibling. This is a somewhat normal response.*
4. *Wrong! Children of this age are learning and making up rules all the time. They also want to be the one to be the leader and it's hard for them to not be the boss sometimes. This commonly occurs and children need to work it out for themselves as much as possible.*

96. A client, 42 years old, is admitted to the psychiatric hospital for the third time with a diagnosis of schizophrenic disorder, paranoid type. During her admission interview, she tells the nurse, "I'm in the hospital because they told lies about me. They are trying to poison my food." This comment is an example of which of the following?

1. A grandiose delusion.
2. An illusion.
3. An auditory hallucination.
4. A persecutory delusion.

1. *This is not correct. A delusion that is grandiose is a belief that one is endowed with a special power or talent or is identified with a famous or powerful person.*
2. *Wrong. An illusion is a sensory misperception. There is no data that the client has misperceived something she has seen or heard.*
3. *Wrong! An auditory hallucination is hearing something that is not present, such as voices talking to her.*
4. ***Correct. The client's statements are delusional and persecutory because they indicate beliefs that some group ("they") is telling lies about her and trying to poison her food.***

97. A nursing mother asks the nurse how she will know if the baby is getting enough milk. The nurse tells the client that the best way to evaluate adequate intake for the newborn is by which of the following methods?

1. Fit of his clothes.
2. Amount of crying he does.
3. Number of wet diapers.
4. Number of hours he sleeps after each feeding.

1. *Incorrect. The fit of clothes is a poor method to assess a newborn's weight gain or loss related to breast feeding.*
2. *Wrong! There are many reasons why an infant cries; hunger is just one.*
3. ***Good choice! In order to void, the infant must have adequate fluid intake. If he is dehydrated his urinary output will decrease.***
4. *Wrong. If the infant breast feeds for a long length of time he may get very tired because of the effort to get food, thus he will sleep after the feeding. If the mother does not have sufficient breast milk he may not have received the necessary calories.*

98. A client, age 25, comes to the health clinic for the results of her HIV testing. When the nurse tells her that the results are negative, the client states, "Thank God that I don't have AIDS!" What would be the nurse's most appropriate response?

1. "Yes, that is good news. You have not been infected with the virus this time. Please be careful in the future."
2. "You are fortunate that you have immunity to the AIDS virus—some people are not so lucky."
3. "The results mean that antibodies to the virus are not present at this time. Use the safe sex guidelines and consider retesting in three months."
4. "This test result indicates that you don't have AIDS now, but the disease may be dormant and become active up to 10 years from now."

1. *Not correct. The client may have been infected with the virus but the antibodies have not appeared yet.*
2. *Incorrect! There is no such thing as "immunity" to the AIDS virus.*
3. **Correct! This response gives the client correct information and reinforces safe health practices.**
4. *Although this statement is partially correct regarding the seropositive conversion of up to 10 years, a negative test does not diagnose the client for AIDS— only for the antibodies to HIV. A client can be seropositive for HIV and not have AIDS.*

99. **A nurse working with a client with agoraphobia recognizes that the most effective technique for treatment of agoraphobia is:**

1. Continual exposure to situations that she fears.
2. Distraction each time she brings up her problem.
3. Teaching relaxation techniques.
4. Gradual desensitization by controlled exposure to the situation she fears.

1. *Wrong. Continual exposure to situations she fears will create even greater anxiety.*
2. *Wrong choice! Distraction will not assist her to overcome her fear and anxiety.*
3. *Teaching relaxation techniques is helpful, but there is a better technique to treat agoraphobia.*
4. **Correct. Desensitization is a type of behavioral therapy. The client is gradually exposed to the feared situation under controlled conditions and learns to overcome the anxious response.**

100. **Which of the following interventions would the nurse anticipate using, following a Shirodkar procedure at 14 weeks of gestation?**

1. Administration of betamethasone.
2. Nonstress testing.
3. Administration of tocolytic drugs.
4. Administration of oxytocic drugs.

1. *No. Betamethasone is a drug given to an expectant mother to cause maturation of fetal lungs and at 14*

weeks would serve no purpose.
2. *No. Nonstress testing is rarely done prior to 28 weeks gestation, which is considered the age of viability. If it is done prior to this gestational age and the results are abnormal, there is little that can be done to save the fetus.*
3. **Good choice! When the client has a Shirodkar procedure there is a risk of preterm labor. Tocolytic drugs are used to achieve or maintain uterine relaxation.**
4. *No, oxytocic drugs cause uterine contractions, which are undesirable at 14 weeks of gestation.*

NCLEX-RN

Test 5

NCLEX-RN TEST 5

1. **A 56-year-old male client has had a CVA and a homonymous hemianopsia. An improvement related to this condition that the nurse might document in a positive evaluation statement would be that the client now:**

   1. Maintains communication with others.
   2. Walks with a cane.
   3. Has frequent episodes of crying.
   4. Visually scans while eating.

2. **A 78-year-old is admitted to the hospital for an exploratory laparotomy. The client anxiously says to the nurse, "Do you think that the doctor can fix whatever is wrong with me?" Which response by the nurse would be best initially?**

   1. "That question can only be answered after your surgery."
   2. "People your age frequently have problems that can be corrected by surgery."
   3. "You need to get more information from your doctor."
   4. "You must be worried about what the doctor might find."

3. **The nurse would avoid including which information in the teaching plan for a client who is using eye medications for glaucoma?**

   1. Instill the drops without touching the dropper to the eye.
   2. Store the medication at the proper temperature, refer to the directions.
   3. Vision may become blurred after instillation, the client needs to use precautions.
   4. The medication is taken for two to three weeks and then discontinued.

4. **During a preoperative interview for a seven-year-old female, the child's mother requests information to prepare her daughter for hospitalization. The interview is being conducted three days prior to admission for a tonsillectomy. The child was hospitalized last year for a fractured femur. Which of the following would best meet this child's needs for preparation?**

   1. Suggest a role play, and provide materials.
   2. Remind the child of the experience of her past hospitalization.

   3. Read her a story about another child having a similar operation.
   4. Tell her she is only going in to have her throat checked.

5. **In contrast to clients with anorexia nervosa, the nurse knows that which of the following characteristics are common among clients with bulimia?**

   1. Recognize their eating behavior is abnormal.
   2. Rarely suffer serious medical consequences.
   3. Have positive feelings about their eating patterns.
   4. Vomit after eating or use laxatives to purge the food.

6. **A client questions the nurse concerning the usual course of multiple sclerosis. What would be the most appropriate response by the nurse?**

   1. "Each client is different, we cannot tell what will happen."
   2. "I can see that you are worried, but it's too soon to predict what will happen."
   3. "Usually, acute episodes are followed by remissions, which may last a long time."
   4. "It's too early to think about the future; let's focus on the present and go day-by-day."

7. **Following a colostomy, a client and his wife have been taught to perform a colostomy irrigation. Which behavior would best indicate readiness for discharge?**

   1. The client's wife verbalizes all steps in the irrigation procedure.
   2. The client performs the irrigation following written instructions.
   3. The client and his wife attend all classes given about colostomy care.
   4. The client asks appropriate questions about irrigations.

8. **A client, 34, is admitted for the third time to a psychiatric hospital with a diagnosis of schizophrenia. The police found her wandering along the highway. When questioned, she was not able to give a coherent answers to any questions. During the admission procedure, the nurse notices that her appearance is unkempt and she appears to be actively hallucinating. The initial nursing priority is to assess which of the following?**

   1. Her mental status.
   2. Her ability to follow directions.

3. Her perception of reality.
4. Her physical health needs.

9. A client gave birth to a six-pound baby boy. The Apgar score was nine at one minute. In the delivery room, the nurse administered parenteral vitamin K (Aquamephyton) to the baby. The nurse understands that the best rationale for giving the baby vitamin K is that:

1. Infants are usually born with vitamin K deficiency unless large doses are given to the mother prenatally.
2. Vitamin K is poorly absorbed from the gastrointestinal tract and must be given parenterally.
3. Vitamin K is normally produced by bacteria in the intestine. Infants are born with a sterile intestine.
4. There is no infant formula available that contains significant quantities of vitamin K.

10. A client does not return her mother's greeting and instead lies down on the bed and curls up in the fetal position. The nurse observes the behavior and concludes the defense mechanism that the client is displaying is:

1. Fixation.
2. Symbolization.
3. Repression.
4. Regression.

11. The nurse discovers that the wrong medication was given to a confused client, who had answered to an incorrect name. The physician is notified and states that the medication that the client received will not harm him and nothing needs to be done. Which of the following is the best nursing action following this incident?

1. Apologize to the client involved.
2. Make out an incident report documenting the occurrence.
3. Try to avoid being responsible for administering medications again, since this could have been a terrible situation.
4. Realize that everyone makes mistakes and continue on with administering the rest of the medications to the other clients.

12. A client's urinary tract infection does not improve, and he is admitted to the hospital. His prescription is for sulfamethoxazole with trimethoprim (Bactrim). The nurse knows that over a period of 24 hours his urine output should be at least:

1. 500 mL.
2. 700 mL.
3. 1500 mL.
4. Over 2000 mL.

13. The nurse understands that the client with angina pectoris demonstrates pain that has which of the following characteristics, least likely associated with the pain of myocardial infarction?

1. It is relieved by rest.
2. It is substernal or retrosternal.
3. It does not radiate.
4. It is described as tightness or heaviness in the chest.

14. A nephrectomy is scheduled tomorrow on a three-year-old client. Which of the following is an appropriate preparatory nursing order?

1. Demonstrate by pointing on the child's body where the incision will be made the evening before the procedure.
2. Give the preoperative sedation as ordered with a small needle so that a bandaid will not be needed.
3. Ask the child's parents to leave the room while the preoperative medication is administered.
4. Explain the procedure to the child in simple sentences just before giving the preoperative sedation.

15. A 23-year-old gravida 1, para 0 is admitted to the hospital at 38 weeks with pregnancy induced hypertension. The physician orders bed rest, IV of 1000 mL Ringers lactate, four grams of magnesium sulfate bolus followed by a continuous infusion of two grams of magnesium sulfate in 1000 mL Ringers lactate. During the admission assessment, the nurse notes which finding that the nurse knows is inconsistent with the diagnosis of pregnancy induced hypertension:

1. Three plus protein in the urine.
2. Deep tendon reflexes of plus one.
3. Blood pressure of 148/98.
4. Plus one pitting sacral edema.

16. Three days following a left simple mastectomy, the nurse finds the client crying and withdrawn after her physician has changed the dressing. Which is the best initial response to this situation?

1. "Would you like me to show you some samples of breast prostheses?"
2. "Would you like me to contact the Reach to Recovery visitor?"
3. "Are you angry about the loss of your breast?"
4. "I've seen a lot of women who've had mastectomies and they do just fine and you will, too."

17. The nurse would expect a client with hyperthyroidism to report which of the following symptoms?

1. Weight gain of 10 lbs in three weeks.
2. Constipation.
3. Sensitivity to cold.
4. Flushed, moist skin.

18. The **nurse knows that which of the following actions is the most common cause of invasion of a client's privacy?**

    1. Over-exposing a client during a treatment or examination.
    2. Failing to pull the curtain while performing a treatment or examination.
    3. Talking about the client to other staff members who are not involved with the care of the client.
    4. Helping an elderly client with a tub bath.

19. **A client has sustained a gunshot wound to her left side and has a closed water seal drainage system attached to a chest tube. The nurse notices continuous bubbling in the water seal collection immediately after insertion of the chest tube. Which of the following actions should the nurse take?**

    1. Notify the physician immediately.
    2. Clamp the chest tube.
    3. Continue to monitor for continuous bubbling.
    4. Reposition the client.

20. **An emergency room nurse takes a telephone call from a woman who reports she has just taken 100 amitriptyline (Elavil) tablets to kill herself. The woman is crying and says, "I want to die. I have no reason to live." Which of the following responses by the nurse is most therapeutic?**

    1. "Let me help you. I'm sure things are not as bad as they seem to you now."
    2. "Is there anyone with you now?"
    3. "How do you feel about what you have just done?"
    4. "I'm glad you called, because I can help you. What is your name and your address?"

21. **Occasionally a client forgets to take her ibuprofen (Motrin). When this occurs the nurse would suggest to the client that she do which of the following?**

    1. Double the next dose.
    2. Take the medication as soon as she remembers and then continue the same dose schedule even if doses are close together.
    3. Resume the usual dosing interval.
    4. Take half the dose as soon as it is remembered, then continue the dose schedule.

22. **During a nursing staff meeting, what information about safety for hospitalized suicidal clients is most important for the nurse to emphasize?**

    1. The more specific the plan, the more likely the client will attempt suicide.
    2. Inhospital suicides are more likely to occur closely following admission than at any other time during the hospitalization.
    3. Inhospital suicides are more likely to occur at changes of shifts or on weekends.
    4. The person who makes a suicide attempt and fails probably will not try again.

23. **A client is a truck driver who sits for hours in his truck while driving. He has a swollen and inflamed right calf and is diagnosed with thrombophlebitis. He is hospitalized immediately, placed on bed rest and started on a continuous heparin infusion. He asks the nurse how long it will take for the heparin to dissolve his clot. What is the best response by the nurse?**

    1. "It usually takes two to three days for heparin to work."
    2. "I'm not sure, ask your doctor."
    3. "Heparin begins to work immediately, but it actually does not dissolve clots. It prevents new clots from forming, and the present one from getting bigger."
    4. "Heparin thins the blood quickly."

24. **A 22-year-old sustained a fracture of the tibia and fibula while playing football. A long leg cast has been applied, and the client is admitted to the orthopedic unit. In providing nursing care for the client, which of the following is a vital consideration?**

    1. Elevation of the leg in the cast on a pillow will minimize edema.
    2. Healing of a fractured bone requires an extended period of time.
    3. A long period of immobility may lead to atrophy of the muscle.
    4. Analgesics may be needed for pain associated with the fracture.

25. **The nurse administering acetaminophen (Tylenol) knows that it is used primarily for which of its clinical properties?**

    1. Analgesic and antipyretic.
    2. Anti-inflammatory and antirheumatic.
    3. Antiplatelet aggregation.
    4. Antileukocytic migration.

26. The nurse knows that which of the following events is outside the scope of those required to be reported to appropriate agencies?

 1. Births.
 2. Child abuse.
 3. Marital quarrels.
 4. Typhoid fever.

27. Which statement by a 14-year-old female would the nurse consider least attributable to normal adolescent development?

 1. "I haven't gotten my period yet, and all my friends have theirs."
 2. "None of the kids at this school like me and I don't like them either."
 3. "My parents treat me like a baby sometimes."
 4. "There's a big pimple on my face and I worry that everyone will notice it."

28. When conducting a nursing interview with a client admitted with Cushing's syndrome, which of the following symptoms would the nurse expect the client to report?

 1. Weight loss.
 2. Diarrhea.
 3. Double vision.
 4. Increased bruising.

29. A client is admitted to the emergency room with an overdose of acetaminophen (Tylenol). The nurse would expect to give immediate consideration to which of the following?

 1. Slow respiratory rate.
 2. Nausea, vomiting and abdominal discomfort.
 3. Decreased urine output.
 4. Convulsions.

30. A 25-year-old female client being treated with a cesium implant is found crying in her room. Which is the best response?

 1. "I will come and spend ten minutes with you each hour."
 2. "Let's see if we can get a phone installed in your room."
 3. "We'll plan to admit someone to your room for company."
 4. "You will be discharged in two days, try to enjoy the peace and quiet."

31. A 46-year-old client is two days postoperative following an abdominal aneurysm repair. Which nursing intervention will help to prevent the development of postoperative thrombophlebitis?

 1. Have the client sit with his feet touching the floor.
 2. Apply gentle leg massage.
 3. Encourage the client to ambulate.
 4. Place pillows under the client's knees.

32. In assessing a newborn for congenital dislocation of the hip, the nurse should be alert for which of the following?

 1. Symmetrical gluteal folds.
 2. Absence of Ortolani click on abduction.
 3. Limited abduction of one hip.
 4. Flexion of one leg while extending other leg.

33. The client has privacy rights that the nurse must not overlook. The nurse knows that the client's privacy rights include all of the following except:

 1. The right not to have a gunshot wound reported.
 2. The right to refuse to receive visitors.
 3. The right generally to wear one's own clothing.
 4. The right to request the presence of a member of the same sex during a physical examination.

34. A client is having a nonstress test. The fetal heart rate is 130-150 bpm, but there has been no fetal movement for 15 minutes. Which of the following is the most appropriate nursing response?

 1. Encourage her to walk around the monitoring unit for 10 minutes, then resume monitoring.
 2. Immediately report the situation to her physician and prepare her for induction of labor.
 3. Offer her a snack of orange juice and crackers.
 4. Turn her on her left side and attempt to auscultate fetal heart sounds with a doppler.

35. An 82-year-old widow is admitted to the hospital for hip replacement surgery. She appears alert and cooperative, although in great pain. While doing an assessment, the nurse learns she is disoriented to time and believes she is in a hotel. The nurse identifies acute confusion as a nursing problem and realizes the client's confusion could be the result of any of the following except:

 1. Her age.
 2. Relocation to the hospital.
 3. Her physical pain.
 4. Bed confinement.

36. A client has been taking morphine for several weeks to relieve her cancer pain. During the last two home health visits, she has complained that her dose does not seem to be working. What could explain the client's complaint?

1. She has finally become addicted to her morphine.
2. She is becoming confused and probably is not taking her medications properly.
3. A tolerance to the medication has developed.
4. The pain medications are being abused, and the client needs counseling about her addiction.

37. **Which instruction would be least appropriate for the nurse to include in discharge teaching for a client who had a vasectomy?**

    1. Wait 24 hours to bathe.
    2. Apply ice bags to the incision for the first 24 hours.
    3. Resume sexual activity without contraceptive measures within two to three days.
    4. Wear a scrotal support for the first few days.

38. **During the early phase of alcohol withdrawal, what is the primary focus of nursing care?**

    1. Rest and nutrition.
    2. Assessing coping skills.
    3. Confronting the use of denial and other defense mechanisms.
    4. Education about alcohol abuse and treatment.

39. **A 13-year-old boy is admitted for an emergency appendectomy. While doing the preoperative teaching, he asks, "Will I have a large scar from the surgery?" The nurse's best response is which of the following statements?**

    1. "Most scars from appendectomies are not very large."
    2. "That isn't our biggest concern right now, let's get you well first."
    3. "Don't worry, scars fade a lot in just a few months."
    4. "It will be small enough so it won't show with bathing trunks on."

40. **A client is admitted to the hospital following an automobile accident. The client is to have a Foley catheter inserted. The initial nursing action when implementing this procedure is which of the following?**

    1. Using sterile technique during this procedure.
    2. Checking the client's identification.
    3. Placing all necessary equipment within easy reach.
    4. Explaining the procedure to the client.

41. **A client is being treated with pilocarpine (Pilocar) for his glaucoma. He complains of blurred vision after administration of his drops. Which of the following is the best explanation by the nurse of this side effect?**

1. The client is not using the eye drops correctly.
2. Pilocarpine (Pilocar) causes the pupil to constrict, making the eye accommodate for near vision. Therefore, objects far away seem blurred.
3. When the pupil is dilated, it is more difficult to adjust vision.
4. Pilocarpine irritates the lining of the eye and causes blurring and inflammation.

42. **An 11-year-old female has suddenly developed a voracious appetite and has outgrown her clothes in six months. The mother is concerned and seeks the nurse's advice. The best response by the nurse would be which of the following statements?**

    1. "Being overweight as a child can mean problems later on."
    2. "What kinds of foods has she been eating?"
    3. "The growth spurt does not occur until adolescence; let's check her weight."
    4. "This is often the time when a growth spurt occurs. Let's talk some more."

43. **In preparing to administer a medication to a confused elderly client, the nurse discovers that the client does not have her identification bracelet on. The client states that she has already taken her medication. Which of the following nursing actions provides for the client's safety?**

    1. Ask the client if she might be confused about taking her medication.
    2. Identify the client based upon which bed she occupies in the room.
    3. Check the client's chart and ask another health care worker to identify the client.
    4. Ask the client to identify herself, and obtain an identification bracelet for her.

44. **At 12 hours of age, an infant's respiratory rate is 44 per minute. Her respirations are shallow with periods of apnea lasting up to five seconds. Based upon this assessment data, the nurse should do which of the following?**

    1. Activate respiratory arrest procedures.
    2. Call the physician immediately and report the assessment.
    3. Continue routine monitoring.
    4. Request an order for supplemental oxygen.

45. **The nurse demonstrates accurate knowledge of the administration of a Mantoux skin test for TB by:**

    1. Inserting the needle with the bevel up.
    2. Administering 0.1 ml of PPD on the outer surface of the arm.

3. Using a 21 or 22 gauge needle.
4. Massaging the area after administration of the medication.

46. **An eight-year-old male child has had successful corrective surgery for a ventricular septal defect. The child's mother says, "My son really wants to join the swim club, but I know that is not a possibility for him." Which of the following is the most therapeutic response by the nurse?**

1. "Would you like me to tell his doctor that you have a question?"
2. "Do you think he is aware of his limitations?"
3. "Would you like me to encourage him toward another school activity?"
4. "Do you think there should be limits on his activity?"

47. **A mother speaks with the nurse about her three-month-old son. She says that he was well until two weeks ago. At this time he has been spitting up after he eats. Now the vomit "shoots across the room." As soon as he vomits, he cries and acts very hungry. The best response by the nurse is which of the following statements?**

1. "You need to burp him more frequently."
2. "Have him drink Pedialyte."
3. "Let his stomach rest for two hours."
4. "Perhaps the doctor should examine him."

48. **Which of the following actions would the nurse implement initially for a client in panic?**

1. Determine the source of his anxiety by asking the client to describe the events before the anxiety occurred.
2. Provide privacy for the client by moving him to a quiet area away from other people, and leaving him alone so he can regain control.
3. Help the client describe his feelings, to begin to diagnose the problem as anxiety.
4. Provide a sense of safety and security by remaining with the client, speaking in a calm manner and offering sedation if needed.

49. **The morning of the client's surgery for repair of an abdominal aortic aneurysm, the nurse should do which of the following first?**

1. Administer pre-anesthetic medications.
2. Remove the client's watch and rings.
3. Check that the operative permit is signed.
4. Discuss the postoperative complications with the client's family.

50. **A client is taking furosemide (Lasix) 60 mg p.o. twice a day. The nurse is teaching the client methods to decrease the incidence of orthostatic hy-**

potension. **Which of the following statements is probably least appropriate for the nurse to include in this teaching?**

1. "You should rise slowly when you change positions from lying to standing."
2. "It would be helpful for you reduce, or eliminate, your alcohol intake."
3. "Try to avoid exercising in hot weather."
4. "Eat foods high in sodium to prevent dehydration."

51. **A client's bloodwork reveals the following: Coombs positive, Rh negative blood type, Rh (D) antibody titer negative. Her infant's blood type is Rh positive. Which of the following nursing actions is indicated for the client?**

1. Give her RHoGAM while she is in the hospital.
2. Tell her sensitization has occurred and she will not receive RHoGAM.
3. Tell her she will not receive RHoGAM because of the positive Coombs.
4. Tell her she will not receive RHoGAM because of the bolus blood type.

52. **A client is post-craniotomy and is progressing well. While he is sitting in a chair, the nurse notices he begins to experience a grand mal seizure. The most important nursing action is to:**

1. Provide oxygen.
2. Restrain the client.
3. Insert an airway.
4. Lower the client to the floor.

53. **A client is to receive eye drops. Which of the following actions taken by the nurse best prevents injury to the eye during administration?**

1. Apply gentle pressure over the opening to the nasolacrimal duct.
2. Hold the tip of the container above the conjunctival sac.
3. Instruct the client to look upward.
4. Deposit the drops into the conjunctival sac.

54. **A newly diagnosed diabetic is receiving instructions regarding dietary management of his disease. In providing information, the nurse is aware that the most important objective in the dietary management of diabetes mellitus is:**

1. Control of the total calorie intake in the proper proportions to attain or maintain ideal weight.
2. An accurate distribution of calories from carbohydrates, protein, and fat.
3. Weight reduction to reverse the hyperglycemia.
4. Meeting energy needs while decreasing blood lipid levels.

55. **In caring for a seven-year-old child who has lice, the nurse should instruct family members to do which of the following?**

    1. Throw out all combs the child used.
    2. Isolate the child with the lice in his room.
    3. Remove all nits with a fine tooth comb.
    4. Keep others away from the child as lice can jump.

56. **When changing dressings for an HIV positive client, in addition to proper handwashing the nurse should do which the following?**

    1. Wear a mask.
    2. Wear gloves.
    3. Maintain strict isolation.
    4. Wear a gown and gloves.

57. **In planning activities for depressed clients during their early stages of hospitalization, the nurse's best choice is to implement which of the following plans?**

    1. Provide one activity a day to avoid fatigue.
    2. Let the client choose an activity that is appealing.
    3. Provide a structured daily program of activities for the client.
    4. Wait until the client's mood improves and he or she indicates an interest in productive activity.

58. **A six-month-old infant with sudden, severe colic and vomiting has been admitted for testing to rule out intussusception. In planning teaching for the parents of the infant, the nurse would include information on which likely treatment?**

    1. Barium enema.
    2. Manual reduction
    3. High dose steroids
    4. Double barrel colostomy

59. **The physician has prescribed ciprofloxacin (Cipro) 200 mg IV every 12 hours for a client diagnosed with osteomyelitis of the left knee. The nurse should monitor the client for which of the following adverse drug reactions?**

    1. Hypotension.
    2. Bronchospasm.
    3. Diarrhea.
    4. Leukopenia.

60. **A client is scheduled for surgery. When the transporter arrives to take the client to the operating room, the client is sitting in a chair. The best action to get the client onto the stretcher is which of the following?**

    1. Assist the client to get back into bed, and then move her across to the stretcher with the help of a drawsheet.
    2. Have the client first stand on the chair and then get onto the stretcher.
    3. Assist the client to hop up onto the stretcher.
    4. Together with the transporter, lift the client onto the stretcher, keeping a wide stance and a straight back.

61. **A non-pregnant woman is diagnosed with trichomoniasis and metronidazole (Flagyl) is ordered. Which of the following instructions would the nurse appropriately give to the client regarding the treatment plan?**

    1. Both partners need to take the drug and abstain from intercourse until cultures are negative.
    2. Only the client needs to take the Flagyl, but she should not have intercourse until her culture is negative.
    3. If both partners are treated simultaneously they may continue sexual intercourse.
    4. The male partner needs to be cultured and be treated with Flagyl only if his cultures are positive.

62. **A 70-year-old client is diagnosed with benign prostatic hypertrophy. Which of the following nursing interventions is contraindicated following a prostatectomy?**

    1. Administration of analgesics as ordered.
    2. Notify the physician of excessive clots.
    3. Irrigation of the Foley catheter as ordered and p.r.n.
    4. Rectal temperatures taken every four hours for the first 24 hours.

63. **A client has been taking phenytoin (Dilantin) for several years for her epilepsy. She has recently married and wants to start a family. What advice should the nurse give her about her medication usage?**

    1. Epilepsy should not interfere with her pregnancy or medicine regime.
    2. She will have to be more careful regarding her weight gain while on Dilantin.
    3. There is an increased association with birth defects born to mothers who use anticonvulsants.
    4. She will need to increase her dose of Dilantin during her pregnancy.

64. **When caring for a client using a cane, which nursing action would be most appropriate?**

    1. Schedule physical therapy visits to strengthen muscle mass.
    2. Remind the client to place the cane on the strong side.

3. Remove the rubber tips to enhance ambulation.
4. Place the cane safely in the closet at nap and bed-time.

65. A client is admitted with a complaint of weight loss of 12 pounds in the last two months despite increased appetite. She is also experiencing increased perspiration, fatigue, and restlessness. A diagnosis of hyperthyroidism is made. Which of the following measures is it essential that the nurse include in her plan of care to prevent thyrotoxic crisis?

1. Provide a quiet, low stimulus environment.
2. Administer aspirin as ordered for any sign of hyperthermia.
3. Maintain the client's NPO status until her anorexia subsides.
4. Observe the client carefully for signs of hypocalcemia.

66. A client is in the seventh month of pregnancy and has symptoms of preeclampsia. When discussing diet, the nurse instructs her to eat a high protein diet and to avoid foods that have a high sodium content. Which of the following, if selected, would indicate an understanding of the dietary instructions?

1. Creamed chipped beef on dry toast.
2. Cheese sandwich on wholewheat toast.
3. Frankfurter on a roll.
4. Tomato stuffed with diced chicken.

67. Which of the following statements made by a female client indicates to the nurse that she has an adequate understanding concerning the administration of nitroglycerin tablets?

1. "I will only have to take these pills for a few weeks."
2. "I should take a pill after strenuous exercise to prevent an angina attack."
3. "If I get a headache, I should stop taking the pills."
4. "This drug is not habit-forming, so I don't have to worry about addiction."

68. A client is taking methyldopa (Aldomet) 500 mg p.o. every eight hours. When monitoring the client, which side effect is the nurse least likely to observe?

1. Headache.
2. Sedation.
3. Tachycardia.
4. Weakness.

69. In planning the care for a child in Bryant's traction, the nurse will include measures to avoid which major complication?

1. Sacral decubitus.
2. Inflammation at pin sites.
3. Circulation impairment.
4. Lack of adequate countertraction.

70. A 24-year-old client is taking amphotericin B (Fungizone) as treatment for histoplasmosis. The nurse ensures that the medication is to be infused slowly over six hours. If the Fungizone were to infuse too rapidly, the client would be at greatest risk for which of the following?

1. Fluid overload.
2. Fever and chills.
3. Cardiovascular collapse.
4. Extravasation.

71. The nurse notes that a client frequently makes delusional statements. The nurse understands that the delusional statements are an indication the client is using which ego-defense mechanism?

1. Projection.
2. Dissociation.
3. Displacement.
4. Regression.

72. During a postpartum assessment, one hour following delivery, the nurse finds a large amount of continuous rubra lochia with several moderate sized clots. The fundus is midline and firm at the umbilicus. In regard to these findings, which of the following is the most therapeutic nursing action?

1. Reassure the client that this is normal in the first hours after delivery.
2. Notify the physician who delivered this client of the clinical findings.
3. Massage the uterus frequently to contract the uterus.
4. Increase the rate of the IV bag containing Pitocin.

73. A client is admitted for fluid replacement. A diagnosis of hepatitis A virus is made. It is most important for the nurse to maintain which of the following measures in the client's plan of care?

1. Strict bed rest.
2. Universal precautions.
3. Patency of the T tube.
4. A low protein, high fat diet.

74. A biophysical profile is done and the client is told the score was 10, the highest score possible. She asks what this means. The best nursing response is which of the following?

1. The fetus is in immediate danger; more tests need to be done.

2. The fetus is certainly mature and can be delivered at any time.

3. The fetus is healthy and may remain in utero safely at this time.

4. The score is appropriate for gestational age (AGA) of the fetus at this time.

75. **A client appears apprehensive and says to the nurse, "One of the men in my office died last week from a heart attack." Which of the following responses by the nurse would be most therapeutic?**

   1. "Tell me more about what you are feeling."
   2. "Are you thinking the same thing might happen to you?"
   3. "Your physician will not let that happen. This test will tell him how to best treat your condition."
   4. "Has anyone in your family had a heart attack?"

76. **Which of the following precautions is appropriate for the nurse to give a client who is taking clonidine (Catapres)?**

   1. You will need to be weaned off of this drug if the physician decides to discontinue it.
   2. Light-headedness is rarely a problem with this antihypertensive medication.
   3. You will need to have someone check your blood pressure each day while taking this medication.
   4. Try to include more salt in your diet because this drug can deplete your body's supply.

77. **Prednisone is ordered for a two-year-old client with nephrotic syndrome. The nurse can confirm the effectiveness of the prednisone therapy by noting which finding?**

   1. The child's weight drops 500 grams.
   2. The child's food intake increases.
   3. The child's respiratory rate decreases from 25 to 16 breaths per minute.
   4. The child's rectal temperature returns to 37° C.

78. **The nurse knows that the discharge teaching is successful for a client with hepatitis A virus if the client indicates she will refrain from which of the following activities?**

   1. Donating blood.
   2. Eating fried foods.
   3. Vacationing in a foreign country.
   4. Ordering a salad in a restaurant.

79. **How should the nurse respond to the anxious client who states, "I feel like I am going to die. Am I having a heart attack?"**

   1. Reassure the client that nothing bad is going to happen to him.

2. Encourage him to reduce his anxiety by a physical activity such as pacing or trying some other relief behavior.

3. Respond to the fear he has expressed by stating that he is not having a heart attack and will not be left alone until he is feeling more comfortable.

4. Inform him, "No, your problem is severe anxiety."

80. **A client will be having an amniocentesis. The nurse asks the client to explain what the health care provider told her about the risks of this procedure. Which of the following responses indicates a proper understanding of the procedure by the client?**

   1. "I might go into labor early."
   2. "It could produce a congenital defect in my baby."
   3. "Actually, there are no real risks to this procedure."
   4. "The test could stunt my baby's growth."

81. **In a long-term care facility, the nurse finds an elderly client on the floor. After having the client examined by the physician, the most important nursing action would be which of the following?**

   1. Call the family and ask them to stay with the client.
   2. Provide for the safety and protection of the client.
   3. Apply wrist and leg restraints to prevent the client from falling from the bed.
   4. Obtain an order for medication to sedate the client.

82. **A client taking lithium is discharged. After five days, she is still having difficulty with hyperactivity. She asks how long it will take for her lithium to be effective. The best explanation the nurse can give is:**

   1. "Each person is different. Lithium usually takes one to two weeks to be effective."
   2. "We are monitoring your blood level to see when it is in the therapeutic range. At that point your symptoms should be controlled."
   3. "You should see an immediate improvement. I will call the office so your psychiatrist can increase your dose."
   4. "You will begin to see some improvement when your blood level reaches the therapeutic range, but it still may be a while before your symptoms are controlled."

83. **A client has a fractured right tibia. The nurse knows that, immediately following cast application, the priority is which of the following?**

   1. Perform a complete neurovascular assessment.
   2. Encourage adequate nutritional intake of calcium.

3. Air dry the cast.
4. Monitor drainage through the cast.

84. **A 56-year-old client, admitted with hypertension and a baseline blood pressure of 160/98, is started on guanethidine (Ismelin) 10 mg p.o. every day. Which of the following findings by the nurse would require notification of the physician?**

1. Blood pressure of 134/62.
2. Apical pulse of 52.
3. Serum sodium of 144 mEq/L.
4. Serum potassium of 4.8 mEq/L.

85. **Which of the following vital sign assessments would indicate to the nurse that a client may be in cardiogenic shock after a myocardial infarction?**

1. BP - 180/100, P - 90, irregular.
2. BP - 130/80, P - 100 regular.
3. BP - 90/50, P - 50 regular.
4. BP - 80/60, P - 110, irregular.

86. **A client is to be up in a chair three times a day. He is paralyzed from the waist down. What is the best nursing approach when transferring the client from a bed into a wheelchair?**

1. Place the wheelchair close to the foot of the bed.
2. Utilize the principles of body mechanics while providing a safe transfer for the client.
3. Slide the client to the edge of the bed, keeping the nurse's back straight and using a rocking motion to pull the client.
4. Place the nurse's arms under the client's axillae from the back of the client.

87. **Which of the following enzyme studies should the nurse recognize as the most reliable indicator of acute myocardial damage?**

1. Lactic dehydrogenase isoenzyme LDH1.
2. Lactic dehydrogenase isoenzyme LDH2.
3. Creatine kinase CPK-MB.
4. Creatine kinase CPK.

88. **A client is about to be discharged from the hospital on phenytoin (Dilantin). What comment should alert the nurse that further teaching is needed?**

1. "I will notify my dentist that I am taking this medication."
2. "I'll be glad when I am free of seizures, so I can stop taking this medicine."
3. "I know that I cannot substitute other brands of this medication."
4. "I will notify my doctor before taking any other medications."

89. **A client has a tracheostomy tube in place following a complete laryngectomy. Which of the following correctly describes an aspect of tracheostomy suctioning by the nurse?**

1. Apply suction for 10 to 15 seconds while withdrawing the catheter.
2. Hyperoxygenate for several deep breaths with the ambu bag after each procedure.
3. Maintain clean technique at all times while suctioning.
4. Suction the oral cavity prior to suctioning the tracheostomy tube.

90. **A gestational diabetic had a baby who weighs 4200 grams. It is estimated to be a 40-week LGA baby. The mother has heard that "fat" babies are not healthy. She asks that the baby receive only sterile water in the nursery and wants to limit the frequency of breastfeeding to every three to four hours from birth. The best response from the nurse would be based on which rationale?**

1. Due to maternal gestational diabetes, the infant experiences hyperinsulinemia, and more frequent feedings and/or glucose water may be needed to prevent hypoglycemia.
2. Being larger than normal, LGA babies should be limited in their intake from birth so they do not continue to be "fat" babies.
3. Being larger than normal, LGA babies are hungrier and should be allowed to eat all they want.
4. Due to maternal gestational diabetes, the infant experiences hyperglycemia immediately after birth due to excessive glucose passing the placental barrier, so the mother's request is appropriate.

91. **The nurse provides preoperative teaching for a client. Which of the following statements by the client indicates an understanding of the information?**

1. "Coughing and deep breathing will probably be painful after surgery."
2. "Since I don't smoke, I probably won't have to deep breathe and cough after surgery."
3. "Show my daughter, so she can help me after surgery."
4. "I should move as little as possible to decrease any pain from the incision."

92. **A client had a mitral commissurotomy yesterday. Which of the following lab values gives the nurse the best indication of his renal function?**

1. Blood urea nitrogen (BUN).
2. Serum creatinine.

3. Urine specific gravity.
4. Serum albumin.

93. **When assessing a child with a cast, which of the following observations would be of most immediate concern to the nurse?**

   1. Itching at the cast site.
   2. Indentations in the cast.
   3. Swelling distal to the cast.
   4. "Hot spots" on the cast.

94. **An emergency room nurse admits a three-year-old girl with a two-day history of a sore throat. The child is pale in color, drooling, and very restless. Which of the following orders would the nurse question as inappropriate?**

   1. Place the head of bed up 90 degrees.
   2. Remain with the client at all times.
   3. Obtain a throat culture specimen.
   4. Keep a tracheostomy set at the bedside.

95. **Which of the following statements, if made by a female client taking hydralazine (Apresoline), would indicate to the nurse that the client understands the instructions given about the medication regimen?**

   1. "I'll take my blood pressure daily and report any change to the physician."
   2. "I'll weigh myself once a month and report a gain of five pounds to the physician."
   3. "I have to stop eating canned vegetables and sandwich meats like bologna."
   4. "I'll be glad when I can stop taking this medication. I can't wear my wedding ring because of the swelling in my hands."

96. **The nurse understands that all of the following statements about reality testing are accurate except:**

   1. It is an ego function.
   2. It is the capacity to distinguish thoughts, feelings, fantasies, and other experiences that originate inside the individual from those which are part of the outside environment.
   3. It is impaired in psychotic individuals.
   4. It is impaired in persons who are mentally retarded.

97. **A client is admitted in hypertensive crisis due to a pheochromocytoma. The physician orders nitroprusside (Nitropress) IV at 3 mcg/kg/min. In addition to the routine assessments, which of the following interventions is most critical for the nurse to include in her plan of care?**

   1. Place the client in modified Trendelenburg position.
   2. Prepare the client for an arterial line (A-line) insertion.
   3. Provide a darkened, quiet environment for the client.
   4. Obtain an infusion pump for the Nitropress.

98. **The nurse understands that all of the following statements about the "dopamine hypothesis" in schizophrenia are accurate except?**

   1. Most antipsychotic drugs block the effects of dopamine and receptor sites in the brain.
   2. Amphetamine enhances dopamine activity in the brain and can cause a psychotic response that is indistinguishable from paranoid schizophrenia.
   3. The potency of antipsychotic drugs seems to be related to their antidopamine action.
   4. Schizophrenic clients excrete excessive amounts of dopamine in their urine.

99. **A client, age 68, is admitted with possible rheumatic endocarditis. Which of the following, if found in her medical history, would help to confirm this diagnosis?**

   1. Congestive heart failure.
   2. Tuberculosis.
   3. Strep throat.
   4. Coronary artery disease.

100. **A client with obsessive-compulsive disorder asks the nurse if he will ever be able to "live like a normal person?" Which of the following responses is most therapeutic by the nurse?**

   1. "You definitely can be helped with family and individual therapy."
   2. "It's not always possible to free a person from his symptoms."
   3. "You sound pretty discouraged. Is that how you are feeling?"
   4. "That goal is within your reach, although it will require a lot of hard work."

NOTES

NCLEX-RN

Test 5

Questions with Rationales

NCLEX-RN TEST 5 WITH RATIONALES

1. A 56-year-old male client has had a CVA and a homonymous hemianopsia. An improvement related to this condition that the nurse might document in a positive evaluation statement would be that the client now:

   1. Maintains communication with others.
   2. Walks with a cane.
   3. Has frequent episodes of crying.
   4. Visually scans while eating.

   1. *Incorrect. This would be appropriate if the case scenario had stated aphasia as the dysfunction.*
   2. *Incorrect. Did you think the case scenario read "hemiplegia?"*
   3. *No, hemianopsia doesn't mean labile emotions.*
   4. ***Very good! You knew that the hemianopsia is a defect in the visual field.***

2. A 78-year-old is admitted to the hospital for an exploratory laparotomy. The client anxiously says to the nurse, "Do you think that the doctor can fix whatever is wrong with me?" Which response by the nurse would be best initially?

   1. "That question can only be answered after your surgery."
   2. "People your age frequently have problems that can be corrected by surgery."
   3. "You need to get more information from your doctor."
   4. "You must be worried about what the doctor might find."

   1. *Wrong. The client's words and actions indicate that he is anxious. The key word in this question is "initially." The nurse should initially focus on the client's feelings. This statement puts the client's concern on hold.*
   2. *Wrong. This kind of a generalization devalues the client's feelings.*
   3. *No, because the nurse is putting the client's concern on hold. Whenever this type of "pass the buck" answer appears, the astute test-taker looks for something that the nurse should do before, or instead of, referring to the doctor. The key word in this question is "initially." The nurse should first focus on the client's feelings.*
   4. ***Correct. The client's words and actions indicate that he is anxious. The key word in the stem of this question is "initially." The nurse should first focus on the client's feelings. In this response, the nurse uses the therapeutic communication tool of empathy. This response focuses on***

   the client's feelings and encourages him to more clearly state what he is feeling. After his feelings have been addressed, the client may be ready for additional information.

3. The nurse would avoid including which information in the teaching plan for a client who is using eye medications for glaucoma?

   1. Instill the drops without touching the dropper to the eye.
   2. Store the medication at the proper temperature, refer to the directions.
   3. Vision may become blurred after instillation, the client needs to use precautions.
   4. The medication is taken for two to three weeks and then discontinued.

   1. *Incorrect choice. Proper instillation is necessary to prevent infections, and to get the best results. This is a false response question and the correct option is one that is not accurate.*
   2. *Wrong choice! Eye medications must be stored properly. Some need refrigeration and all must be checked for expiration dates.*
   3. *Incorrect choice! Blurring of vision is very likely. If this happens, the client may fall or have an accident. Remember, this question has a false response stem and is asking for a response that is not accurate.*
   4. ***Correct. This statement is not accurate and does not need to be taught to clients. Glaucoma medications will be taken for life.***

4. During a preoperative interview for a seven-year-old female, the child's mother requests information to prepare her daughter for hospitalization. The interview is being conducted three days prior to admission for a tonsillectomy. The child was hospitalized last year for a fractured femur. Which of the following would best meet this child's needs for preparation?

   1. Suggest a role play, and provide materials.
   2. Remind the child of the experience of her past hospitalization.
   3. Read her a story about another child having a similar operation.
   4. Tell her she is only going in to have her throat checked.

   1. ***Yes, concrete experiences are the most meaningful learning for the school age child. This is the rationale for pediatric orientation programs. Even***

if there is inadequate time for her to participate in such a program, a shortened version where she could practice with a mask and other equipment in a non-threatening environment, would be helpful.

2. *No. Past experiences, especially traumatic ones may not have been positive.*

3. *No, this isn't the best response. This is somewhat abstract, and abstract thinking is not highly developed in the seven-year-old child. Think about how you learned what an operation was really like for a client.*

4. *Wrong! Never lie to a child. This is inappropriate under any circumstances.*

5. **In contrast to clients with anorexia nervosa, the nurse knows that which of the following characteristics are common among clients with bulimia?**

    1. Recognize their eating behavior is abnormal.
    2. Rarely suffer serious medical consequences.
    3. Have positive feelings about their eating patterns.
    4. Vomit after eating or use laxatives to purge the food.

    1. *Correct. Bulimic clients are aware that their eating behavior is abnormal, and during binges fear that they won't be able to stop eating voluntarily. Anorexic clients typically deny that they have an eating disorder.*

    2. *This is not an accurate statement. Bulimia is associated with many medical problems and some can become life-threatening. The most common problems are menstrual irregularities, enlarged parotid glands, dental caries, esophagitis, tears or rupture of the esophagus, hypokalemia, and aspiration pneumonia.*

    3. *This is not an accurate statement. Bulimics often suffer from depression and are self-critical and intensely ashamed of their eating behavior. In contrast, anorexics often express a sense of pride about their eating behavior and loss of weight.*

    4. *This is not an accurate statement. Both bulimic and anorexic clients terminate their eating binges by self-induced vomiting or laxative use.*

6. **A client questions the nurse concerning the usual course of multiple sclerosis. What would be the most appropriate response by the nurse?**

    1. "Each client is different, we cannot tell what will happen."
    2. "I can see that you are worried, but it's too soon to predict what will happen."
    3. "Usually, acute episodes are followed by remissions, which may last a long time."
    4. "It's too early to think about the future; let's focus on the present and go day-by-day."

1. *Wrong response. This provides no information to the client and blocks further communication.*

2. *Incorrect. The nurse acknowledges the client's feelings, but then blocks communication by not providing any information to help address her fears.*

3. **Good choice! The nurse provides factual information while giving the client some realistic hope.**

4. *Incorrect. Remember that giving advice is a block to communication and will stop the client from feeling free enough to express concerns and fears.*

7. **Following a colostomy, a client and his wife have been taught to perform a colostomy irrigation. Which behavior would best indicate readiness for discharge?**

    1. The client's wife verbalizes all steps in the irrigation procedure.
    2. The client performs the irrigation following written instructions.
    3. The client and his wife attend all classes given about colostomy care.
    4. The client asks appropriate questions about irrigations.

    1. *No, this is not the best response. Consider teaching/learning theory and how readiness is best evaluated.*

    2. **Yes, this is right. The client has demonstrated ability to perform the skill using the instructions that he will have when he is at home.**

    3. *Sounds good, but this doesn't prove competence in the skill.*

    4. *No, this demonstrates involvement and effort, but not skill in the procedure.*

8. **A client, 34, is admitted for the third time to a psychiatric hospital with a diagnosis of schizophrenia. The police found her wandering along the highway. When questioned, she was not able to give a coherent answers to any questions. During the admission procedure, the nurse notices that her appearance is unkempt and she appears to be actively hallucinating. The initial nursing priority is to assess which of the following?**

    1. Her mental status.
    2. Her ability to follow directions.
    3. Her perception of reality.
    4. Her physical health needs.

    1. *Wrong! This is important but it is not the highest priority initially.*

    2. *No. This is important because it is part of the assessment of her mental status but it is not the highest initial priority.*

    3. *Her perception of reality is important for setting realistic goals and determining safety needs, but it is not the initial priority.*

4. Correct. The client's problems may be due to a physical illness or injury, or to fluid and electrolyte imbalance. Assessing her physical health needs should be the initial priority for the nurse.

9. A client gave birth to a six-pound baby boy. The Apgar score was nine at one minute. In the delivery room, the nurse administered parenteral vitamin K (Aquamephyton) to the baby. The nurse understands that the best rationale for giving the baby vitamin K is that:

1. Infants are usually born with vitamin K deficiency unless large doses are given to the mother prenatally.
2. Vitamin K is poorly absorbed from the gastrointestinal tract and must be given parenterally.
3. Vitamin K is normally produced by bacteria in the intestine. Infants are born with a sterile intestine.
4. There is no infant formula available that contains significant quantities of vitamin K.

1. Wrong! Large doses of vitamin K are not routinely given to mothers prenatally. Vitamin K is normally produced by bacteria in the intestine. Since infants are born without bacteria in their intestines, they cannot initially produce this vitamin. It is administered in the delivery room to assure the infant's ability to form blood clots.

2. This statement is false. Vitamin K can be given either orally or parenterally. Vitamin K is normally produced by bacteria in the intestine. Since infants are born without bacteria in their intestines, they cannot initially produce this vitamin. It is administered in the delivery room to ensure that the infant is able to form blood clots.

3. Good choice! Vitamin K is normally produced by bacteria in the intestine. Since infants are born without bacteria in their intestines, they cannot initially produce this vitamin. It is administered in the delivery room to assure the infant's ability to form blood clots.

4. Wrong! Vitamin K is normally produced by bacteria in the intestine. Since infants are born without bacteria in their intestines, they cannot initially produce this vitamin. It is administered in the delivery room to assure the infant's ability to form blood clots.

10. A client does not return her mother's greeting and instead lies down on the bed and curls up in the fetal position. The nurse observes the behavior and concludes the defense mechanism that the client is displaying is:

1. Fixation.
2. Symbolization.
3. Repression.
4. Regression.

1. This is not correct. Fixation means not progressing beyond a given level of development.

2. Wrong. Symbolization occurs when one idea or object comes to stand for another.

3. Wrong choice! Repression is unconsciously removing something from one's awareness.

4. Correct. Regression represents a dysfunctional attempt to reduce anxiety and conflict by returning to less mature behaviors that help the client better tolerate the anxiety.

11. The nurse discovers that the wrong medication was given to a confused client, who had answered to an incorrect name. The physician is notified and states that the medication that the client received will not harm him and nothing needs to be done. Which of the following is the best nursing action following this incident?

1. Apologize to the client involved.
2. Make out an incident report documenting the occurrence.
3. Try to avoid being responsible for administering medications again, since this could have been a terrible situation.
4. Realize that everyone makes mistakes and continue on with administering the rest of the medications to the other clients.

1. No. Since the client is confused, he will not know what the apology is about. This action may make the nurse feel better but will not be of any value to the client.

2. Best choice! An incident report should be initiated whenever an error is made involving a client. If an adverse effect results and the caregiver needs to remember the events at a later date, the documentation will be available to refresh the memory. The incident reports are also used for statistical purposes in determining the types of incidents that occur. They help administrators to recognize when a particular problem occurs and if problem-solving will assist in preventing reoccurrences.

3. No. Refusing to administer any more medications is not realistic or practical. Although the outcome could have been terrible, accepting responsibility for the error and learning from the situation is important.

4. No. Although no one is perfect, the fact that the error was made should be acknowledged through documentation. The error may have been made because of understaffing or a variety of other factors that need to be addressed by administration. The error may have been carelessness on the part of the caregiver, which may be a pattern of behavior that needs to be changed for safe client care.

12. A client's urinary tract infection does not improve, and he is admitted to the hospital. His prescription is for sulfamethoxazole with trimethoprim (Bactrim). The nurse knows that over a period of 24 hours his urine output should be at least:

1. 500 mL.
2. 700 mL.
3. 1500 mL.
4. Over 2000 mL.

1. *This is incorrect. An output of 500 mL is too low for proper kidney function.*
2. *Wrong! 700 mL is too low for proper functioning of the kidneys.*
3. ***This is correct. At least 1500 mL output is necessary for the hospitalized client, in order to avoid a serious problem with renal toxicity.***
4. *Wrong! Rather than being related to the client's urinary tract infection and medication, 2000 mL would be considered polyuria, which may indicate diabetes insipidus.*

13. The nurse understands that the client with angina pectoris demonstrates pain that has which of the following characteristics, least likely associated with the pain of myocardial infarction?

1. It is relieved by rest.
2. It is substernal or retrosternal.
3. It does not radiate.
4. It is described as tightness or heaviness in the chest.

1. ***Correct! Anginal pain is usually relieved by rest and/or nitroglycerine, which is not the case with MI pain.***
2. *No, both types of pain may be substernal or retrosternal.*
3. *Incorrect! Anginal pain can also radiate to the neck, jaw or arms.*
4. *No. Both anginal and MI pain can be described in this way! MI pain is often described as crushing or viselike and is often more severe than angina.*

14. A nephrectomy is scheduled tomorrow on a three-year-old client. Which of the following is an appropriate preparatory nursing order?

1. Demonstrate by pointing on the child's body where the incision will be made the evening before the procedure.
2. Give the preoperative sedation as ordered with a small needle so that a bandaid will not be needed.
3. Ask the child's parents to leave the room while the preoperative medication is administered.
4. Explain the procedure to the child in simple sentences just before giving the preoperative sedation.

1. *Incorrect! This is too long before the procedure to explain to a three-year-old and it will increase anxiety.*
2. *No. The child does need a bandaid, because at the age of three the child has fears of mutilation.*
3. *No. The child needs the parents for support during the pain of the injection and for immediate comfort following it. Parents should only leave the room if that is their preference.*
4. ***Correct! The child should receive an explanation at an age appropriate level just before you are going to follow through. This approach promotes trust and avoids unnecessary anxiety.***

15. A 23-year-old gravida 1, para 0 is admitted to the hospital at 38 weeks with pregnancy induced hypertension. The physician orders bed rest, IV of 1000 mL Ringers lactate, four grams of magnesium sulfate bolus followed by a continuous infusion of two grams of magnesium sulfate in 1000 mL Ringers lactate. During the admission assessment, the nurse notes which finding that the nurse knows is inconsistent with the diagnosis of pregnancy induced hypertension:

1. Three plus protein in the urine.
2. Deep tendon reflexes of plus one.
3. Blood pressure of 148/98.
4. Plus one pitting sacral edema.

1. *Wrong! Symptoms of pregnancy induced hypertension include proteinuria, edema, and elevated blood pressure. Three plus protein in the urine would be consistent with the diagnosis of pregnancy induced hypertension. Because this question has a false response stem, the correct answer is something that the nurse would NOT expect to find in an assessment.*
2. ***Good! In pregnancy induced hypertension, the nurse would expect to find an increased deep tendon reflex, not a decreased deep tendon reflex.***

> **STRATEGY ALERT!** *Because this question has a false response stem, the correct answer is something the nurse would NOT expect to find in an assessment.*

3. *No! Symptoms of pregnancy induced hypertension include proteinuria, edema, and elevated blood pressure. Blood pressure of 148/98 is elevated and would be consistent with the diagnosis of pregnancy induced hypertension. Because this question has a false response stem, the correct answer is something the nurse would NOT expect to find in an assessment.*
4. *Not correct! Symptoms of pregnancy induced hypertension include proteinuria, edema, and elevated blood pressure. Plus one pitting sacral edema would be consistent with the diagnosis of pregnancy*

induced hypertension. Because this question has a false response stem, the correct answer is something the nurse would NOT expect to find in an assessment.

16. **Three days following a left simple mastectomy, the nurse finds the client crying and withdrawn after her physician has changed the dressing. Which is the best initial response to this situation?**

    1. "Would you like me to show you some samples of breast prostheses?"
    2. "Would you like me to contact the Reach to Recovery visitor?"
    3. "Are you angry about the loss of your breast?"
    4. "I've seen a lot of women who've had mastectomies and they do just fine and you will, too."

    1. *No, too early for this. You're skipping an important issue.*
    2. *Incorrect. This is part of the rehabilitation of the mastectomy client, but not the best response at this time.*
    3. *Great!! You weren't fooled into a teaching intervention before you deal with feelings. This is a fundamental principle of teaching/learning theory. If you felt uncomfortable about this direct approach, it is a question and at least opens the door for exploring emotions.*
    4. *Think about this one again. This statement is like telling the client that her feelings are inappropriate. This will limit the nurse's therapeutic interventions with this client.*

17. **The nurse would expect a client with hyperthyroidism to report which of the following symptoms?**

    1. Weight gain of 10 lbs in three weeks.
    2. Constipation.
    3. Sensitivity to cold.
    4. Flushed, moist skin.

    1. *No. Hyperthyroidism causes an increased rate of body metabolism, so the client will experience a weight loss.*
    2. *Incorrect. Hyperthyroidism is a hypermetabolic state. The client will have increased peristalsis diarrhea, not constipation.*
    3. *No. Clients with hyperthyroidism have an increased metabolic rate and are always "warm," due to the energy expenditure. They have heat intolerance.*
    4. *Correct! Clients with hyperthyroidism tolerate heat poorly and perspire unusually freely. The skin is flushed continuously, with a characteristic salmon color, and is likely to be warm, soft, and moist.*

18. **The nurse knows that which of the following actions is the most common cause of invasion of a client's privacy?**

    1. Over-exposing a client during a treatment or examination.
    2. Failing to pull the curtain while performing a treatment or examination.
    3. Talking about the client to other staff members who are not involved with the care of the client.
    4. Helping an elderly client with a tub bath.

    1. *Wrong choice! It is true that only the body part that is involved in an examination or treatment should be exposed in order to provide as much privacy as possible for the client. But this is not the most common violation of privacy.*
    2. *Wrong choice! It is true that the curtain should be closed whenever a client is to have a treatment or examination that may expose body parts. This is not, however, the most common violation of privacy.*
    3. *Correct! No information about the client, including personal concerns, diagnosis, and treatment, should be discussed with anyone who is not involved in the care of the client. Talking about the client is the most common cause of invasion of privacy in the health care setting. The nurse should take special care not to compromise this right by discussing client care in such places as elevators, restaurants, or other areas that are accessible to the public and where the discussion might be overheard.*
    4. *Although there is loss of privacy for the client when assisting with a tub bath, this is not the most common invasion of privacy.*

19. **A client has sustained a gunshot wound to her left side and has a closed water seal drainage system attached to a chest tube. The nurse notices continuous bubbling in the water seal collection immediately after insertion of the chest tube. Which of the following actions should the nurse take?**

    1. Notify the physician immediately.
    2. Clamp the chest tube.
    3. Continue to monitor for continuous bubbling.
    4. Reposition the client.

    1. *Incorrect choice, because bubbling that occurs immediately after insertion is normal.*
    2. *False. This prevents external air from entering pleural space. It is not necessary based on the facts in this scenario because bubbling that occurs immediately after insertion is normal.*
    3. *Good job! Fluid and air initially rush out from the intrapleural space under high pressure, so the nurse would watch for continuous bubbling.*
    4. *Not the best choice! This would not have any effect on leakage from the chest tube.*

20. An emergency room nurse takes a telephone call from a woman who reports she has just taken 100 amitriptyline (Elavil) tablets to kill herself. The woman is crying and says, "I want to die. I have no reason to live." Which of the following responses by the nurse is most therapeutic?

1. "Let me help you. I'm sure things are not as bad as they seem to you now."
2. "Is there anyone with you now?"
3. "How do you feel about what you have just done?"
4. "I'm glad you called, because I can help you. What is your name and your address?"

1. *This is not correct because the nurse's response is demeaning and condescending. Also, the nurse fails to acknowledge the caller is in a life-threatening situation. Tricyclics, taken in overdose, are highly lethal drugs.*
2. *This is a good response, but it is not the best option.*
3. *This is not correct. The nurse must prioritize nursing actions, and safety needs are more important than emotional needs for this client.*
4. *Correct. The nurse expresses her interest in helping the caller and also attempts to find out her location so she can get help to her as quickly as possible. This is a priority when the client's life is in jeopardy such as when she has taken an overdose of a potentially lethal substance. The nurse will then focus on keeping the client on the telephone until the emergency team arrives.*

21. Occasionally a client forgets to take her ibuprofen (Motrin). When this occurs the nurse would suggest to the client that she do which of the following?

1. Double the next dose.
2. Take the medication as soon as she remembers and then continue the same dose schedule even if doses are close together.
3. Resume the usual dosing interval.
4. Take half the dose as soon as it is remembered, then continue the dose schedule.

1. *Since there are so many side effects, the medication should not be doubled.*
2. *This is incorrect. She should space the medication to avoid gastrointestinal complications.*
3. *You are correct. If a client omits a dose, wait for the next scheduled dose, rather than taking the pill late; then resume the usual schedule.*
4. *This is incorrect. Since there are so many side effects, the medication should not be taken at too frequent intervals.*

22. During a nursing staff meeting, what information about safety for hospitalized suicidal clients is most important for the nurse to emphasize?

1. The more specific the plan, the more likely the client will attempt suicide.
2. Inhospital suicides are more likely to occur closely following admission than at any other time during the hospitalization.
3. Inhospital suicides are more likely to occur at changes of shifts or on weekends.
4. The person who makes a suicide attempt and fails probably will not try again.

1. *This is not the best option because it is not the most important safety factor for hospitalized suicidal clients.*
2. *Not correct. Suicidal persons may attempt suicide at any time during the hospitalization. The risk varies and should be evaluated on a daily basis.*
3. *Correct. Risk of suicide increases during periods when there is a decreased number of staff or at times when the staff are distracted, such as at changes of shifts. Close supervision of suicidal clients is vitally important at these times.*
4. *Incorrect. Persons with prior suicide attempts are at higher risk for suicide. Most successful suicides are committed by persons who have made previous suicide attempts.*

23. A client is a truck driver who sits for hours in his truck while driving. He has a swollen and inflamed right calf and is diagnosed with thrombophlebitis. He is hospitalized immediately, placed on bed rest and started on a continuous heparin infusion. He asks the nurse how long it will take for the heparin to dissolve his clot. What is the best response by the nurse?

1. "It usually takes two to three days for heparin to work."
2. "I'm not sure, ask your doctor."
3. "Heparin begins to work immediately, but it actually does not dissolve clots. It prevents new clots from forming, and the present one from getting bigger."
4. "Heparin thins the blood quickly."

1. *This response is not accurate. Heparin starts to work immediately. Coumadin takes two to three days to begin working.*
2. *No, this response is not appropriate because the nurse can answer this question.*
3. *Correct. Heparin does start to work immediately and does not actually dissolve clots. He will be on heparin for as long as a week and then go home on anticoagulants. It will be a while before he can return to work.*
4. *No, many times we hear of heparin thinning the blood, but this is not really its function.*

24. **A 22-year-old sustained a fracture of the tibia and fibula while playing football. A long leg cast has been applied, and the client is admitted to the orthopedic unit. In providing nursing care for the client, which of the following is a vital consideration?**

    1. Elevation of the leg in the cast on a pillow will minimize edema.
    2. Healing of a fractured bone requires an extended period of time.
    3. A long period of immobility may lead to atrophy of the muscle.
    4. Analgesics may be needed for pain associated with the fracture.

    1. *Excellent! When caring for a client with a newly applied cast, it is important to keep the affected extremity elevated to reduce swelling. Note that the words "leg" and "cast" appear in the question as well as in this option.*
    2. *While this is an accurate statement, it does not answer the question asked in the stem. The issue is a newly applied cast, and the stem asks you to select an option that is a vital consideration.*
    3. *While this is an accurate statement, it does not address the question asked in the stem. The issue is a newly applied cast, and the stem asks you to select an option that is a vital consideration.*
    4. *While this is an accurate statement, it does not address the question asked in the stem. The issue is a newly applied cast, and the stem asks you to select an option that is a vital consideration.*

25. **The nurse administering acetaminophen (Tylenol) knows that it is used primarily for which of its clinical properties?**

    1. Analgesic and antipyretic.
    2. Anti-inflammatory and antirheumatic.
    3. Antiplatelet aggregation.
    4. Antileukocytic migration.

    1. *Correct! Acetaminophen has analgesic and antipyretic properties equivalent to aspirin.*
    2. *This is incorrect. Tylenol does not have clinical usefulness as an anti-inflammatory or antirheumatic.*
    3. *Incorrect! Tylenol does not have clinical usefulness in preventing clotting.*
    4. *No. Leukocytic migration is an inflammatory response and Tylenol does not have clinical usefulness as an anti-inflammatory.*

26. **The nurse knows that which of the following events is outside the scope of those required to be reported to appropriate agencies?**

    1. Births.
    2. Child abuse.
    3. Marital quarrels.
    4. Typhoid fever.

    1. *This is not correct. Births are required to be reported. The nurse should follow the institution's procedures.*
    2. *This is not correct. Child abuse must be reported, and the nurse should follow the institution's procedures.*
    3. *Very good! Marital quarrels are not subject to reporting requirements. This client data is protected by the client's right to privacy.*
    4. *Typhoid fever, a communicable disease, must be reported.*

27. **Which statement by a 14-year-old female would the nurse consider least attributable to normal adolescent development?**

    1. "I haven't gotten my period yet, and all my friends have theirs."
    2. "None of the kids at this school like me and I don't like them either."
    3. "My parents treat me like a baby sometimes."
    4. "There's a big pimple on my face and I worry that everyone will notice it."

    1. *Wrong. Adolescents constantly compare themselves to their peers and feel very isolated if there are any differences. The nurse would want to discuss this concern with this adolescent female. Most likely there is not a physical problem, just a difference in maturation.*
    2. *Yes. This is of great concern as the peer group is critical to adolescent development and sense of self-esteem. This needs to be explored in greater depth as this child could be at risk for many problems.*
    3. *Wrong. Adolescence is a time of struggle between independence and dependence. The same struggle also goes on with parents. It is a difficult time for both, and the nurse can be of assistance. It is a normal response.*
    4. *Wrong. Young adolescents especially think that everyone is looking at them and seeing all their imperfections. It is difficult for them to learn to deal with this and can be a major crisis for them as they learn to deal with acceptance of themselves.*

28. **When conducting a nursing interview with a client admitted with Cushing's syndrome, which of the following symptoms would the nurse expect the client to report?**

    1. Weight loss.
    2. Diarrhea.
    3. Double vision.
    4. Increased bruising.

1. *No, the client with Cushing's syndrome will have a weight gain due to overproduction of adrenal cortical hormone.*
2. *Incorrect. The gastrointestinal disturbances found in Cushing's syndrome are minimal. The major concern is for complications of peptic ulcer and pancreatitis secondary to glucocorticoid therapy.*
3. *No, there is no evidence of this visual disturbance in Cushing's syndrome. The only eye complications may be glaucoma or corneal lesions.*
4. ***Good choice! You remembered that clients with Cushing's syndrome have thin skin, which is fragile and easily traumatized; ecchymoses and striae will often develop.***

29. **A client is admitted to the emergency room with an overdose of acetaminophen (Tylenol). The nurse would expect to give immediate consideration to which of the following?**

    1. Slow respiratory rate.
    2. Nausea, vomiting and abdominal discomfort.
    3. Decreased urine output.
    4. Convulsions.

    1. *Although acetaminophen affects the central nervous system by blocking prostaglandins, it does not depress respiration.*
    2. ***Excellent! The principal feature of a Tylenol overdose is hepatic necrosis, which is manifested by these early symptoms.***
    3. *Wrong! Hepatic failure is the major concern in Tylenol overdose, not renal failure.*
    4. *Wrong choice! Coma may occur as a late symptom but is not one of the immediate symptoms for which the nurse would be watching.*

30. **A 25-year-old female client being treated with a cesium implant is found crying in her room. Which is the best response?**

    1. "I will come and spend ten minutes with you each hour."
    2. "Let's see if we can get a phone installed in your room."
    3. "We'll plan to admit someone to your room for company."
    4. "You will be discharged in two days, try to enjoy the peace and quiet."

    1. *Inappropriate. This would be considered a hazard to the well-being of the nurse, since limiting time with the client is necessary to control exposure to the radiation.*
    2. ***Great! This response recognizes the client's sense of social isolation and provides an appropriate, safe means of meeting her needs for contact.***
    3. *Wrong. Persons with radiation implants are placed in isolation. Time and distance are the factors that reduce exposure.*

4. *No, this response is saying that the client's feelings are not valid.*

31. **A 46-year-old client is two days postoperative following an abdominal aneurysm repair. Which nursing intervention will help to prevent the development of postoperative thrombophlebitis?**

    1. Have the client sit with his feet touching the floor.
    2. Apply gentle leg massage.
    3. Encourage the client to ambulate.
    4. Place pillows under the client's knees.

    1. *Wrong, because this position will help to prevent orthostatic hypotension, not thrombophlebitis.*
    2. *No. This is contraindicated since it may cause a thrombus to become an embolus.*
    3. ***Yes! Early ambulation promotes optimal cardiovascular function and helps to prevent thrombus formation.***
    4. *No. Pillows under the knees (popliteal area) will impede circulation. Pressure here should be avoided.*

32. **In assessing a newborn for congenital dislocation of the hip, the nurse should be alert for which of the following?**

    1. Symmetrical gluteal folds.
    2. Absence of Ortolani click on abduction.
    3. Limited abduction of one hip.
    4. Flexion of one leg while extending other leg.

    1. *Wrong! Symmetrical folds are a normal finding and indicate absence of hip dislocation.*
    2. *Sorry, this is not correct! The Ortolani click is heard when the head of the femur slips in the acetabulum. Absence of this sign indicates normal hip placement.*
    3. ***Correct! Limited abduction indicates that the head of the femur may have slipped out of the acetabulum. This is a sign of hip dislocation.***
    4. *Not correct! Flexion of one leg while extending the other is a normal newborn reflex.*

33. **The client has privacy rights that the nurse must not overlook. The nurse knows that the client's privacy rights include all of the following except:**

    1. The right not to have a gunshot wound reported.
    2. The right to refuse to receive visitors.
    3. The right generally to wear one's own clothing.
    4. The right to request the presence of a member of the same sex during a physical examination.

    1. ***Good work! Gunshot wounds must be reported. The nurse should follow the institution's procedures.***

> **TEST-TAKING TIP:** *This question has a false response stem and is asking you to identify the option that is false.*

2. *The client has the right to maintain privacy by choosing their company and may choose not to receive visitors.*
3. *The client has the right to wear personal clothing unless it interferes with medical procedures. An example of a situation where personal clothing would interfere is surgery.*

> **TEST-TAKING TIP:** *Words like "generally" tend to make a statement accurate. This question has a false response stem and is asking you to identify the option that is false.*

4. *The client does have this right, and such a request should be respected by the nurse.*

34. **A client is having a nonstress test. The fetal heart rate is 130-150 bpm, but there has been no fetal movement for 15 minutes. Which of the following is the most appropriate nursing response?**

    1. Encourage her to walk around the monitoring unit for 10 minutes, then resume monitoring.
    2. Immediately report the situation to her physician and prepare her for induction of labor.
    3. Offer her a snack of orange juice and crackers.
    4. Turn her on her left side and attempt to auscultate fetal heart sounds with a doppler.

    1. *No. A nonstress test depends upon fetal movement. Walking the mother is not likely to achieve this result.*
    2. *Incorrect. Failure of the fetus to move could mean fetal sleep or another benign reason. There are several nursing interventions that can be employed to awake a sleeping fetus.*
    3. ***Good choice! Most fetuses are more active after meals due to the high blood sugar in the mother. Giving the mother a snack will promote fetal movement.***
    4. *Wrong! Turning the client on the left side increases the placental perfusion of oxygen to the fetus but the fetal heart rate of 130-150 is not indicative of fetal distress. Since the nurse is able to hear the fetal heart with the fetal monitor there is no reason to try to auscultate with a doppler.*

35. **An 82-year-old widow is admitted to the hospital for hip replacement surgery. She appears alert and cooperative, although in great pain. While doing an assessment, the nurse learns she is disoriented to time and believes she is in a hotel. The nurse identifies acute confusion as a nursing problem and realizes the client's confusion probably could be the result of any of the following except:**

    1. Her age.
    2. Relocation to the hospital.
    3. Her physical pain.
    4. Bed confinement.

    1. ***Correct. Although acute confusion commonly occurs in persons over the age of 80, the condition is caused by physical and psychological problems that occur in advanced old age, not age itself. Acute confusion can be successfully resolved by diagnosing and treating the underlying problem(s).***
    2. *No, relocation to a new environment, particularly when the move is sudden or unplanned, can result in a period of acute confusion for an elderly person.*
    3. *No, pain or discomfort from unmet physical needs is often the cause of acute confusion in persons of any age, including the elderly.*
    4. *No, bed confinement, especially in a horizontal position, is often associated with acute confusion because the individual does not have access to the full range of visual cues needed to maintain good orientation.*

36. **A client has been taking morphine for several weeks to relieve her cancer pain. During the last two home health visits, she has complained that her dose does not seem to be working. What could explain the client's complaint?**

    1. She has finally become addicted to her morphine.
    2. She is becoming confused and probably is not taking her medications properly.
    3. A tolerance to the medication has developed.
    4. The pain medications are being abused, and the client needs counseling about her addiction.

    1. *Wrong. Addiction may occur; but with cancer pain and long-term use, the medication is still needed to relieve the pain. It would not be helpful to discuss this with the client.*
    2. *Incorrect. Not enough information is given to support this answer.*
    3. ***Excellent choice! Tolerance is an undesirable side effect of narcotic analgesics. It occurs when a larger dose is needed to produce the same response. Tolerance, however, does not occur for every client. It is unpredictable and sporadic.***
    4. *Not enough information is given to assume this answer.*

37. **Which instruction would be least appropriate for the nurse to include in discharge teaching for a client who had a vasectomy?**

    1. Wait 24 hours to bathe.
    2. Apply ice bags to the incision for the first 24 hours.
    3. Resume sexual activity without contraceptive measures within two to three days.

4. Wear a scrotal support for the first few days.

1. *No, it is appropriate for the nurse to include this instruction. The dressing must be kept clean and dry for the first 24 hours. Remember, this is a negative response stem question.*
2. *This is an appropriate instruction. Ice bags will help decrease edema. Remember, this is a negative response stem question, so the correct option is a statement that is NOT appropriate.*
3. ***Excellent choice! This instruction is inappropriate because contraceptive measures must be used after a vasectomy until sperm analysis is negative. This analysis is done five to six weeks after surgery or after l5 ejaculations.***
4. *The is an appropriate instruction. Scrotal support reduces discomfort and minimizes movement of the scrotum to decrease swelling.*

38. **During the early phase of alcohol withdrawal, what is the primary focus of nursing care?**

    1. Rest and nutrition.
    2. Assessing coping skills.
    3. Confronting the use of denial and other defense mechanisms.
    4. Education about alcohol abuse and treatment.

    1. ***Correct. Rest is important for two reasons. Alcohol abuse disrupts normal sleep patterns and alcohol withdrawal or detoxification is often associated with increased restlessness and agitation. Also, alcoholism depletes the body stores of B-complex vitamins and is often accompanied by poor eating habits. Restoring fluid and electrolyte balance, preventing dehydration, and improving nutritional status are other important goals during detoxification.***
    2. *This is not correct. The primary focus of detoxification is managing the client's physical withdrawal from alcohol. Meeting the client's physical needs are a priority until he completes the detoxification phase of treatment.*
    3. *This is not correct. The nursing priorities during detoxification are managing the client's physical withdrawal from alcohol.*
    4. *This is not correct. Education about alcohol abuse and treatment options is always important, but the primary focus of detoxification is managing the client's physical and medical needs.*

39. **A 13-year-old boy is admitted for an emergency appendectomy. While doing the preoperative teaching, he asks, "Will I have a large scar from the surgery?" The nurse's best response is which of the following statements?**

    1. "Most scars from appendectomies are not very large."
    2. "That isn't our biggest concern right now, let's get you well first."

3. "Don't worry, scars fade a lot in just a few months."
4. "It will be small enough so it won't show with bathing trunks on."

1. *Wrong. Although this isn't wrong, it's not the best answer. He may not even know where the incision is likely to be made. Think about the self-esteem issues appropriate to a 13-year-old.*
2. *No!! This response essentially says to the client that his concerns are of no value. Is that the message you really meant to convey?*
3. *Not right. If he has no experience with surgical scars, he doesn't know what it will look like initially. Besides, for the adolescent, "months" is a lifetime.*
4. ***Great! This includes concrete location, and allays fears that this will be visible to the world. You have recognized that his concern is body image. A large, highly visible scar would distinguish him from the "all-important" peer group.***

40. **A client is admitted to the hospital following an automobile accident. The client is to have a Foley catheter inserted. The initial nursing action when implementing this procedure is which of the following?**

    1. Using sterile technique during this procedure.
    2. Checking the client's identification.
    3. Placing all necessary equipment within easy reach.
    4. Explaining the procedure to the client.

    1. *Although sterile technique is used for insertion of a Foley catheter, the question asks about the initial nursing action.*
    2. ***Good! Identifying the client should be done before any of the other options. If the nurse approaches the wrong client, then none of the other options apply.***
    3. *Placing equipment within easy reach is recommended for any procedure, but it is not the correct initial action.*
    4. *The nurse should explain a procedure to the client before beginning it; however, this is not the initial action.*

41. **A client is being treated with pilocarpine (Pilocar) for his glaucoma. He complains of blurred vision after administration of his drops. Which of the following is the best explanation by the nurse of this side effect?**

    1. The client is not using the eye drops correctly.
    2. Pilocarpine (Pilocar) causes the pupil to constrict, making the eye accommodate for near vision. Therefore, objects far away seem blurred.
    3. When the pupil is dilated, it is more difficult to adjust vision.

4. Pilocarpine irritates the lining of the eye and causes blurring and inflammation.

1. *Incorrect. This would not be the best explanation. The client needs more facts.*
2. ***Correct. Pilocarpine is a miotic, which makes the eye adapt to near vision.***
3. *Wrong choice. Pilocarpine does not dilate the pupil. Reread the options.*
4. *Incorrect. Blurred vision is caused by pupil changes.*

42. **An 11-year-old female has suddenly developed a voracious appetite and has outgrown her clothes in six months. The mother is concerned and seeks the nurse's advice. The best response by the nurse would be which of the following statements?**

1. "Being overweight as a child can mean problems later on."
2. "What kinds of foods has she been eating?"
3. "The growth spurt does not occur until adolescence; let's check her weight."
4. "This is often the time when a growth spurt occurs. Let's talk some more."

1. *While this may be accurate, it is too early in the assessment to decide this. Explaining it in this manner may not be helpful to either the child or parent.*
2. *Wrong choice! This may be a piece of assessment data that may be valuable to have, but it would not necessarily be the first thing the nurse would ask. It does not focus on the mother's concerns as well as other responses would.*
3. *No! A growth spurt often occurs at around age 10 years for girls and 12 years for boys. It usually occurs two years before puberty.*
4. ***Yes! This statement is accurate and the nurse encourages the mom to share what is of most concern to her at the present time, which will yield the best assessment data.***

43. **In preparing to administer a medication to a confused elderly client, the nurse discovers that the client does not have her identification bracelet on. The client states that she has already taken her medication. Which of the following nursing actions provides for the client's safety?**

1. Ask the client if she might be confused about taking her medication.
2. Identify the client based upon which bed she occupies in the room.
3. Check the client's chart and ask another health care worker to identify the client.
4. Ask the client to identify herself, and obtain an identification bracelet for her.

1. *No! The client may not be correct in stating that she has already taken a medication, and this action by the nurse does not identify the client. This action does not provide for the client's safety.*
2. This is not correct, because the client may be occupying the wrong bed.
3. Very good! This action provides for the client's safety. The chart will contain other identifying information about the client and will indicate which medications have been administered. Staff members who have cared for the client are capable of identifying her.
4. No! The question states that the client is confused and that there is no identification bracelet. To provide for the client's safety, the nurse should take some other action to be sure that the client is correctly identified.

44. **At 12 hours of age, an infant's respiratory rate is 44 per minute. Her respirations are shallow with periods of apnea lasting up to five seconds. Based upon this assessment data, the nurse should do which of the following?**

1. Activate respiratory arrest procedures.
2. Call the physician immediately and report the assessment.
3. Continue routine monitoring.
4. Request an order for supplemental oxygen.

1. *Incorrect. This description of respirations is normal for an infant at 12 hours of age.*
2. *No, there is no need to call the physician. This assessment indicates normal respiratory function.*
3. ***Correct! This infant's assessments indicate normal adaptation of the respiratory system to extrauterine life. Continued monitoring is indicated.***
4. *Wrong. This infant's respiratory system is functioning correctly and there is no clinical indication for supplemental oxygen.*

45. **The nurse demonstrates accurate knowledge of the administration of a Mantoux skin test for TB by:**

1. Inserting the needle with the bevel up.
2. Administering 0.1 mL of PPD on the outer surface of the arm.
3. Using a 21 or 22 gauge needle.
4. Massaging the area after administration of the medication.

1. ***Correct. The tuberculin syringe should be held close to the skin, so that the hub of the needle touches it as the needle is introduced, bevel up. This reduces the needle angle at the skin surface and facilitates the injection of tuberculin just beneath the surface of the skin, to form a wheal.***

2. *No. The dosage listed is correct, but the injection is made on the inner aspect of the forearm.*

3. *Incorrect. A tuberculin syringe with a 26 or 27 gauge needle must be used.*

4. *No, the area should not be massaged after an intradermal injection. A wheal should form for accurate determination of a skin reaction within 48 to 72 hours.*

46. **An eight-year-old male child has had successful corrective surgery for a ventricular septal defect. The child's mother says, "My son really wants to join the swim club, but I know that is not a possibility for him." Which of the following is the most therapeutic response by the nurse?**

    1. "Would you like me to tell his doctor that you have a question?"
    2. "Do you think he is aware of his limitations?"
    3. "Would you like me to encourage him toward another school activity?"
    4. "Do you think there should be limits on his activity?"

    1. *This is not the best response. The nurse can deal with this.*
    2. *No, the expectation for corrective surgery for VSD is that the client's activity would not be limited.*
    3. *Incorrect. The child should be encouraged to engage in physical activities. Swimming is not a bad choice.*
    4. ***Good job! This question didn't fool you! The mother may be having difficulty adjusting to having a "well child." The nurse explores her expectations and concerns with this initial response.***

47. **A mother speaks with the nurse about her three-month-old son. She says that he was well until two weeks ago. At this time he has been spitting up after he eats. Now the vomit "shoots across the room." As soon as he vomits, he cries and acts very hungry. The best response by the nurse is which of the following statements?**

    1. "You need to burp him more frequently."
    2. "Have him drink Pedialyte."
    3. "Let his stomach rest for two hours."
    4. "Perhaps the doctor should examine him."

    1. *Wrong! More frequent burping and checking on the amount being fed at one time could help with some spitting up problems. The projectile vomiting should make the nurse concerned about pyloric stenosis. The infant should be seen by the doctor.*
    2. *Wrong! Pedialyte is an oral rehydrating solution that is excellent for infants and young children because it contains electrolytes. These symptoms*

sound like possible pyloric stenosis. The infant needs to be examined.

3. *Try again. Allowing the stomach to rest for two hours is good for vomiting associated with a viral infection. This infant has symptoms that sound like possible pyloric stenosis. This condition needs to ruled out through examination.*

4. ***This is the best answer. The symptoms of worsening "projectile" vomiting and the child acting hungry afterwards are suspicious for pyloric stenosis. The baby needs to be examined by a physician.***

48. **Which of the following actions would the nurse implement initially for a client in panic?**

    1. Determine the source of his anxiety by asking the client to describe the events before the anxiety occurred.
    2. Provide privacy for the client by moving him to a quiet area away from other people, and leaving him alone so he can regain control.
    3. Help the client describe his feelings, to begin to diagnose the problem as anxiety.
    4. Provide a sense of safety and security by remaining with the client, speaking in a calm manner and offering sedation if needed.

    1. *Incorrect! Assisting the client to determine the source of his anxiety is appropriate in mild to moderate levels of anxiety, but the client with a panic level of anxiety needs immediate relief from his overwhelming feelings.*
    2. *Incorrect option! A client in panic should not be left alone.*
    3. *Incorrect! The client in panic will not be able to deal coherently with his feelings until his level of anxiety is lower.*
    4. ***Correct. The initial goal for a client in panic is to obtain relief. Staying with the client, speaking in a calm manner and offering sedation are the best initial actions for the nurse.***

49. **The morning of the client's surgery for repair of an abdominal aortic aneurysm, the nurse should do which of the following first?**

    1. Administer pre-anesthetic medications.
    2. Remove the client's watch and rings.
    3. Check that the operative permit is signed.
    4. Discuss the postoperative complications with the client's family.

    1. *No. The nurse would not administer preoperative medications unless the surgical consent form has been signed.*
    2. *No. This is not necessary if the consent form is not signed.*

3. *Good choice! Informed consent is necessary to protect the surgeon and hospital staff from legal suit.*

4. *No. This should have been discussed with the client during preoperative teaching.*

50. **A client is taking furosemide (Lasix) 60 mg p.o. twice a day. The nurse is teaching the client methods to decrease the incidence of orthostatic hypotension. Which of the following statements is probably least appropriate for the nurse to include in this teaching?**

1. "You should rise slowly when you change positions from lying to standing."
2. "It would be helpful for you reduce, or eliminate, your alcohol intake."
3. "Try to avoid exercising in hot weather."
4. "Eat foods high in sodium to prevent dehydration."

1. *No, this is an accurate statement and would not require further teaching. Orthostatic hypotension occurs when the blood pressure drops significantly after an upright posture is assumed, especially if the client changes positions suddenly. Intravascular volume depletion should be suspected as a cause of orthostatic hypotension after diuretic therapy.*

2. *Incorrect. This is appropriate information to give the client. The client should be cautioned that the use of alcohol, which can lead to dehydration, may enhance orthostatic hypotension.*

3. *Wrong. This is an appropriate instruction. The client should be instructed to avoid exercising in hot weather as this activity may increase the chance of orthostatic hypotension secondary to dehydration. Remember that this sudden drop in blood pressure when an upright position is assumed is often caused by intravascular volume depletion.*

4. *Correct choice! If the client is taking diuretics to decrease fluid volume, it would not be appropriate to have the client increase sodium intake, which increases fluid retention. This action would negate the desired effect of the diuretic.*

51. **A client's bloodwork reveals the following: Coombs positive, Rh negative blood type, Rh (D) antibody titer negative. Her infant's blood type is Rh positive. Which of the following nursing actions is indicated for the client?**

1. Give her RHoGAM while she is in the hospital.
2. Tell her sensitization has occurred and she will not receive RHoGAM.
3. Tell her she will not receive RHoGAM because of the positive Coombs.
4. Tell her she will not receive RHoGAM because of the bolus blood type.

1. *Great job! The Rh negative mother giving birth to an Rh positive infant is at risk for Rh sensitization. The positive Coombs indicates that there is an antibody in the mother's blood but the negative Rh (D) antibody titer rules out the specific Rh antibody. Administration of RHoGAM to this mother will prevent antibody formation in the event any Rh positive red blood cells entered her system at the time of delivery.*

2. *Incorrect. The negative Rh (D) antibody titer rules out Rh sensitization in this woman.*

3. *Wrong. The positive Coombs means that there is an antibody present in this mother's blood, but the negative Rh (D) titer confirms that it is not the Rh antibody specific to Rh sensitization.*

4. *Wrong. This option does not make sense. There is no such thing as a blood bolus.*

52. **A client is post-craniotomy and is progressing well. While he is sitting in a chair, the nurse notices he begins to experience a grand mal seizure. The most important nursing action is to:**

1. Provide oxygen.
2. Restrain the client.
3. Insert an airway.
4. Lower the client to the floor.

1. *Not the first priority. Oxygen is provided if needed, but only if the client becomes hypoxic.*

2. *Never! Restraints are contraindicated as they may cause the client to harm himself. Resistance against strong muscle contractions may cause injury.*

3. *Never! Forcing the jaw apart while a client is experiencing a seizure can cause permanent damage to teeth and gums.*

4. *Correct! When a client begins a seizure in a chair, the nurse should gently lower him to the floor to protect him from injury.*

53. **A client is to receive eye drops. Which of the following actions taken by the nurse best prevents injury to the eye during administration?**

1. Apply gentle pressure over the opening to the nasolacrimal duct.
2. Hold the tip of the container above the conjunctival sac.
3. Instruct the client to look upward.
4. Deposit the drops into the conjunctival sac.

1. *Wrong. Occlusion of the nasal lacrimal ducts prevents systemic absorption, but does not protect the eye from injury.*

2. *Correct. The tip of the container can injure the client's eye and should not come in contact with the eye.*

3. *Incorrect! Having the client look up decreases the likelihood of a blink reflex but does not protect the eye from injury.*

4. *Wrong! Depositing the drop into the conjunctival sac helps to distribute the medication throughout the eye, but does not protect the eye from injury.*

54. **A newly diagnosed diabetic is receiving instructions regarding dietary management of his disease. In providing information, the nurse is aware that the most important objective in the dietary management of diabetes mellitus is:**

1. Control of the total calorie intake in the proper proportions to attain or maintain ideal weight.

2. An accurate distribution of calories from carbohydrates, protein, and fat.

3. Weight reduction to reverse the hyperglycemia.

4. Meeting energy needs while decreasing blood lipid levels.

1. *Excellent! Success of this goal alone is often associated with reversal of the hyperglycemia in type II diabetic clients. In a young client with type I diabetes, priority should be given to providing a diet with enough calories to maintain normal growth and development.*

2. *Although this is a focus of the diabetic meal plan, it is too limited in scope to be the major objective in the dietary treatment of diabetes.*

3. *Incorrect. Weight reduction may be an effect of the dietary management of type II diabetes, but it's not the major goal for all clients. Some clients may be underweight at the onset of type I diabetes because of rapid weight loss from severe hyperglycemia. The goal for these clients may be to help them regain lost weight.*

4. *Not the best choice. These are both goals of nutritional management of diabetes mellitus for selected clients, but are not the most important objectives. Look for a more global response!*

55. **In caring for a seven-year-old child who has lice, the nurse should instruct family members to do which of the following?**

1. Throw out all combs the child used.

2. Isolate the child with the lice in his room.

3. Remove all nits with a fine tooth comb.

4. Keep others away from the child as lice can jump.

1. *Not necessary. The combs that the child has used need to properly disinfected, but do not need to be thrown away.*

2. *Not necessary. The child does not need to be isolated in his room. He probably feels alienated enough with the stigma that lice infestation often brings. He should not share combs or hats, but*

can be around others, as long as his hair does not make contact with another's until after a lice-killing shampoo has been used.

3. ***You are right! It's important to remove all nits after using the lice-killing shampoo. The nits are eggs that can hatch into lice. The child will be reinfested with lice if this is not done.***

4. *Wrong! It's a commonly held myth that lice can jump. They cannot. Lice is spread by sharing combs, hats, or by having children's heads come in contact with each other. It can also be spread by sharing pillows that are infested.*

56. **When changing dressings for an HIV positive client, in addition to proper handwashing the nurse should do which the following?**

1. Wear a mask.

2. Wear gloves.

3. Maintain strict isolation.

4. Wear a gown and gloves.

1. *Incorrect. Masks are not necessary. Goggles should be used if splatter is likely.*

2. ***Correct! Gloves are necessary, and after handwashing, are the best protection from HIV clients.***

3. *Incorrect. Universal precautions are required to care for HIV positive clients, not strict isolation.*

4. *Incorrect. This is necessary only if the nurse's clothing may become contaminated.*

57. **In planning activities for depressed clients during their early stages of hospitalization, the nurse's best choice is to implement which of the following plans?**

1. Provide one activity a day to avoid fatigue.

2. Let the client choose an activity that is appealing.

3. Provide a structured daily program of activities for the client.

4. Wait until the client's mood improves and he or she indicates an interest in productive activity.

1. *Providing only one activity a day will reinforce the client's feelings of inadequacy and withdrawal. This is not the correct option.*

2. *Wrong. The depressed person has great difficulty making decisions, so this is not the correct option.*

3. ***A regular schedule provides structure for the depressed client who has difficulty making decisions and providing structure for himself. This is the correct option.***

4. *This is not a recommended approach because inactivity reinforces a depressed mood by preventing satisfaction and social recognition. This is not the correct option.*

58. **A six-month-old infant with sudden, severe colic and vomiting has been admitted for testing to rule out intussusception. In planning teaching for the parents of the infant, the nurse would include information on which likely treatment?**

1. Barium enema.
2. Manual reduction
3. High dose steroids
4. Double barrel colostomy

1. *Excellent choice! A barium enema is used to definitively diagnose intussusception. In addition, the pressure created by the barium enema may force the bowel to resume a normal configuration. Most children are treated with the barium enema and do not require surgical intervention.*
2. *Wrong! Manual examination is unlikely to reduce intussusception. Most intussusceptions occur at the ileocecal valve, far too high to be affected by manual endeavor.*
3. *Wrong! Intussusception is not an inflammatory process, but a mechanical obstruction; therefore, high doses of steroids would not treat the condition.*
4. *Wrong! In the event of surgical intervention, the nonviable portion of the bowel is removed and the bowel is anastomosed. There is no need to create any colostomy.*

59. **The physician has prescribed ciprofloxacin (Cipro) 200 mg IV every 12 hours for a client diagnosed with osteomyelitis of the left knee. The nurse should monitor the client for which of the following adverse drug reactions?**

1. Hypotension.
2. Bronchospasm.
3. Diarrhea.
4. Leukopenia.

1. *No, Cipro has no adverse effect upon the cardiovascular system.*
2. *Incorrect. Quinolones produce few adverse reactions, affecting only three body systems. The respiratory system is not one of them!*
3. *Good job! The most common reactions to Cipro involve the GI tract (2-10% of clients) with signs/ symptoms such as nausea/vomiting, diarrhea, and abdominal pain.*
4. *Wrong! Cipro may rarely cause eosinophilia secondary to hypersensitivity reactions—not leukopenia.*

60. **A client is scheduled for surgery. When the transporter arrives to take the client to the operating room, the client is sitting in a chair. The best action to get the client onto the stretcher is which of the following?**

1. Assist the client to get back into bed, and then move her across to the stretcher with the help of a drawsheet.
2. Have the client first stand on the chair and then get onto the stretcher.
3. Assist the client to hop up onto the stretcher.
4. Together with the transporter, lift the client onto the stretcher, keeping a wide stance and a straight back.

1. *Very good. The client should first get back onto the bed. Then, with the bed and stretcher at the same height, the client should slide across to the stretcher. This is the safest option for the client and staff in preventing a fall or back injury.*
2. *The purpose of a chair is for sitting, not standing. This is unsafe. A client could fall when climbing onto or standing on a chair, or the chair could slide out from under the client during the transfer to the stretcher. The client is at risk for a fall.*
3. *Wrong! The client could miss the edge of the stretcher and fall, which could result in an injury.*
4. *Wrong! Clients should be lifted only when necessary, to avoid a potential fall for the client and back injuries to the staff.*

61. **A non-pregnant woman is diagnosed with trichomoniasis and metronidazole (Flagyl) is ordered. Which of the following instructions would the nurse appropriately give to the client regarding the treatment plan?**

1. Both partners need to take the drug and abstain from intercourse until cultures are negative.
2. Only the client needs to take the Flagyl, but she should not have intercourse until her culture is negative.
3. If both partners are treated simultaneously they may continue sexual intercourse.
4. The male partner needs to be cultured and be treated with Flagyl only if his cultures are positive.

1. *Correct. When a woman is diagnosed with trichomoniasis both she and her sexual partner need to be treated. Abstinence from sexual intercourse until both cultures are negative will prevent reinfection to and from both partners.*
2. *Incorrect. Unless both partners are treated, the male will very likely reinfect the female.*
3. *Wrong, because the length of treatment may vary from partner to partner. Both partners need to be negative before sexual intercourse may be resumed.*
4. *Incorrect, because treatment of the male partner is done without a culture if his female partner has trichomonas. A culture is done on both partners following treatment.*

62. A 70-year-old client is diagnosed with benign prostatic hypertrophy. Which of the following nursing interventions is contraindicated following a prostatectomy?

    1. Administration of analgesics as ordered.
    2. Notify the physician of excessive clots.
    3. Irrigation of the Foley catheter as ordered and p.r.n.
    4. Rectal temperatures taken every four hours for the first 24 hours.

    1. *This is not contraindicated. Postoperative pain is usually mild, but expected. A non-narcotic analgesic is usually ordered.*
    2. *This is not contraindicated. Bright red bleeding or excessive clots could indicate hemorrhage, in which case the physician should be notified.*
    3. *This is not contraindicated. Irrigation of the catheter will ensure patency by preventing clots from blocking the catheter, thereby causing bladder distension and possibly fresh bleeding*
    4. *Correct choice! This is contraindicated. Rectal temperatures are not taken because of the close proximity of the prostate and rectum, and the potential of causing damage.*

63. A client has been taking phenytoin (Dilantin) for several years for her epilepsy. She has recently married and wants to start a family. What advice should the nurse give her about her medication usage?

    1. Epilepsy should not interfere with her pregnancy or medicine regime.
    2. She will have to be more careful regarding her weight gain while on Dilantin.
    3. There is an increased association with birth defects born to mothers who use anticonvulsants.
    4. She will need to increase her dose of Dilantin during her pregnancy.

    1. *This is incorrect. There is evidence that pregnant women who take Dilantin have a greater risk for infants with birth defects.*
    2. *Wrong! Dilantin has no bearing on weight gain.*
    3. *Correct! Birth defects are more common when the mother uses Dilantin, and this needs to be communicated to the client.*
    4. *This is incorrect. Dilantin would not be increased due to the greater likelihood of birth defects.*

64. When caring for a client using a cane, which nursing action would be most appropriate?

    1. Schedule physical therapy visits to strengthen muscle mass.
    2. Remind the client to place the cane on the strong side.
    3. Remove the rubber tips to enhance ambulation.
    4. Place the cane safely in the closet at nap and bedtime.

    1. *Wrong. While it may be tempting to try to strengthen the client's muscle mass, that decision is within the physician's domain and would require a physician's order.*
    2. *This is correct. The cane should always be placed on the client's strong side.*
    3. *This is not a correct nursing action. Any ambulation aid needs to have rubber tips on the end to prevent slipping. Removing the rubber tips places the client at risk for falls.*
    4. *This is not a correct nursing action. If the client has to go look for the cane, the client is in danger of falling.*

65. A client is admitted with a complaint of weight loss of 12 pounds in the last two months despite increased appetite. She is also experiencing increased perspiration, fatigue, and restlessness. A diagnosis of hyperthyroidism is made. Which of the following measures is it essential that the nurse include in her plan of care to prevent thyrotoxic crisis?

    1. Provide a quiet, low stimulus environment.
    2. Administer aspirin as ordered for any sign of hyperthermia.
    3. Maintain the client's NPO status until her anorexia subsides.
    4. Observe the client carefully for signs of hypocalcemia.

    1. *Good choice! Thyrotoxic crisis usually occurs in response to a stressor, and the client should not be exposed to other clients in the room who are very sick. Visitors should maintain a calm environment.*
    2. *Incorrect. Although fever is an additional stressor, aspirin is contraindicated since it displaces the thyroid hormone from plasma proteins and results in active thyroid hormone in the blood, which may exacerbate a thyrotoxic crisis.*
    3. *Incorrect. Anorexia, nausea, and vomiting may precede thyrotoxic crisis. The client should be encouraged to eat a high protein, high caloric diet to maintain weight and prevent negative nitrogen balance.*
    4. *Incorrect. Hypocalcemia is a clinical finding in hypoparathyroidism, and does not play a role in preventing thyroid storm.*

66. A client is in the seventh month of pregnancy and has symptoms of preeclampsia. When discussing diet, the nurse instructs her to eat a high protein diet and to avoid foods that have a high sodium content. Which of the following, if selected, would indicate an understanding of the dietary instructions?

1. Creamed chipped beef on dry toast.
2. Cheese sandwich on wholewheat toast.
3. Frankfurter on a roll.
4. Tomato stuffed with diced chicken.

1. *Wrong. Creamed chipped beef is very high in sodium.*
2. *No. Processed cheese is very high in sodium.*
3. *Wrong choice. Frankfurters are very high in sodium.*
4. *Correct choice! Diced chicken is high in protein and low in sodium. The fresh tomato provides a low sodium vegetable.*

67. **Which of the following statements made by a female client indicates to the nurse that she has an adequate understanding concerning the administration of nitroglycerin tablets?**

    1. "I will only have to take these pills for a few weeks."
    2. "I should take a pill after strenuous exercise to prevent an angina attack."
    3. "If I get a headache, I should stop taking the pills."
    4. "This drug is not habit-forming, so I don't have to worry about addiction."

    1. *Incorrect. The client will need to take the nitroglycerin tablets whenever she has an attack of angina. Angina is a chronic condition and will not disappear within a few weeks.*
    2. *No, the client should take a nitroglycerin tablet BEFORE strenuous activity. The client should be instructed that, whenever the client anticipates that activities or situations may precipitate an attack, the nitroglycerin should be taken sublingually, before chest pain begins. Because sublingual administration works fast, this route is ideal for short-term prophylaxis when exertion is anticipated.*
    3. *Wrong. Headache is an adverse side effect of nitroglycerin therapy, but it does not mean that the client should stop taking the medication. Lying down in a cool environment and resting may help relieve the headache; over-the-counter analgesic preparations may help.*
    4. *Correct. Nitroglycerin tablets are not habit-forming and can be taken as needed. It should be stressed to the client, however, that if chest pain becomes severe or is not relieved with nitroglycerin, the physician should be notified.*

68. **A client is taking methyldopa (Aldomet) 500 mg p.o. every eight hours. When monitoring the client, which side effect is the nurse least likely to observe?**

    1. Headache.
    2. Sedation.
    3. Tachycardia.
    4. Weakness.

1. *Incorrect. Headache is a common side effect due to vasodilation of the cerebral vessels. A headache usually occurs early in treatment and is transient (goes away after four to six weeks of treatment).*
2. *No. Drowsiness and sedation are common side effects of Aldomet, a central acting sympatholytic agent. The client should avoid driving a car or engaging in tasks that require alertness while experiencing these symptoms.*
3. *Right! The side effect that the nurse would expect to observe would be bradycardia; not tachycardia. Remember that the vasodilating effect of certain antihypertensives will lower blood pressure and also slow the pulse.*
4. *Wrong choice. Weakness is a common side effect when the client begins treatment with Aldomet. It usually goes away as the client continues to take the medication.*

69. **In planning the care for a child in Bryant's traction, the nurse will include measures to avoid which major complication?**

    1. Sacral decubitus.
    2. Inflammation at pin sites.
    3. Circulation impairment.
    4. Lack of adequate countertraction.

    1. *No. Prevention of skin breakdown is a necessary general care measure with children who are immobilized. The buttocks are slightly off the bed in Bryant's traction, however, so the likelihood of sacral decubitus is small.*
    2. *Incorrect. Bryant's traction is a form of skin traction. The weight is applied by adhesive traction strips. There are no skeletal pins.*
    3. *Yes, you are correct! Circulation impairment is a major concern with children in Bryant's traction for a number of reasons. The lower extremities are elevated 90 degrees perpendicular to the body, the traction bandages can have a tourniquet effect, and the traction may cause vasospasms. Routine neurovascular checks will indicate any possible complication.*
    4. *Wrong. Lack of adequate countertraction can present a problem for the child in Bryant's traction. A vest restraint can be used to maintain the proper amount of weight. This is a problem in setting up the traction, however, not a complication occurring from the use of the traction.*

70. **A 24-year-old client is taking amphotericin B (Fungizone) as treatment for histoplasmosis. The nurse ensures that the medication is to be infused slowly over six hours. If the Fungizone were to infuse too rapidly, the client would be at greatest risk for which of the following?**

1. Fluid overload.
2. Fever and chills.
3. Cardiovascular collapse.
4. Extravasation.

1. Incorrect. For IV administration, amphotericin B is mixed in 250 mL of dextrose 5% in water. A rapid infusion of this amount of fluid would not put a 24-year-old client at high risk for fluid overload.

2. No, fever and chills occur even with slow infusion of amphotericin B. Fever may appear in one to two hours, but should subside within four hours of discontinuing the drug. The client is usually premedicated with acetaminophen.

3. Correct. Rapid infusion may cause cardiovascular collapse. The medication is never given in less than two hours; the usual time frame is four to six hours. Vital signs are monitored every 30 minutes for the first four hours of infusion to detect early signs of hypotension or arrhythmias.

4. No, a too rapid infusion would not necessarily put the client at high risk for extravasation, since a large vein would have been accessed for administration of this irritant drug.

71. **The nurse notes that a client frequently makes delusional statements. The nurse understands that the delusional statements are an indication the client is using which ego-defense mechanism?**

1. Projection.
2. Dissociation.
3. Displacement.
4. Regression.

*1. **Correct. In projection, a person attributes his or her own unacceptable emotions and qualities to others. This is the defense mechanism that is operative in delusional thinking.***

2. This is not correct. In dissociation, a person detaches emotional or behavioral processes from his or her usual conscious behavior patterns or identity. The client does not have amnesia or problems remembering who or where she is.

3. This is not correct. In displacement, the person redirects an emotion from the original object to a more acceptable substitute. Displacement is not the defense mechanism used in delusional thinking.

4. Regression is a defense mechanism used by persons with psychotic disorders. It is not, however, the defense mechanism associated with delusional thinking.

72. **During a postpartum assessment, one hour following delivery, the nurse finds a large amount of continuous rubra lochia with several moderate sized clots. The fundus is midline and firm at the**

umbilicus. **In regard to these findings, which of the following is the most therapeutic nursing action?**

1. Reassure the client that this is normal in the first hours after delivery.
2. Notify the physician who delivered this client of the clinical findings.
3. Massage the uterus frequently to contract the uterus.
4. Increase the rate of the IV bag containing Pitocin.

1. Incorrect! The assessments are not normal, the lochia should be intermittent associated with uterine contractions. Small clots are common in rubra lochia but moderate sized clots are a cause for concern.

*2. **Correct! Abnormal lochia in the presence of a firm fundus indicates that there may be a laceration somewhere in the birth canal. The only way to control this bleeding is to locate the laceration and surgically repair it. Since this is a physician responsibility the nurse needs to notify the physician.***

3. Incorrect. The fundus is already firm. Massage is not indicated in this situation.

4. Incorrect. Pitocin is used to treat uterine atony, but this is not the cause of the client's bleeding, as evidenced by the firm fundus.

73. **A client is admitted for fluid replacement. A diagnosis of hepatitis A virus is made. It is most important for the nurse to maintain which of the following measures in the client's plan of care?**

1. Strict bedrest.
2. Universal precautions.
3. Patency of the T tube.
4. A low protein, high fat diet.

1. Wrong. The client's activity level should be maintained. This is done through promotion of rest to prevent undue fatigue and decrease metabolic demands. Rarely is strict bedrest necessary. The client usually has bathroom privileges.

*2. **Good choice! Since the mode of transmission of this virus is the fecal oral route, universal precautions will prevent contamination of the nurse and others.***

3. Incorrect. A T-tube is not warranted for treatment of hepatitis A virus. A T-tube is utilized when the common bile duct is edematous and prevents the flow of bile.

4. Incorrect. Nutritional deficits can easily occur due to increased metabolic demands. In hepatitis A virus, there is an altered metabolism of fats, and fats are usually not well tolerated. A high protein diet is recommended to promote liver healing and improve activity tolerance.

74. **A biophysical profile is done and the client is told the score was 10, the highest score possible. She asks what this means. The best nursing response is which of the following?**

1. The fetus is in immediate danger; more tests need to be done.
2. The fetus is certainly mature and can be delivered at any time.
3. The fetus is healthy and may remain in utero safely at this time.
4. The score is appropriate for gestational age (AGA) of the fetus at this time.

1. *Incorrect! A score of 10 on a biophysical profile is indicative of fetal well-being.*
2. *Wrong! The score of 10 is indicative of fetal well-being but has no relationship to fetal maturity.*
3. ***Yes, best choice! A score of 10 is the best score possible, confirming a healthy fetus.***
4. *Wrong choice. This assessment is made only after the fetus is delivered using birth weight and gestational age.*

75. **A client appears apprehensive and says to the nurse, "One of the men in my office died last week from a heart attack." Which of the following responses by the nurse would be most therapeutic?**

1. "Tell me more about what you are feeling."
2. "Are you thinking the same thing might happen to you?"
3. "Your physician will not let that happen. This test will tell him how to best treat your condition."
4. "Has anyone in your family had a heart attack?"

1. ***Correct. This question will help the nurse and the client learn more about the specific reasons for his anxiety. Also, expressing his feelings is the best way to begin to deal constructively with his anxiety.***
2. *This question can be answered with a "yes" or "no" answer and is unlikely to provide any information about how the client really feels.*
3. *No, the nurse has not yet assessed the source of the client's anxiety. This response serves as a communication block since it offers false reassurance.*
4. *This question ignores how the client feels by changing the topic to an assessment of risk factors. It will not help him deal more effectively with his anxiety.*

76. **Which of the following precautions is appropriate for the nurse to give a client who is taking clonidine (Catapres)?**

1. You will need to be weaned off of this drug if the physician decides to discontinue it.

2. Light-headedness is rarely a problem with this antihypertensive medication.
3. You will need to have someone check your blood pressure each day while taking this medication.
4. Try to include more salt in your diet because this drug can deplete your body's supply.

1. ***Correct choice. Catapres, like all central acting sympatholytics, should not be stopped abruptly. Therapy should be discontinued gradually by reducing the dosage over two to four days to avoid rebound hypertension, restlessness, and anxiety.***
2. *No. Catapres reduces blood pressure by vasodilation, which can cause orthostatic hypotension (dizziness and light-headedness when rising quickly from a lying to a standing position).*
3. *Incorrect. Although blood pressure monitoring is an important component of antihypertensive therapy, daily monitoring is usually not necessary. Clients can be taught to monitor blood pressure at home two to three times a week and to bring the log to the physician's office at the next scheduled appointment.*
4. *Absolutely not! The client is instructed to restrict intake of sodium (salt) because Catapres can cause sodium and water retention. Central acting sympatholytics are used cautiously in clients with a history of congestive heart failure or cardiac disease.*

77. **Prednisone is ordered for a two-year-old client with nephrotic syndrome. The nurse can confirm the effectiveness of the prednisone therapy by noting which finding?**

1. The child's weight drops 500 grams.
2. The child's food intake increases.
3. The child's respiratory rate decreases from 25 to 16 breaths per minute.
4. The child's rectal temperature returns to 37° C.

1. ***Excellent choice! In nephrotic syndrome, prednisone acts on the body to decrease the excretion of protein and thus help fluids shift back to their normal spaces. The extra fluid is excreted in the urine. A decrease in edema can be measured by weight loss.***
2. *Wrong. The child's food intake may increase as the internal edema of the intestines subsides, but this is not the most direct way to assess the effectiveness of the prednisone.*
3. *Wrong. A normal two-year-old may breathe at 25 breaths per minute. Reduction in respiratory rate does not indicate a therapeutic action.*
4. *Temperature elevations are not common with nephrotic syndrome unless there is something else going on, or a complication. The body temperature is not in direct relation to the administration of the prednisone.*

78. **The nurse knows that the discharge teaching is successful for a client with hepatitis A virus if the client indicates she will refrain from which of the following activities?**

    1. Donating blood.
    2. Eating fried foods.
    3. Vacationing in a foreign country.
    4. Ordering a salad in a restaurant.

    1. *Correct. Once a person has been infected with hepatitis A virus, they can never donate blood.*
    2. *Incorrect. Although dietary fat is not contraindicated, it may not be well tolerated. The client should recover and be able to tolerate fats within two months.*
    3. *Incorrect. It is not necessary for the client to refrain from vacationing. This itself has no direct correlation to hepatitis A virus.*
    4. *Incorrect, although the fear is real if the initial infection of hepatitis A was acquired through eating at a restaurant. It is not necessary for the client to refrain from eating in restaurants forever.*

79. **How should the nurse respond to the anxious client who states, "I feel like I am going to die. Am I having a heart attack?"**

    1. Reassure the client that nothing bad is going to happen to him.
    2. Encourage him to reduce his anxiety by a physical activity such as pacing or trying some other relief behavior.
    3. Respond to the fear he has expressed by stating that he is not having a heart attack and will not be left alone until he is feeling more comfortable.
    4. Inform him, "No, your problem is severe anxiety."

    1. *Wrong! The client is in a state of terror and fears he will die. This response is ignoring the urgency he feels at this time.*
    2. *Wrong. The client with a panic level of anxiety is immobilized. Relief behaviors are only helpful for lower levels of anxiety.*
    3. *Correct. The nurse should respond to the client's expressed fear and then offer to stay with him. Clients in panic need to feel that someone understands what is happening to them and they will not be left alone.*
    4. *Wrong. The client is in a state of terror. This answer provides him with information but does not address his overwhelming emotions. There is a better option.*

80. **A client will be having an amniocentesis. The nurse asks the client to explain what the health care provider told her about the risks of this procedure. Which of the following responses indicates a proper understanding of the procedure by the client?**

    1. "I might go into labor early."
    2. "It could produce a congenital defect in my baby."
    3. "Actually, there are no real risks to this procedure."
    4. "The test could stunt my baby's growth."

    1. *Correct! The client needs to be aware that there is a risk of preterm labor following amniocentesis. With this in mind, the benefits of amniocentesis should outweigh the risks for it to be indicated.*
    2. *No. Amniocentesis is not done until after the 14th week. The fetus is fully formed at this time; any congenital defects are already present.*
    3. *Wrong choice! There are risks associated with amniocentesis such as labor, infection, bleeding and fetal injury.*
    4. *No, there is no correlation between amniocentesis and the growth of the fetus.*

81. **In a long-term care facility, the nurse finds an elderly client on the floor. After having the client examined by the physician, the most important nursing action would be which of the following?**

    1. Call the family and ask them to stay with the client.
    2. Provide for the safety and protection of the client.
    3. Apply wrist and leg restraints to prevent the client from falling from the bed.
    4. Obtain an order for medication to sedate the client.

    1. *Having a member of the family stay with the client may be a possibility if it can be arranged. This provides for the client's safety and allows some mobility for the client while in bed but it is not the best option. Read all the options and select again.*
    2. *Excellent! This option in effect includes providing all appropriate interventions that address the safety needs of the client.*

    > **TEST-TAKING TIP:** *This is the global response option. It is a more comprehensive statement about providing for the client's safety.*

    3. *Incorrect! Applying wrist and leg restraints is not the first nursing action. Application of a vest restraint may be appropriate to ensure the safety of the client, since it provides mobility for the client, and is less likely to cause agitation of the client. Try again.*
    4. *Sedating a client often makes the client more confused and more likely to behave inappropriately. Other measures should take priority over sedation.*

82. **A client taking lithium is discharged. After five days, she is still having difficulty with hyperactivity. She asks how long it will take for her lithium to be effective. The best explanation the nurse can give is:**

1. "Each person is different. Lithium usually takes one to two weeks to be effective."
2. "We are monitoring your blood level to see when it is in the therapeutic range. At that point your symptoms should be controlled."
3. "You should see an immediate improvement. I will call the office so your psychiatrist can increase your dose."
4. "You will begin to see some improvement when your blood level reaches the therapeutic range, but it still may be a while before your symptoms are controlled."

1. *This is a possibility, because it is an accurate statement, but there is a better answer. Read the other options.*
2. *This is not accurate. Symptoms only begin to remit after the blood level reaches the therapeutic range. It can take up to two weeks for the client to achieve maximum effect.*
3. *This statement is not correct. Lithium dosage is prescribed based on the client's blood level, not clinical signs and symptoms.*
4. *Correct. There is a lag time between when the lithium level is within the normal range and the manic episode is under control. The length of time this takes varies among clients.*

83. **A client has a fractured right tibia. The nurse knows that, immediately following cast application, the priority is which of the following?**

1. Perform a complete neurovascular assessment.
2. Encourage adequate nutritional intake of calcium.
3. Air dry the cast.
4. Monitor drainage through the cast.

1. *Good choice! Neurovascular compromises must be detected in the early stages to avoid irreversible and permanent damage.*
2. *Incorrect. General good dietary habits are encouraged rather than just calcium intake, even though calcium promotes healing and bone repair.*
3. *Incorrect. Using unnatural ways to dry the cast is contraindicated. Drying of the cast does not take priority.*
4. *Incorrect. Monitoring of drainage is important to validate the amount, but it is not a priority.*

84. **A 56-year-old client, admitted with hypertension and a baseline blood pressure of 160/98, is started on guanethidine (Ismelin) 10 mg p.o. every day. Which of the following findings by the nurse would require notification of the physician?**

1. Blood pressure of 134/62.
2. Apical pulse of 52.
3. Serum sodium of 144 mEq/L.
4. Serum potassium of 4.8 mEq/L.

1. *Incorrect. This blood pressure is within normal limits and is the expected outcome when a client is placed on antihypertensive medication therapy. Recall that the normal adult values for blood pressure range from 100/60 to 140/90.*
2. *Right. Bradycardia (pulse rate less than 60) is a side effect of peripherally acting anti-adrenergics such as Ismelin. Remember that these drugs cause vasodilation by decreasing norepinephrine, resulting in a decrease in cardiac output.*
3. *No, this serum sodium level is within normal limits (135-145 mEq/L), which indicates that the client's electrolyte balance has not been disturbed.*
4. *Wrong. A serum potassium of 4.8 mEq/L is within normal limits (3.5-5.5 mEq/L). The client has no electrolyte imbalance at this time.*

85. **Which of the following vital sign assessments would indicate to the nurse that a client may be in cardiogenic shock after a myocardial infarction?**

1. BP - 180/100, P - 90, irregular.
2. BP - 130/80, P - 100 regular.
3. BP - 90/50, P - 50 regular.
4. BP - 80/60, P - 110, irregular.

1. *Incorrect. These vital signs are not seen in a shock-like state.*
2. *No, these vital signs are within normal limits.*
3. *Incorrect. The client in cardiogenic shock will be hypotensive, but the client will not have bradycardia.*
4. *Good choice! The classic signs of cardiogenic shock are low blood pressure, rapid and weak pulse, cold, clammy skin, decreased urinary output, and cerebral hypoxia.*

86. **A client is to be up in a chair three times a day. He is paralyzed from the waist down. What is the best nursing approach when transferring the client from a bed into a wheelchair?**

1. Place the wheelchair close to the foot of the bed.
2. Utilize the principles of body mechanics while providing a safe transfer for the client.
3. Slide the client to the edge of the bed, keeping the nurse's back straight and using a rocking motion to pull the client.
4. Place the nurse's arms under the client's axillae from the back of the client.

1. *This is not correct. The wheelchair should be placed as close to the position of the client's buttocks as possible for a safe and easy transfer. The wheelchair should not be placed at the foot of the bed.*
2. *Very good! The nurse is in control of the nurse's own body and the client's movement during the transfer. Providing for the safety of the client, and utilizing the principles of body mechanics to*

provide safety for the nurse and the client, is the best nursing approach.

> **TEST-TAKING TIP:** Options 3 and 4 describe specific actions that are correct in transferring a client, but Option 2 is the best option because it is a more comprehensive or global statement.

3. *This is an appropriate nursing action that addresses the safety of the nurse and client. Positioning the client near the edge of the bed will reduce the energy required to move the client to the wheelchair, and the nurse's back will be protected by using leg and arm muscles to move the client to the edge of the bed. There is another option, however, that better describes the best nursing approach in transferring this client.*

4. *This is a correct action that helps provide for the nurse's and the client's safety. Supporting the upper portion of the client's body helps to place the weight of the client over the nurse's center of gravity. There is another option, however, that better describes the best nursing approach in transferring this client.*

87. **Which of the following enzyme studies should the nurse recognize as the most reliable indicator of acute myocardial damage?**

    1. Lactic dehydrogenase isoenzyme LDH1.
    2. Lactic dehydrogenase isoenzyme LDH2.
    3. Creatine kinase CPK-MB.
    4. Creatine kinase CPK.

    1. *No, LDH1 is not the most reliable indicator of acute myocardial damage. This enzyme peaks later and is elevated longer than others; therefore, it's useful for diagnosing clients who may have had a MI but delayed admission to the hospital.*

    2. *Incorrect. LDH2 is not a reliable indicator of acute myocardial damage. It peaks later and is useful in diagnosing MI clients who delayed admission to the hospital.*

    3. ***Good job! CPK-MB is the most specific indicator for the diagnosis of acute myocardial infarction. It is always increased in cases of severe angina pectoris, coronary insufficiency, and acute MI.***

    4. *No, although CPK is a sensitive and reliable indicator of myocardial damage, it is not the most cardiac-specific enzyme.*

88. **A client is about to be discharged from the hospital on phenytoin (Dilantin). What comment should alert the nurse that further teaching is needed?**

    1. "I will notify my dentist that I am taking this medication."
    2. "I'll be glad when I am free of seizures, so I can stop taking this medicine."
    3. "I know that I cannot substitute other brands of this medication."

    4. "I will notify my doctor before taking any other medications."

    1. *No, the client understands that Dilantin causes an overgrowth of the gums; therefore, oral hygiene is emphasized and dental monitoring is important. You are looking for a sign of NOT having understood the effects of phenytoin.*

    2. ***Correct! This medication should not be stopped without the advice of a physician.***

    3. *Wrong choice! The client correctly understands that bioavailability varies with different brands so no substitutions should be made. You are looking for a statement that indicates the client does NOT understand the implications of use of Dilantin.*

    4. *Wrong choice. Many drug interactions can occur with Dilantin. You are looking for signs that the client does NOT understand the use of the medicine.*

89. **A client has a tracheostomy tube in place following a complete laryngectomy. Which of the following correctly describes an aspect of tracheostomy suctioning by the nurse?**

    1. Apply suction for 10 to 15 seconds while withdrawing the catheter.
    2. Hyperoxygenate for several deep breaths with the ambu bag after each procedure.
    3. Maintain clean technique at all times while suctioning.
    4. Suction the oral cavity prior to suctioning the tracheostomy tube.

    1. ***Correct choice! The client can become hypoxic and develop dysrhythmias if suctioning is performed for more than 15 seconds at a time.***

    2. *Incorrect. The client should be hyperoxygenated for several deep breaths with an ambu bag both before and after the procedure.*

    3. *No! All equipment that comes into direct contact with the client's lower airway must be sterile to prevent overwhelming pulmonary and systemic infections.*

    4. *No. Remember that the basic principle of asepsis is clean to dirty. The sterile trachea should be suctioned prior to the mouth.*

90. **A gestational diabetic had a baby who weighs 4200 grams. It is estimated to be a 40-week LGA baby. The mother has heard that "fat" babies are not healthy. She asks that the baby receive only sterile water in the nursery and wants to limit the frequency of breastfeeding to every three to four hours from birth. The best response from the nurse would be based on which rationale?**

1. Due to maternal gestational diabetes, the infant experiences hyperinsulinemia, and more frequent feedings and/or glucose water may be needed to prevent hypoglycemia.
2. Being larger than normal, LGA babies should be limited in their intake from birth so they do not continue to be "fat" babies.
3. Being larger than normal, LGA babies are hungrier and should be allowed to eat all they want.
4. Due to maternal gestational diabetes, the infant experiences hyperglycemia immediately after birth due to excessive glucose passing the placental barrier, so the mother's request is appropriate.

1. Correct. The infant born to a diabetic mother is at high risk for hypoglycemia in the period following birth. This is a result of large amounts of insulin production in utero to meet the high glucose levels the fetus received from the mother. This increased production does not stop spontaneously at birth so these infants need extra glucose to prevent hypoglycemia.
2. No. Limiting intake would be detrimental to the LGA infant's health.
3. Wrong. An LGA baby often is a poor eater and may need gavage of intravenous fluids to prevent hypoglycemia.
4. No. LGA babies experience hypoglycemia, not hyperglycemia. All LGA babies (born to diabetics or otherwise) need to be observed for signs and symptoms of hypoglycemia.

91. The nurse provides preoperative teaching for a client. Which of the following statements by the client indicates an understanding of the information?

1. "Coughing and deep breathing will probably be painful after surgery."
2. "Since I don't smoke, I probably won't have to deep breathe and cough after surgery."
3. "Show my daughter, so she can help me after surgery."
4. "I should move as little as possible to decrease any pain from the incision."

1. Excellent choice! This response by the client indicates that the client understands what is expected by the nurse and also that it may be painful. It also implies that the client is motivated to perform the breathing exercises. Learning theory emphasizes the importance of motivation for successful learning to occur. This question reflects the evaluation phase of the nursing process.
2. Wrong! This response by the client indicates that breathing and coughing is not important or necessary because the client doesn't smoke. The client does not understand that the breathing and coughing are needed because of the effects of general anesthesia.

3. Incorrect. This response puts the responsibility of the breathing and coughing on the daughter and indicates that the client is not motivated to learn this task.
4. This option indicates that the client does not understand the information that was provided by the nurse in the preoperative teaching. Clients are encouraged to move following surgery to increase circulation and prevent complications caused by stasis of body fluids.

92. A client had a mitral commissurotomy yesterday. Which of the following lab values gives the nurse the best indication of his renal function?

1. Blood urea nitrogen (BUN).
2. Serum creatinine.
3. Urine specific gravity.
4. Serum albumin.

1. No, the BUN is used as a gross index of glomerular function and the production and excretion of urea. Rapid protein catabolism will also result in an elevated BUN. There is a more sensitive indicator of renal function.
2. Excellent! A disorder of kidney function reduces the excretion of creatinine, resulting in increased levels of blood creatinine. Creatinine is a more specific and sensitive indicator of kidney function than BUN.
3. Incorrect. Specific gravity is a means by which the kidney's ability to concentrate urine is measured; it correlates roughly with osmolality. It is not a test of glomerular function.
4. Wrong choice. Albumin is a protein, formed in the liver, that helps to maintain normal distribution of water in the body colloidal osmotic pressure. Although decreased albumin levels are seen in nephrosis, the serum albumin level is not the test ordered to monitor renal function.

93. When assessing a child with a cast, which of the following observations would be of most immediate concern to the nurse?

1. Itching at the cast site.
2. Indentations in the cast.
3. Swelling distal to the cast.
4. "Hot spots" on the cast.

1. Itching may become a concern if the child scratches under the cast, particularly with a sharp object. Client education may avoid this problem. It is not, however, of immediate concern.
2. A wet cast should be handled by the palms rather than the fingertips in order to avoid indentations that can create pressure areas. Indentations in the cast of a child who is asymptomatic, however, are not of immediate concern.

3. *Correct! When there is edema and swelling in the casted extremity, the cast may act as a tourniquet, cutting off circulation. Neurovascular damage can quickly occur. In order to avoid this damage, the nurse elevates the casted extremity, monitors for edema, and reports swelling promptly.*

4. *Incorrect! "Hot spots" on a cast can indicate infection. Often, a window is cut so that the area can drain. While this is an important assessment to make and report, it is not as high a priority as assessing for potential neurovascular impairment.*

94. **An emergency room nurse admits a three-year-old girl with a two-day history of a sore throat. The child is pale in color, drooling, and very restless. Which of the following orders would the nurse question as inappropriate?**

1. Place the head of bed up 90 degrees.
2. Remain with the client at all times.
3. Obtain a throat culture specimen.
4. Keep a tracheostomy set at the bedside.

1. *This is appropriate because the child is exhibiting classic symptoms of epiglottitis, which can obstruct the upper airway. In order to maximize oxygenation, the head of the bed should be upright.*

2. *Monitoring this child is appropriate because the child is exhibiting classic symptoms of epiglottitis. Because complete airway obstruction can occur, the child should be monitored at all times.*

3. *You are correct! This child is exhibiting symptoms of epiglottitis. Reaction to a tongue depressor or culture swab can cause increased airway obstruction and should be avoided.*

4. *Keeping a tracheostomy set at the bedside is appropriate. This child is exhibiting classic symptoms of epiglottis. Airway obstruction can be rapid, with fatal consequences.*

95. **Which of the following statements, if made by a female client taking hydralazine (Apresoline), would indicate to the nurse that the client understands the instructions given about the medication regimen?**

1. "I'll take my blood pressure daily and report any change to the physician."
2. "I'll weigh myself once a month and report a gain of five pounds to the physician."
3. "I have to stop eating canned vegetables and sandwich meats like bologna."
4. "I'll be glad when I can stop taking this medication. I can't wear my wedding ring because of the swelling in my hands."

1. *Incorrect. This is not an accurate statement, and would require further teaching by the nurse. Blood*

pressure is normally variable and does not stay fixed at one number. Daily monitoring with reporting of small fluctuations would not be appropriate. Changes which reflect a move toward hypotension (B/P less than 100/60) or hypertension (B/P greater than 140/90) should be reported to the physician.

2. *Wrong. The client should weigh herself at least once a week and report a gain of two to three pounds to the physician. Apresoline can cause sodium and water retention. Remember that a gain or loss of one kilogram (2.2 lbs) is equal to a gain or loss of one liter of fluid.*

3. *Yes! This statement is correct and indicates that the client knows some of the dietary modifications necessary to decrease the in take of sodium (salt). Other high sodium products such as bacon, processed foods, potato chips, pretzels, cheese, and crackers should be limited.*

4. *No. This is not an accurate statement and would require further teaching by the nurse. Antihypertensive medications will need to be taken for life in order to control hypertension. Another issue: the swelling in the hands indicates edema and should be reported to the physician.*

96. **The nurse understands that all of the following statements about reality testing are accurate except?**

1. It is an ego function.
2. It is the capacity to distinguish thoughts, feelings, fantasies, and other experiences that originate inside the individual from those which are part of the outside environment.
3. It is impaired in psychotic individuals.
4. It is impaired in persons who are mentally retarded.

1. *Incorrect choice. Reality testing is an important ego function that refers to the capacity to distinguish inner experiences from those that occur in the environment and to have intact ego boundaries. The stem is asking for the option that is INACCURATE.*

2. *This is accurate, so it is not the correct option. Select the option that is INACCURATE.*

3. *Wrong choice. In psychotic disorders, the individual can no longer tell whether his or her own thoughts and feelings come from within, but instead may experience them as hallucinations and delusions originating from elsewhere. The stem is asking for an option that is false.*

4. *Good, you spotted the inaccurate statement. Reality testing is not impaired in persons who are mentally retarded unless they are also psychotic.*

97. **A client is admitted in hypertensive crisis due to a pheochromocytoma. The physician orders nitroprusside (Nitropress) IV at 3 mcg/kg/min. In**

addition to the routine assessments, which of the following interventions is most critical for the nurse to include in her plan of care?

1. Place the client in modified Trendelenburg position.
2. Prepare the client for an arterial line (A-line) insertion.
3. Provide a darkened, quiet environment for the client.
4. Obtain an infusion pump for the Nitropress.

1. *Not necessary. The modified Trendelenburg position is used when the client is in shock (hypotensive): the extremities are elevated 20 degrees, knees are straight, trunk horizontal and head slightly elevated.*
2. *Wrong. It is not essential for blood pressure to be monitored directly. The client's pressure will be monitored extremely closely (every two to three minutes) because a precipitous drop in blood pressure can occur and action must be taken immediately to prevent shock. Nitroprusside has an immediate vasodilating action that is short-lived: it's a potent antihypertensive drug.*
3. *Incorrect. Although this action is appropriate for a client who is hypertensive, it's not as critical as another option listed. Always think of client safety: the NEED to do versus the NICE to do.*
4. ***Absolutely. Because Nitropress is a potent vasodilator with immediate onset of action, it must be administered via an infusion pump to ensure an accurate dosage rate.***

98. **The nurse understands that all of the following statements about the "dopamine hypothesis" in schizophrenia are accurate except?**

1. Most antipsychotic drugs block the effects of dopamine and receptor sites in the brain.
2. Amphetamine enhances dopamine activity in the brain and can cause a psychotic response that is indistinguishable from paranoid schizophrenia.
3. The potency of antipsychotic drugs seems to be related to their antidopamine action.
4. Schizophrenic clients excrete excessive amounts of dopamine in their urine.

1. *Wrong choice. This is an accurate statement and this negative response stem is asking for an option that is INACCURATE.*
2. *Wrong choice. This is an accurate statement and this negative response stem is asking for an option that is INACCURATE.*
3. *Wrong choice. This is an accurate statement. Remember, this question is a negative response stem and is asking for an option that is INACCURATE.*
4. ***Yes, this statement is not accurate because schizophrenic clients do not excrete excessive amounts***

of dopamine in their urine. The dopamine hypothesis refers to the theory that an excess of brain dopamine may be the cause of schizophrenia.

99. **A client, age 68, is admitted with possible rheumatic endocarditis. Which of the following, if found in her medical history, would help to confirm this diagnosis?**

1. Congestive heart failure.
2. Tuberculosis.
3. Strep throat.
4. Coronary artery disease.

1. *Incorrect. A history of congestive heart failure has no correlation with rheumatic endocarditis. Try to recall the pathophysiology of the disease process.*
2. *No, there is no connection between TB and rheumatic endocarditis.*
3. ***Excellent! You recall that a streptococcal infection, usually group A beta-hemolytic streptococcus, is a major cause of endocarditis.***
4. *No, there is no connection between coronary artery disease and rheumatic endocarditis, which affects the heart's inner lining and valves.*

100. **A client with obsessive-compulsive disorder asks the nurse if he will ever be able to "live like a normal person?" Which of the following responses is most therapeutic by the nurse?**

1. "You definitely can be helped with family and individual therapy."
2. "It's not always possible to free a person from his symptoms."
3. "You sound pretty discouraged. Is that how you are feeling?"
4. "That goal is within your reach, although it will require a lot of hard work."

1. *This is not an accurate statement. Behavior therapy, sometimes combined with medication, is the treatment of choice for obsessive-compulsive disorder.*
2. *This is not accurate and does not convey any hope for the client. Current treatment frees most persons of their obsessive-compulsive symptoms. Even persons with particularly severe forms of this disorder can be substantially helped.*
3. ***Correct. The nurse is acknowledging his feelings. This is the first step in helping the client. When he has dealt with his feelings, he will be able to continue to work on his treatment goals.***
4. *This is not an incorrect statement, but it is not the best initial response to the client's questions.*

NOTES

NCLEX-RN

Test 6

NCLEX-RN TEST 6

1. A client was admitted for a severe episode of gastrointestinal bleeding. Prior to discharge, which of the following statements by the client would indicate to the nurse a need for further instruction?

   1. "If my arthritis bothers me, I'll take Tylenol."
   2. "It's a good thing I gave up drinking five years ago."
   3. "It will sure be good to have my morning coffee."
   4. "I'll take my Tagamet before I eat and at bedtime."

2. A client, age 65, is receiving doxycycline (Vibramycin) for actinomycosis (fungal infection). The nurse should observe the client for which of the following side effects?

   1. Photosensitivity.
   2. Constipation.
   3. Ototoxicity.
   4. Permanent discoloration of teeth.

3. A client is in labor and is admitted with a blood pressure of 86/52. She is four centimeters dilated and uncomfortable. The nurse should give immediate consideration to which of the following nursing actions?

   1. Call the physician to report the blood pressure.
   2. Turn the client on her side and retake her blood pressure.
   3. Reassure the client that everything is all right.
   4. Ask the client if she would like some pain medication.

4. A client received a large contusion on the head and a fracture of the femur. The nurse must be alert for possible complications. Which of the following signs and symptoms indicates a serious complication?

   1. An oral temperature change from 98.8° F to 98.2° F.
   2. A blood pressure decrease from 122/88 to 110/72.
   3. Increased pain at the site of the femur fracture.
   4. A change in respiratory rate from 18 to 32, with increased restlessness.

5. The client's mother brings clean clothing and toilet articles to the hospital. When the client sees her, she does not return her greeting and lies down on the bed curling up into a fetal position. Her mother responds by becoming visibly upset. Outside the room she asks the nurse, "Do you think I should not visit again until she is better?" Which of the following statements is the most therapeutic response by the nurse?

   1. "It is important for the client to maintain contact with her family. Continue to make brief visits, every day if you can."
   2. "This has been an upsetting experience for you. Let's go into the lounge where we can talk privately for a few minutes."
   3. "I think that might be best. I will stay with the client until she seems to feel better."
   4. "Do you have any idea why your daughter responded as she did?"

6. The nurse understands which of the following is a goal of remotivation therapy in long-term care facilities?

   1. To stimulate and encourage social participation.
   2. To reorient clients with cognitive problems.
   3. To share memories of past experiences and events.
   4. To resolve emotional problems.

7. The nurse understands that epinephrine (Epifrin) can be used for open angle glaucoma because of which of the following effects?

   1. Pupil dilatation.
   2. Pupil constriction.
   3. Reducing the aqueous formation and enhancing outflow.
   4. Increasing aqueous formation.

8. A client is admitted in acute renal failure and undergoes peritoneal dialysis. Immediately after infusing 2,000 mL of 2.5% Dialysate, the nurse should do which of the following first?

   1. Clamp the inflow tubing.
   2. Monitor the client's vital signs.
   3. Assess the outflow fluid.
   4. Weigh the client.

9. A client will go home on warfarin (Coumadin). What is important for the nurse to include in the teaching plan for the client?

1. The client should carry an ID card with him at all times.
2. The client should take only aspirin for headaches.
3. The client should eat lots of foods high in vitamin K, like broccoli, liver and spinach.
4. The client should avoid any exercise.

10. **The nurse is preparing medications for administration in a pediatric unit. Which of the following actions by the nurse is least appropriate?**

    1. Prepare medications for one client at a time.
    2. Calculate proper drug dosage.
    3. Open unit dose tablets and place medications in medication cup.
    4. Avoid touching or fingering any tablets or capsules.

11. **The nurse in a mental health clinic is concluding an interview with a depressed client. He suddenly tells the nurse that no one can help him, and that he is going to kill himself by using his 38 caliber gun. Which of the following nursing actions would be best initially?**

    1. Since you have been unable to help the client, arrange for him to meet with another nurse tomorrow.
    2. Ask an aide to remain with the client while you notify the physician to arrange for temporary hospitalization.
    3. Realize that this type of statement is expected of a depressed client, and maintain a nonjudgmental attitude.
    4. Call the client's family and ask them to search his belongings for a 38 caliber gun.

12. **The nurse knows that atropine is contraindicated in people with glaucoma because of which of the following side effects?**

    1. Pupil constriction (miosis).
    2. Decreased production of aqueous humor.
    3. Pupil dilatation (mydriasis).
    4. Decreases in intraocular pressure.

13. **While assessing a newborn at two days of age, the nurse finds a soft spot on the left side of his head. Careful inspection reveals a bluish discoloration with edema that does not cross the suture line. What information should be given to the mother?**

    1. "This will resolve within two to three days without treatment."
    2. "This will resolve within two to six weeks without treatment."
    3. "I will tell the doctor to examine his head carefully this morning."
    4. "Don't worry about it, it's normal."

14. **On the psychiatric unit a nurse observes a client standing at the window in her room and touching the glass. She also mutters to herself from time to time. Which comment by the nurse indicates the best understanding of the client's behavior?**

    1. "Why are you standing by the window and touching the glass?"
    2. "There you are. I came to see if you wanted to see the video we are showing on the unit."
    3. "What are you looking at through the window?"
    4. "Are you hearing voices or seeing things?"

15. **The nursing staff decide to develop a behavioral program to help an anorexic client gain weight. The least appropriate intervention for the nursing staff to include in the program is:**

    1. Provide positive reinforcement for each pound that she gains.
    2. Permit her to spend some quiet time in her room after each meal.
    3. Allow her to select her meals from the same daily menu offered to all clients.
    4. Refrain from commenting about her eating during meal times.

16. **A client is seen in the health clinic with symptoms of urinary burning and urgency. Which of the following diagnostic tests can the nurse anticipate will be ordered to diagnose the possibility of a urinary tract infection?**

    1. Clean-catch midstream urine.
    2. Catheterized urine.
    3. Intravenous pyelogram (IVP).
    4. Random urine specimen.

17. **The nurse assigned to care for a child with cerebral palsy should obtain information concerning his abilities, limitations, interests and habits because the aim of therapy is to:**

    1. Assess the child's assets and potentialities and capitalize on these in the habilitative process, while ignoring limitations.
    2. Reverse abnormal functioning and restore brain damage through rehabilitation.
    3. Provide a therapeutic program that avoids subjecting the child to frustrating experiences that decrease his achievement.
    4. Develop an individualized therapeutic program that utilizes the child's assets and abilities, and provides experiences that permit him to achieve success as well as to cope with frustration and failure.

18. **The nurse enters a new mother's room to check on her during an infant feeding and finds her in tears. She explains that her sister has a mentally retarded child who is two years old. The mother is**

upset because her baby's eyes roll around just like her niece's and she is afraid of retardation in her own baby. Which of the following statements would be the most therapeutic response by the nurse?

1. "All newborns lack the necessary muscle control to regulate eye movement. It is normal in all infants at this age."
2. "I will return the baby to the nursery and observe him carefully."
3. "I will call your pediatrician and report your concerns."
4. "Lack of muscle control in a newborn is a cause for concern but it doesn't necessarily mean the child is retarded."

19. A client has blastomycosis and is being treated with amphotericin B (Fungizone). Which of the following statements made by the client indicates to the nurse that she has an accurate understanding of the administration of amphotericin B (Fungizone)?

1. "The nurse told me that the drug is destroyed by light, so I'll be getting the medicine on the 11:00 pm to 7:00 am shift."
2. "It sure would be nice if they used my Hickman catheter for administration of this medicine, but I guess the medicine is too irritating to the material in the catheter."
3. "I'm glad that I'll only have to take this medicine for 10 days because of the numerous side effects."
4. "I'll be given some Tylenol before the medicine is given to help decrease the fever that I'll probably get when the medicine is being given."

20. A client with a new colostomy has been given instructions about the irrigation of his ostomy. Which action by the client would indicate to the nurse that the teaching plan has to be reviewed?

1. Used 500 mL of irrigating solution.
2. Used warm tap water to irrigate the ostomy.
3. Inserted a lubricated cone tip into the ostomy stoma to begin the irrigation.
4. Positioned the irrigating solution bag 30 inches above the stoma.

21. In caring for an elderly or debilitated client on piperacillin (Pipracil), the nurse should give immediate attention to which of the following?

1. Unusual weight loss, abdominal cramps.
2. Blurred vision.
3. Prolonged prothrombin time.
4. Skin rashes.

22. A nurse observes a client on the psychiatric unit muttering to herself and standing near a window. The client states, "The voices are telling me to jump. They say test the glass and then jump through." What is the best nursing response to this statement?

1. "Where are these voices coming from? Do you recognize them as belonging to anyone that you know?"
2. "I think you are hallucinating. The only voices in this room are yours and mine."
3. "Tell the voices that you are not going to listen to them."
4. "You say you are hearing voices that make you feel like jumping through the window. I understand the voices are frightening to you, but I want you to know that I do not hear any voices."

23. The wife of an alcoholic client says to the nurse, "I told my husband I would leave him if he did not get into treatment. Now that he is here, I feel differently. What can I do to help him?" Which of the following statements is the most therapeutic nursing response?

1. "You should attend an Al-Anon meeting. The group can teach you how to best help him stay sober."
2. "You have already done a great deal by getting him to come into treatment. Now it is up to him to make the best use of his time here."
3. "Are you feeling some responsibility for his drinking?"
4. "Tell me more about the kind of help you feel you are able to provide at this time."

24. A client who has a broken leg is to be discharged from the hospital after crutch training by physical therapy. His friend brings in a pair of crutches for him to use. What is the best nursing action?

1. If the client has used crutches before, cancel the physical therapy order and allow him to go home.
2. Inform the client that crutches are custom fit for each client, and that he cannot use his friend's crutches.
3. Have the client try the crutches to see if they are the right size.
4. Send the crutches to physical therapy with the client for evaluation by that department.

25. The mother of a two-month-old infant with hydrocephalus calls the nurse at the health center. Which statement by the mother should alert the nurse to a potential problem?

1. "My baby cries all the time and I can't seem to comfort him."
2. "My baby spits up after each feeding."
3. "My baby doesn't smile at me yet."
4. "My baby jumps at sudden noises."

26. **An elderly client is able to walk with a cane and enjoys ambulating in the hall. Since he has memory problems, he has great difficulty remembering which room is his. What nursing action would best alleviate this problem?**

    1. Assign him a room close to the nursing station so staff members will be available to help him.
    2. Assign him to a room with a roommate who can watch out for him.
    3. Do not allow him to leave his room unaccompanied.
    4. Put his picture and his name written in large letters on the door to his room.

27. **Amoxicillin (Amoxil) is absorbed more effectively when the nurse administers it with which of the following?**

    1. Orange juice or grapefruit juice.
    2. Milk or Amphojel.
    3. A complete meal.
    4. A full glass of water on an empty stomach.

28. **The orthopedic nurse admitting a client with osteoarthritis, would expect the client to report all of the following symptoms, specific only to rheumatoid arthritis, except:**

    1. Joint pain.
    2. Joint stiffness in the morning.
    3. Presence of Heberden's nodes on the fingers.
    4. Remissions and exacerbations of symptoms.

29. **The nurse finds an elderly client with her IV pulled out, standing next to her bed with the side rails in the up position. The client is confused, does not have an identification bracelet on, and cannot remember her name. What should the nurse do first?**

    1. Help the client into bed, and remind her to call the nurse when she wants to get out of bed.
    2. Help the client into bed, and then restart the IV.
    3. Place a restraining vest on the client.
    4. Put an identification bracelet on the client and help her back to bed.

30. **A penicillin-allergic client has been prescribed cefoperazone (Cefobid). The nurse should give priority which complication?**

    1. Drug resistance.
    2. Hypersensitivity reactions.

3. Drug tolerance.
4. Interactions with other drugs.

31. **A physician orders a body magnetic resonance imaging (MRI) for diagnostic purposes. It would be most important for the nurse to tell the client that the procedure:**

    1. Takes 15 to 30 minutes.
    2. Involves injection of a contrast dye.
    3. Is painless, except for the discomfort of lying still.
    4. Uses only small amounts of radiation.

32. **A three-month-old client is in respiratory isolation. Which of the following nursing actions will most effectively prevent the spread of pathogens via droplet infection?**

    1. Wearing a gown and mask when feeding the client.
    2. Using sterile gloves when changing her diapers.
    3. Having the baby wear a mask when in the playroom.
    4. Using enteric precautions when caring for the baby.

33. **A 53-year-old client with Type I, Insulin Dependent Diabetes Mellitus (IDDM) usually walks two miles each day after breakfast. She is planning to participate in a Walk-a-Thon in which she may walk as much as six miles. Which of the following statements by the nurse would be best in preparing the client for the Walk-a-Thon?**

    1. "Participating in a Walk-a-Thon is much too strenuous for you."
    2. "Ask your doctor to increase your insulin dose the day of the Walk-a-Thon."
    3. "Test your blood glucose immediately following the Walk-a-Thon."
    4. "Eat some additional carbohydrates before you begin the Walk-a-Thon."

34. **A client with a history of bleeding esophageal varices is concerned about preventing further episodes of bleeding. What caution should the nurse give to the client?**

    1. Include high fiber and roughage in your diet.
    2. Avoid drinking hot liquids.
    3. Restrict activities and exercise in warm weather.
    4. Avoid bearing down when having a bowel movement.

35. **A 47-year-old client has pancytopenia and is placed on protective precautions for infection. Which of the following comments by the client would indicate to the nurse that she understands her condition and the precautions?**

    1. "I have never been so aware that germs are everywhere around us."

2. "I didn't realize that I am so contagious that I need a private room."

3. "Everyone who touches me washes their hands like I am really contaminated."

4. "I might make my sister's baby sick, so I told her not to visit."

36. In addition to the electrocardiogram (ECG), which of the following should the nurse monitor most closely during the IV administration of verapamil (Calan) to a client with a supraventricular tachycardia?

   1. Blood pressure.
   2. Respiratory rate.
   3. Urine output.
   4. Level of consciousness.

37. The nurse knows that which of the following signs/symptoms is considered the earliest indication of increased intracranial pressure (ICP)?

   1. Ipsilateral pupil dilation.
   2. Restlessness.
   3. Lethargy.
   4. Bradycardia.

38. A 10-year-old male client is in skeletal traction for the treatment of a fractured femur. This is his fifth day post-pinning. At the change of shift the nurse finds the client crying in pain and the right foot is pale and pulseless. Which of the following is the most appropriate interpretation of this assessment?

   1. Severe pain is to be expected; pain medication should be given.
   2. This client has a low pain tolerance and needs appropriate distraction.
   3. The traction may be pulling too hard and should be released.
   4. This is an abnormal finding and the physician should be notified.

39. The nurse must lift a heavy object found in the hallway. What is the proper technique for the nurse to use in lifting a heavy object?

   1. Lift the object at arm's length so all of the arm muscles are being used.
   2. Bend from the waist, using a wide stance, so that the leg muscles are used.
   3. Maintain good body alignment and use the large muscles of the body while lifting an object.
   4. Bend at the knees and use the large leg muscles when lifting the object.

40. An unconscious 18-year-old man is brought to the emergency room by two friends, who report that he took an overdose of heroin. A narcotic antagonist, naloxone (Narcan), is administered. After giving the medication, the nurse should monitor him closely for signs of:

   1. Respiratory depression.
   2. Seizure activity.
   3. Nausea.
   4. Kidney failure.

41. A client is admitted to the hospital with a diagnosis of myasthenia gravis. Because of the varying degrees of muscle weakness, the nursing priority should be to carefully observe for:

   1. Symptoms of increased ICP.
   2. Confusion and disorientation.
   3. Respiratory difficulty.
   4. Diplopia.

42. After one week in the hospital, a client's condition has improved and she and the nurse are talking regularly. She reports that she had stopped taking her medication several weeks before she was admitted to the hospital, "because I wanted to make it on my own without pills." Which of the following is the most therapeutic response by the nurse?

   1. "You know now that you cannot stop the pills or you'll get sick again. Please don't do it again."
   2. "You're a smart girl. You know what will happen to you if you stop your pills again."
   3. "I know you get tired of taking the meds, especially when you are doing well. Was there any special reason you decided to stop them when you did?"
   4. "This experience taught you that you can't stop your medication. Next time you are tempted to do so, remember how upset your parents were when you had to be re-hospitalized."

43. The nurse takes precautions to prevent constipation and fecal impaction in an immobilized client. The nurse is aware that if a client develops a fecal impaction, what serious complication could result?

   1. Intestinal obstruction.
   2. Bowel perforation.
   3. Peritonitis.
   4. Rectal bleeding.

44. A client develops a fecal impaction. Before digital removal of the mass, what type of enema is usually given by the nurse to loosen the feces?

    1. Fleets.
    2. Oil retention.
    3. Soap suds.
    4. Tap water.

45. The physician has ordered a sputum specimen to be collected for culture and sensitivity. The nurse is aware that the preferable time to collect this specimen is:

    1. In the morning.
    2. In the evening, after forcing fluids all day.
    3. After antibiotics have been started.
    4. After the client has taken an expectorant.

46. A client has been receiving moxalactam (Moxam) 800 mg IV for septicemia. He is now ready for discharge. Which of the following discharge instructions would be most appropriate for the nurse to give?

    1. Do not drink any alcohol for at least three days after discharge.
    2. Report any shortness of breath to your physician immediately.
    3. Be sure to continue taking the Moxam (p.o.) until the entire prescription is gone.
    4. Drink extra fluids for at least one week to help prevent kidney damage from the IV Moxam.

47. An eight-month-old child screams when his mother leaves the room. The mother begins to cry and says, "I don't understand why he is so upset, no one has hurt him." Choose the best response for the nurse, which would reflect the proper interpretation of the infant's behavior.

    1. "This is a response to an over-stimulating environment, he is tired."
    2. "This is a reaction to overexposure to caregivers."
    3. "He probably remembers you were gone two hours the last time you left."
    4. "This is a normal reaction for a child of his age."

48. A client is scheduled for a sigmoidoscopy. The nurse should advise the client that, during the procedure, he will be placed in which position?

    1. Supine.
    2. Prone.
    3. Left lateral.
    4. Semi-Fowler's.

49. A client, age 10, is recovering following an appendectomy. He is ambulatory and goes to the day room with his parents. While changing the linen on the client's bed, the nurse should handle the linen by which of the following methods?

    1. Hold it close to the body to avoid dropping it.
    2. Place the soiled linen on the chair until done making the bed.
    3. Hold the linen away from the body and uniform.
    4. Shake the clean linen to unfold it to provide ease in making the bed.

50. A client's son is distressed over his mother's crying and saying that she wants to die. He asks the nurse to help him "calm her down." The nurse's best response to his request is:

    1. "All right, I'll talk with her and see if I can comfort her."
    2. "If you just sit quietly with her, I'm sure she will calm down when she gets these feelings out."
    3. "It's hard to see her so upset, but she needs to let these feelings out; we can both stay with her."
    4. "This seems to bother you more than it does her."

51. A client is scheduled for surgery this morning. The preoperative checklist has been completed, and the nurse has just administered the preoperative injection. Which nursing action should be implemented next?

    1. Take the client to the bathroom to void.
    2. Dim the overhead and bedside lights.
    3. Review deep breathing and coughing exercises.
    4. Put the side rails up on both sides of the bed.

52. A client had a right lobectomy yesterday and has a chest tube connected to suction at 20 cm of water pressure. Upon assessment of the client this morning, the nurse notes that there is no fluctuation in the water-seal chamber. What would be the nurse's immediate action?

    1. Increase the suction until fluctuation reappears.
    2. Observe for kinks in the tubing.
    3. Elevate the head of the bed to 80 degrees.
    4. No action is necessary, since the lung has most likely re-expanded.

53. A seven-year-old boy is brought to the physician's office with complaints of a sore throat. As the nurse prepares to collect a throat culture, the mother states, "I don't know why you can't just give him antibiotics and be done with it." The nurse's best response is which of the following statements?

1. "This could be a virus. If it is, antibiotics would not be effective."
2. "Antibiotics have dangerous side effects. Let's see which one he really needs."
3. "Insurance companies require a throat culture before antibiotics can be ordered."
4. "This is the physician's order. Would you like me to call him for you?"

54. **Initially, which of the following actions will the nurse most likely consider in dealing with the ritualistic behaviors of a client with obsessive-compulsive disorder?**

1. Confront the client about the senseless nature of the ritualistic behaviors.
2. Set strict limits on the behaviors so the client can better conform to the unit rules and schedules.
3. Isolate the client for a period of time to lower his anxiety about offending others.
4. Plan the client's schedule to allow extra time to perform the rituals to keep his anxiety within manageable levels.

55. **All of the following nursing interventions aid in the prevention of hyperbilirubinemia except:**

1. Early and frequent feedings.
2. Promotion of adequate hydration.
3. Prevention of cold stress.
4. Early administration of parenteral Vitamin K.

56. **A toddler in the pediatrics ward is to be placed in a highchair for a meal. After placing the client in the highchair, which nursing action is most appropriate initially?**

1. Pour a small amount of milk into the glass.
2. Ask the mother to feed the child, since she is present.
3. Belt the child securely to the chair.
4. Cut the child's food into bite size pieces.

57. **An eight-year-old child is admitted to the hospital with swollen, painful joints, fatigue, and weight loss. He is diagnosed with rheumatic fever. When the parents ask what can lead to rheumatic fever, the nurse's best response is based on what knowledge?**

1. There is no known etiology for rheumatic fever.
2. Rheumatic fever is an opportunistic disease.
3. Rheumatic fever often occurs in children with congenital heart defects.
4. Rheumatic fever is almost always preceded by a streptococcal infection.

58. **A client has just returned to the unit after a right pneumonectomy. The nurse should position him on his:**

1. Right side.
2. Left side or back.
3. Back only.
4. Right side or left side.

59. **A client's son remarks to the nurse, "My father has been dead for six months now. I think my mother needs to get on with her life." What is the best response for the nurse to make to this statement?**

1. "A death is usually a crisis for the whole family. How has your father's death affected you?"
2. "I agree. How can you help her find more pleasure in her life?"
3. "I think it would be helpful if you could give her more support."
4. "Perhaps she needs more time. Grieving often takes a year or more to complete."

60. **The nurse understands that which of the following statements about mourning is inaccurate?**

1. It is a normal response to loss.
2. It functions to free the individual from an attachment to the lost object so future relationships can be established.
3. It is accompanied by a growing realization that the loss has occurred.
4. Mourning occurs only in humans.

61. **Following a gastric resection, a client is taught nutritional habits that will slow gastric emptying, helping to decrease the incidence of the "dumping syndrome." Which foods selected by the client indicate to the nurse that he understands the instructions given?**

1. Ice cream.
2. Oranges.
3. Wheat bread.
4. Turkey.

62. **A client is admitted to the hospital with a diagnosis of active pulmonary tuberculosis. An immediate goal is controlling the spread of infection. To achieve this, the nurse would:**

1. Wear a gown and mask when caring for the client.
2. Recommend that the client wear a mask when she has visitors.
3. Teach the client how to cover her nose and mouth when she coughs or sneezes.
4. Use blood and needle precautions.

63. **A three-month-old infant has undergone a colos-**

tomy for Hirschsprung's disease. When the mother questions the nurse about her child's prognosis, the nurse's most helpful response is:

1. "Corrective surgery is a three-step approach. Let's wait and talk about the second stage when your child is ready for it."
2. "Most colostomies are temporary and can be reversed when the child is older."
3. "You're upset by your child's appearance, aren't you?"
4. "An enterostomal therapist can provide you with information on the management of a colostomy."

64. A 48-year-old woman is admitted to the psychiatric unit with a diagnosis of depression. Her husband reports that she had seemed despondent since their youngest child left for college two months before. She had become progressively more withdrawn, refused food, lost 20 pounds and neglected her appearance. During the admission interview, the client asks the nurse not to bother with her because "I am totally worthless." The nurse's best response to this statement is which of the following statements?

1. "I have seen many valuable things about you."
2. "You feel worthless now because you are so depressed. You will feel differently when you begin to recover."
3. "You have been feeling very sad and alone for some time now."
4. "You really have a great deal to live for."

65. In preparation for a sigmoid colon resection, a client is receiving instructions about the colostomy that will be performed. Which instruction given by the nurse will require further clarification?

1. "Your colostomy will begin to function seven to ten days after surgery."
2. "The stoma of your colostomy will appear large at first, but it will shrink over the next few weeks."
3. "You will have to wear a colostomy bag at all times to prevent accidental leakage of stool."
4. "Your diet will not have to change dramatically. You can use a trial-and-error method to see which foods will not agree with you."

66. In performing ileostomy care, the nurse measures the circumference of the collection device opening so that it is at least how much larger than the stoma circumference?

1. 1/8 inch.
2. 1/4 inch.
3. 1/2 inch.

4. 3/4 inch.

67. Which of the following findings by the nurse would the nurse understand to be consistent with a diagnosis of endometriosis:

1. Menses-linked symptoms that worsen over time.
2. Abdominal bloating starting seven to 10 days before menses.
3. Previous pregnancy loss one year previously.
4. Maternal history of pelvic inflammatory disease (PID).

68. A client is scheduled for ECT in the morning. The nurse's responsibility in preparation for this procedure include all of the following except:

1. Explaining the procedure, including its risks and benefits, and obtaining the client's signature on the consent form.
2. Instructing the client to empty his bladder before the treatment.
3. Maintaining NPO status from midnight the night before the treatment.
4. Removing dentures, contact lenses, and other prosthetics before the treatment.

69. A client has had a right total hip replacement and is three days postoperative. When the nurse and nursing assistant are transferring her to a chair, she cries out in pain. Which observation by the nurse would lead to the suspicion of a dislocated hip prosthesis:

1. Shortening of the right leg.
2. Bulging in the right hip area.
3. Adduction of the left leg.
4. Loose hip joint movement on the right side.

70. After her first night in the hospital, a depressed client complains of feeling too tired to get out of bed in the morning. In planning how to deal therapeutically with this, the nurse is guided by the knowledge that:

1. Helping to mobilize the client physically will also help to improve her emotional state.
2. Most people do require more rest when they are depressed.
3. It is best to wait until the client indicates she is ready to participate in structured activities.
4. Encouraging the client to get up and come out on the ward will only increase her feelings of worthlessness and guilt.

71. A seven-month-old will be admitted for bacterial

meningitis. The physician orders the following: blood culture, stat; prepare for a spinal tap; Ancef 250 mg IV, stat; continue the current IV at 25 mL/ hour. (The IV was started in the emergency room at KVO.) Which of the following is the first priority of the nurse who will be admitting the child?

1. Regulate the IV flow rate to avoid overhydration.
2. After the blood work is drawn, administer the antibiotic to treat the meningitis.
3. Arrange for the child to be in isolation, to protect others from infection.
4. Assess the child, including vital signs and history of allergy.

72. A client is instructed to test her urine for the presence of luteinizing hormone. The nurse explains that the test is useful for:

1. Prediction of ovulation.
2. Assessment of hormonal balance necessary for ovulation.
3. Prediction of normal menstrual function.
4. Assessment of the pH of cervical mucosa.

73. A client is ambulating down the tile hallway in her stocking covered feet. Which of the following is the priority nursing action?

1. Remind the client to avoid any wet spots on the floor.
2. Tell the client that she should always wear slippers or shoes when ambulating.
3. Get the client's slippers and have her put them on.
4. No intervention is necessary since the client has her feet covered.

74. A concerned mother calls the physician's office. Her child has a respiratory infection and a temperature of 39° C orally. She needs to give her son 240 mg of acetaminophen (Tylenol). The label on her bottle at home reads 160 mg/5 mL. The nurse's most helpful response is which of the following statements?

1. Give 1/2 teaspoon.
2. Give 1 1/2 teaspoons.
3. Give 1 1/2 mL.
4. Give 15 mL.

75. Which of the following diagnostic procedures is considered invasive and requires a special consent form?

1. Magnetic resonance imaging (MRI).
2. Cerebral arteriogram.
3. Computed tomography (CT scan).
4. Echoencephalography.

76. An elderly widower with depression complains of

not sleeping at all the first two nights in the hospital. The primary nurse notes the night nurses charted he was frequently awake when they made rounds. Which measure would be least appropriate to include in the nursing care plan to help him with his sleep problem?

1. Spending time with him when he awakens at night to explore what seems to be interfering with his sleep.
2. Providing a soothing nighttime routine, such as a warm bath and backrub, to promote relaxation and sleep.
3. Limiting intake of caffeinated beverages in the late afternoon and evening.
4. Discouraging napping during the day.

77. A client has just received the diagnosis of endometrial cancer. In taking a nursing history, which of the following symptoms is most likely to be reported by this client?

1. An abnormal Papanicolaou (Pap) smear.
2. Post menopausal bleeding.
3. Recurrent backache.
4. Uterine enlargement.

78. A client is being treated with nystatin (Mycostatin) oral suspension for a candida oropharyngeal infection. How should the nurse instruct the client to use this medication?

1. Swallow the solution quickly, to avoid burning the throat.
2. Take the medication with a glass of water.
3. Swish the solution around in the mouth, then hold it there for as long as possible.
4. Take the medication on an empty stomach.

79. Thirty minutes after receiving Valium, a client reports that he is feeling much calmer. "I can't believe how scared I was when I came in. I will do anything to avoid having another panic attack." The nurse realizes the most important information to give him at this time is which of the following?

1. Advise him to admit himself to the psychiatric unit where he can have a comprehensive evaluation in a protected setting.
2. Reduce the amount of stress in his life.
3. Make an appointment for outpatient psychotherapy to receive help with any emotional issues that might be responsible for his panic attacks.
4. Tell him he can always return to the emergency room if he should have another panic attack.

80. A client, age 31, is brought to the emergency room

after an automobile accident. She is conscious upon admission. A physical examination and x-rays reveal a transection of the spinal cord at T4. The nurse should give the highest priority to which of the following?

1. The client has an allergy to iodine.
2. The client last voided seven hours ago.
3. The client smokes two packs of cigarettes a day.
4. The client is menstruating.

81. A visitor asks the nurse about the client in the next room, who has metastatic cancer and cries out frequently. "That person must have a terrible disease. What is the matter with him?" The most appropriate response by the nurse would be which of the following?

1. "That client has cancer and is quite uncomfortable."
2. "Mr. Jones is being kept as comfortable as possible."
3. "That person is quite uncomfortable. Does his crying out bother you?"
4. "I cannot reveal anything about his diagnosis. Why don't you ask his family when they visit? I'm sure they would appreciate your concern."

82. A client has been depressed and took too many sleeping pills. She is admitted to the psychiatric unit after being treated for the drug overdose. Which of the following nursing actions is NOT a priority?

1. Remove objects such as the client's personal razor and fingernail scissors from her room.
2. Allow the client to spend most of the day in bed, since she is very depressed.
3. Spend time with the client, in an effort to establish a therapeutic relationship.
4. Introduce the client to other clients and members of the health care team.

83. A client is very irritable at breakfast. When asked if there is a problem, the client states that he was unable to sleep because of noise made by the staff on the night shift. The best initial response by the nurse is which of the following?

1. "It must be very distressing to be unable to sleep at night. Would you like to take a nap this morning?"
2. "I'll report that to the supervisor."
3. "Maybe we can move you to a room further from the nurses' station when one of those rooms becomes available."
4. "Why don't you close your door at night? Sometimes the nurses make noise and don't realize it."

84. Following cervical x-rays and a CT scan, a client

is found to have a spinal cord transection at T2-T3 vertebrae. Nursing staff can anticipate that the client's nursing care will be planned for which type of paralysis:

1. Hemiplegia.
2. Paraplegia.
3. Quadriplegia.
4. Paresthesia.

85. A client is admitted to a long-term care facility. She requires total care. In providing mouth care to the client, the nurse should do which of the following?

1. Place the client on her back, with a pillow under her head.
2. Use her thumb and index finger to keep the client's mouth open.
3. Use a stiff toothbrush to clean the client's teeth.
4. Place the client on her side before starting mouth care.

86. A client had a BKA as a result of chronic diabetes mellitus. Postoperatively, the best position for the client to maintain is which of the following?

1. Prone for at least 15 minutes daily.
2. Prone with pillows under the affected leg for four days postoperatively.
3. Supine with the knee in full extension.
4. Semi-Fowler's with two pillows under the stump.

87. A client is receiving magnesium sulfate for severe PIH. Which of the following clinical findings would warrant use of the antidote, calcium gluconate?

1. Rapid rise in blood pressure.
2. Rapid respiratory rate - above 40/min.
3. Urinary output 90 mL in two hours.
4. Absent patellar reflexes.

88. The physician has ordered an indwelling urinary catheter for a male client. Where should the nurse tape the catheter to prevent pressure on the urethra at the penoscrotal junction?

1. Medial thigh.
2. Upper abdomen.
3. Mid-abdominal region.
4. Lateral thigh.

89. Shortly after passing out the 9:00 a.m. medications, the nurse realizes that another nurse had given digoxin (Lanoxin) 0.125 mg instead of the prescribed furosemide (Lasix) 2.5 mg, to an eight-year-old client. What is the most appropriate initial response?

1. Assess apical pulse, BP, and respirations.

2. Call the doctor to get orders.
3. Notify the supervisor of the error.
4. Document the error in the chart and complete an incident report.

90. **A client, age 83, develops acute pulmonary edema secondary to congestive heart failure. The physician orders rotating tourniquets. Which action taken by the nurse demonstrates accurate understanding of this procedure?**

    1. The nurse places the client flat in bed with a small pillow.
    2. Tourniquets are applied to each extremity for 15 minutes and then released.
    3. The nurse checks for the presence of an arterial pulse in the extremity after applying a tourniquet.
    4. When the procedure is completed, the tourniquets are released in a clockwise manner, one every five minutes.

91. **The nurse is counseling a parent about the management of her five-year-old child who has pinworms. The nurse should consider the teaching effective if the parent makes which of the following statements?**

    1. "I will change her underwear twice a day."
    2. "I will give her the mebendazole (Vermox) today and again next week."
    3. "I will keep her out of school until I don't see the pinworms any more."
    4. "I will discard the sheets on her bed."

92. **A child with a rectal temperature of 39° C has an order for acetaminophen (Tylenol) 280 mg by mouth. The label on the bottle reads 160 mg/5 mL. How many mL's should the nurse dispense to the child?**

    1. 8.8 mL.
    2. 1.8 mL.
    3. 6.4 mL.
    4. 9.8 mL.

93. **The nurse, in caring for psychiatric clients, knows that tardive dyskinesia:**

    1. It is a movement disorder caused by antipsychotic drugs.
    2. It occurs within the first few days of treatment in most clients.
    3. It improves rapidly if the offending drug is discontinued.
    4. It is treated with antiparkinsonian drugs.

94. **A client is admitted to the ER with a sharp object**

in his right eye. What is the most important action for the nurse to take immediately?

1. Remove the foreign object.
2. Irrigate the eye with copious amounts of normal saline.
3. Carefully place sterile gauze over the object to cover the eye.
4. Instill a topical anesthetic to reduce his pain.

95. **A 67-year-old widow is brought to the clinic by her son, who found her at home crying. She said that she "could not go on alone." He tells the nurse that when his father died six months earlier the family was amazed at his mother's fortitude during and immediately after the funeral. She did not cry or seem unduly upset. The nurse recognizes that his mother had dealt with her husband's death by using which of the following defense mechanisms?**

    1. Denial.
    2. Repression.
    3. Introjection.
    4. Sublimation.

96. **A 42-year-old female is admitted with right-sided weakness and slurred speech. Which diagnostic tests should the nurse be prepared to instruct the client/family about?**

    1. EEG and MRI.
    2. Angiography and EMG.
    3. PET and pneumoencephalogram.
    4. CT scan and lumbar puncture.

97. **A client on the psychiatric unit attends activity therapy and is encouraged to pound designs into a leather belt. This intervention is based on which model of depression?**

    1. Behavioral.
    2. Cognitive.
    3. Aggression-turned-inward.
    4. Learned helplessness

98. **A 60-year-old client has advanced cancer of the lung, with metastasis. His wife says to the nurse, "I know my husband is in severe pain. I wish I could do something to make him feel better." Which of the following comments by the nurse would be most therapeutic for the wife?**

    1. "It must be very difficult for you to see your husband suffering."
    2. "I wish there was more that I could do to relieve

his pain, too."

3. "I'm sure he will begin to feel better after his next pain medication."

4. "Your husband tries hard not to show the pain when you are with him."

99. **The nurse should assess an immobilized client for symptoms of a fecal impaction, the most definitive of which is:**

1. The absence of bowel sounds.
2. Diarrhea stools with abdominal cramping.
3. A rigid board-like abdomen.
4. Constipation with liquid fecal seepage.

100. **A 56-year-old woman is being discharged after a simple mastectomy. She will begin radiation therapy as an outpatient tomorrow. Which of the following instructions, directed at maintaining skin integrity, should be given by the nurse?**

1. Wear a good support bra and use ice for any swelling.
2. Use of a heating pad is contraindicated.
3. Skin breakdown is common and should be treated with antibiotic ointment.
4. Keep skin lubricated to prevent dryness.

NCLEX-RN

Test 6

Questions with Rationales

NCLEX-RN TEST 6 WITH RATIONALES

1. **A client was admitted for a severe episode of gastrointestinal bleeding. Prior to discharge, which of the following statements by the client would indicate to the nurse a need for further instruction?**

   1. "If my arthritis bothers me, I'll take Tylenol."
   2. "It's a good thing I gave up drinking five years ago."
   3. "It will sure be good to have my morning coffee."
   4. "I'll take my Tagamet before I eat and at bedtime."

   1. *The client understands that Tylenol is appropriate, although any aspirin-related drug would be contraindicated because it causes GI bleeding. This option is a distractor, because this question has a false response stem. The answer will be a statement which indicates that the client does NOT understand how to care for his health problem.*
   2. *The client understands that he should avoid alcohol, which stimulates the GI tract. This question has a false response stem, so the answer will be a statement which indicates that the client does NOT understand how to care for his health problem.*
   3. *Good! This response shows that the client "needs further instruction," because coffee stimulates the GI tract and should be avoided.*
   4. *The client is correctly taking Tagamet before eating and at bedtime. This drug is used in treatment of peptic ulcers to inhibit the secretion of histamine. This is a distractor, since this question has a false response stem. The answer will be a statement which indicates that the client does NOT understand how to care for his health problem.*

2. **A client, age 65, is receiving doxycycline (Vibramycin) for actinomycosis (fungal infection). The nurse should observe the client for which of the following side effects?**

   1. Photosensitivity.
   2. Constipation.
   3. Ototoxicity.
   4. Permanent discoloration of teeth.

   1. *Correct! Photosensitivity is an adverse effect of tetracyclines, in which the skin reacts abnormally to light, especially ultraviolet radiation or sunlight. The result is an intense sunburn reaction with erythema, macules and gray-blue patches. Prevention involves avoiding direct exposure to sunlight and ultraviolet light and using a sunscreen with a sun protection factor (SPF) of 15 or greater.*

   2. *No. Clients on tetracycline therapy often experience GI distress, manifested by anorexia, nausea/vomiting and diarrhea.*
   3. *Incorrect. Ototoxicity is a concern when clients are on aminoglycosides or on minocycline (Minocin). It has not been reported as an adverse reaction to Vibramycin.*
   4. *No. Although permanent discoloration of the teeth is an adverse reaction, it only affects the neonate in the last half of pregnancy and children under eight years of age. This client is 65 years old.*

3. **A client is in labor and is admitted with a blood pressure of 86/52. She is four centimeters dilated and uncomfortable. The nurse should give immediate consideration to which of the following nursing actions?**

   1. Call the physician to report the blood pressure.
   2. Turn the client on her side and retake her blood pressure.
   3. Reassure the client that everything is all right.
   4. Ask the client if she would like some pain medication.

   1. *Wrong! Calling the physician may be appropriate, however, the need for adequate blood pressure is a physiological need that requires immediate intervention. Look for an option that more immediately addresses this need.*
   2. *Good choice! Supine hypotension is a frequent cause of low blood pressure in pregnant clients. By turning the client on her side and retaking the blood pressure, the nurse is attempting to correct the low blood pressure and then re-assessing. The need for adequate blood pressure is a physiological need that requires immediate intervention. Maslow's Hierarchy of Needs indicates that physiological needs should receive priority.*
   3. *No. Reassuring the client that everything is all right is not a priority action and may be false reassurance. The need for adequate blood pressure is a physiological need that requires immediate intervention. Maslow's Hierarchy of Needs indicates that physiological needs should receive priority.*
   4. *The issue in this question is labor and low blood pressure. The need for adequate blood pressure is a physiological need that requires immediate intervention. This option is focused on the client's discomfort, which is not life-threatening. The client's comfort should be addressed as soon as the nurse has determined that the blood pressure is stable.*

4. A client received a large contusion on the head and a fracture of the femur. The nurse must be alert for possible complications. Which of the following signs and symptoms indicates a serious complication?

   1. An oral temperature change from 98.8° F to 98.2° F.
   2. A blood pressure decrease from 122/88 to 110/72.
   3. Increased pain at the site of the femur fracture.
   4. A change in respiratory rate from 18 to 32, with increased restlessness.

   1. *Incorrect choice! This change in temperature is not significant; both values are in the normal range.*
   2. *Incorrect. This change in blood pressure is not significant; both values are within the normal range.*
   3. *Wrong. Pain at the fracture site is expected. Even though the word "fracture" also appears in the case scenario, this option is a distractor. The strategy of looking for similar words should only be used when you do not know the answer. It is very important to know the ranges for normal vital signs.*
   4. ***Correct! Increased respiratory rate and increased restlessness are symptoms that indicate possible fat embolism. Fat embolism is a serious complication following the type of fracture sustained by the client. Fat emboli may be trapped in lung tissue, leading to respiratory symptoms and mental disturbances.***

   > **STRATEGY ALERT:** Note that the word "fracture" appears in the stem of the question and in Option 3 -- which is a distractor. Knowing the ranges for normal vital signs is very important. You should always use your nursing knowledge first, and use strategies only when you do not know the answer.

5. The client's mother brings clean clothing and toilet articles to the hospital. When the client sees her, she does not return her greeting and lies down on the bed curling up into a fetal position. Her mother responds by becoming visibly upset. Outside the room she asks the nurse, "Do you think I should not visit again until she is better?" Which of the following statements is the most therapeutic response by the nurse?

   1. "It is important for the client to maintain contact with her family. Continue to make brief visits, every day if you can."
   2. "This has been an upsetting experience for you. Let's go into the lounge where we can talk privately for a few minutes."
   3. "I think that might be best. I will stay with the client until she seems to feel better."
   4. "Do you have any idea why your daughter responded as she did?"

   1. *In general, it is best to encourage family members to visit and telephone often to demonstrate their*

   continued interest in the client. However, this is not the most therapeutic response for the nurse to make initially to the client's mother.
   2. ***Correct! The nurse is acknowledging the mother's feelings and being available to explore them further. This response recognizes that the client's mother has unmet needs. Also it would provide the nurse an opportunity to gather additional assessment data.***
   3. *Staying away would further disrupt the client's relationship with her mother. Also, the nurse has ignored the mother's feelings and has only responded to the overt content of her statement.*
   4. *This is not correct. The mother is having a problem, but the nurse has ignored her and focused instead on the client. This is not a therapeutic response by the nurse.*

6. The nurse understands which of the following is a goal of remotivation therapy in long-term care facilities?

   1. To stimulate and encourage social participation.
   2. To reorient clients with cognitive problems.
   3. To share memories of past experiences and events.
   4. To resolve emotional problems.

   1. ***Correct. The goals of remotivation therapy are to stimulate and encourage social participation using structured group approaches.***
   2. *This is not correct. Reality orientation programs are designed to reorient clients with cognitive deficits.*
   3. *This is not correct. Reminiscence therapy is used to encourage the sharing of memories of past experiences and events.*
   4. *This is not correct. Psychotherapy, either individual or group, is used to assist clients to resolve emotional and psychological difficulties.*

7. The nurse understands that epinephrine (Epifrin) can be used for open angle glaucoma because of which of the following effects?

   1. Pupil dilatation.
   2. Pupil constriction.
   3. Reducing the aqueous formation and enhancing outflow.
   4. Increasing aqueous formation.

   1. *Epinephrine does cause the pupil to dilate, but dilatation alone is contraindicated for glaucoma.*
   2. *Incorrect. The pupil is dilated with epinephrine, not constricted.*
   3. ***Great work! Epinephrine can be used with glaucoma because it reduces aqueous production and enhances outflow.***
   4. *Wrong. If aqueous production was increased, glaucoma would get worse.*

8. **A client is admitted in acute renal failure and undergoes peritoneal dialysis. Immediately after infusing 2,000 mL of 2.5% Dialysate, the nurse should do which of the following first?**

1. Clamp the inflow tubing.
2. Monitor the client's vital signs.
3. Assess the outflow fluid.
4. Weigh the client.

1. **Correct! With the tubing clamped, air will not enter the peritoneal cavity and cause complications.**
2. Incorrect. Although careful monitoring is necessary to detect such complications as peritonitis, pneumonia and fluid overload, it should be done after the inflow tubing has been clamped.
3. Incorrect. This should be done to determine fluid balance after dwell time and outflow has occurred.
4. Incorrect. Baseline data is necessary and the client should be weighed daily, but it is not necessary to weigh the client immediately after infusion of Dialysate.

9. **A client will go home on warfarin (Coumadin). What is important for the nurse to include in the teaching plan for the client?**

1. The client should carry an ID card with him at all times.
2. The client should take only aspirin for headaches.
3. The client should eat lots of foods high in vitamin K, like broccoli, liver and spinach.
4. The client should avoid any exercise.

1. **Correct. The client must be able to alert anyone to his anticoagulant use in case of an emergency.**
2. No, aspirin or the NSAIDs will prolong clotting times and potentiate the effects of Coumadin. Try again.
3. No, broccoli, liver, and spinach have high amounts of vitamin K in them, this may decrease the effects of coumadin. Try again.
4. No, avoiding any exercise will lead to venous stasis and thrombophlebitis. This would not be a wise thing to do.

10. **The nurse is preparing medications for administration in a pediatric unit. Which of the following actions by the nurse is least appropriate?**

1. Prepare medications for one client at a time.
2. Calculate proper drug dosage.
3. Open unit dose tablets and place medications in medication cup.
4. Avoid touching or fingering any tablets or capsules.

1. Preparing medications for one client at a time is appropriate. It helps prevent preparation errors such as inadvertently placing one client's medication into another client's medication cup.
2. No! Calculation of drug dosage should be done prior to administration, when the information from the drug label is readily available. Look for an action that is NOT appropriate.
3. **Right! Unit dose medications should remain in their wrappers to maintain cleanliness, for identification of medication and for avoidance of waste if the medication is not given.**
4. No, it is appropriate to avoid touching the tablets or capsules. Using aseptic technique maintains cleanliness of the medications and prevents possible absorption through contact with the skin.

11. **The nurse in a mental health clinic is concluding an interview with a depressed client. He suddenly tells the nurse that no one can help him, and that he is going to kill himself by using his 38 caliber gun. Which of the following nursing actions would be best initially?**

1. Since you have been unable to help the client, arrange for him to meet with another nurse tomorrow.
2. Ask an aide to remain with the client while you notify the physician to arrange for temporary hospitalization.
3. Realize that this type of statement is expected of a depressed client, and maintain a nonjudgmental attitude.
4. Call the client's family and ask them to search his belongings for a 38 caliber gun.

1. No. The issue in this question is depression. If the nurse does not assure the client's safety immediately, he may make a suicide attempt. Meeting with another nurse tomorrow does not assure his safety today. Maslow's Hierarchy of Needs identifies safety as the priority when no physiological need exists.
2. **Correct. The issue in this question is depression. The depressed client's safety should receive priority. The nurse assures his immediate safety by asking an aide to remain with the client now. The client's continued safety is assured by arranging for the client to be hospitalized. Maslow's Hierarchy of Needs indicates that safety needs receive priority when no physiological need exists.**
3. Incorrect! Not all depressed clients are suicidal. When a client verbalizes a plan for suicide, the client's safety is the nurse's priority. Maintaining a nonjudgmental attitude does not assure the client's safety.
4. This action is not appropriate. Client confidentiality becomes an issue with this action. Also, the nurse must provide for the client's safety while the nurse is making the phone call.

12. **The nurse knows that atropine is contraindicated in people with glaucoma because of which of the following side effects?**

    1. Pupil constriction (miosis).
    2. Decreased production of aqueous humor.
    3. Pupil dilatation (mydriasis).
    4. Decreases in intraocular pressure.

    1. *Incorrect. Atropine causes the eye to dilate, not constrict.*
    2. *Incorrect. Atropine does not decrease aqueous humor.*
    3. ***Correct. Atropine causes the eye to dilate and the ciliary body blocks the canal of Schlemm, which prevents the outflow of aqueous humor. This would be a severe reaction for a client with glaucoma.***
    4. *No. Atropine does not decrease the pressure.*

13. **While assessing a newborn at two days of age, the nurse finds a soft spot on the left side of his head. Careful inspection reveals a bluish discoloration with edema that does not cross the suture line. What information should be given to the mother?**

    1. "This will resolve within two to three days without treatment."
    2. "This will resolve within two to six weeks without treatment."
    3. "I will tell the doctor to examine his head carefully this morning."
    4. "Don't worry about it, it's normal."

    1. *Wrong. The findings on the infant's head are a cephalohematoma which will not resolve in two to three days.*
    2. ***Correct! When an infant develops a cephalohematoma the parents need to be aware that it could take up to six weeks for the edema and discoloration to disappear. There is no need for treatment; it will resolve spontaneously with no complications.***
    3. *Wrong! The assessment of the head can be made by the nurse, who should be knowledgeable about the difference between cephalohematoma and caput succedaneum, which resolves spontaneously within two to three days.*
    4. *No. Although caput succedaneum and cephalohematoma are relatively common in newborns, the parents need information about them.*

14. **On the psychiatric unit a nurse observes a client standing at the window in her room and touching the glass. She also mutters to herself from time to time. Which comment by the nurse indicates the best understanding of the client's behavior?**

    1. "Why are you standing by the window and touching the glass?"
    2. "There you are. I came to see if you wanted to see the video we are showing on the unit."
    3. "What are you looking at through the window?"
    4. "Are you hearing voices or seeing things?"

    1. ***Correct. The client's behavior indicates that she may be actively hallucinating, but the nurse does not know this for sure until the client validates that impression. This question states what the nurse has observed while asking the client to tell more about what she is experiencing.***
    2. *This comment does not reflect the nurse's observation and does not seek any data from the client about her experience. This is not correct because it ignores data that could be important for the nursing assessment.*
    3. *This comment is a possibility, but it is not the best option because it is not asking the client to talk about what she is experiencing.*
    4. *Asking clients whether they hear voices or see things may produce a negative response. There is a better option.*

15. **The nursing staff decide to develop a behavioral program to help an anorexic client gain weight. The least appropriate intervention for the nursing staff to include in the program is:**

    1. Provide positive reinforcement for each pound that she gains.
    2. Permit her to spend some quiet time in her room after each meal.
    3. Allow her to select her meals from the same daily menu offered to all clients.
    4. Refrain from commenting about her eating during meal times.

    1. *This is an appropriate intervention. Privileges are used to reinforce weight gain. This question is asking for the response that is NOT appropriate.*
    2. ***Correct choice. Clients are monitored for 90 minutes after eating to ensure they do not go to the bathroom and purge the food they have just ingested. Since this is inappropriate, it is the correct response to this question.***
    3. *This is an appropriate intervention. An important focus of treatment is to develop independence in eating behavior. Selecting food from a menu is one way for the client to develop more of a sense of her own autonomy.*
    4. *This is an appropriate plan. Mealtime conversation focuses on the client as a person and not on her eating behaviors. This approach is often a change from family patterns that focused on urging her to eat and reinforced her eating difficulties by rewarding them with attention.*

16. **A client is seen in the health clinic with symptoms of urinary burning and urgency. Which of the following diagnostic tests can the nurse anticipate will be ordered to diagnose the possibility of a urinary tract infection?**

   1. Clean-catch midstream urine.
   2. Catheterized urine.
   3. Intravenous pyelogram (IVP).
   4. Random urine specimen.

   1. *Correct! A clean-catch urine specimen is the routine test of choice to diagnose a urinary tract infection. It is designed to eliminate as much external contamination of the specimen as possible by cleansing of the labia and midstream collection into a sterile container.*
   2. *No, this technique is too invasive, uncomfortable, and expensive for the diagnosis of a urinary tract infection.*
   3. *Incorrect. The IVP is a radiologic test that visualizes the urinary tract. It is ordered in suspected disease or urinary tract dysfunction. It is not used to diagnose a urinary tract infection.*
   4. *No, this collection of urine may result in external contamination of the specimen.*

17. **The nurse assigned to care for a child with cerebral palsy should obtain information concerning his abilities, limitations, interests and habits because the aim of therapy is to:**

   1. Assess the child's assets and potentialities and capitalize on these in the habilitative process, while ignoring limitations.
   2. Reverse abnormal functioning and restore brain damage through rehabilitation.
   3. Provide a therapeutic program that avoids subjecting the child to frustrating experiences that decrease his achievement.
   4. Develop an individualized therapeutic program that utilizes the child's assets and abilities, and provides experiences that permit him to achieve success as well as to cope with frustration and failure.

   1. *This answer is wrong because of the word "ignoring." The nurse should not ignore the child's limitations, but should consider his limitations when preparing his plan of care.*
   2. *Wrong! Medical science does not have the necessary knowledge and ability to accomplish this. Brain damage cannot be reversed.*
   3. *No! This answer indicates that the therapeutic program should avoid frustrating the child. The therapeutic program is rehabilitation. For a child with cerebral palsy, learning new skills through rehabilitation is frustrating. Without frustration, no progress can occur. The nurse should not seek to avoid frustration, but should assist the child in coping with the inevitable frustration.*

   4. *Correct! This option describes the overall aim of therapy for a client with cerebral palsy.*

18. **The nurse enters a new mother's room to check on her during an infant feeding and finds her in tears. She explains that her sister has a mentally retarded child who is two years old. The mother is upset because her baby's eyes roll around just like her niece's and she is afraid of retardation in her own baby. Which of the following statements would be the most therapeutic response by the nurse?**

   1. "All newborns lack the necessary muscle control to regulate eye movement. It is normal in all infants at this age."
   2. "I will return the baby to the nursery and observe him carefully."
   3. "I will call your pediatrician and report your concerns."
   4. "Lack of muscle control in a newborn is a cause for concern but it doesn't necessarily mean the child is retarded."

   1. *Good choice! This mother needs reassurance that all infants lack eye muscle control at this young age. The response does not give her reassurance about retardation, but it informs her that the lack of eye muscle control is normal.*
   2. *Wrong response. This option implies that the infant requires close observation due to this lack of eye muscle control.*
   3. *Wrong choice! This statement infers that the pediatrician needs to be notified about this lack of eye muscle control, when all infants lack eye muscle control at this young age.*
   4. *Incorrect! The lack of eye muscle control is not a cause for concern but a normal finding in a newborn infant.*

19. **A client has blastomycosis and is being treated with amphotericin B (Fungizone). Which of the following statements made by the client indicates to the nurse that she has an accurate understanding of the administration of amphotericin B (Fungizone)?**

   1. "The nurse told me that the drug is destroyed by light, so I'll be getting the medicine on the 11:00 pm to 7:00 am shift."
   2. "It sure would be nice if they used my Hickman catheter for administration of this medicine, but I guess the medicine is too irritating to the material in the catheter."
   3. "I'm glad that I'll only have to take this medicine for 10 days because of the numerous side effects."
   4. "I'll be given some Tylenol before the medicine is given to help decrease the fever that I'll probably get when the medicine is being given."

1. *Incorrect. Although amphotericin B is light sensitive, no significant deterioration occurs within the six to eight hours required for infusion of a single dose. It's not standard practice to protect the medicine from light as it once was.*

2. *No!! Amphotericin B should be given through a central venous access device if one is available in order to maximize the dilution of the medicine as it enters the systemic circulation. A Hickman catheter is a central access device and the chance of extravasation is minimal with this method of IV delivery.*

3. *Incorrect. Amphotericin B therapy must be continued for long periods, perhaps several months, to create the possibility of a cure for disseminated fungal disease. Administering the drug on alternate days and over a six-hour period may reduce the incidence of side effects.*

4. **Correct. The client understands this premedication protocol to help decrease the side effect of fever. The client may also be premedicated with an antiemetic or antihistamine to decrease other side effects of chills, nausea/vomiting, headache and anorexia. These symptoms typically subside within the first four hours of administration.**

20. **A client with a new colostomy has been given instructions about the irrigation of his ostomy. Which action by the client would indicate to the nurse that the teaching plan has to be reviewed?**

    1. Used 500 mL of irrigating solution.
    2. Used warm tap water to irrigate the ostomy.
    3. Inserted a lubricated cone tip into the ostomy stoma to begin the irrigation.
    4. Positioned the irrigating solution bag 30 inches above the stoma.

    1. *Incorrect choice. The correct amount of solution to be used for irrigation is 500-1,000 mL, so the client's choice is appropriate.*

    2. *Wrong choice. Tap water can be used, and it should feel warm to the client's wrist. Water that is too cool can cause cramping; water that is too hot may burn the mucosal lining of the colon.*

    3. *Wrong selection. This is proper procedure for beginning the irrigation. The lubricated cone tip is inserted approximately one inch, and the solution is allowed to flow in slowly.*

    4. **Yes! You have identified the incorrect action. This means that the client needs further teaching. The irrigating bag should be positioned 18 to 20 inches above the height of the stoma, not 30 inches. This height can cause too much pressure in the line and force the irrigating solution in too rapidly, causing abdominal cramping.**

21. **In caring for an elderly or debilitated client on piperacillin (Pipracil), the nurse should give immediate attention to which of the following?**

    1. Unusual weight loss, abdominal cramps.
    2. Blurred vision.
    3. Prolonged prothrombin time.
    4. Skin rashes.

    1. **Very good! Elderly clients are very prone to superinfections and pseudomembranous colitis. A superinfection occurs when the normal flora are eliminated by the antibiotic, making the internal environment susceptible to undesirable bacteria, yeasts, or fungi. Weight loss, abdominal cramps, diarrhea, discolored tongue, and sore mouth are symptoms of pseudomembranous colitis.**

    2. *Changes in the eyes are not related to penicillins.*

    3. *This is not correct. Some penicillins are metabolized up to 50% in the liver, but most excretion is via the kidney.*

    4. *Wrong! Skin rashes should be observed for in all clients, regardless of age, although it is true that elderly clients are more likely to be hypersensitive to skin rashes from penicillin. You are to look for a symptom that would be particularly threatening for an elderly or debilitated client.*

22. **A nurse observes a client on the psychiatric unit muttering to herself and standing near a window. The client states, "The voices are telling me to jump. They say test the glass and then jump through." What is the best nursing response to this statement?**

    1. "Where are these voices coming from? Do you recognize them as belonging to anyone that you know?"
    2. "I think you are hallucinating. The only voices in this room are yours and mine."
    3. "Tell the voices that you are not going to listen to them."
    4. "You say you are hearing voices that make you feel like jumping through the window. I understand the voices are frightening to you, but I want you to know that I do not hear any voices."

    1. *This is not correct because the nurse is conveying the belief that the hallucinations are real.*

    2. *This statement is not correct because it denies the validity of the client's perceptions. Attempts to reason with the client, argue about, or challenge the perceptions will only tend to further reinforce them.*

    3. *This is not correct because the nurse is supporting the client's belief in the voices. The nurse's role is to provide a link with reality.*

    4. **Good choice! Hearing voices telling her to jump from the window is a very unsafe situation for the client, who might carry out these "commands." It is important for the nurse to acknowledge the client's perceptions while also casting doubt on them by stating clearly that the nurse does not share them. Additional measures may have to be taken to ensure this client's safety.**

23. The wife of an alcoholic client says to the nurse, "I told my husband I would leave him if he did not get into treatment. Now that he is here, I feel differently. What can I do to help him?" Which of the following statements is the most therapeutic nursing response?

   1. "You should attend an Al-Anon meeting. The group can teach you how to best help him stay sober."

   2. "You have already done a great deal by getting him to come into treatment. Now it is up to him to make the best use of his time here."

   3. "Are you feeling some responsibility for his drinking?"

   4. "Tell me more about the kind of help you feel you are able to provide at this time."

   1. Incorrect. Al-Anon is a support group that primarily benefits the family members. The program provides information on enabling behaviors and how to cope more effectively with the person who drinks. Members also are supported to focus more closely on meeting their own needs and less on those of the alcoholic.

   2. This is not correct. Alcoholism is a family disease in that each member is affected by the drinking behavior. Most programs include the family in aspects of the treatment process.

   3. This is not correct. The nurse is assuming information that the wife has not presented.

   4. Correct. This comment will help the wife clarify what assistance she can realistically provide without sacrificing the meeting of her own needs in the process.

24. A client who has a broken leg is to be discharged from the hospital after crutch training by physical therapy. His friend brings in a pair of crutches for him to use. What is the best nursing action?

   1. If the client has used crutches before, cancel the physical therapy order and allow him to go home.

   2. Inform the client that crutches are custom fit for each client, and that he cannot use his friend's crutches.

   3. Have the client try the crutches to see if they are the right size.

   4. Send the crutches to physical therapy with the client for evaluation by that department.

   1. Wrong. This option is not appropriate because of the risk of falling if the crutches are used incorrectly. Before discharge, the client must be evaluated for his understanding and correct usage of crutches.

   2. No. Although crutches are sized and adjusted for proper fit for each client, crutches are not customized for each individual. The client may be able to use his friend's crutches if both men are similar in size.

   3. Wrong. Merely trying out the crutches is not sufficient. A client must be instructed in proper use of crutches in order to avoid potential falls.

   4. Correct! It may be possible for the client to use his friend's crutches, and it is most appropriate to have them evaluated by physical therapy personnel during crutch training.

25. The mother of a two-month-old infant with hydrocephalus calls the nurse at the health center. Which statement by the mother should alert the nurse to a potential problem?

   1. "My baby cries all the time and I can't seem to comfort him."

   2. "My baby spits up after each feeding."

   3. "My baby doesn't smile at me yet."

   4. "My baby jumps at sudden noises."

   1. Correct! A high-pitched cry, or constant crying, indicates irritability that could be caused by increased intracranial pressure or infection.

   2. Wrong choice! Frequent or projectile vomiting might indicate increased intracranial pressure; however, it is a normal characteristic for infants to spit up small amounts after feedings.

   3. Wrong choice! Although most babies smile by two months, lack of a social smile by this time does not necessarily indicate a complication.

   4. Wrong choice! The startle reflex is normal in newborns and usually disappears by four months.

26. An elderly client is able to walk with a cane and enjoys ambulating in the hall. Since he has memory problems, he has great difficulty remembering which room is his. What nursing action would best alleviate this problem?

   1. Assign him a room close to the nursing station so staff members will be available to help him.

   2. Assign him to a room with a roommate who can watch out for him.

   3. Do not allow him to leave his room unaccompanied.

   4. Put his picture and his name written in large letters on the door to his room.

   1. Incorrect. This action is not feasible in most settings and, even if it were, would only serve to make him more dependent on the nursing staff.

   2. Incorrect. This just makes him dependant on his roommate. There is a better option.

   3. Incorrect. This action would foster increasing dependency and loss of a sense of control.

   4. Correct. This is an orienting tactic that would allow the client to locate his room independently.

27. **Amoxicillin (Amoxil) is absorbed more effectively when the nurse administers it with which of the following?**

   1. Orange juice or grapefruit juice.
   2. Milk or Amphojel.
   3. A complete meal.
   4. A full glass of water on an empty stomach.

   1. *This is incorrect. Citrus juices destroy oral penicillins.*
   2. *Antacids or milk should not be needed. If gastrointestinal upset occurs, pseudomembranous colitis should be suspected.*
   3. *This is incorrect. Absorption of many penicillins decreases when taken with food.*
   4. ***That's right! Oral penicillins should be given on an empty stomach because they bind to food and are poorly absorbed in the acid media of the stomach.***

28. **The orthopedic nurse admitting a client with osteoarthritis, would expect the client to report all of the following symptoms, specific only to rheumatoid arthritis, except:**

   1. Joint pain.
   2. Joint stiffness in the morning.
   3. Presence of Heberden's nodes on the fingers.
   4. Remissions and exacerbations of symptoms.

   1. *No. Both osteoarthritis and rheumatoid arthritis cause joint pain, although it tends to be more generalized in rheumatoid states.*
   2. *Incorrect. Both types of arthritis have joint stiffness in the morning. In rheumatoid arthritis, the stiffness does decrease with moderate activity, whereas the stiffness of osteoarthritis gets worse after exercise.*
   3. *No, Heberden's nodes are bony nodes on the distal interphalangeal joints that are characteristic of osteoarthritis only.*
   4. ***Correct! Rheumatoid arthritis, a chronic systemic disease of unknown etiology, is characterized by exacerbations and remissions. Osteoarthritis is characterized by a progressive loss of joint cartilage with joint degeneration.***

29. **The nurse finds an elderly client with her IV pulled out, standing next to her bed with the side rails in the up position. The client is confused, does not have an identification bracelet on, and cannot remember her name. What should the nurse do first?**

   1. Help the client into bed, and remind her to call the nurse when she wants to get out of bed.
   2. Help the client into bed, and then restart the IV.
   3. Place a restraining vest on the client.

   4. Put an identification bracelet on the client and help her back to bed.

   1. *Wrong. Reminding a confused client to use a call light is not an appropriate nursing action. The case scenario tells you that the client cannot remember her name, so she will probably not remember to use a call light.*
   2. *Wrong. The case scenario does not tell you whether the IV has life-saving medications or fluids infusing, so you cannot assume that the IV is a physiological need. Do not "read into" the question! Since a physiological need is not identified, the safety of the client is the most important nursing consideration at this time.*
   3. ***Excellent! The case scenario tells you that the client got out of a bed that had the side rails up. This is an unsafe situation, since the client is at risk of falling. Such a fall could result in a life-threatening injury. Placing a restraining vest on the client will provide for her safety. In fact, this is the only option that provides for the client's immediate safety.***
   4. *The client's lack of an identification bracelet is an important safety concern, however, the case scenario tells you that the client got out of a bed that had the side rails up. This is an unsafe situation, since the client is at risk for falling. Such an injury can be life-threatening. After the immediate physical safety of the client is assured, an identification bracelet can be obtained.*

30. **A penicillin-allergic client has been prescribed cefoperazone (Cefobid). The nurse should give priority which complication?**

   1. Drug resistance.
   2. Hypersensitivity reactions.
   3. Drug tolerance.
   4. Interactions with other drugs.

   1. *Wrong choice! Drug resistance is always possible, but this is not the highest priority.*
   2. ***You are correct! Cephalosporins are chemical modifications of penicillins. The possibility of a cross-reaction is five to 10 percent.***
   3. *This is incorrect. Drug tolerance does not develop with antibiotics.*
   4. *Wrong! While this may be true in general, no other drugs are mentioned in this case. Look for a complication related to penicillin itself.*

31. **A physician orders a body magnetic resonance imaging (MRI) for diagnostic purposes. It would be most important for the nurse to tell the client that the procedure:**

   1. Takes 15 to 30 minutes.
   2. Involves injection of a contrast dye.
   3. Is painless, except for the discomfort of lying still.
   4. Uses only small amounts of radiation.

1. *Incorrect. It takes 60 to 90 minutes for body imagery.*
2. *No, an MRI does not require contrast dye. This is a noninvasive procedure.*
3. **Correct! No discomfort is felt during the test. A tingling sensation may be felt in metal fillings, and the client may experience discomfort from remaining motionless, but there is no pain.**
4. *Incorrect choice. An MRI does not require ionizing radiation.*

32. A three-month-old client is in respiratory isolation. Which of the following nursing actions will most effectively prevent the spread of pathogens via droplet infection?

1. Wearing a gown and mask when feeding the client.
2. Using sterile gloves when changing her diapers.
3. Having the baby wear a mask when in the playroom.
4. Using enteric precautions when caring for the baby.

1. *Yes! This question seeks to identify the main threat to the general population from this client's infection. To prevent the spread of pathogens to other clients, the nurse must ensure that respiratory secretions are not transmitted. When feeding and burping the infant, the respiratory secretions will become mixed with the formula. When the baby burps, there is risk of spreading the pathogens via droplet as well as by contact with the nurse's uniform. Wearing a gown and mask will decrease the probability of transmitting the organisms.*
2. *Wearing gloves to change her diapers will not prevent the transmission of respiratory secretions.*
3. *A three-month-old in respiratory isolation should not leave the room. Taking the baby to the playroom is inappropriate.*
4. *Enteric precautions will not prevent the transmission of respiratory secretions. They are not appropriate for a baby in respiratory isolation.*

33. A 53-year-old client with Type I, Insulin Dependent Diabetes Mellitus (IDDM) usually walks two miles each day after breakfast. She is planning to participate in a Walk-a-Thon in which she may walk as much as six miles. Which of the following statements by the nurse would be best in preparing the client for the Walk-a-Thon?

1. "Participating in a Walk-a-Thon is much too strenuous for you."
2. "Ask your doctor to increase your insulin dose the day of the Walk-a-Thon."
3. "Test your blood glucose immediately following the Walk-a-Thon."
4. "Eat some additional carbohydrates before you begin the Walk-a-Thon."

1. *Incorrect. The client walks regularly. There is no data to support the idea that a Walk-a-Thon is too strenuous for her.*
2. *Incorrect! Since insulin acts more quickly when the injection is followed by vigorous exercise, an increased dose of insulin on the day of the Walk-a-Thon may cause a hypoglycemic reaction.*
3. *This is not correct. Blood glucose should be monitored before meals and at bedtime.*
4. *Exercise causes increased utilization of carbohydrates. Prior to unusual exercise, an insulin dependent diabetic should consume an extra amount of complex carbohydrates to prevent a hypoglycemic reaction.*

34. A client with a history of bleeding esophageal varices is concerned about preventing further episodes of bleeding. What caution should the nurse give to the client?

1. Include high fiber and roughage in your diet.
2. Avoid drinking hot liquids.
3. Restrict activities and exercise in warm weather.
4. Avoid bearing down when having a bowel movement.

1. *No, absolutely not! Esophageal varices can often bleed after irritation of the dilated vessels by poorly chewed foods or irritating fluids. Foods that are high in fiber and roughage can also mechanically irritate the varices, causing them to bleed.*
2. *No, not necessary. There is no indication that drinking hot liquids will cause varices to bleed.*
3. *No, not necessary. There is no connection between exercise in warm weather and bleeding esophageal varices. Look for an option that may increase portal pressure.*
4. *Yes! The client should avoid all maneuvers that increase intra-abdominal or intrathoracic pressure: straining, coughing, sneezing, bending over, etc.*

35. A 47-year-old client has pancytopenia and is placed on protective precautions for infection. Which of the following comments by the client would indicate to the nurse that she understands her condition and the precautions?

1. "I have never been so aware that germs are everywhere around us."
2. "I didn't realize that I am so contagious that I need a private room."
3. "Everyone who touches me washes their hands like I am really contaminated."
4. "I might make my sister's baby sick, so I told her not to visit."

1. *Yes. This comment indicates an understanding of the need for protective precautions.*
2. *No. This comment indicates that the client does not understand her condition or the need for precau-*

tions. Pancytopenia is not contagious. Protective precautions are implemented to protect the client from infection, not to prevent the spread of a contagious disease.

3. *Incorrect. This comment indicates that the client does not understand her condition or the need for precautions. The client is not contaminated with a contagious disease. Strict hand washing is done to protect the client from infection.*

4. *No, this comment indicates that the client does not understand her condition or the need for precautions. Pancytopenia is not contagious. The sister and her baby are not at risk for developing an illness as a result of visiting the client.*

36. **In addition to the electrocardiogram (ECG), which of the following should the nurse monitor most closely during the IV administration of verapamil (Calan) to a client with a supraventricular tachycardia?**

    1. Blood pressure.
    2. Respiratory rate.
    3. Urine output.
    4. Level of consciousness.

    1. ***Correct choice! Calan is a calcium channel blocker that can be used to control supraventricular tachyarrhythmias. It also decreases blood pressure and acts as a coronary vasodilator and antianginal agent: it has many uses! A major side effect is hypotension; therefore, the blood pressure and pulse must be monitored before and frequently during parenteral administration of Calan.***

    2. *Wrong. Calan does not cause respiratory depression when given IV, although it may precipitate respiratory muscle failure if the client has Duchenne's muscular dystrophy. The only side effect related to the respiratory system is pulmonary edema, which does not often occur.*

    3. *Incorrect. Calan does not affect the kidneys: remember that this drug is a calcium channel blocker, inhibiting calcium transport into myocardial and vascular small muscle cells, resulting in slowed electrical conduction.*

    4. *No. Calan is a calcium channel blocker and may cause dizziness as a side effect, but no change in level of consciousness.*

37. **The nurse knows that which of the following signs/symptoms is considered the earliest indication of increased intracranial pressure (ICP)?**

    1. Ipsilateral pupil dilation.
    2. Restlessness.
    3. Lethargy.
    4. Bradycardia.

    1. *No, pupil dilation occurs when increasing pressure displaces the brain against the optic nerve. It is not an early sign of increased ICP.*

    2. *Incorrect. Restlessness can be an early sign of tissue hypoxia, but not necessarily of increasing ICP.*

    3. ***Correct! The earliest sign of increasing ICP is lethargy. It's important to remember that the level of responsiveness/consciousness is one of the most important indicators of a client's condition.***

    4. *Wrong choice. Alterations in vital signs may be a late sign of increased ICP.*

38. **A 10-year-old male client is in skeletal traction for the treatment of a fractured femur. This is his fifth day post-pinning. At the change of shift the nurse finds the client crying in pain and the right foot is pale and pulseless. Which of the following is the most appropriate interpretation of this assessment?**

    1. Severe pain is to be expected; pain medication should be given.
    2. This client has a low pain tolerance and needs appropriate distraction.
    3. The traction may be pulling too hard and should be released.
    4. This is an abnormal finding and the physician should be notified.

    1. *No. By the fifth day it is not expected that acute pain would be found on assessment, and pain medication will only mask the problem. This assessment requires a different interpretation.*

    2. *Incorrect. Even if the nurse has reason to believe that this client is crying because he has a low pain tolerance, there is other data that has not been correctly interpreted.*

    3. *No. The weight of the pull should not cause increasing pain. If the traction were released, this is most apt to cause increased pressure on the blood and nerve supply and allow movement of the fractured bone.*

    4. ***Yes, you're right! These symptoms indicate compartment syndrome. This is an emergency, and the physician should be notified immediately.***

39. **The nurse must lift a heavy object found in the hallway. What is the proper technique for the nurse to use in lifting a heavy object?**

    1. Lift the object at arm's length so all of the arm muscles are being used.
    2. Bend from the waist, using a wide stance, so that the leg muscles are used.
    3. Maintain good body alignment and use the large muscles of the body while lifting an object.
    4. Bend at the knees and use the large leg muscles when lifting the object.

1. *Wrong. When lifting an object at arm's length, the muscles in the arm are stretched, which fatigues the muscles quickly. This position also results in poor balance, because the heavy object is outside the body's base of support.*

2. *Wrong. Bending from the waist results in the use of the small back muscles, which become stretched and easily injured.*

3. ***Right! Using good body alignment and large muscles provides a good base of support, which reduces back strain and helps maintain balance. Note that this option includes or encompasses the correct idea in Option 4. Option 3 is more global, making it the best option.***

4. *Not the best choice. Bending at the knees and using the large leg muscles to lift provides decreased risk for musculoskeletal strain. Although this is a correct action, one of the other options is a more global statement that includes this action. Read the options again and try to identify the more global statement.*

40. **An unconscious 18-year-old man is brought to the emergency room by two friends, who report that he took an overdose of heroin. A narcotic antagonist, naloxone (Narcan), is administered. After giving the medication, the nurse should monitor him closely for signs of:**

    1. Respiratory depression.
    2. Seizure activity.
    3. Nausea.
    4. Kidney failure.

    1. ***Congratulations. Naloxone displaces the opioid from the receptor sites in neurons and dramatically reverses the effects of the drug overdose. The client still must be monitored closely, however, because naloxone has a short duration of action and its effect may wear off before the overdosed drug has been sufficiently eliminated. If the client returns to a coma, naloxone must be given again.***

    2. *This is not correct. Seizure activity is not associated with either heroin overdose or the use of naloxone.*

    3. *This is not correct. Nausea is not associated with either heroin overdose or the use of naloxone. Nausea is, however, one of the late developing symptoms of heroin withdrawal.*

    4. *This is not correct. Kidney failure is not associated with either heroin overdose or the use of naloxone.*

41. **A client is admitted to the hospital with a diagnosis of myasthenia gravis. Because of the varying degrees of muscle weakness, the nursing priority should be to carefully observe for:**

    1. Symptoms of increased ICP.
    2. Confusion and disorientation.
    3. Respiratory difficulty.
    4. Diplopia.

    1. *Incorrect. Myasthenia gravis affects neuromuscular transmission of the voluntary muscles of the body. It does not affect pressure within the brain.*

    2. *No, confusion and disorientation are not characteristics of myasthenia gravis.*

    3. ***Excellent choice! Progressive weakness of the diaphragmatic and intercostal muscles may produce respiratory distress or predispose the client to respiratory infections. This is always a nursing priority.***

    4. *Wrong choice. Although diplopia is an early symptom of myasthenia gravis due to involvement of the ocular muscles, another assessment is more life-threatening.*

42. **After one week in the hospital, a client's condition has improved and she and the nurse are talking regularly. She reports that she had stopped taking her medication several weeks before she was admitted to the hospital, "because I wanted to make it on my own without pills." Which of the following is the most therapeutic response by the nurse?**

    1. "You know now that you cannot stop the pills or you'll get sick again. Please don't do it again."
    2. "You're a smart girl. You know what will happen to you if you stop your pills again."
    3. "I know you get tired of taking the meds, especially when you are doing well. Was there any special reason you decided to stop them when you did?"
    4. "This experience taught you that you can't stop your medication. Next time you are tempted to do so, remember how upset your parents were when you had to be re-hospitalized."

    1. *Reminding the client of her relapse because she stopped taking medication is appropriate, but this is not the most therapeutic option.*

    2. *This response is an effort to provide positive feedback, but it is done in a condescending manner. There is another option that is more therapeutic.*

    3. ***Correct. The nurse restated the client's feelings and then went on to help her assess more fully what might have motivated her to stop her medication when she did. After obtaining more information from the client, the nurse can help her plan how to handle similar situations in the future to hopefully prevent further relapses.***

    4. *This response is reinforcing the importance of taking medication, but the nurse's comment about her parents' distress is inappropriate because it inflicts guilt. Select the option that is most therapeutic.*

43. The nurse takes precautions to prevent constipation and fecal impaction in an immobilized client. The nurse is aware that if a client develops a fecal impaction, what serious complication could result?

1. Intestinal obstruction.
2. Bowel perforation.
3. Peritonitis.
4. Rectal bleeding.

1. *Yes. A fecal impaction is the presence of either hardened or putty-like feces in the rectum and sigmoid colon. If the condition is not relieved, intestinal obstruction can occur.*
2. *Wrong. Although this complication could occur during digital removal of the fecal impaction, it is not a complication of the impaction itself.*
3. *Wrong. Peritonitis is an inflammation of the peritoneum caused by the introduction of bacteria into the abdominal cavity. A fecal impaction is contained within the bowel and therefore cannot cause peritonitis.*
4. *Wrong. Rectal bleeding is seen in clients with hemorrhoids or certain types of bowel pathology, but a fecal impaction does not cause rectal bleeding.*

44. A client develops a fecal impaction. Before digital removal of the mass, what type of enema is usually given by the nurse to loosen the feces?

1. Fleets.
2. Oil retention.
3. Soap suds.
4. Tap water.

1. *Incorrect. A Fleets enema, which is a hypertonic solution, is given to cleanse the bowel. It is usually given after digital removal of the impaction.*
2. *Correct. Before digital removal of the fecal mass, an oil retention enema is often given to soften the stool. This makes the digital removal less painful for the client.*
3. *No. A soap suds enema acts as an irritant to increase peristalsis and thus facilitate the removal of stool. The soap suds enema is usually given after the fecal impaction has been digitally removed in order to completely cleanse the bowel.*
4. *Wrong. Tap water enemas were previously used to cleanse the bowel, but are now contraindicated because of the possibility of fluid and electrolyte imbalances. Tap water, which is hypotonic, can be drawn into the cells, causing a fluid overload (hypervolemic state).*

45. The physician has ordered a sputum specimen to be collected for culture and sensitivity. The nurse is aware that the preferable time to collect this specimen is:

1. In the morning.
2. In the evening, after forcing fluids all day.
3. After antibiotics have been started.
4. After the client has taken an expectorant.

1. *Correct! Generally, the deepest specimens are obtained in the early morning. The client is instructed to rinse his mouth prior to expectorating into the sterile container; therefore, it's preferable to collect the specimen before breakfast.*
2. *No. Although forcing fluids (especially clear liquids) will help to thin the secretions, the evening hours are not the best time.*
3. *Incorrect choice! Recall that any specimen ordered for culture and sensitivity should be obtained before antibiotic therapy is started in order to prevent interference with test results.*
4. *No, this is not the best time. Expectorants can contaminate the specimen.*

46. A client has been receiving moxalactam (Moxam) 800 mg IV for septicemia. He is now ready for discharge. Which of the following discharge instructions would be most appropriate for the nurse to give?

1. Do not drink any alcohol for at least three days after discharge.
2. Report any shortness of breath to your physician immediately.
3. Be sure to continue taking the Moxam (p.o.) until the entire prescription is gone.
4. Drink extra fluids for at least one week to help prevent kidney damage from the IV Moxam.

1. *Good job!! You remembered that alcohol may cause a disulfiram-like reaction when taken with certain cephalosporins: Cefobid, Mandol, Cefotan, and Moxam. Symptoms include stomach pain, n/v, headaches, hypotension, flushing of the face, and tachycardia. Clients are to avoid alcohol-containing beverages, medications and OTC medications containing alcohol during administration of these meds and for three days after the medicine is discontinued.*
2. *Incorrect choice. Although dyspnea is significant, this symptom, often associated with bronchospasm secondary to anaphylaxis, would most likely occur during the first administration of this drug—not after discharge.*
3. *No. Moxam is not absorbed from the GI tract and must be given parenterally (IV or IM only).*
4. *Incorrect. Although cephalosporins are excreted via the kidneys and should be used cautiously in clients with renal impairment, there is no indication for the client to drink extra fluids for a week after the medication is discontinued.*

47. An eight-month-old child screams when his mother leaves the room. The mother begins to cry and says, "I don't understand why he is so upset, no one has hurt him." Choose the best response for the nurse, which would reflect the proper interpretation of the infant's behavior.

    1. "This is a response to an over-stimulating environment, he is tired."
    2. "This is a reaction to overexposure to caregivers."
    3. "He probably remembers you were gone two hours the last time you left."
    4. "This is a normal reaction for a child of his age."

    1. *No, not the best answer. Yes, a hospital can be over-stimulating, and he may be tired, but this response is likely to occur even if he has just awakened.*
    2. *No. The child isn't responding to too much attention, the stem states he "screams when the mother leaves the room."*
    3. *Incorrect. Eight-month-olds have little sense of time. This is not the reason for the child's response.*
    4. **Yes, absolutely. The eight-month-old is responding to separation from the primary caregiver, his mom, by protesting loudly. Explaining this to the mother may help her cope with feelings of guilt when she needs to leave the child's room.**

48. A client is scheduled for a sigmoidoscopy. The nurse should advise the client that, during the procedure, he will be placed in which position?

    1. Supine.
    2. Prone.
    3. Left lateral.
    4. Semi-Fowler's.

    1. *Incorrect. This position would not allow for proper insertion of the sigmoidoscope and could cause bowel perforation.*
    2. *No. This position is not used because it does not provide the client with adequate lung aeration during the procedure and does not allow for proper insertion of the sigmoidoscope, following the natural curvature of the bowel.*
    3. **Good choice. The left lateral, or Sim's position, is the preferred position, just as for enema administration. It provides the most comfort for the client and allows the scope to be inserted along the natural curvature of the sigmoid colon.**
    4. *Absolutely not! This position is never used for colonoscopic examinations. It offers no visibility of the rectal opening and is dangerous for the client; it would dramatically increase the possibility of bowel perforation.*

49. A client, age 10, is recovering following an appendectomy. He is ambulatory and goes to the day room with his parents. While changing the linen on the client's bed, the nurse should handle the linen by which of the following methods?

    1. Hold it close to the body to avoid dropping it.
    2. Place the soiled linen on the chair until done making the bed.
    3. Hold the linen away from the body and uniform.
    4. Shake the clean linen to unfold it to provide ease in making the bed.

    1. *Wrong! Holding the clean linen next to the body can transfer organisms from the uniform to the clean linen. Holding dirty linen next to the body can transfer organisms from the soiled linen to the uniform. Either action results in contamination and transfer of organisms.*
    2. *Wrong! Soiled linen is contaminated and will further contaminate the surfaces of the chair. The soiled linen should be placed directly into the laundry hamper in order to prevent contamination of other surfaces.*
    3. **Right! The linen should be held away from the uniform. Since the nurse must go from client to client, any organisms present on the uniform can be transferred from one client to another.**
    4. *Opening linens by shaking them causes movement of air. Air currents can carry dust and organisms about the room, resulting in potential infection.*

50. A client's son is distressed over his mother's crying and saying that she wants to die. He asks the nurse to help him "calm her down." The nurse's best response to his request is:

    1. "All right, I'll talk with her and see if I can comfort her."
    2. "If you just sit quietly with her, I'm sure she will calm down when she gets these feelings out."
    3. "It's hard to see her so upset, but she needs to let these feelings out; we can both stay with her."
    4. "This seems to bother you more than it does her."

    1. *This is not the best option because the nurse is ignoring the son's feelings of distress. The nurse's response is not based on an understanding of the grief process.*
    2. *This option is partially correct in that the nurse recognizes his mother has a need to express her feelings through crying. The response does not recognize, however, that the son is having difficulty with his feelings and his understanding of the grief process.*
    3. **Correct. The nurse's response acknowledges the son's feelings while also informing him of his mother's need to express her feelings through crying. This response also uses the communication tool of offering self.**
    4. *This is flippant and untrue. It is not the correct option.*

51. A client is scheduled for surgery this morning. The preoperative checklist has been completed, and the nurse has just administered the preoperative injection. Which nursing action should be implemented next?

    1. Take the client to the bathroom to void.
    2. Dim the overhead and bedside lights.
    3. Review deep breathing and coughing exercises.
    4. Put the side rails up on both sides of the bed.

    1. *Incorrect. The client should have voided before being given the injection. Now that he has been given preoperative medication he is at a higher risk for a fall.*
    2. *This is an appropriate action, but it is not the priority at this time. The client is at risk for a fall.*
    3. *This action is an important part of preoperative teaching. It is inappropriate at this time, however, because of the preoperative injection.*
    4. ***Very good! The client is at a greater risk of falling because of the injection. This action ensures the client's safety.***

52. A client had a right lobectomy yesterday and has a chest tube connected to suction at 20 cm of water pressure. Upon assessment of the client this morning, the nurse notes that there is no fluctuation in the water-seal chamber. What would be the nurse's immediate action?

    1. Increase the suction until fluctuation reappears.
    2. Observe for kinks in the tubing.
    3. Elevate the head of the bed to 80 degrees.
    4. No action is necessary, since the lung has most likely re-expanded.

    1. *No. This action will have no effect upon the water-seal compartment. Recall that the amount of suction is controlled by the water level in the suction-control bottle (i.e., 20 cm level). Turning up the suction will only increase the bubbling!*
    2. ***Good choice! Fluctuation of the water level in the tube shows that there is effective communication between the pleural cavity and the drainage bottle. A decrease in fluctuation on the first postoperative day most likely means that the tubing is obstructed by blood clots, fibrin, or kinking.***
    3. *No, elevating the head of the bed will not affect the water-seal bottle. An absence of fluctuation indicates a problem within the system.*
    4. *Highly unlikely! Lung re-expansion will not occur within 24 hours after a lobectomy. It will take at least two to three days, and needs to be confirmed by a chest x-ray.*

53. A seven-year-old boy is brought to the physician's office with complaints of a sore throat. As the nurse prepares to collect a throat culture, the mother states, "I don't know why you can't just give him antibiotics and be done with it." The nurse's best response is which of the following statements?

    1. "This could be a virus. If it is, antibiotics would not be effective."
    2. "Antibiotics have dangerous side effects. Let's see which one he really needs."
    3. "Insurance companies require a throat culture before antibiotics can be ordered."
    4. "This is the physician's order. Would you like me to call him for you?"

    1. ***Best choice! Most upper respiratory infections are caused by viruses. It is important to rule out bacterial agents, but antibiotics are generally not considered until the causative agent is identified as bacterial.***
    2. *Wrong choice! This statement is a poor choice because it alarms the mother unnecessarily and it is inaccurate. Most respiratory infections are caused by viruses, against which no antibiotic will be effective.*
    3. *Wrong choice! This statement does not educate the client's family to the need for a throat culture, and to the action of the medication. Moreover, it is inaccurate and implies that medication protocols are set by insurance companies.*
    4. *Wrong! Referring this client to the physician would be inappropriate. The answer to this question is within the realm of the nurse's practice.*

54. Initially, which of the following actions will the nurse most likely consider in dealing with the ritualistic behaviors of a client with obsessive-compulsive disorder?

    1. Confront the client about the senseless nature of the ritualistic behaviors.
    2. Set strict limits on the behaviors so the client can better conform to the unit rules and schedules.
    3. Isolate the client for a period of time to lower his anxiety about offending others.
    4. Plan the client's schedule to allow extra time to perform the rituals to keep his anxiety within manageable levels.

    1. *Wrong! Most clients with rituals recognize the senselessness of their behaviors, but they cannot control them.*
    2. *Wrong. Strict limit setting will increase the client's anxiety, especially when he is first beginning treatment.*
    3. *Wrong. Isolating the client will increase anxious behavior.*

4.   Correct. It is important that sufficient time be allotted for the client to perform his rituals early in his treatment. This will help him keep his anxiety level manageable.

55.   **All of the following nursing interventions aid in the prevention of hyperbilirubinemia except:**

1.   Early and frequent feedings.
2.   Promotion of adequate hydration.
3.   Prevention of cold stress.
4.   Early administration of parenteral Vitamin K.

1.   Incorrect choice. Early and frequent feedings promote the excretion of bilirubin by promoting urine and bowel elimination. This question has a false response stem, so you are looking for an INEFFECTIVE intervention.
2.   Wrong choice! Good hydration of the newborn is effective in promoting excretion of bilirubin from the body. Look for an intervention that is INEFFECTIVE.
3.   No, preventing hypothermia actually does help prevent hyperbilirubinemia. Hypothermia in the newborn results in decreased GI mobility, which interferes with the excretion of bilirubin.
4.   Correct. Administration of vitamin K to newborn infants promotes normal blood coagulation but it has no effect on bilirubin levels.

56.   **A toddler in the pediatrics ward is to be placed in a highchair for a meal. After placing the client in the highchair, which nursing action is most appropriate initially?**

1.   Pour a small amount of milk into the glass.
2.   Ask the mother to feed the child, since she is present.
3.   Belt the child securely to the chair.
4.   Cut the child's food into bite size pieces.

1.   This is an appropriate action but not the most appropriate action initially. Never fill a glass or cup more than half full.
2.   This is an appropriate action, but it is not the most appropriate action initially. Toddlers have severe separation anxiety, and having mother feed the child will decrease their fear and increase their intake of food.
3.   Very good! This is a prioritizing question, and the priority in this case scenario is safety. The nurse should assess this potentially unsafe situation and make the appropriate changes to provide a safe environment. The toddler is at immediate risk of falling.
4.   This is appropriate, however, it is not the most appropriate action initially. A toddler should always have small pieces of food that can be picked up with the fingers.

57.   **An eight-year-old child is admitted to the hospital**

with swollen, painful joints, fatigue, and weight loss. He is diagnosed with rheumatic fever. When the parents ask what can lead to rheumatic fever, the nurse's best response is based on what knowledge?

1.   There is no known etiology for rheumatic fever.
2.   Rheumatic fever is an opportunistic disease.
3.   Rheumatic fever often occurs in children with congenital heart defects.
4.   Rheumatic fever is almost always preceded by a streptococcal infection.

1.   This is incorrect. Rheumatic fever is precipitated by Group A beta-hemolytic strep, which releases proteins that initiate an autoimmune process. In almost all cases, there is a known etiology.
2.   Incorrect! Rheumatic fever is an autoimmune process, but not a disease that strictly affects those with impaired immune systems.
3.   Incorrect! Rheumatic fever can cause cardiac damage; however, congenital defects do not predispose a child to rheumatic fever.
4.   Correct. In almost all cases, the child with rheumatic fever has had a recent history of a streptococcal infection. Prevention of rheumatic fever is aimed at early treatment of strep infections.

58.   **A client has just returned to the unit after a right pneumonectomy. The nurse should position him on his:**

1.   Right side.
2.   Left side or back.
3.   Back only.
4.   Right side or left side.

1.   Excellent choice! After a pneumonectomy, the operative side should be dependent so that fluid in the pleural space remains below the level of the bronchial stump, and the inoperative side can fully expand.
2.   No, positioning the client on his left side, the inoperative side, may compromise complete ventilation of the only lung that the client has.
3.   Incorrect. There is another position available that will not compromise the client's respirations.
4.   No, the nurse would not want to position the client in such a way as to impair his gas exchange. Think through the surgical results!

59.   **A client's son remarks to the nurse, "My father has been dead for six months now. I think my mother needs to get on with her life." What is the best response for the nurse to make to this statement?**

1.   "A death is usually a crisis for the whole family. How

has your father's death affected you?"

2. "I agree. How can you help her find more pleasure in her life?"
3. "I think it would be helpful if you could give her more support."
4. "Perhaps she needs more time. Grieving often takes a year or more to complete."

1. *This response does not address the son's question, so it is not the correct option. This might be an appropriate question after the nurse has responded to the son's question.*
2. *This response is not appropriate based on what is known about the grief process.*
3. *This response does not recognize the nature of the grief process. It also is not helpful to the son because the nurse does not explain what is meant by support.*
4. *Correct. This response indicates an understanding that acute grieving, such as would result from the loss of a spouse or other loved one, often takes one to two years to complete.*

60. **The nurse understands that which of the following statements about mourning is inaccurate?**

1. It is a normal response to loss.
2. It functions to free the individual from an attachment to the lost object so future relationships can be established.
3. It is accompanied by a growing realization that the loss has occurred.
4. Mourning occurs only in humans.

1. *No. The process of mourning or grieving is a normal response to a loss.*
2. *No. The final goal of mourning is to free the individual from too close an attachment to the lost object. Completing the process of mourning permits the person to move on and establish new relationships.*
3. *No. The initial phase of the grief process is usually shock and denial. This is followed by a growing realization that the loss has occurred. Remember, this question is asking for an option that is NOT accurate.*
4. *Correct! Mourning does not only occur in humans. Other animals also can experience mourning. Particularly those animals, such as primates and household pets, that form individual attachments.*

61. **Following a gastric resection, a client is taught nutritional habits that will slow gastric emptying, helping to decrease the incidence of the "dumping syndrome." Which foods selected by the client indicate to the nurse that he understands the instructions given?**

1. Ice cream.

2. Oranges.
3. Wheat bread.
4. Turkey.

1. *Correct. Foods that are high in fat are recommended, because fat tends to slow down gastric emptying.*
2. *Incorrect. Oranges, or any fruit, are not useful in helping to delay gastric emptying.*
3. *No, wheat bread or high fiber foods are not known to slow gastric emptying. The bulk provided by these foods helps to increase peristaltic activity and thus prevent constipation, but not the "dumping syndrome".*
4. *No. Turkey is a high protein food but has not been identified as producing the desired effect of delayed or slowed gastric emptying.*

62. **A client is admitted to the hospital with a diagnosis of active pulmonary tuberculosis. An immediate goal is controlling the spread of infection. To achieve this, the nurse would:**

1. Wear a gown and mask when caring for the client.
2. Recommend that the client wear a mask when she has visitors.
3. Teach the client how to cover her nose and mouth when she coughs or sneezes.
4. Use blood and needle precautions.

1. *No. The mask would be appropriate, but there is no need for a gown.*
2. *Incorrect. The right procedure would be for visitors, as well as all health care providers, to wear a mask when in the room.*
3. *Good choice! Teaching this, along with proper hand washing, will help prevent the spread of the infection by droplet nuclei.*
4. *No, tuberculosis is not transmitted via blood.*

63. **A three-month-old infant has undergone a colostomy for Hirschsprung's disease. When the mother questions the nurse about her child's prognosis, the nurse's most helpful response is:**

1. "Corrective surgery is a three-step approach. Let's wait and talk about the second stage when your child is ready for it."
2. "Most colostomies are temporary and can be reversed when the child is older."
3. "You're upset by your child's appearance, aren't you?"
4. "An enterostomal therapist can provide you with information on the management of a colostomy."

1. *Incorrect! Delaying discussion of the treatment process does not answer the mother's question. It may also increase the mother's anxiety to hear of further stages without explanation.*
2. *This is correct! The most helpful response ad-*

dresses the client's question and answers it simply and with accurate information. This information is in the realm of client teaching and also may allay some of the mother's concerns.

3. *Incorrect! Reflection is a useful therapeutic communication device; however, the mother has asked an information question rather than stated a concern. The nurse is most helpful when supplying the requested information. Assessment of the mother's emotions may be included after the question has been answered.*

4. *Wrong! It is inappropriate to refer the client for teaching when the mother has asked about prognosis. At a later time, referral for management might be appropriate, but at this time, the mother's request for information needs to be addressed by the nurse.*

64. **A 48-year-old woman is admitted to the psychiatric unit with a diagnosis of depression. Her husband reports that she had seemed despondent since their youngest child left for college two months before. She had become progressively more withdrawn, refused food, lost 20 pounds and neglected her appearance. During the admission interview, the client asks the nurse not to bother with her because "I am totally worthless." The nurse's best response to this statement is which of the following statements?**

1. "I have seen many valuable things about you."
2. "You feel worthless now because you are so depressed. You will feel differently when you begin to recover."
3. "You have been feeling very sad and alone for some time now."
4. "You really have a great deal to live for."

1. *This statement sounds like an attempt to raise self-esteem. It is not the best response because clients with low self-esteem do not benefit from feedback that they do not perceive is justified. There is a better option.*

2. *This statement is a possibility because it is teaching the client about the symptoms of her depression. However, the nurse cannot assure her she will feel better when she recovers. This is not the correct option.*

3. **Correct. This response reflects the client's feelings in a nonjudgmental way that indicates the nurse is willing to listen and accept what she is expressing. This will help the client feel more comfortable expressing feelings to the nurse.**

4. *No. This response would block further comments by the client because the nurse, in an effort to help, is really belittling the client's perceptions.*

65. **In preparation for a sigmoid colon resection, a**

client is receiving instructions about the colostomy that will be performed. Which instruction given by the nurse will require further clarification?

1. "Your colostomy will begin to function seven to ten days after surgery."
2. "The stoma of your colostomy will appear large at first, but it will shrink over the next few weeks."
3. "You will have to wear a colostomy bag at all times to prevent accidental leakage of stool."
4. "Your diet will not have to change dramatically. You can use a trial-and-error method to see which foods will not agree with you."

1. *No, this statement does not require further clarification. Because of the lack of bowel peristalsis after surgery and the client's NPO status, it is not unusual to see only mucous drain from the ostomy until approximately a week after surgery.*

2. *No, this statement does not require further clarification. The stoma will be edematous at first because of the trauma of surgery and manipulation of the colon, but the stoma will shrink to a "rosebud" size within a few weeks after surgery.*

3. **Good work -- this statement does require further clarification. Clients with a sigmoid colostomy may gain control of elimination and will only need to wear a small dressing over the site once they know their pattern of elimination. The lower the colostomy can be placed on the colon, the more control the client may have and the less need for the constant wearing of an ostomy bag.**

4. *No, this statement would not need further clarification. Most clients have no change in their diet patterns: what bothered them before surgery (gas-producing foods) will probably bother them after surgery. Clients are instructed to "try" foods and evaluate their effect upon the GI tract.*

66. **In performing ileostomy care, the nurse measures the circumference of the collection device opening so that it is at least how much larger than the stoma circumference?**

1. 1/8 inch.
2. 1/4 inch.
3. 1/2 inch.
4. 3/4 inch.

1. **Correct. The 1/8 inch edge around the stoma opening means that as little skin as possible is exposed to the irritating drainage from the ileostomy.**

2. *No, this is not the correct amount of peristomal skin to be exposed to the irritating effects of the ileostomy drainage.*

3. *Incorrect. The amount of skin to be exposed to the irritating effects of the ileostomy drainage is less than this.*

4. *Wrong. This amount of skin exposed to the ileo-*

stomy drainage will lead to peristomal skin irritation.

67. Which of the following findings by the nurse would the nurse understand to be consistent with a diagnosis of endometriosis:

1. Menses-linked symptoms that worsen over time.
2. Abdominal bloating starting seven to 10 days before menses.
3. Previous pregnancy loss one year previously.
4. Maternal history of pelvic inflammatory disease (PID).

1. Correct choice! The client with endometriosis complains of dysmenorrhea that increases in severity over time.

2. Wrong. Abdominal bloating is not a symptom of endometriosis.

3. Wrong. Pregnancy loss is not related to endometriosis; inability to conceive is common in these women.

4. No. A history of PID is not related to the diagnosis of endometriosis.

68. A client is scheduled for ECT in the morning. The nurse's responsibility in preparation for this procedure include all of the following except:

1. Explaining the procedure, including its risks and benefits, and obtaining the client's signature on the consent form.
2. Instructing the client to empty his bladder before the treatment.
3. Maintaining NPO status from midnight the night before the treatment.
4. Removing dentures, contact lenses, and other prosthetics before the treatment.

1. Correct! The psychiatrist is responsible for explaining the procedure, including its risks and benefits, and obtaining the client's signature on the consent form.

2. The nurse is responsible for ensuring that routine preoperative care is performed prior to ECT because the client will receive general anesthesia during the treatment.

3. Wrong. The nurse is responsible for ensuring that the client maintains NPO status from midnight the night before the treatment.

4. The nurse is responsible for ensuring that dentures, contact lenses, and other prosthetics are removed before the treatment.

69. A client has had a right total hip replacement and is three days postoperative. When the nurse and nursing assistant are transferring her to a chair, she cries out in pain. Which observation by the nurse would lead to the suspicion of a dislocated hip prosthesis:

1. Shortening of the right leg.
2. Bulging in the right hip area.
3. Adduction of the left leg.
4. Loose hip joint movement on the right side.

1. Correct choice! One of the classic indicators of prosthetic dislocation is shortening of the affected leg, along with inability to move it, abnormal rotation, and increased discomfort.

2. Incorrect. Dislocation of the prosthesis will not result in any visible bulging in the surgical area.

3. No. A prosthetic dislocation will not result in changes to the unaffected leg.

4. Incorrect choice. Dislocation of the prosthesis will result in inability to move the affected leg.

70. After her first night in the hospital, a depressed client complains of feeling too tired to get out of bed in the morning. In planning how to deal therapeutically with this, the nurse is guided by the knowledge that:

1. Helping to mobilize the client physically will also help to improve her emotional state.
2. Most people do require more rest when they are depressed.
3. It is best to wait until the client indicates she is ready to participate in structured activities.
4. Encouraging the client to get up and come out on the ward will only increase her feelings of worthlessness and guilt.

1. Correct. Mobilizing persons who are depressed helps to demonstrate that it is possible to change and thus counter feelings of hopelessness. Also, activity helps shift the client's preoccupation with self to interests in the outside world.

2. This is not correct. Persons who are depressed lack energy and often sleep excessively, but the sleep and rest are not restorative, like they would be for the nondepressed person.

3. Depressed persons are reluctant to initiate any activity on their own. This cannot be the correct option.

4. No. There is no such causal relationship.

71. A seven-month-old will be admitted for bacterial meningitis. The physician orders the following: blood culture, stat; prepare for a spinal tap; Ancef 250 mg IV, stat; continue the current IV at 25 mL/hour. (The IV was started in the emergency room at KVO.) Which of the following is the first priority of the nurse who will be admitting the child?

1. Regulate the IV flow rate to avoid overhydration.
2. After the blood work is drawn, administer the antibiotic to treat the meningitis.
3. Arrange for the child to be in isolation, to protect others from infection.
4. Assess the child, including vital signs and history of allergy.

1. No. You've missed an earlier intervention. Also,

note that there really isn't a change in the rate ordered for the IV.

2. *No. It did say stat, but before the antibiotic is given the spinal tap would also be performed. Think about the nurse's role in primary prevention.*

3. ***Yes, this is the nurse's first responsibility. This needs to be addressed before the child arrives on the unit. Children with bacterial meningitis must be treated as highly contagious.***

4. *No. Assessment and history are important, but they do not require the nurse's first intervention.*

72. **A client is instructed to test her urine for the presence of luteinizing hormone. The nurse explains that the test is useful for:**

    1. Prediction of ovulation.
    2. Assessment of hormonal balance necessary for ovulation.
    3. Prediction of normal menstrual function.
    4. Assessment of the pH of cervical mucosa.

    1. ***Correct! A surge of luteinizing hormone predicts ovulation within 24 hours. Clients begin urine testing several days prior to their predicted date of ovulation.***

    2. *Incorrect. The presence or absence of LH in urine does not evaluate hormonal balance.*

    3. *Wrong. Testing for LH in urine does not predict normal menstrual function.*

    4. *Wrong choice. Testing for LH in the urine does not assess the cervical mucosa pH.*

73. **A client is ambulating down the tile hallway in her stocking covered feet. Which of the following is the priority nursing action?**

    1. Remind the client to avoid any wet spots on the floor.
    2. Tell the client that she should always wear slippers or shoes when ambulating.
    3. Get the client's slippers and have her put them on.
    4. No intervention is necessary since the client has her feet covered.

    1. *Although telling the client to avoid wet spots may help to prevent a fall, it is not the priority nursing action. Stocking feet are very slippery on a tile floor, and this situation needs to be addressed first.*

    2. *The client should be instructed in proper footwear to avoid falling. This action alone, however, will not prevent this client from slipping on the tile floor.*

    3. ***You're right! Making sure that slippers or shoes are worn by the client is the priority action, since it addresses the immediate problem of slipping on the tile floor.***

    4. *This option is incorrect. The client should have footwear that protects the client from slipping and falling.*

74. **A concerned mother calls the physician's office. Her child has a respiratory infection and a temperature of 39° C orally. She needs to give her son 240 mg of acetaminophen (Tylenol). The label on her bottle at home reads 160 mg/5 mL. The nurse's most helpful response is which of the following statements?**

    1. Give 1/2 teaspoon.
    2. Give 1 1/2 teaspoons.
    3. Give 1 1/2 mL.
    4. Give 15 mL.

    1. *Wrong.*
    2. *Correct! Here's the math: 240 mg/160 mg x 5 mL = 7.5 mL. There are 5 mL in a teaspoon so: 7.5 mL/5 mL x 1 tsp = 1 1/2 tsp.*
    3. *Wrong.*
    4. *Wrong.*

75. **Which of the following diagnostic procedures is considered invasive and requires a special consent form?**

    1. Magnetic resonance imaging (MRI).
    2. Cerebral arteriogram.
    3. Computed tomography (CT scan).
    4. Echoencephalography.

    1. *No, the MRI is a noninvasive and painless procedure that uses a powerful magnetic field to obtain images of different body areas.*

    2. *Yes! A cerebral arteriogram is considered invasive, with the injection of contrast material into a selected artery to study the cerebral circulation. A consent is required.*

    3. *Incorrect. The CT scan makes use of a narrow beam of x-ray to scan the body in successive layers. CT is a noninvasive and painless procedure.*

    4. *No. Echoencephalography is the recording of sound waves in response to ultrasound signals created by a transducer positioned over specific areas of the head. It is a noninvasive test.*

76. **An elderly widower with depression complains of not sleeping at all the first two nights in the hospital. The primary nurse notes the night nurses charted he was frequently awake when they made rounds. Which measure would be least appropriate to include in the nursing care plan to help him with his sleep problem?**

    1. Spending time with him when he awakens at night to explore what seems to be interfering with his sleep.
    2. Providing a soothing nighttime routine, such as a warm bath and backrub, to promote relaxation and sleep.
    3. Limiting intake of caffeinated beverages in the late afternoon and evening.

4. Discouraging napping during the day.

1. *Correct. Talking with the client for long periods during the night should be avoided because it can be stimulating as well as counterproductive. Long interactions reward the client for not sleeping by giving him additional attention. Interactions at night should be kept brief to reinforce the expectation that the client will sleep.*
2. *No, this would be appropriate to include in the nursing care plan. A soothing nighttime routine can promote relaxation and rest.*
3. *No, this would be appropriate to include in the nursing care plan. It is important to limit the intake of caffeine, which is a stimulant.*
4. *No, this would be appropriate to include in the nursing care plan. Taking naps during the day will make it more difficult for the client to sleep at night.*

77. **A client has just received the diagnosis of endometrial cancer. In taking a nursing history, which of the following symptoms is most likely to be reported by this client?**

1. An abnormal Papanicolaou (Pap) smear.
2. Post menopausal bleeding.
3. Recurrent backache.
4. Uterine enlargement.

1. *Wrong. An abnormal Pap smear is found in the client with cervical cancer.*
2. *Best choice! Most clients who have endometrial cancer report having post menopausal bleeding.*
3. *No. Recurrent backache is not related to endometrial cancer.*
4. *Wrong. Uterine enlargement is not found in the client with endometrial cancer.*

78. **A client is being treated with nystatin (Mycostatin) oral suspension for a candida oropharyngeal infection. How should the nurse instruct the client to use this medication?**

1. Swallow the solution quickly, to avoid burning the throat.
2. Take the medication with a glass of water.
3. Swish the solution around in the mouth, then hold it there for as long as possible.
4. Take the medication on an empty stomach.

1. *This is incorrect. Nystatin should not be swallowed quickly.*
2. *This is incorrect. Water will wash away the medication.*
3. *Correct. The medication is not absorbed from the stomach. It provides a local antifungal effect, so it needs to be in contact with the fungus for as long as possible.*
4. *Incorrect. An empty stomach is not necessary.*

79. **Thirty minutes after receiving Valium, a client reports that he is feeling much calmer. "I can't believe how scared I was when I came in. I will do anything to avoid having another panic attack." The nurse realizes the most important information to give him at this time is which of the following?**

1. Advise him to admit himself to the psychiatric unit where he can have a comprehensive evaluation in a protected setting.
2. Reduce the amount of stress in his life.
3. Make an appointment for outpatient psychotherapy to receive help with any emotional issues that might be responsible for his panic attacks.
4. Tell him he can always return to the emergency room if he should have another panic attack.

1. *This is not correct. There is no data to support his need for inpatient treatment. Panic disorder is usually treated in an outpatient setting.*
2. *This statement is correct, but it is not the best option for this question because stress reduction alone will not prevent future panic attacks.*
3. *Excellent! Panic attacks occur when the individual's defense mechanisms fail to contain his anxiety. Psychotherapy will help him learn to identify and resolve his emotional issues and conflicts and thereby prevent future panic attacks.*
4. *Wrong! This is not a helpful comment because the client wants to prevent future panic attacks.*

80. **A client, age 31, is brought to the emergency room after an automobile accident. She is conscious upon admission. A physical examination and x-rays reveal a transection of the spinal cord at T4. The nurse should give the highest priority to which of the following?**

1. The client has an allergy to iodine.
2. The client last voided seven hours ago.
3. The client smokes two packs of cigarettes a day.
4. The client is menstruating.

1. *Incorrect. Although this information may be important later, especially if any diagnostic tests using dye contrast media are ordered, it is not a priority at this time.*
2. *Excellent priority setting! A distended bladder is the most common cause of autonomic dysreflexia, an acute emergency that occurs as a result of exaggerated autonomic responses. It is characterized by severe, pounding headache with paroxysmal hypertension, profuse sweating, and bradycardia. Because this is an emergency situation, the objective is to remove the triggering stimulus as soon as possible.*
3. *Incorrect choice. This assessment is certainly important to validate the high risk for respiratory complications secondary to smoking; however, it's*

> *not the priority observation at this time. Look for an option that can be life-threatening to the client in this immediate situation.*
>
> 4. *No. The fact that the client is menstruating does not constitute an immediate emergency situation.*

81. A visitor asks the nurse about the client in the next room, who has metastatic cancer and cries out frequently. "That person must have a terrible disease. What is the matter with him?" The most appropriate response by the nurse would be which of the following?

1. "That client has cancer and is quite uncomfortable."
2. "Mr. Jones is being kept as comfortable as possible."
3. "That person is quite uncomfortable. Does his crying out bother you?"
4. "I cannot reveal anything about his diagnosis. Why don't you ask his family when they visit? I'm sure they would appreciate your concern."

1. *Wrong! Identifying the client in the next room and revealing his diagnosis is an invasion of the client's privacy.*
2. *Wrong! Identifying the client in the next room by name is a breach of confidentiality.*
3. ***Correct! This option states the obvious and focuses on the client's feelings, rather than on confidential information concerning the uncomfortable person.***
4. *This option does not address the immediate concern of the client, and it ignores the family's right to privacy.*

82. A client has been depressed and took too many sleeping pills. She is admitted to the psychiatric unit after being treated for the drug overdose. Which of the following nursing actions is NOT a priority?

1. Remove objects such as the client's personal razor and fingernail scissors from her room.
2. Allow the client to spend most of the day in bed, since she is very depressed.
3. Spend time with the client, in an effort to establish a therapeutic relationship.
4. Introduce the client to other clients and members of the health care team.

1. *Wrong. The client's razor and fingernail scissors could be used in another suicide attempt. These objects should be removed from her room as a safety measure. The stem of this question asks you to identify a nursing action that is NOT a priority.*
2. ***Allowing the client to spend most of the day in bed is not therapeutic. She is depressed and may feel tired, but for her own safety she should not be***

allowed to be alone most of the day. She should be with a member of the health care team who can monitor her activities to assure her safety. Maslow's Hierarchy of Needs indicates that when no physiological need exists, safety needs get priority. This is the answer, since the stem of this question asks you to select an option that does not represent a priority nursing action.

3. *Wrong. The stem of this questions asks you to identify a nursing action that is not a priority. Developing a therapeutic relationship is important in the care of clients with mental health problems. Low self-esteem is a critical aspect of depression. Spending time and developing a therapeutic relationship with the client is very important in helping the client reestablish self-esteem. Spending time with a depressed client is also important as a safety measure.*
4. *Incorrect. Introducing the client to other clients and members of the health care team will help to get her involved in unit activities. The stem of this question asks for a nursing action that is NOT a priority.*

83. A client is very irritable at breakfast. When asked if there is a problem, the client states that he was unable to sleep because of noise made by the staff on the night shift. The best initial response by the nurse is which of the following?

1. "It must be very distressing to be unable to sleep at night. Would you like to take a nap this morning?"
2. "I'll report that to the supervisor."
3. "Maybe we can move you to a room further from the nurses' station when one of those rooms becomes available."
4. "Why don't you close your door at night? Sometimes the nurses make noise and don't realize it."

1. ***Excellent! Addressing the client's feelings is the first action by the nurse. This response lets the client know that his feelings are important and need to be addressed. This response also addresses the client's need for sleep. Sleep-deprived clients are at risk for injury related to decreased judgment, slower response time, and slower reflexes.***
2. *Although reporting the situation to the supervisor may be appropriate, this response by the nurse is not therapeutic because it does not address the client's feelings or the problem of sleep deprivation.*
3. *Moving the client when a room becomes available does not address the client's present problem of sleep deprivation.*
4. *This response is not therapeutic, because it is defensive and attempts to provide justification for the noise. The client, for safety and health reasons, has the right to uninterrupted sleep if the physician's orders don't require that the client be awakened during the night.*

84. Following cervical x-rays and a CT scan, a client is found to have a spinal cord transection at T2-T3 vertebrae. Nursing staff can anticipate that the client's nursing care will be planned for which type of paralysis:

1. Hemiplegia.
2. Paraplegia.
3. Quadriplegia.
4. Paresthesia.

1. *Incorrect. Hemiplegia, paralysis of an arm and leg on the same side of the body, is seen after a cerebral vascular accident.*
2. **Correct! Paraplegia, paralysis of both legs, is seen after a spinal cord transection below T1.**
3. *Wrong choice. Quadriplegia, paralysis of all four extremities, is seen with spinal cord transections in the cervical vertebrae above C4. An injury at C2-3 is usually rapidly fatal.*
4. *No. Paresthesia is burning or tingling sensations due to pressure on nerves or circulatory impairment. It is not a form of paralysis.*

85. A client is admitted to a long-term care facility. She requires total care. In providing mouth care to the client, the nurse should do which of the following?

1. Place the client on her back, with a pillow under her head.
2. Use her thumb and index finger to keep the client's mouth open.
3. Use a stiff toothbrush to clean the client's teeth.
4. Place the client on her side before starting mouth care.

1. *Wrong. Placing the client on her back during mouth care could result in aspiration of fluid into the lungs.*
2. *Wrong. A padded tongue blade--not a thumb or index finger--should be used to keep the client's mouth open.*
3. *No. A soft toothbrush should be used, not a stiff one.*
4. **This is correct, because placing the client on her side encourages fluids to run out of her mouth.**

86. A client had a BKA as a result of chronic diabetes mellitus. Postoperatively, the best position for the client to maintain is which of the following?

1. Pronc for at least 15 minutes daily.
2. Prone with pillows under the affected leg for four days postoperatively.
3. Supine with the knee in full extension.
4. Semi-Fowler's with two pillows under the stump.

1. *Incorrect. This position is promoted for clients with AKA amputations.*

2. *Incorrect. Pillows are contraindicated for AKA and BKA amputations after 48 hours.*
3. **Correct. With a BKA amputation, the client must be encouraged to maintain the supine position with the knee in full extension. This prevents contractures.**
4. *Incorrect. Pillows are contraindicated for AKA and BKA amputations after 48 hours.*

87. A client is receiving magnesium sulfate for severe PIH. Which of the following clinical findings would warrant use of the antidote, calcium gluconate?

1. Rapid rise in blood pressure.
2. Rapid respiratory rate - above 40/min.
3. Urinary output 90 mL in two hours.
4. Absent patellar reflexes.

1. *Wrong! Rapid rise in blood pressure indicates an acceleration of the PIH, but does NOT indicate hypermagnesemia, which would warrant administration of calcium. Hypotension would be seen in clients with hypermagnesemia.*
2. *Wrong! Respiratory rate is one of the critical assessments used to determine the need for calcium gluconate, but in hypermagnesemia it would be low (16/min or lower), not rapid.*
3. *No. Urinary output is used as a critical evaluation of the body's ability to excrete magnesium. An output above 25 mL per hour is usually considered acceptable. Therefore, this clinical finding does not warrant administration of calcium gluconate.*
4. **Correct! Absence of patellar reflexes is seen in clients who have hypermagnesemia, which requires administration of calcium gluconate.**

88. The physician has ordered an indwelling urinary catheter for a male client. Where should the nurse tape the catheter to prevent pressure on the urethra at the penoscrotal junction?

1. Medial thigh.
2. Upper abdomen.
3. Mid-abdominal region.
4. Lateral thigh.

1. *No, taping in this area would not eliminate the penoscrotal angle and could lead to a fistula.*
2. *Incorrect. This section of the abdomen would not be possible to reach without putting undo pressure on the catheter and the retention balloon.*
3. *No. The mid-abdominal region would not be comfortable for the client, nor would it allow for the downward flow of urine via gravity into the drainage bag. This is not the preferred taping site.*
4. **Correct! The lateral thigh or lower abdomen are the recommended sites to eliminate the penoscrotal angle and prevent the formation of a urethrocutaneous fistula.**

89. Shortly after passing out the 9:00 a.m. medications, the nurse realizes that another nurse had given digoxin (Lanoxin) 0.125 mg instead of the prescribed furosemide (Lasix) 2.5 mg, to an eight-year-old client. What is the most appropriate initial response?

1. Assess apical pulse, BP, and respirations.
2. Call the doctor to get orders.
3. Notify the supervisor of the error.
4. Document the error in the chart and complete an incident report.

1. *Correct answer! The nurse needs this information to be able to give a complete picture to the physician, so that orders will be based on the client's current status.*
2. *This isn't the first priority. How is the physician going to decide what needs to be done?*
3. *No, not first. The supervisor does need to be notified, but will this action help correct the error or prevent further injury?*
4. *No, this is not the priority. Documentation of the error can be completed after having administered any corrective action. An accurate record is essential, but the nurse's first obligation is to the client's safety.*

90. A client, age 83, develops acute pulmonary edema secondary to congestive heart failure. The physician orders rotating tourniquets. Which action taken by the nurse demonstrates accurate understanding of this procedure?

1. The nurse places the client flat in bed with a small pillow.
2. Tourniquets are applied to each extremity for 15 minutes and then released.
3. The nurse checks for the presence of an arterial pulse in the extremity after applying a tourniquet.
4. When the procedure is completed, the tourniquets are released in a clockwise manner, one every five minutes.

1. *No! Remember that the client is in the ultimate stage of pulmonary congestion and feels as if she is suffocating. She should be positioned upright, with legs and feet down if possible.*
2. *Incorrect. Tourniquets are applied to three of four extremities and rotated every 15 minutes in a clockwise pattern.*
3. *Correct! The tourniquets are applied to three of four extremities securely enough to impede venous return to the heart but not so tightly that they interfere with arterial flow to each extremity.*
4. *No. When the procedure is finished, the tourniquets are released in a clockwise pattern, one every 15 minutes. This slow release allows for gradual return of blood from the extremities back into the general circulation.*

91. The nurse is counseling a parent about the management of her five-year-old child who has pinworms. The nurse should consider the teaching effective if the parent makes which of the following statements?

1. "I will change her underwear twice a day."
2. "I will give her the mebendazole (Vermox) today and again next week."
3. "I will keep her out of school until I don't see the pinworms any more."
4. "I will discard the sheets on her bed."

1. *Wrong! The pinworms come out to the anus at night to lay their eggs. Showering in the morning is advised. Underwear is changed at this time with the child standing. Changing the underwear twice a day is not necessary.*
2. *Yes! Vermox is used to treat pinworms. It is given in two separate doses spaced out one week apart.*
3. *No. The child does not need to stay out of school. Good handwashing, keeping her nails short, and good morning hygiene will contain the spread of pinworms. Sometimes the pinworms are not visible at all and are detected by a simple lab test called the pinworm paddle. Also, frequent checking would be invasive for the child who may already be upset about having pinworms.*
4. *No. Sheets and other bed linens need to be washed in hot soapy water to get rid of the pinworms. They do not need to be discarded.*

92. A child with a rectal temperature of 39° C has an order for acetaminophen (Tylenol) 280 mg by mouth. The label on the bottle reads 160 mg/5 mL. How many cc's should the nurse dispense to the child?

1. 8.8 mL.
2. 1.8 mL.
3. 6.4 mL.
4. 9.8 mL.

1. *Good work! Use the formula: Desired (280 mg) divided by amount on hand (160 mg) multiplied by the volume (5 mL).*
2. *Wrong. This number is too low. Use the formula: Desired divided by amount on hand, multiplied by volume.*
3. *Wrong. This amount is too low. Use the formula: Desired divided by amount on hand, multiplied by volume.*
4. *Wrong. This amount is too high. Use the formula: Desired divided by the amount on hand, multiplied by volume.*

93. The nurse, in caring for psychiatric clients, knows that tardive dyskinesia:

1. It is a movement disorder caused by antipsychotic drugs.
2. It occurs within the first few days of treatment in most clients.
3. It improves rapidly if the offending drug is discontinued.
4. It is treated with antiparkinsonian drugs.

1. **Correct! Tardive dyskinesia is a serious movement disorder caused by treatment with antipsychotic drugs.**
2. Wrong. Most clients with tardive dyskinesia develop the condition after taking antipsychotics for many years. It rarely occurs shortly after beginning antipsychotic drug therapy.
3. Tardive dyskinesia occurs because antipsychotics block the transmission of dopamine in the basal ganglia. When the dosage of antipsychotic medication is reduced, or the drug discontinued, dopamine is again released and floods the neurons, which demonstrate a supersensitivity to its presence.
4. Not correct. There currently is no treatment for tardive dyskinesia.

94. **A client is admitted to the ER with a sharp object in his right eye. What is the most important action for the nurse to take immediately?**

1. Remove the foreign object.
2. Irrigate the eye with copious amounts of normal saline.
3. Carefully place sterile gauze over the object to cover the eye.
4. Instill a topical anesthetic to reduce his pain.

1. Incorrect. Removal of a sharp object by the nurse is contraindicated since more damage can be done. An ophthalmologist should be notified immediately.
2. Incorrect. Copious irrigation with normal saline is the treatment of choice for chemical burns to the eye, not for a puncture wound.
3. **Correct. Sterile gauze should be placed carefully to absorb the drainage and to protect the eye from infection.**
4. Incorrect. Although a topical anesthetic is often instilled in the eye to reduce pain during eye examination, it is not the most important action initially.

95. **A 67-year-old widow is brought to the clinic by her son, who found her at home crying. She said that she "could not go on alone." He tells the nurse that when his father died six months earlier the family was amazed at his mother's fortitude during and immediately after the funeral. She did not cry or seem unduly upset. The nurse recognizes that his mother had dealt with her husband's death by using which of the following defense mechanisms?**

1. Denial.
2. Repression.
3. Introjection.
4. Sublimation.

1. **Correct. Denial is a component of the grief process. This woman's emotional response to her husband's death has been delayed, but she now is experiencing the depressive phase of the grief process.**
2. Repression is the involuntary forgetting or banishment of unacceptable ideas or feelings into the unconscious. This cannot be the correct option because the stem does not state that this woman forgot that her husband died.
3. No. Introjection is adopting characteristics of a loved one.
4. No. Sublimation is the diversion of unacceptable drives into socially sanctioned activities.

96. **A 42-year-old female is admitted with right-sided weakness and slurred speech. Which diagnostic tests should the nurse be prepared to instruct the client/family about?**

1. EEG and MRI.
2. Angiography and EMG.
3. PET and pneumoencephalogram.
4. CT scan and lumbar puncture.

1. Incorrect. EEG is not initially useful. EEG would be abnormal, but wouldn't provide specific information about the type and amount of damage. This information is most useful in diagnosis of seizure disorders. MRI would be appropriate.
2. Incorrect. EMG is electromyography, which measures muscle potentials. Although cerebral angiography will detect cerebral vascular disorders, it is not usually used initially.
3. No. The pneumoencephalogram is an x-ray of the cerebral ventricles. While it is useful in the diagnosis of cerebral malformations, it is very painful. PET would be appropriate.
4. **Correct. The CT scan may show areas of hematoma or infarct, with distortion or shift of ventricles. The lumbar puncture may be useful if there is a subarachnoid hemorrhage.**

97. **A client on the psychiatric unit attends activity therapy and is encouraged to pound designs into a leather belt. This intervention is based on which model of depression?**

1. Behavioral.
2. Cognitive.
3. Aggression-turned-inward.
4. Learned helplessness

1. Incorrect! There is no behavioral model of depression.

2. *No. The cognitive model of depression proposes that people experience depression because their thinking is dominated by a negative evaluation of self, the world and the future.*

3. **Correct. The aggression-turned-inward model views depression as the turning of anger and aggression inward towards the self instead of directing it outward at the appropriate object.**

4. *The learned helplessness model views depression as the belief that one has no control over the important outcomes in one's life.*

98. **A 60-year-old client has advanced cancer of the lung, with metastasis. His wife says to the nurse, "I know my husband is in severe pain. I wish I could do something to make him feel better." Which of the following comments by the nurse would be most therapeutic for the wife?**

    1. "It must be very difficult for you to see your husband suffering."
    2. "I wish there was more that I could do to relieve his pain, too."
    3. "I'm sure he will begin to feel better after his next pain medication."
    4. "Your husband tries hard not to show the pain when you are with him."

    1. **This answer is correct. The wife is the client in this question. The nurse is responding to her feelings. The response is therapeutic and illustrates the communication tool of empathy.**
    2. *Wrong! This option focuses on the nurse rather than the client and is not therapeutic.*
    3. *This choice illustrates the non-therapeutic communication block of false reassurance.*
    4. *The client in this question is the wife. The response in this option is incorrect because it focuses on the husband. It might also cause the wife to feel guilty.*

99. **The nurse should assess an immobilized client for symptoms of a fecal impaction, the most definitive of which is:**

    1. The absence of bowel sounds.
    2. Diarrhea stools with abdominal cramping.
    3. A rigid board-like abdomen.
    4. Constipation with liquid fecal seepage.

    1. *No. Absence of bowel sounds is seen in a paralytic ileus when peristalsis has stopped. That is not the problem with a fecal impaction.*
    2. *Incorrect. Diarrhea stools with abdominal cramping are often caused by gastroenteritis. Although both signs and symptoms may be present in the case of a fecal impaction, they are not the most definitive assessments that can be made.*

3. *Wrong choice. A rigid, board-like abdomen is seen in peritonitis, an inflammation of the peritoneum. As the affected area of the abdomen becomes extremely tender, the muscles become rigid, giving the board-like appearance to the abdomen.*

4. **Yes, these are the classic symptoms of a fecal impaction. Other symptoms of a fecal impaction include painful defecation, feeling of fullness in the rectum, abdominal distention, and sometimes cramps and watery stools. Very often, liquid fecal material may bypass the hardened mass.**

100. **A 56-year-old woman is being discharged after a simple mastectomy. She will begin radiation therapy as an outpatient tomorrow. Which of the following instructions, directed at maintaining skin integrity, should be given by the nurse?**

    1. Wear a good support bra and use ice for any swelling.
    2. Use of a heating pad is contraindicated.
    3. Skin breakdown is common and should be treated with antibiotic ointment.
    4. Keep skin lubricated to prevent dryness.

    1. *No, both are contraindicated as they may cause increased irritation.*
    2. **Terrific! This is the only instruction that is certain to help avoid tissue damage. Radiated tissue becomes thinner and may lack tissue receptors which would normally alert the client to a potential burn.**
    3. *Incorrect. Skin breakdown may occur, but ointments should only be used with specific instructions from the physician responsible for the radiation therapy.*
    4. *Not correct. This implies that creams should be used routinely. Discharge instructions should state that the skin is to be kept clean and dry.*

NOTES

NCLEX-RN

Test 7

NCLEX-RN TEST 7

1. **A 58-year-old client is receiving nasal oxygen postoperatively. Which of the following laboratory findings would indicate to the nurse that the oxygen therapy is effective?**

    1. PaO_2 of 56 mm Hg.
    2. PaO_2 of 85 mm Hg.
    3. PaO_2 of 90 mm Hg.
    4. PaO_2 of 97 mm Hg.

2. **A 29-year-old diabetic is admitted to the hospital for dialysis because of poor renal function. He says to the nurse, "I don't even know why I'm doing this. There is no cure." Which of the following statements is the most appropriate nursing response?**

    1. "There is always a chance that, through research, a cure will be found."
    2. "Dialysis will help you live longer."
    3. "You shouldn't complain! You are fortunate to be in this good a shape, considering the type of diabetes you have."
    4. "It sounds as though you have given up on life."

3. **While working the night shift, the nurse notices a mouse running down the hallway of the clinical unit. The best initial action is which of the following?**

    1. Place rat poison in the vicinity where the mouse was seen.
    2. Set some mouse traps to catch the mouse, and then dispose of it in a plastic bag labeled as contaminated.
    3. Notify the supervisor of the problem.
    4. Call the environmental health department of the hospital, and report the incident.

4. **In which of the following situations would the nurse expect administration of naloxone (Narcan) be indicated?**

    1. Mother ready to deliver who received meperidine (Demerol) IM four and one-half hours ago.
    2. Mother experiencing hypotension following epidural anesthesia.
    3. Mother ready to deliver who received butorphanol (Stadol) IV five minutes ago.
    4. A drug addicted mother about to deliver who received Demerol IM one-half hour ago.

5. **When taking a nursing history, the primary nurse learns an elderly client has had difficulty sleeping at night for several months. In evaluating his sleep disturbance, the nurse should remember which of the following facts?**

    1. Elderly people have an increase in Stages 3 and 4 sleep.
    2. Elderly people seldom awake at night once they have fallen asleep.
    3. Anxiety and depression frequently cause disturbed sleep patterns.
    4. Elderly people require much less sleep than younger adults.

6. **A 62-year-old client comes to the emergency room with a temperature of 102° F, blood pressure of 150/110, and tachycardia. She has been taking haloperidol (Haldol) 5 mg t.i.d. for the past three months. The nurse knows that these symptoms indicate a diagnosis of:**

    1. Neuroleptic malignant syndrome (NMS).
    2. Agranulocytosis.
    3. Hypertensive crisis.
    4. Tardive dyskinesia.

7. **The nurse enters the room and finds a mother crying. Her son has been diagnosed with leukemia and is currently receiving chemotherapy. The mother says, "I just can't believe he's going to lose all his beautiful blonde hair!" Which response by the nurse is most justifiable?**

    1. "Sometimes the hair only thins."
    2. "You're feeling a lot of loss right now."
    3. "Remember, hair loss means the chemotherapy is working!"
    4. "Kids love to wear the special baseball caps we have."

8. **A couple is in the hospital because of a fetal death at 37 weeks gestation. Which of the following is an appropriate response by the nurse?**

    1. "You are both young and you can have other children."
    2. "It is God's will, and it must be accepted."
    3. "It must be very difficult for you both. I will be available if you need anything."
    4. "I think you should call your minister. He can help comfort you."

9. A newborn infant has just returned from surgery for correction of a cleft lip. Which nursing interventions are indicated?

    1. Arm restraints, postural drainage and oral irrigations.
    2. Cleansing suture line, arm restraints, and supine or side lying position.
    3. Prone or side lying position, cleansing suture line, and oral irrigations.
    4. Side lying position, use specially designed nipple and arm restraints.

10. When counseling a client who is taking isosorbide dinitrate (Isordil) for angina, which of the following side effects can the nurse anticipate will occur least often?

    1. Hypotension.
    2. Headache.
    3. Bradycardia.
    4. Weakness.

11. A child is to receive 400 mL of IV fluid over an eight-hour shift. The drip factor on the IV tubing is 60 drops/mL. How many drops/minute will deliver the proper amount?

    1. 12.5 drops/minute.
    2. 16 drops/minute.
    3. 50 drops/minute.
    4. 63 drops/minute.

12. A confused, elderly client has wet herself and is standing in the hospital corridor in a puddle of urine. She looks ashamed and says to the nurse, "I want to go outside for a walk now." What would be the most appropriate response by the nurse at this time?

    1. "Before we go for a walk, perhaps we can make a list that will help you make your bathroom trips easier."
    2. "Right now, let me wipe up the urine on the floor, and let's get a change of clothing for you. I am sure that this problem is upsetting for you."
    3. "This has been a problem for you. Let's see if we can find a solution together."
    4. "Wetting yourself is very upsetting. Yes, let's take a walk."

13. The nurse learns that an elderly client's sleeping problems began six months before, when his physician diagnosed prostatic cancer. Prior to that time, he had enjoyed good physical health. She also learned that his wife of 50 years had died one year ago. One day the client tells the nurse, "I'd be better off dead because I am totally worthless." The nurse's most therapeutic response is which of the following remarks?

    1. "I have seen some very valuable things about you."
    2. "You feel worthless now because you are so depressed. You will feel differently when you depression begins to improve."
    3. "You really have a great deal to live for."
    4. "You have been feeling very sad and alone for some time now."

14. The nurse is working in an acute care pediatric unit. One of the LPN's has assessments on four postoperative clients. Which client requires the nurse's most immediate attention?

    1. A 12-year-old appendectomy, two days postoperative and refusing to ambulate.
    2. An 8-year-old tonsillectomy, just returned from the recovery room, having frequent swallowing.
    3. Possible peripheral IV infiltration (rate 50 mL/hr) on a 15-year-old herniorrhaphy.
    4. An 18-month-old one day postoperative for cleft palate repair with a pulse of 120 beats per minute.

15. Soon after being admitted to a rehabilitation unit, a chronic alcoholic says to the nurse, "I don't really need to be here. My wife and family make me drink. My wife spends all my money. My kid just had an accident with his car that will cost me a fortune in repairs." The most appropriate response by the nurse at this time would be:

    1. "Tell me more about how your wife is spending all your money."
    2. "Could you tell me more about why your child's car accident cost you money?"
    3. "It sounds like you are having a great deal of financial difficulty."
    4. "Tell me more about your feelings about being here in the hospital."

16. A vest restraint is placed on a confused elderly client who is at high risk for falling. He is partially paralyzed and is at risk for developing pressure sores. How should the nurse handle the linen when changing this client's bed?

    1. When removing the linen from the bed, hold it close to the body to avoid dropping it.
    2. After removing the linen from the bed, place it on the floor until finished making the bed.
    3. When removing the linen from the bed, hold it away from the uniform.
    4. Shake the clean linen to unfold it, before making the bed.

17. The client is transferred to the recovery room after a colon resection for adenocarcinoma. Which of the following body system adaptations would the nurse expect to see initially if the client were to develop internal abdominal bleeding postoperatively?

1. Tachycardia.
2. Oliguria.
3. Hyperthermia.
4. Bradypnea.

18. **A 66-year-old client is receiving hemodialysis via left internal angioaccess for management of chronic renal disease. Which of the following should the nurse include when teaching this client?**

    1. Check the access hourly for patency.
    2. Maintain skin integrity through frequent cleansing and application of lotion over the site.
    3. Avoid tight clothing around the access site.
    4. Sleep on his left side to maintain patency of access site.

19. **The physician has ordered extremity restraints for safety reasons for a confused, elderly client. After placing the client in extremity restraints, the priority nursing action is which of the following?**

    1. Release each extremity every two hours for range of motion exercises.
    2. Discuss the rationale for the restraints with the family members.
    3. Reduce the client's distress by dimming the lights and closing the door.
    4. Tie the restraints to the side rails using a half bow knot.

20. **The nurse is admitting a client who is suspected of having diabetes mellitus. Which of the following characteristics would the nurse expect to observe?**

    1. Shallow, labored respirations.
    2. Increased blood pressure associated with slight periorbital edema.
    3. Periods of altered pulse rate.
    4. Increased urinary output.

21. **The physician has determined that the client is extremely dehydrated and in need of intravenous fluids. The client is confused, and has pulled out one intravenous catheter and caused another intravenous site to become infiltrated. The nurse restarts the intravenous in the client's left arm. An order for restraints is given. Which of the following is the best action by the nurse?**

    1. Apply a vest restraint and extremity restraints to ensure that the intravenous site will be protected.
    2. Apply a restraint to the left arm.
    3. Apply a restraint to the right arm.
    4. Apply restraints to the right and left arms.

22. **On the second day after hip surgery, an elderly client is awake for brief periods of time. During the evening, she becomes restless and begins to pull at her IV tubing. The most appropriate nursing action when she pulls at the tubing is to:**

    1. Maintain steady pressure on her arm to prohibit her from dislodging the tubing, while continuing to speak gently to her until she lets go of the tubing.
    2. Speak in a loud, clear way telling her to stop pulling on the IV, while gently trying to pry her fingers from around the tubing.
    3. Explain that she has an IV for fluid replacement and offer to show it to her when she lets go of the tubing.
    4. Call for help and prepare to apply soft wrist restraints so she will not be able to grab the tubing again.

23. **A 16-year-old client has left her used insulin syringe on the bedside table. What is the best action by the nurse to help prevent spread of infection by way of the contaminated needle?**

    1. Explain to the client that the syringe should be disposed of in the garbage can to avoid a potential needle stick by someone providing care for the client.
    2. Cap the syringe and take to the needle disposal container.
    3. Place the uncapped syringe in the needle disposal container.
    4. Have the nurse administer the injection, since the client is not responsible enough to follow through with the proper procedure.

24. **A general anesthesia has been given for multiple tooth extractions on a three-year-old child. He returns crying but awake from the recovery room. What approach is most likely to be successful?**

    1. Examine the mouth first.
    2. Leave the mouth until last.
    3. It really makes no difference what is done first.
    4. Medicate the child for pain first.

25. **The night nurse complains that an elderly client on the surgical unit has started to have periods of agitation at night that include screaming out loudly for help. The primary nurse suggests several interventions to diminish this behavior. Which of the following interventions should the nurse avoid?**

    1. Remaining calm and encouraging the client to express her fears so the nurse will have a better understanding of how to help.
    2. Requesting an order for a sedative medication.
    3. Keeping a nightlight on in her room.

4. Assessing her level of pain or the presence of other physical discomfort.

26. **Which of the following statements, if made by a male client who has a prescription for nitroglycerin (Nitrostat) tablets, would <u>indicate</u> to the nurse that he needs further teaching?**

    1. "I'll make sure that the medication container is kept tightly sealed."
    2. "I'm lucky I have a prescription plan that allows me to buy pills in bulk quantities."
    3. "I'll keep my pills in the medicine cabinet when I'm home."
    4. "I know that I should go to the hospital emergency room if my chest pain doesn't go away."

27. **A 12-year-old boy has been recently diagnosed with diabetes. In order to minimize his anxiety, which nursing action would be most appropriate?**

    1. Provide a toy ""Doctor's Kit" to play with.
    2. Keep all syringes and needles out of sight until the last moment.
    3. Explain to the child that his parents will administer all of the medications.
    4. Allow the child to manipulate a syringe and give himself injections.

28. **While caring for a client, the nurse notices that the call light cord is frayed. At this time, which of the following nursing actions would be most important?**

    1. Tell the client not to use the call light until it is fixed.
    2. Remove the call light, and report the problem to the supervising nurse immediately.
    3. Tape up the cord until the maintenance people can fix it, so the client will have a call light.
    4. Tell the client to call out if he needs help, and to use the call light only in an emergency.

29. **After detoxification, the client begins the rehabilitation phase of treatment. He tells the nurse that he cannot imagine living his life without alcohol. The nurse's best response is based on what knowledge?**

    1. He will be more successful if he focuses on goals for short periods of time such as "today" or "this week".
    2. He is likely to drink again when under stress.
    3. He will not be successful if he is not strongly motivated.
    4. He may require treatment with Antabuse to maintain sobriety.

30. **A six-year-old female is admitted with rheumatic fever. She has painful joints and a temperature of 103° F. Bedrest is ordered. What is the primary rationale for bedrest?**

    1. The workload of the heart is decreased by bedrest.
    2. Bedrest will limit the joint pain.
    3. Permanent arthritic changes of the joints will be prevented.
    4. BMR (basal metabolic rate) will be decreased, which will decrease the elevated temperature.

31. **A psychiatric client is receiving chlorpromazine (Thorazine) and is doing well. The unit is planning an outdoor activity for Saturday. The weather has been warm and sunny. What information should the nurse give the client about the side effects of Thorazine before he leaves the unit?**

    1. Wear a hat and a long-sleeved shirt.
    2. Watch for signs of jaundice.
    3. Drink plenty of fluids to replace any he might lose by sweating in the sun.
    4. Don't drink more than one beer.

32. **An unconscious 18-year-old man is brought to the emergency room. Friends report that he took an overdose of heroin. After the client regains consciousness, he is transferred to the substance abuse treatment unit. The signs and symptoms of heroin withdrawal are written in the nursing care plan. Which of the following behaviors could the nurse anticipate to occur early in the withdrawal process?**

    1. Vomiting and diarrhea.
    2. Sneezing and rhinorrhea.
    3. Restlessness and irritability.
    4. Yawning and diaphoresis.

33. **Two days after a psychiatric client begins taking fluphenazine (Prolixin), she comes to the nursing station. The nurse observes that the client is very frightened. Her head is twisted to one side, her back is arched, and her eyes are rolled up. The nurse recognizes these symptoms as indicative of:**

    1. Parkinsonian syndrome.
    2. Akathisia.
    3. Impending seizure.
    4. Dystonic reaction.

34. **A client with a history of angina is to take isosorbide dinitrate (Isordil) 10 mg p.o. every six hours. When the client asks how the drug works, the nurse's reply is based upon the understanding that the primary action of Isordil is to:**

1. Reduce cardiac preload and afterload.
2. Dilate the coronary blood vessels.
3. Increase the heart's oxygen consumption.
4. Decrease myocardial circulation.

35. A psychotic client receiving chlorpromazine (Thorazine) tried to "cheek" the medication so he could later spit it out. The nurse correctly decides to request that the physician change the order from the tablet form to a form that will prevent this from happening. Which of the following choices would be best?

    1. Liquid concentrate.
    2. Capsule.
    3. Suppository.
    4. Intramuscular injection.

36. Family therapy is scheduled for an anorexic client and her family. Her parents ask how the family therapy will help their daughter's eating problem. The best nursing response is to state that the focus of the therapy will be primarily on which of the following?

    1. Their daughter's eating behavior.
    2. The parents and how their behavior may be causing their daughter to starve herself.
    3. Increasing communication between the family members.
    4. Teaching family members to better meet each other's needs.

37. A client, newly diagnosed with angina, is instructed to take one nitroglycerin (Nitrostat) tablet sublingual at the first sign of an anginal attack, waiting five minutes before taking another tablet. The nurse explains this waiting period to the client, based upon the rationale that:

    1. Absorption of the drug is slower via the sublingual route.
    2. The client will need to monitor the blood pressure between dosages.
    3. The client would demonstrate a potential allergic reaction within the first five minutes of drug administration.
    4. Nitrates can lower the blood pressure very quickly.

38. A child, three months of age, has been admitted with a tentative diagnosis of intussusception. The parents ask the nurse how the diagnosis is made. Based on an understanding of the diagnostic evaluation for intussusception, what should the nurse say to the parents?

    1. "A small amount of tissue from the colon will be biopsied."
    2. "Genotyping can identify this condition."

3. "A barium enema will be given to visualize the obstruction."
4. "An upper GI series should identify the area involved."

39. While the nurse is caring for a client, the intravenous tubing becomes disconnected from the intravenous catheter, resulting in the client's blood spilling onto the sides of the bed and floor. Which of the following solutions are recommended for disinfection of blood spills?

    1. Betadine solution.
    2. Alcohol.
    3. Soap and water.
    4. Sodium hypochlorite or chlorine bleach solution.

40. A six-month-old is in the pediatric clinic. The nurse practitioner ordered a DPT vaccine to be administered. Which of the following assessments would cause the nurse to question the administration of the DPT vaccine?

    1. Previous evidence of sensitivity to egg antigens.
    2. High fever and high-pitched cry following last DPT.
    3. Current temperature of 100° F.
    4. Currently receiving steroid therapy.

41. A client, 64 years old, is hospitalized with chronic obstructive pulmonary disease. Oxygen per nasal cannula at two liters per minute is initiated. When the nurse made an assessment at 3:00 p.m., the client appeared to have made a good adjustment to hospitalization. At 5:00 p.m., upon entering the room to bring the client his dinner tray, the nurse finds the oxygen cannula on the floor. The client is angry and says, "It's about time you got here. Where am I? Where is my breakfast?" The nurse should give immediate consideration to which of the following?

    1. Has the oxygen cannula been off long enough to cause hypoxia?
    2. Is the client's anger related to being hospitalized again?
    3. Does the client need a clock in the room to keep track of the time?
    4. Is the client accustomed to eating meals at unusual times?

42. In treating diabetic ketoacidosis (DKA), the nurse is aware that a goal of treatment is to correct which of the following imbalances?

    1. Hypoglycemia.
    2. Dehydration.
    3. Hyperkalemia.
    4. Respiratory acidosis.

43. A client, age 65, is receiving doxycycline (Vibramycin) for actinomycosis (fungal infection). The nurse should observe the client for which of the following side effects?

    1. Photosensitivity.
    2. Constipation.
    3. Ototoxicity.
    4. Permanent discoloration of teeth.

44. To assess for proper placement of a nasogastric tube, the nurse should:

    1. Instill 30 mL of saline into the tube to assess client tolerance.
    2. Instill 10 mL of air into the tube and listen for gurgling sounds with a stethoscope over the gastric area.
    3. Aspirate stomach contents with a syringe.
    4. Place the end of the tube in water to assess for bubbling.

45. While caring for a client receiving fluids using an IV pump plugged into an electrical outlet, the nurse should avoid which action?

    1. Palpate the client's IV site while resetting the pump for the next bag of IV solution.
    2. Assess the IV site visually and by palpation.
    3. Change the tubing according to hospital protocol.
    4. Observe the pump for correct operation.

46. A client is admitted with end stage cirrhosis of the liver. Which of the following measures would the nurse expect to decrease the serum ammonia level?

    1. Administration of vitamin K.
    2. Increased fluid intake.
    3. Administration of diuretics.
    4. Offer low-protein, high-calorie diet.

47. A 10-year-old is recovering following an appendectomy. While changing the linens on the client's bed, the nurse notes that drainage from an infected wound has soiled the bed sheet. Which of the following is the best method to use when changing the soiled bed linens?

    1. Carefully place the soiled sheet in the cloth linen bag and label it as contaminated.
    2. Spray the soiled area with a bleach solution prior to placing it in the linen bag.
    3. Carefully place the soiled sheet in a moisture-resistant plastic linen bag designated for soiled articles.
    4. Discard the sheet into a plastic trash bag.

48. A client is recovering from surgery. He has in place a urinary catheter that needs to be irrigated. The best intervention by the nurse to prevent injury to the mucosa of the bladder is which of the following?

    1. Gently compress the ball of the syringe to instill the irrigating solution.
    2. Quickly instill the irrigating solution using some pressure to loosen any clots or mucus.
    3. After instilling the solution, apply gentle pressure to remove the irrigating solution from the bladder.
    4. Place a sterile cap on the end of the drainage tubing to protect it from contamination.

49. A client is receiving combination chemotherapy for breast cancer. Her most recent complete blood count (CBC) shows the following: Hgb 12.2, Hct 36%, WBC 2.3/cu mm, and platelets 150,000. Which of the following goals should be given priority by the nurse in planning care?

    1. Prevention of infection.
    2. Maintenance of tissue integrity.
    3. Prevention of injury.
    4. Maintenance of tissue perfusion.

50. Which of the following instructions is appropriate for the nurse to give a client who is to take nitroglycerin (Nitrostat) tablets sublingual for angina pain?

    1. Take your blood pressure prior to administration of Nitrostat. If the diastolic is less than 80, do not take the pill.
    2. Take the Nitrostat with a full glass of water.
    3. Sit or lie down prior to taking the medication.
    4. Notify the physician immediately if you feel dizzy or get a headache after taking the Nitrostat.

51. While transferring a client with left-leg weakness from the bed to a wheelchair, the best nursing action is to do which of the following?

    1. Have the seat of the wheelchair at a right angle to the bed.
    2. Lock the wheels on the bed and the wheelchair.
    3. Allow the client to do as much as possible to increase his sense of independence.
    4. Have the client lock his hands around the nurse's neck to provide the client with a sense of security.

52. The nurse initiates a diversional activity for a nine-year-old female client who is hospitalized with osteomyelitis. The activity is writing a story about the hospitalization experience. Which statement reflects a positive outcome of this activity?

1. The client was actively engaged in writing for one-half hour.
2. During one-half hour of activity, the client put the light on six times.
3. The client told her mother she likes her nurse.
4. Correct grammar was demonstrated when writing the story.

53. **In planning for the care of a 45-year-old woman diagnosed with Addison's disease, which of the following nursing diagnoses would be most appropriate?**

    1. Fluid volume excess related to sodium retention.
    2. Activity intolerance related to muscular weakness and fatigue.
    3. Impaired skin integrity related to pigmentation changes and lesions.
    4. Body image disturbance related to virilization of feminine features.

54. **A client is admitted to the hospital with cirrhosis of the liver and possible bleeding esophageal varices. Which of the following symptoms, if observed by the nurse, would help to validate the esophageal varices?**

    1. Swelling in the neck area.
    2. Painless hematemesis.
    3. A dry, hacking cough.
    4. Hemoptysis with chest pain.

55. **A 10-year-old client is recovering following an appendectomy. The nurse changes the bed linens and notes that drainage from an infected wound has soiled the bed sheet. A 13-year-old client with a newly applied full leg cast is to share the room. Which of the following best describes the nurse's role in infection control?**

    1. Hand washing.
    2. Using gloves when in contact with blood and body fluids.
    3. Proper disposal of contaminated dressings.
    4. Preventing the onset and spread of infection.

56. **A male nurse received a doctor's order to catheterize one of his female clients. The client says, "I'm not going to allow a male nurse to catheterize me." Which of the following statements is most appropriate by the nurse?**

    1. "Your doctor is a male. Would you let him catheterize you?"
    2. "I've done this many times with no problems."
    3. "You can explain to your doctor why the catheter wasn't inserted."
    4. "You appear to be upset. Let me find a female nurse to help with the procedure."

57. **The client has just returned from the x-ray department after undergoing an upper GI series. Which of the following interventions by the nurse would be appropriate at this time?**

    1. Keep him NPO until the gag reflex returns.
    2. Administer a cleansing enema.
    3. Monitor his vital signs every 15 minutes for one hour or until stable.
    4. Give milk of magnesia 30 mL p.o.

58. **A client is being sent home on isoxsuprine (Vasodilan) for treatment of premature labor. Which of the following actions need to be included in her discharge teaching plan?**

    1. Technique for taking oral temperature.
    2. How to assess her radial pulse.
    3. Procedure to assess her blood sugar.
    4. How to assess fetal heart rate.

59. **A male client, admitted with a myocardial infarction (MI) two days ago, develops paroxysmal atrial tachycardia (PAT). The physician orders quinidine sulfate (Quinatime) 300 mg p.o. every three hours until the arrhythmia is terminated. Which baseline data should the nurse obtain prior to starting the quinidine?**

    1. Serum creatinine.
    2. Q-T interval.
    3. Abdominal girth.
    4. Cardiac ejection fraction.

60. **An 18-year-old hemophiliac is scheduled for wisdom teeth extractions. Which of the following can the nurse anticipate will be given prior to the dental procedure?**

    1. Packed red blood cells.
    2. Prophylactic antibiotics.
    3. Fresh frozen plasma.
    4. Factor VIII concentrate.

61. **When a client is taking nifedipine (Procardia), the nurse must be aware of the potential for:**

    1. Hallucinations.
    2. Peripheral edema.
    3. Hyperglycemia.
    4. Photophobia.

62. **The nurse is counseling a parent about the management of her six-year-old child who has chickenpox. Which statement by the parent indicates that the teaching by the nurse has been ineffective?**

1. "I will keep my child's fingernails cut short."
2. "I will keep my child out of school for five days."
3. "If any of the chickenpox become swollen and ooze yellow drainage, I will call the doctor."
4. "I will give my child diphenhydramine (Benadryl) if the itching becomes severe."

63. A four-year-old recently diagnosed with AIDS is due for his preschool immunizations. His immunizations have previously been up to date. Which immunizations would be most appropriate for this client at this time?

    1. MMR and OPV.
    2. DTP and Hib.
    3. None required.
    4. DTP, IPV and MMR.

64. The nurse knows that which of the following is accurate regarding ECT?

    1. Usually requires 10 days to three weeks before depression is noticeably improved.
    2. Results in a high incidence of chronic memory problems.
    3. Is effective for 60% of persons who receive it.
    4. Is used for persons who have not responded to antidepressants.

65. A 17-year-old client is brought to the emergency room with right lower quadrant pain. He has a low grade fever, nausea, and a WBC of 18,000. The nurse is aware that the client's symptoms are indicative of which of the following conditions?

    1. Hepatitis.
    2. Appendicitis.
    3. Peritonitis.
    4. Gastritis.

66. A 48-year-old male's EKG shows a flattening of the T wave. He was admitted for congestive heart failure. Which of the following laboratory results would the nurse anticipate as most likely to occur with this EKG change?

    1. Hgb of 9.8 gm.
    2. Digitalis toxicity.
    3. K+ 2.8 mEq/liter.
    4. Serum Ca++ 8.0 mg %.

67. A 43-year-old female client has had a total abdominal hysterectomy and bilateral salpingo-oophorectomy for stage III uterine cancer. Which instructions would the nurse anticipate providing?

    1. Estrogen therapy will alleviate the discomfort of surgical menopause.
    2. A Papanicolaou smear should be performed every six months.
    3. Lubrication can be used to treat vaginal itching and burning.
    4. Vaginal intercourse will no longer be possible.

68. A client, age 46, is admitted to the hospital with a diagnosis of acute pancreatitis. In assessing the client's condition, the nurse should expect to find an elevation in which of the following serum levels?

    1. Amylase.
    2. Bilirubin.
    3. Cholesterol.
    4. Gastrin.

69. A 32-year-old client is admitted to the emergency room with a respiratory rate of seven per minute. ABG's reveal the following values: pH 7.22; pCO_2 68 mm Hg; HCO_3 28 mEq/L. Which is the proper analysis of this assessment?

    1. Respiratory alkalosis.
    2. Metabolic acidosis.
    3. Metabolic alkalosis.
    4. Respiratory acidosis.

70. An 83-year-old confused client has wrist restraints for safety reasons. Which of the following nursing interventions is necessary to provide for the client's safety?

    1. Check the pulse, color, and temperature of extremities every shift and report these findings.
    2. Make sure the call light is within the client's reach.
    3. Notify the client's family of the restraints and explain the rationale for their use.
    4. Remove the restraints at night while the client is sleeping.

71. A client, age 83, is admitted to the hospital with complaints of abdominal pain and distention. He has a history of no bowel movement for the past 10 days. After a diagnostic evaluation, it is determined that the client has a fecal impaction. Which of the following treatments can the nurse anticipate will be ordered initially?

    1. Soap suds enemas until clear.
    2. Bisacodyl (Dulcolax) suppository.
    3. Oil retention enema.
    4. Tap water enema.

72. The nurse is aware that which of the following effects will occur when the client is taking quinidine (Quinatime) and digoxin (Lanoxin) at the same time?

    1. Elevated quinidine levels.
    2. Decreased quinidine levels.
    3. Elevated digoxin levels.
    4. Decreased digoxin levels.

73. In assessing an adult client with diabetes mellitus, the nurse would expect to observe all of the following characteristics except:

    1. Possible increased body weight.
    2. Increased urinary output.
    3. Periods of polydypsia.
    4. Periods of altered pulse rate.

74. A six-year-old male is admitted with a spiral fracture of the humerus and multiple bruises of the forearm. The physician states abuse is suspected. The nurse's initial goal is which of the following?

    1. Prevent further abuse of the client.
    2. Encourage the client to express his feelings.
    3. Determine who is responsible for the abuse.
    4. Teach the parents appropriate methods of discipline.

75. A 25-year-old man was admitted one week ago with a diagnosis of schizophrenia, paranoid type. Since his admission, he has had several verbal outbursts of anger but has not been violent. A staff member tells the nurse that the client is pacing up and down the hall very rapidly and muttering to himself in an angry manner. Which of the following is the best initial nursing action?

    1. Prepare an intramuscular injection of haloperidol (Haldol) to give him p.r.n.
    2. Observe the client's behavior and approach him in a non-threatening manner.
    3. Gather several staff members and approach the client together.
    4. Contact the client's psychiatrist and request an order to place him in seclusion.

76. A 12-year-old child is being discharged from the hospital with a diagnosis of asthma. She will be maintained on metered dose inhalers at home. The nurse is preparing a care plan on the use of cromolyn sodium (Intal). Which information would the nurse avoid including in the care plan?

    1. Intal will decrease the inflammation in your child's bronchioles.
    2. Do not rely on Intal for relief of an acute attack.
    3. Have your child rinse her mouth after using the puffer.
    4. Your child should breathe more easily after a dose of Intal.

77. A client, age 20, has been admitted to the hospital after having two tonic-clonic seizures at work. She suddenly gives a short cry and stiffens. What is the initial nursing action?

    1. Make a mental notation of the time after looking at a watch.
    2. Place an oral airway in the client's mouth.
    3. Loosen the clothing around the neck.
    4. Turn her head to the side.

78. A 25-year-old client was admitted to the hospital with newly diagnosed diabetes mellitus. She is very concerned about being placed on a calorie-controlled diet, since she has been losing weight even though she has been eating more food. Which of the following statements is the most therapeutic response by the nurse?

    1. "You won't have to worry about weight loss once your sugar is regulated."
    2. "The doctor will order enough food for you."
    3. "Your body has not been producing the insulin necessary to utilize the calories you were eating. Once you start receiving insulin, you will once again be able to use the calories you eat and a calorie-controlled diet will be recommended to help maintain your weight."
    4. "You probably needed to lose some weight to decrease your need for insulin."

79. A client has returned to the ambulatory surgery unit after undergoing a bronchoscopy. She complains of a sore throat. Which of the following nursing measures would be most appropriate after the cough reflex returns?

    1. Ice chips.
    2. Warm saline gargle.
    3. Tepid clear liquids.
    4. Viscous Xylocaine mouth swishes p.r.n.

80. The nurse's neighbor has a baby who is four weeks old. She tells the nurse that the hospital just called to ask her to bring her baby in to repeat the PKU test done at 24 hours of age. What is the nurse's best response?

1. "This is quite unusual, I will go with you."
2. "A second specimen is always done to guarantee the child does not have PKU."
3. "Results of early PKU testing are often inconclusive due to inadequate nutritional intake."
4. "I think you should call your pediatrician to be sure he thinks this repeat test is necessary."

81. **A child, 11 years old, is to receive 400 mL of IV fluid in an eight-hour shift. The IV drip factor is 60. What is the IV rate that will deliver this amount?**

1. 66 mL/hour.
2. 40 mL/hour.
3. 24 mL/hour.
4. 50 mL/hour.

82. **A 55-year-old client has been taking trifluoperazine (Stelazine) for five years to control her paranoid thoughts. When the client's brother comes to visit, he tells the nurse that he strongly believes all psychiatric medications are a form of "chemical mind control." The nurse understands which of the following regarding antipsychotics?**

1. They act directly on specific neurotransmitters in the brain to control the client's psychotic symptoms.
2. They act to sedate the client so she cannot engage in behavior that will cause difficulty for either herself or others.
3. They are a cure for psychotic disorders, like schizophrenic reactions, and are therefore an important part of his sister's treatment plan.
4. They have been in use for close to 30 years and are safe and effective drugs for clients who have problems like his sister's.

83. **A 24-year-old college student is admitted to the emergency room. She is hysterical and states that she was sexually assaulted 20 minutes ago. Which of the following should be the nurse's first priority in this situation?**

1. Remove her clothes carefully, so as not to destroy any evidence.
2. Vaginal exam with lubricant to decrease the pain involved.
3. Place the client in a private room and leave her alone to grieve.
4. Encourage the client to relate what happened and make decisions about the order of examination.

84. **A client is addicted to cocaine and is in labor at 35 weeks gestation. She has heard about a drug that will reverse the effects of narcotics, and wants it given to her newborn after delivery. Which of the**

following statements is the best response by the nurse regarding administration of the naloxone (Narcan)?

1. "I will notify the neonatologist immediately, so it will be available."
2. "The drug does not reverse the effects of cocaine, so it is not indicated for your baby."
3. "Let's wait and evaluate the condition of your baby before we decide to use this drug."
4. "Giving this drug to your baby will cause immediate withdrawal. It is not indicated."

85. **In preparing a client for D&C in an outpatient surgery clinic, the nurse must start an intravenous infusion. Each of the following veins is a possible site for the IV. Which would be the best choice initially?**

1. The great saphenous vein on the ankle.
2. The metacarpal vein on the back of the hand.
3. The median basilic vein in the antecubital fossa.
4. The cephalic vein on the forearm.

86. **Calcium gluconate is being administered to a client with pregnancy induced hypertension. Which of the following actions must the nurse include in the plan of care throughout injection of the drug?**

1. Ventilator assistance.
2. CVP readings.
3. Continuous CPR.
4. EKG tracings.

87. **The mother of two children tells the nurse during a clinic visit that her older son, age nine, has been acting up since his younger sibling's diagnosis of cerebral palsy. Which of the following would best help the nine-year-old?**

1. Suggest ways that the parents may spend time meeting the needs of the nine-year-old.
2. Explain to the older child that expressions of anger are inappropriate ways of dealing with his emotions.
3. Provide information to the nine-year-old on his sibling's condition as soon as he requests it.
4. Tell the parents that they should not expect their nine-year-old to understand the needs of the disabled child.

88. **Betamethasone (Celestone) is administered at 30 weeks gestation to reduce the risk of RDS in a neonate. The infant is born after two injections are given. As the nurse is planning care for the infant, which of the following should be anticipated as a result of the administration of betamethasone to the mother?**

1. Rapid pulse rate.
2. Sternal retractions.
3. Hypoglycemia.
4. Hypothermia.

89. **Which of the following situations warrant an injection of RHoGAM to an Rh negative woman?**

    1. Vaginal bleeding at 24 weeks and following a voluntary termination of pregnancy at 12 weeks gestation .
    2. An episode of flu at 24 weeks gestation and after surgery for an ectopic pregnancy.
    3. At 28 weeks gestation and after blood transfusions during pregnancy.
    4. While the client is in labor and following the delivery of an Rh positive neonate.

90. **The client's psychiatrist orders fluphenazine (Prolixin) 10 mg b.i.d. Before the first dose, the client asks the nurse what the medicine is supposed to do. Which response by the nurse would be most therapeutic for a suspicious client?**

    1. "It will help you feel less anxious."
    2. "It is to help make your thinking clearer and decrease your fears."
    3. "This medication will help you maintain self-control."
    4. "This medication will help you get better."

91. **A nurse on the psychiatric unit poses a question to a client who either does not respond or mumbles incoherently. The nurse will best deal with the client's communication problems by which of the following actions?**

    1. Sitting quietly with the client during their scheduled times without attempting to verbalize until the client indicates a willingness to talk.
    2. Continuing to speak with the client using short, clear statements or open-ended questions about topics that may interest the client.
    3. Continuing to encourage the client to talk by asking direct questions.
    4. Filling silent periods by talking about topics interesting to the nurse.

92. **The nurse learns that a depressed client is an expert at crewel embroidery. The nurse buys embroidery materials and asks the client if she will teach crewel work to the nurse. Which of the following is the best rationale for this nursing intervention?**

    1. To assess the client's ability to communicate clearly.
    2. To distract the client from thinking about her problems.

    3. To reinforce the client's identity as a homemaker.
    4. To use the client's strengths to build self-esteem.

93. **The nurse notices a fire in the linen room. Which type of extinguisher should be used?**

    1. Dry powder.
    2. Water.
    3. Dry chemical.
    4. Carbon dioxide.

94. **The nurse expects that betamethasone (Celestone) would be used with caution in which of the following antepartum clients?**

    1. Primigravida with mild PIH.
    2. Multigravida with diabetes.
    3. Primigravida with AIDS.
    4. Multigravida with renal disease.

95. **A depressed client's progress improves and she now attends group therapy daily. The nurse understands that the most important benefit of group therapy is:**

    1. The opportunity to develop social skills.
    2. Improving the client's orientation to reality.
    3. Gaining support and encouragement from other persons.
    4. Developing greater insight into herself and her problems through the feedback provided by the other members.

96. **A 17-year-old client is recovering from an appendectomy. When the nurse offers her meperidine (Demerol), she says, "No, I don't want to get hooked." Which of the following is the best initial nursing response?**

    1. "You are right. Why take a chance?"
    2. "Tell me what you mean by getting hooked."
    3. "You will not get addicted for the short amount of time that you will be in the hospital."
    4. "The Demerol will make you more comfortable, not make you an addict."

97. **In addition to the prophylactic use of nitrates, the nurse can encourage the client to perform which of the following activities, without increasing the risk of an angina attack?**

    1. Eating large meals.
    2. Smoking cigarettes.
    3. Walking a treadmill.
    4. Shoveling snow.

98. **Which of the following lab findings are consistent with a mother to whom the nurse will expect to administer RHoGAM following delivery?**

    1. Mother Rh negative with a negative Coombs, father Rh positive, baby Rh negative.
    2. Mother Rh negative with a positive Rh antibody titer, father Rh positive, baby Rh positive.
    3. Mother Rh negative with a negative Coombs, father Rh positive, baby Rh positive.
    4. Mother Rh negative with a positive Coombs, father Rh negative, baby Rh negative.

99. **Following a total hip replacement, the nurse takes precautions to ensure that the affected hip is flexed no more than:**

    1. 25 degrees.
    2. 60 degrees.
    3. 75 degrees.
    4. 90 degrees.

100. **A 10-year-old girl is admitted with the hospital unit with cystic fibrosis. It is appropriate for the nurse to administer her pancrelipase (Pancrease) at which time?**

    1. One hour before meals.
    2. With meals.
    3. One-half hour after meals.
    4. On an empty stomach.

NCLEX-RN

Test 7

Questions with Rationales

NCLEX-RN TEST 7 WITH RATIONALES

1. A 58-year-old client is receiving nasal oxygen postoperatively. Which of the following laboratory findings would indicate to the nurse that the oxygen therapy is effective?

   1. PaO_2 of 56 mm Hg.
   2. PaO_2 of 85 mm Hg.
   3. PaO_2 of 90 mm Hg.
   4. PaO_2 of 97 mm Hg.

   1. *Incorrect. In a normal adult, PaO_2 is 95 to 100 mg Hg. This result is very low.*
   2. *Incorrect. This result is quite low.*
   3. *Not quite. This result is slightly low.*
   4. ***Correct. The PaO_2 in a normal adult is 95 to 100 mg Hg. This result is within normal limits.***

2. A 29-year-old diabetic is admitted to the hospital for dialysis because of poor renal function. He says to the nurse, "I don't even know why I'm doing this. There is no cure." Which of the following statements is the most appropriate nursing response?

   1. "There is always a chance that, through research, a cure will be found."
   2. "Dialysis will help you live longer."
   3. "You shouldn't complain! You are fortunate to be in this good a shape, considering the type of diabetes you have."
   4. "It sounds as though you have given up on life."

   1. *Wrong! This statement is an example of a cliché and false reassurance. The client has expressed his feelings to the nurse. Instead of helping the client deal with his feelings, the nurse focuses on the possibility of a future cure.*
   2. *This statement is true, but it does not address the client's feelings. The client has just expressed his feelings to the nurse. To be therapeutic, the nurse's response should focus on the client's feelings.*
   3. *No. This statement expresses the nurse's disapproval of the client's feelings, and devalues his concerns about the future. This response blocks communication and is not appropriate in the nurse-client relationship.*
   4. ***Great work! The nurse is using the communication tool of restatement to encourage the expression of feelings, which is therapeutic for the client. The nurse must maintain a nonjudgmental attitude so that the client will feel free to express his feelings. Note that Option 3 blocks communication by expressing the nurse's disapproval of the client's feelings.***

3. While working the night shift, the nurse notices a mouse running down the hallway of the clinical unit. The best initial action is which of the following?

   1. Place rat poison in the vicinity where the mouse was seen.
   2. Set some mouse traps to catch the mouse, and then dispose of it in a plastic bag labeled as contaminated.
   3. Notify the supervisor of the problem.
   4. Call the environmental health department of the hospital, and report the incident.

   1. *Wrong! Poison should not be placed in an area that clients, staff and visitors utilize, because of the risk of accidental exposure or poisoning.*
   2. *It is not the nurse's responsibility to catch mice. To prevent infection, however, the problem should be reported to the department responsible for rodent control.*
   3. *The supervisor is not responsible for rodent control. If the nurse has a problem getting the department that is responsible for environmental health to take care of the mouse, then the supervisor may be needed to intervene on behalf of the nurse.*
   4. ***Yes! The department that is responsible for environmental health deals with pest and rodent control and should be notified of this problem.***

4. In which of the following situations would the nurse expect administration of naloxone (Narcan) be indicated?

   1. Mother ready to deliver who received meperidine (Demerol) IM four and one-half hours ago.
   2. Mother experiencing hypotension following epidural anesthesia.
   3. Mother ready to deliver who received butorphanol (Stadol) IV five minutes ago.
   4. A drug addicted mother about to deliver who received Demerol IM one-half hour ago.

   1. *Incorrect. Four and one-half hours is plenty of time for the CNS/respiratory depression related to the administration of Demerol to the laboring woman to be gone. Reversal of the effects is not needed.*
   2. *Wrong answer. The use of Narcan has no effect on the hypotensive reaction to local anesthetics. It will only block the effects of narcotic agents given to a client.*

3. *Good choice! When Stadol is given IV, the effect is immediate and it crosses the placenta rapidly. Giving Narcan to the mother prior to the delivery, or to the neonate after the delivery, will block the effects of the drug on the CNS and respiratory system.*

4. *Sorry, Narcan is always contraindicated in the drug addicted mother since it will cause rapid withdrawal.*

5. **When taking a nursing history, the primary nurse learns an elderly client has had difficulty sleeping at night for several months. In evaluating his sleep disturbance, the nurse should remember which of the following facts?**

1. Elderly people have an increase in Stages 3 and 4 sleep.
2. Elderly people seldom awake at night once they have fallen asleep.
3. Anxiety and depression frequently cause disturbed sleep patterns.
4. Elderly people require much less sleep than younger adults.

1. *Incorrect. Elderly people have markedly reduced Stages 3 and 4 sleep.*

2. *Wrong choice! It is not uncommon for elderly persons to awake several times during the night and then fall back to sleep again without difficulty.*

3. *Correct. The nurse should recall that the sleep patterns of elderly people are different from those of younger adults. However, anxiety and depression often result in sleep disturbances in persons of all ages. This client's sleep problems need to be evaluated further but are most likely the result of his depression.*

4. *This is not correct! The elderly, overall, require as much, or more, sleep than younger persons. They are more likely to obtain some of this sleep in the form of daytime naps, so their sleep at night may be for fewer hours.*

6. **A 62-year-old client comes to the emergency room with a temperature of 102° F, blood pressure of 150/110, and tachycardia. She has been taking haloperidol (Haldol) 5 mg t.i.d. for the past three months. The nurse knows that these symptoms indicate a diagnosis of:**

1. Neuroleptic malignant syndrome (NMS).
2. Agranulocytosis.
3. Hypertensive crisis.
4. Tardive dyskinesia.

1. *Correct. Neuroleptic malignant syndrome is a rare, but potentially fatal, adverse effect of antipsychotics. It requires emergency medical intervention. Other symptoms associated with*

NMS are muscle rigidity, tremor, stupor, incontinence, elevated serum CPK, hyperkalemia and renal failure.

2. *This is not correct. Agranulocytosis is a rare adverse effect of antipsychotics. The WBC falls below 500, causing the client to become susceptible to acute infections. The client does have an elevated temperature, but no other signs of infection.*

3. *This is a possible choice because of the client's elevated blood pressure, however, her other symptoms indicate another diagnosis. Hypertensive crisis is associated with MAO inhibitor antidepressants.*

4. *Incorrect. Tardive dyskinesia, an involuntary muscle movement disorder, is an irreversible adverse effect of antipsychotics. It occurs most often in clients who have been on antipsychotics for a long time; hence the term "tardive" for late onset.*

7. **The nurse enters the room and finds a mother crying. Her son has been diagnosed with leukemia and is currently receiving chemotherapy. The mother says, "I just can't believe he's going to lose all his beautiful blonde hair!" Which response by the nurse is most justifiable?**

1. "Sometimes the hair only thins."
2. "You're feeling a lot of loss right now."
3. "Remember, hair loss means the chemotherapy is working!"
4. "Kids love to wear the special baseball caps we have."

1. *While this could be true, this is not therapeutic for the mother, as it minimizes her concerns and feelings and may cut off further communication.*

2. *Excellent! This statement validates the mother's feelings and encourages further communication.*

3. *This statement is not therapeutic and it is false. Hair loss occurs because chemotherapy destroys rapidly growing cells which include hair, linings of the GI tract, and cancer cells. It is not an indication of the effectiveness of the chemotherapy.*

4. *This statement may be true, but it is not therapeutic because it does not address the mother's feelings and concerns. It is also not helpful to generalize for all children.*

8. **A couple is in the hospital because of a fetal death at 37 weeks gestation. Which of the following is an appropriate response by the nurse?**

1. "You are both young and you can have other children."
2. "It is God's will, and it must be accepted."
3. "It must be very difficult for you both. I will be available if you need anything."
4. "I think you should call your minister. He can help comfort you."

1. *This statement may be true, but the nurse cannot know what will happen in the future. This response does not acknowledge the feelings of the clients and blocks communication. This is an example of a cliché and false reassurance.*
2. *This is a cliché that expresses the nurse's beliefs and values. It is not empathetic and does not recognize the clients' feelings. This is a communication block.*
3. ***Correct! This statement acknowledges the clients' feelings. The nurse is showing empathy, and is also offering self by offering to assist them.***
4. *Wrong! This statement implies that the minister is needed for comforting and that the nurse is not available discuss the clients' feelings. This response is also giving advice to the client. This response is not therapeutic.*

9. **A newborn infant has just returned from surgery for correction of a cleft lip. Which nursing interventions are indicated?**

    1. Arm restraints, postural drainage and oral irrigations.
    2. Cleansing suture line, arm restraints, and supine or side lying position.
    3. Prone or side lying position, cleansing suture line, and oral irrigations.
    4. Side lying position, use specially designed nipple and arm restraints.

    1. *No, for two reasons. Arm restraints are correct, usually elbow would be used. Postural drainage indicates head lower than heart; this would increase swelling to the operative site, which is to be avoided. Irrigations could potentially injure the plastic repair of the lip.*
    2. ***Correct! Cleansing of the suture line is to prevent crusting. Arm restraints prevent the infant from touching the suture line, and the side lying or supine positions are preferred to prevent swelling of the suture line.***
    3. *Incorrect. Prone position increases edema to suture line, and the irrigations may damage the repair. Cleansing of the suture line and the side lying positions are correct.*
    4. *No! Did the "specially designed nipple" attract you? Remember, no nippling is allowed postoperatively, and even immediately preoperatively for cleft lip repair.*

10. **When counseling a client who is taking isosorbide dinitrate (Isordil) for angina, which of the following side effects can the nurse anticipate will occur least often?**

    1. Hypotension.
    2. Headache.
    3. Bradycardia.
    4. Weakness.

1. *Incorrect. Hypotension is one of the most frequent side effects of Isordil. Remember that this medication is a potent vasodilator with hypotension as the most significant side effect.*
2. *Wrong. Headache is a common side effect of nitrate therapy due to vasodilation of the cerebral vessels. The headache should decrease with continued therapy. The client should notify the physician if the headache is persistent or severe and should not alter the dose to avoid a headache.*
3. ***Right choice. Bradycardia does not result from the use of Isordil, a vasodilator. Bradycardia is caused by medications which affect the conduction pathways in the heart (e.g., beta adrenergic blockers).***
4. *No. Weakness is a common side effect of Isordil, which is a potent vasodilator. This symptom may pass as the client adjusts to the medication, but the client should be instructed to change position slowly and to take safety precautions.*

11. **A child is to receive 400 mL of IV fluid over an eight-hour shift. The drip factor on the IV tubing is 60 drops/mL. How many drops/minute will deliver the proper amount?**

    1. 12.5 drops/minute.
    2. 16 drops/minute.
    3. 50 drops/minute.
    4. 63 drops/minute.

    1. *Wrong. This rate is too low. Check your calculations.*
    2. *Wrong. This rate is too low. Check your calculations.*
    3. ***Correct. Figure: 400 mL/8 hours = 50 mL/hour. Then: 50 mL/60 minutes x 60 gtt/min = 50 gtts/min.***
    4. *Wrong. This rate is too high. Check your calculations.*

12. **A confused, elderly client has wet herself and is standing in the hospital corridor in a puddle of urine. She looks ashamed and says to the nurse, "I want to go outside for a walk now." What would be the most appropriate response by the nurse at this time?**

    1. "Before we go for a walk, perhaps we can make a list that will help you make your bathroom trips easier."
    2. "Right now, let me wipe up the urine on the floor, and let's get a change of clothing for you. I am sure that this problem is upsetting for you."
    3. "This has been a problem for you. Let's see if we can find a solution together."
    4. "Wetting yourself is very upsetting. Yes, let's take a walk."

1.   *Wrong! The issue in this question is a wet client standing in a puddle of urine. This response does not address the current problem. Also, since the client is confused, making a list is not appropriate.*

2.   ***Yes, this is the best response! This response deals with the here and now by helping the client focus on her current need, which is dry clothes, and it informs the client that the nurse is going to wipe up the urine off the floor. The nurse is also showing empathy. This response is therapeutic for the client.***

> **STRATEGY ALERT!** Note that the phrase "puddle of urine" in the question is similar to the words "urine on the floor" in this option. This is a clue that this may be the correct answer.

3.   *No. The client is feeling uncomfortable, and her basic needs for dry clothes and a safe environment must be met. Discussing possible solutions to the problem of not getting to the bathroom in time will not help those immediate problem. The client is also confused, and she is feeling ashamed. The correct response addresses the physical, safety and emotional needs of this client.*

4.   *Wrong. In this response, the nurse is showing empathy. However, this response does not address the client's basic need at this time for dry clothes, or the nursing priority of wiping up the urine off the floor.*

13.   **The nurse learns that an elderly client's sleeping problems began six months before, when his physician diagnosed prostatic cancer. Prior to that time, he had enjoyed good physical health. She also learned that his wife of 50 years had died one year ago. One day the client tells the nurse, "I'd be better off dead because I am totally worthless." The nurse's most therapeutic response is which of the following remarks?**

1.   "I have seen some very valuable things about you."
2.   "You feel worthless now because you are so depressed. You will feel differently when you depression begins to improve."
3.   "You really have a great deal to live for."
4.   "You have been feeling very sad and alone for some time now."

1.   *The nurse should accept the client's perceptions without agreeing with his conclusions. There is a better option.*

2.   *This statement is not untrue, but there is a better option.*

3.   *This is not correct because, from the client's point of view, this is not true. There is a better option.*

4.   ***Correct. Depressed persons have great difficulty expressing their feelings. This response by the nurse is a good way to begin to help him become more aware and accepting of his feelings.***

14.   **The nurse is working in an acute care pediatric unit. One of the LPN's has assessments on four postoperative clients. Which client requires the nurse's most immediate attention?**

1.   A 12-year-old appendectomy, two days postoperative and refusing to ambulate.
2.   An 8-year-old tonsillectomy, just returned from the recovery room, having frequent swallowing.
3.   Possible peripheral IV infiltration (rate 50 mL/hr) on a 15-year-old herniorrhaphy.
4.   An 18-month-old one day postoperative for cleft palate repair with a pulse of 120 beats per minute.

1.   *Incorrect! This child should ambulate, but it's not an emergency.*

2.   ***Good! The swallowing may be a sign of bleeding from the surgical site. This requires immediate investigation with a flashlight, and if there is fresh red blood, the surgeon should be notified. Aspiration and/or excessive blood loss are potentially life-threatening.***

3.   *No, not the first priority. This is not a life-threatening situation since it is a peripheral IV. The nurse would certainly want to investigate, unless the LPN can manage IV's in that facility.*

4.   *Not an immediate priority situation. This pulse is within normal limits for an 18-month-old.*

15.   **Soon after being admitted to a rehabilitation unit, a chronic alcoholic says to the nurse, "I don't really need to be here. My wife and family make me drink. My wife spends all my money. My kid just had an accident with his car that will cost me a fortune in repairs." The most appropriate response by the nurse at this time would be:**

1.   "Tell me more about how your wife is spending all your money."
2.   "Could you tell me more about why your child's car accident cost you money?"
3.   "It sounds like you are having a great deal of financial difficulty."
4.   "Tell me more about your feelings about being here in the hospital."

1.   *Wrong choice! The client is a chronic alcoholic who is in denial. ("I don't really need to be here.") Before the client can accept help for his problem, he must examine his feelings and acknowledge that he is an alcoholic who needs help. This option focuses on his financial difficulties rather than his feelings. Note that Options 2 and 3 also focus on financial difficulties; these similar distractors can be eliminated.*

2.   *Wrong choice! The client is a chronic alcoholic who is in denial. This option focuses on his financial difficulties rather than his feelings. Note that Options 1 and 3 also focus on financial difficulties; these similar distractors can be eliminated.*

3. *Wrong! The client is a chronic alcoholic who is in denial. This option focuses on his financial difficulties rather than his feelings. Note that Options 2 and 3 also focus on financial difficulties; these similar distractors can be eliminated.*

4. ***You are correct! The client is a chronic alcoholic who is in denial. ("I don't really need to be here.") Before the client can accept help for his problem, he must examine his feelings and acknowledge that he is an alcoholic who needs help. This option focuses on the client's feelings about being in the hospital.***

> **STRATEGY ALERT!** Note that the other three options all focus on money and financial difficulties. Options that express the same idea can be eliminated.

16. **A vest restraint is placed on a confused elderly client who is at high risk for falling. He is partially paralyzed and is at risk for developing pressure sores. How should the nurse handle the linen when changing this client's bed?**

   1. When removing the linen from the bed, hold it close to the body to avoid dropping it.
   2. After removing the linen from the bed, place it on the floor until finished making the bed.
   3. When removing the linen from the bed, hold it away from the uniform.
   4. Shake the clean linen to unfold it, before making the bed.

   1. *No. The linen will contaminate the nurse's uniform and should be placed in the dirty linen bag immediately.*
   2. *No. The linen will contaminate the nurse's uniform and should be placed in the dirty linen bag immediately.*
   3. ***This choice is correct, because the linen is considered "dirty" and should be held away from the uniform to avoid contaminating it.***
   4. *This is incorrect. Shaking linen spreads bacteria and other harmful organisms.*

17. **The client is transferred to the recovery room after a colon resection for adenocarcinoma. Which of the following body system adaptations would the nurse expect to see initially if the client were to develop internal abdominal bleeding postoperatively?**

   1. Tachycardia.
   2. Oliguria.
   3. Hyperthermia.
   4. Bradypnea.

   1. ***Excellent reasoning! Because of the decreased circulating blood volume due to the internal bleed-***

ing, there is a decreased oxygen carrying capacity of the blood; the body attempts to relieve the hypoxia by increasing the heart rate and cardiac output along with increasing the respiratory rate.

2. *No, this is not an initial sign of hypovolemic shock, although it is part of the clinical picture due to the decreased circulating blood volume through the glomerulus.*

3. *This is not an initial sign of hypovolemic shock. One of the classic signs of shock is cool, moist skin. Hyperthermia is seen in septic shock.*

4. *Incorrect. Initially, in shock, the respirations are deep and rapid, progressing to an even more rapid and then shallow rate as the body attempts to take in more oxygen to reduce the hypoxia.*

18. **A 66-year-old client is receiving hemodialysis via left internal angioaccess for management of chronic renal disease. Which of the following should the nurse include when teaching this client?**

   1. Check the access hourly for patency.
   2. Maintain skin integrity through frequent cleansing and application of lotion over the site.
   3. Avoid tight clothing around the access site.
   4. Sleep on his left side to maintain patency of access site.

   1. *Wrong. It is only necessary to check the access site twice daily for the "buzz" that indicates adequate blood flow. Hourly checks are unnecessary.*
   2. *Wrong. The use of creams or lotions is to be avoided over the access site to prevent infection.*
   3. ***Good work! Tight clothing may decrease the blood flow and cause clotting.***
   4. *Wrong. Sleeping on the side of the access may cause impairment of blood flow and clotting to occur.*

19. **The physician has ordered extremity restraints for safety reasons for a confused, elderly client. After placing the client in extremity restraints, the priority nursing action is which of the following?**

   1. Release each extremity every two hours for range of motion exercises.
   2. Discuss the rationale for the restraints with the family members.
   3. Reduce the client's distress by dimming the lights and closing the door.
   4. Tie the restraints to the side rails using a half bow knot.

   1. ***This is the priority action, because the client with restraints is at risk of circulatory problems and possible permanent injury. Releasing the extrem-***

ity for range of motion exercises addresses this risk, and allows the nurse to assess for possible injury from the restraints.

2. *While it would be important to discuss the use of restraints with the family, it is not a priority action. Actions that ensure the safety of the client take priority.*

3. *The nurse should never isolate a restrained client by dimming the lights and closing the door. The client's distress might be increased. It is also important to visually check on a restrained client frequently.*

4. *The half bow knot is correct, but tying the restraints to the side rails is incorrect. The restraints are tied to the bed frame. Because part of this option is incorrect, this cannot be the correct answer.*

20. **The nurse is admitting a client who is suspected of having diabetes mellitus. Which of the following characteristics would the nurse expect to observe?**

    1. Shallow, labored respirations.
    2. Increased blood pressure associated with slight periorbital edema.
    3. Periods of altered pulse rate.
    4. Increased urinary output.

    1. *This is a good distractor! It is a possibility, because it suggests Kussmaul's breathing, which is a characteristic of ketoacidosis — a complication of diabetes mellitus. Kussmaul's breathing is deep and rapid, however, not shallow and labored. Also, the stem asks for a characteristic of diabetes, not a complication.*

    2. *This is not a characteristic of diabetes. This option is a distractor.*

    3. *Although this may be a sign of ketoacidosis, it is not a characteristic of diabetes. This option is a distractor.*

    4. *Correct! Remember the "three P's" associated with the diagnosis of diabetes mellitus: polyuria, polyphagia and polydypsia.*

21. **The physician has determined that the client is extremely dehydrated and in need of intravenous fluids. The client is confused, and has pulled out one intravenous catheter and caused another intravenous site to become infiltrated. The nurse restarts the intravenous in the client's left arm. An order for restraints is given. Which of the following is the best action by the nurse?**

    1. Apply a vest restraint and extremity restraints to ensure that the intravenous site will be protected.
    2. Apply a restraint to the left arm.
    3. Apply a restraint to the right arm.
    4. Apply restraints to the right and left arms.

    1. *This option completely restrains the client. The clinical situation indicates that only the intrave-*

nous site is in need of being protected. This is an example of over-restraining a client, and is inappropriate.

2. *Restraining the left arm allows the client to reach the intravenous site with the right hand. The intravenous site is not protected.*

3. *Even though the right hand is restrained, the client can move the left hand over to the right side, which will allow the client to disturb the intravenous site.*

4. *This is correct. Applying restraints to both upper extremities provides protection for the intravenous site. The client does not have the opportunity to disturb the site.*

22. **On the second day after hip surgery, an elderly client is awake for brief periods of time. During the evening, she becomes restless and begins to pull at her IV tubing. The most appropriate nursing action when she pulls at the tubing is to:**

    1. Maintain steady pressure on her arm to prohibit her from dislodging the tubing, while continuing to speak gently to her until she lets go of the tubing.
    2. Speak in a loud, clear way telling her to stop pulling on the IV, while gently trying to pry her fingers from around the tubing.
    3. Explain that she has an IV for fluid replacement and offer to show it to her when she lets go of the tubing.
    4. Call for help and prepare to apply soft wrist restraints so she will not be able to grab the tubing again.

    1. *Correct. The nurse should remain calm and gently apply pressure to the client's hand or arm to prevent her from dislodging the IV. If the nurse continues to speak gently and calmly to the client, she will eventually release her hold on the tubing. A person in constant attendance can prevent the client from pulling out tubing. Family members or "sitters" can also be used for this purpose.*

    2. *This is not correct. The nurse must remain calm to avoid causing further agitation in the client. Trying to force the client to let go of tubing usually results in the tubing becoming dislodged.*

    3. *This is not an incorrect statement, but it is not the most appropriate nursing action because it will not prevent the client from dislodging the IV tubing. It is appropriate to show the tubing to the client and let her touch it when she is calm and more able to comprehend what the nurse is telling her.*

    4. *This is not correct. Restraints are only used as a measure of last resort after all other interventions have been tried because restraints cause greater agitation and safety problems.*

23. **A 16-year-old client has left her used insulin syringe on the bedside table. What is the best action by the nurse to help prevent spread of infection by way of the contaminated needle?**

1. Explain to the client that the syringe should be disposed of in the garbage can to avoid a potential needle stick by someone providing care for the client.
2. Cap the syringe and take to the needle disposal container.
3. Place the uncapped syringe in the needle disposal container.
4. Have the nurse administer the injection, since the client is not responsible enough to follow through with the proper procedure.

1. The syringe should not be disposed of in the garbage can, because the employees that take care of the trash can incur a needle stick while handling the trash. Needles and syringes should be incinerated. Therefore, whatever hospital procedure is in effect for contaminated trash should be followed. Note that needles should not be recapped, since there is a potential risk of sticking oneself during this action. The correct action is to place the needle and syringe in a container that protects everyone from potential needle sticks.

2. Wrong! Needles should not be recapped because there is a potential risk of sticking oneself during this action.

3. Correct. Special containers are available for syringe and needle disposal. These containers should be utilized. Remember that needles should not be recapped, however, because there is a potential risk of sticking oneself during this action.

4. The client should be reminded or taught about the potential injuries and infections that can result from a needle stick. The client should continue to administer the insulin, with closer supervision by the nurse concerning disposal of the needle and syringe.

24. **A general anesthesia has been given for multiple tooth extractions on a three-year-old child. He returns crying but awake from the recovery room. What approach is most likely to be successful?**

1. Examine the mouth first.
2. Leave the mouth until last.
3. It really makes no difference what is done first.
4. Medicate the child for pain first.

1. No. Since this is the area of discomfort, this is likely to cause more crying and uncooperative behavior.

2. Good! Leave the most distressing part of an exam on a toddler until the end. You must assess the child before pain medication can be administered.

3. This is not correct! It cannot be the best option.

TEST-TAKING TIP: Try to eliminate the options you know are incorrect. Which options in this question are inappropriate actions?

4. No, this is inappropriate. An assessment is always performed immediately upon transfer from recovery.

25. **The night nurse complains that an elderly client on the surgical unit has started to have periods of agitation at night that include screaming out loudly for help. The primary nurse suggests several interventions to diminish this behavior. Which of the following interventions should the nurse avoid?**

1. Remaining calm and encouraging the client to express her fears so the nurse will have a better understanding of how to help.
2. Requesting an order for a sedative medication.
3. Keeping a nightlight on in her room.
4. Assessing her level of pain or the presence of other physical discomfort.

1. Screaming usually indicates that the client is afraid. The specific fears should be the focus of the nursing intervention, and not the screaming. The nurse must assess the fear so she will know how to better intervene. This is a recommended intervention, so it cannot be the correct option.

2. Correct. Screaming indicates that the client is afraid. Medication may sedate the client but it will not remove her fear. Sedative medication is used very sparingly in a postoperative client of advanced old age who is also on pain medication.

3. This is a recommended intervention, so it cannot be the correct option. A nightlight illuminating the room will help orient the client when she awakens during the night. It will also decrease fears that result from misperceiving the nature of objects in her room.

4. This is a recommended intervention, so it cannot be the correct option. Pain and other types of physical discomfort such as unmet toileting needs are often the cause of a client's fear and agitation.

26. **Which of the following statements, if made by a male client who has a prescription for nitroglycerin (Nitrostat) tablets, would indicate to the nurse that he needs further teaching?**

1. "I'll make sure that the medication container is kept tightly sealed."
2. "I'm lucky I have a prescription plan that allows me to buy pills in bulk quantities."
3. "I'll keep my pills in the medicine cabinet when I'm home."
4. "I know that I should go to the hospital emergency room if my chest pain doesn't go away."

1. *No. This statement does not indicate a need for further teaching. The client should keep the nitroglycerin tablets in a dark, dry place, and in a dark-colored glass bottle with a tight lid. Tablets lose potency in containers made of plastic or cardboard or when mixed with other capsules or tablets.*

2. ***Right choice. This is not a safe practice and would require further teaching. The client should not buy large quantities because this drug does not store well. Nitroglycerin tablets are chemically unstable and can lose effectiveness over time, although they should remain effective for at least six months after the container is first opened. As a rule, nitroglycerin tablets should be discarded after this time.***

3. *Wrong selection. This is an acceptable practice. The client knows to keep the medication in a dark, dry place because exposure to air, heat, and moisture cause loss of potency.*

4. *Incorrect choice. This is a critical teaching point and may save the client's life. The client is instructed to call the physician or go to the nearest emergency room if anginal pain is not relieved by three tablets (taken five minutes apart) in 15 minutes.*

27. **A 12-year-old boy has been recently diagnosed with diabetes. In order to minimize his anxiety, which nursing action would be most appropriate?**

    1. Provide a toy ""Doctor's Kit" to play with.
    2. Keep all syringes and needles out of sight until the last moment.
    3. Explain to the child that his parents will administer all of the medications.
    4. Allow the child to manipulate a syringe and give himself injections.

    1. *A 12-year-old is beyond the age of imitative play. He will not benefit from hospital toys, as it will not meet his need to manipulate the environment and accomplish tasks.*
    2. *Wrong. Hiding the syringes and needles will only increase the child's fear by adding to it the fear of the unknown. This approach decreases the control the child has over his environment.*
    3. *No. A 12-year-old child is at an age where he needs to feel in control of his environment and achieve a sense of accomplishment. By encouraging the parents to carry out all the care, the child is not allowed to achieve mastery over the administration skills.*
    4. ***Yes. Anxiety is best decreased by allowing the child as much control and mastery as is possible. Teaching the child to give himself injections will give the child a sense of accomplishment, which is vital in the school age years.***

28. **While caring for a client, the nurse notices that the call light cord is frayed. At this time, which of the following nursing actions would be most important?**

    1. Tell the client not to use the call light until it is fixed.
    2. Remove the call light, and report the problem to the supervising nurse immediately.
    3. Tape up the cord until the maintenance people can fix it, so the client will have a call light.
    4. Tell the client to call out if he needs help, and to use the call light only in an emergency.

    1. *No. This will not protect the client from potential electrical burns or shocks. A frayed cord is an electrical hazard.*
    2. ***Correct. Removal of a frayed cord is the only way to protect the client from potential electrical burns. The supervising nurse will make arrangements for another call light or system for the client.***
    3. *Wrong. This is not a proper repair, and it will not protect the client from potential electrical burns or shocks. A frayed cord is an electrical hazard.*
    4. *Wrong. This will not protect the client from potential electrical burns or shocks. A frayed cord is an electrical hazard.*

29. **After detoxification, the client begins the rehabilitation phase of treatment. He tells the nurse that he cannot imagine living his life without alcohol. The nurse's best response is based on what knowledge?**

    1. He will be more successful if he focuses on goals for short periods of time such as "today" or "this week".
    2. He is likely to drink again when under stress.
    3. He will not be successful if he is not strongly motivated.
    4. He may require treatment with Antabuse to maintain sobriety.

    1. ***Correct. Clients are less overwhelmed by the thought of sobriety when they set short-term goals that focus on "today" or "this week". Dealing with shorter periods of time is more manageable. The saying by AA "One day at a time" is a reflection of this principle.***
    2. *This could be a true statement, but it is not the best option because it would not be a helpful response for this client.*
    3. *This is not an incorrect statement, but it is not the best option. Motivation, without the development of needed skills, will not help the client to maintain sobriety.*
    4. *This is not a true statement. Antabuse is used for individuals who lack the ability to abstain from*

alcohol without fear of adverse consequences. There is no data to indicate that this client requires Antabuse, since he is just beginning his rehabilitation program.

30.   A six-year-old female is admitted with rheumatic fever. She has painful joints and a temperature of 103° F. Bedrest is ordered. What is the primary rationale for bedrest?

1.   The workload of the heart is decreased by bedrest.
2.   Bedrest will limit the joint pain.
3.   Permanent arthritic changes of the joints will be prevented.
4.   BMR (basal metabolic rate) will be decreased, which will decrease the elevated temperature.

*1.   **Correct! The goal is to protect the heart, since the pathophysiology of rheumatic fever involves cardiac tissue.***
2.   No, not the primary rationale, since bedrest does not reduce the inflammatory response.
3.   Not correct! The painful joints of rheumatic fever are not a precursor to arthritis.
4.   No! It sounds good, but the fever is basically due to the infection. Antibiotic therapy and antipyretics would be ordered for these symptoms.

31.   A psychiatric client is receiving chlorpromazine (Thorazine) and is doing well. The unit is planning an outdoor activity for Saturday. The weather has been warm and sunny. What information should the nurse give the client about the side effects of Thorazine before he leaves the unit?

1.   Wear a hat and a long-sleeved shirt.
2.   Watch for signs of jaundice.
3.   Drink plenty of fluids to replace any he might lose by sweating in the sun.
4.   Don't drink more than one beer.

*1.   **Correct. Photophobic skin reactions and damage to the retina of the eye can occur when the client is outside in direct sunlight. It is important that clients be told to wear protective clothing, apply suntan products that contain a sunblocking agent, and wear sunglasses when they are outside.***
2.   Jaundice is a rare allergic reaction associated with Thorazine. It usually occurs within the first few days of treatment with the medication in sensitive individuals. It is not related to sunlight, so this is not a correct statement.
3.   This is not the best option. While maintaining fluid and electrolyte balance is important for all clients, clients who are on lithium have to be particularly careful about this because electrolyte imbalances will affect serum lithium levels.

4.   Wrong. Clients should completely avoid alcoholic beverages or street drugs for many reasons, among them potentiation of CNS depressant effects and the development of liver problems.

32.   An unconscious 18-year-old man is brought to the emergency room. Friends report that he took an overdose of heroin. After the client regains consciousness, he is transferred to the substance abuse treatment unit. The signs and symptoms of heroin withdrawal are written in the nursing care plan. Which of the following behaviors could the nurse anticipate to occur early in the withdrawal process?

1.   Vomiting and diarrhea.
2.   Sneezing and rhinorrhea.
3.   Restlessness and irritability.
4.   Yawning and diaphoresis.

1.   This is not correct. Vomiting and diarrhea are usually late, rather than early, signs of heroin withdrawal.
2.   This is not correct. Sneezing and rhinorrhea are usually late, rather than early, signs of heroin withdrawal.
*3.   **Correct. Restlessness, irritability, piloerection (gooseflesh), tremors, and loss of appetite are all early signs of heroin withdrawal.***
4.   This is not correct. Yawning and diaphoresis are usually late, rather than early, signs of heroin withdrawal.

33.   Two days after a psychiatric client begins taking fluphenazine (Prolixin), she comes to the nursing station. The nurse observes that the client is very frightened. Her head is twisted to one side, her back is arched, and her eyes are rolled up. The nurse recognizes these symptoms as indicative of:

1.   Parkinsonian syndrome.
2.   Akathisia.
3.   Impending seizure.
4.   Dystonic reaction.

1.   Wrong. Parkinsonian syndrome is an extrapyramidal side effect characterized by behaviors associated with Parkinson's disease, such as mask-like facies, muscle stiffness, shuffling gait, rigid posture and tremors.
2.   Wrong. Akathisia is an extrapyramidal side effect characterized by motor restlessness. The client usually complains of an inability to sit still and paces, shifts her weight from one foot to the other, etc. Akathisia occurs later in the course of therapy, after several weeks of months on the medication, and not within the first few days.

3. *Wrong. Antipsychotics do lower the seizure threshold, so seizures may occur in clients with a preexisting seizure disorder or those taking high doses of antipsychotics. However, the described behavior are not indicative of the typical grand mal seizure that can occur.*

4. ***Correct. Contractions of the neck, back, or extraocular muscles producing torticollis, opisthotonos and oculogyric crisis ("Little Orphan Annie" eyes) are symptoms of a severe distonic reaction, an extrapyramidal side effect of antipsychotic medications. It is often a frightening and painful reaction.***

34. **A client with a history of angina is to take isosorbide dinitrate (Isordil) 10 mg p.o. every six hours. When the client asks how the drug works, the nurse's reply is based upon the understanding that the primary action of Isordil is to:**

1. Reduce cardiac preload and afterload.
2. Dilate the coronary blood vessels.
3. Increase the heart's oxygen consumption.
4. Decrease myocardial circulation.

1. ***Correct! Isordil, a nitrate, is a potent vasodilator of both the venous and arterial systems. If the arterioles are dilated, the blood is moved out with less cardiac effort (decreased afterload). If the venous system is dilated, there is less blood return to the heart (decreased preload).***

2. *Wrong choice. Isordil, a nitrate, will dilate coronary arteries to a some degree (which helps to increase myocardial circulation), but this is not the primary action of the nitrates.*

3. *Incorrect. Isordil, a vasodilator, helps to decrease the heart's oxygen consumption because of its primary action (which you haven't identified yet)!*

4. *No. Isordil, as a vasodilator, will increase coronary blood flow by dilating coronary arteries and improving collateral flow to ischemic regions.*

35. **A psychotic client receiving chlorpromazine (Thorazine) tried to "cheek" the medication so he could later spit it out. The nurse correctly decides to request that the physician change the order from the tablet form to a form that will prevent this from happening. Which of the following choices would be best?**

1. Liquid concentrate.
2. Capsule.
3. Suppository.
4. Intramuscular injection.

1. ***Correct. It is more difficult for the client to avoid swallowing the medication when it is in liquid form. The concentrate form acts more quickly because it reaches the blood stream faster. The dosage, however, remains the same.***

2. *This is not the best choice. The capsule form would not be an improvement over the tablet form for a client who resists swallowing medication.*

3. *This is not the best choice. The suppository form acts too slowly to be effective in a psychotic client.*

4. *This is not the best choice. The intramuscular route is used in emergency situations to rapidly control an agitated client.*

36. **Family therapy is scheduled for an anorexic client and her family. Her parents ask how the family therapy will help their daughter's eating problem. The best nursing response is to state that the focus of the therapy will be primarily on which of the following?**

1. Their daughter's eating behavior.
2. The parents and how their behavior may be causing their daughter to starve herself.
3. Increasing communication between the family members.
4. Teaching family members to better meet each other's needs.

1. *This is not correct. Family therapy does not focus on the problems of any one member, but instead aims at improving the relationships between all the members.*

2. *This is not correct. Family therapy focuses on the relationships among family members but does not try to fix blame on specific individuals. Its aim is to help members learn how to better meet their needs without causing difficulty for others in the family.*

3. ***Correct. Family therapy focuses on improving communication between members so that members can learn to meet their needs in a healthy manner. Families with anorexic members often have difficulty accepting differences of opinion and managing conflict.***

4. *This is not correct. While some teaching does go on during family therapy, its primary focus is on improving the communication relationship patterns among the family members.*

37. **A client, newly diagnosed with angina, is instructed to take one nitroglycerin (Nitrostat) tablet sublingual at the first sign of an anginal attack, waiting five minutes before taking another tablet. The nurse explains this waiting period to the client, based upon the rationale that:**

1. Absorption of the drug is slower via the sublingual route.
2. The client will need to monitor the blood pressure between dosages.
3. The client would demonstrate a potential allergic reaction within the first five minutes of drug administration.
4. Nitrates can lower the blood pressure very quickly.

1. *No. The sublingual route is a faster route of absorption (compared to oral) because of increased vascularity under the tongue. When administered sublingually, nitroglycerin is absorbed directly through the oral mucosa and into the bloodstream. Effects begin rapidly—in one to three minutes—and persist for up to one hour.*

2. *No. Although Nitrostat may result in hypotension as a side effect, it is not necessary, or realistic, for the client to monitor blood pressure between dosages.*

3. *Incorrect. This is not the reason for the five minute waiting period. Some clients do develop a hypersensitivity to the medication, but it would not necessarily occur within the first five minutes of drug administration.*

4. ***Correct! Nitrostat, as a vasodilator, is a potent antihypertensive and will lower the blood pressure very quickly. For that reason, clients must wait five minutes between sublingual doses.***

38. **A child, three months of age, has been admitted with a tentative diagnosis of intussusception. The parents ask the nurse how the diagnosis is made. Based on an understanding of the diagnostic evaluation for intussusception, what should the nurse say to the parents?**

1. "A small amount of tissue from the colon will be biopsied."
2. "Genotyping can identify this condition."
3. "A barium enema will be given to visualize the obstruction."
4. "An upper GI series should identify the area involved."

1. *No, you're probably thinking about Hirschsprung's disease. The pathophysiology of intussusception is not related to a defect of nerve innervation, and the disorder does not always occur in the colon.*

2. *No, genotyping would be used for hereditary disease.*

3. ***Yes. A barium enema is given, which may also treat the condition by nonsurgical means. The telescoping of the bowel, which characterizes intussusception, may be reduced by hydrostatic pressure of the barium enema.***

4. *No, this procedure focuses on an area too high to see intussusception. This is more likely to be used for the diagnosis of peptic ulcer.*

39. **While the nurse is caring for a client, the intravenous tubing becomes disconnected from the intravenous catheter, resulting in the client's blood spilling onto the sides of the bed and floor. Which of the following solutions are recommended for disinfection of blood spills?**

1. Betadine solution.
2. Alcohol.
3. Soap and water.
4. Sodium hypochlorite or chlorine bleach solution.

1. *Wrong! Betadine solution is used for disinfecting skin and is effective after being allowed to dry on the skin surface. It is not appropriate to apply to objects because it stains surfaces that it comes in contact with.*

2. *False! Alcohol is a skin disinfectant. It has not been found to destroy the HIV virus; therefore, it is not effective for blood spills.*

3. *Wrong! Soap and water emulsifies dirt for easy removal of the dirt; however, it is not a disinfectant.*

4. ***Correct! Chlorine acts as a disinfectant and is recommended for cleansing objects. It is recommended for blood spills because it is effective in killing the HIV virus, which is found in body fluids such as blood.***

40. **A six-month-old is in the pediatric clinic. The nurse practitioner ordered a DPT vaccine to be administered. Which of the following assessments would cause the nurse to question the administration of the DPT vaccine?**

1. Previous evidence of sensitivity to egg antigens.
2. High fever and high-pitched cry following last DPT.
3. Current temperature of 100° F.
4. Currently receiving steroid therapy.

1. *No, not for this vaccine. Severe anaphylactic egg sensitivity would represent a contraindication to administration of measles and mumps vaccine.*

2. ***Yes, most definitely! These are both symptoms of untoward responses to DPT, and are indicative of neurologic reaction. If a full dose of pertussis vaccine were to be given again it might cause a serious or even life-threatening adverse reaction.***

3. *No, mild fever, in the absence of other symptoms is not a reason to withhold DPT vaccine.*

4. *No. OPV is the vaccine that should be withheld if the child is receiving steroid therapy, since it is a live vaccine, and the child may respond in an unpredictable manner.*

41. **A client, 64 years old, is hospitalized with chronic obstructive pulmonary disease. Oxygen per nasal cannula at two liters per minute is initiated. When the nurse made an assessment at 3:00 p.m., the client appeared to have made a good adjustment to hospitalization. At 5:00 p.m., upon entering the room to bring the client his dinner tray, the nurse finds the oxygen cannula on the floor. The client is angry and says, "It's about time you got here. Where am I? Where is my breakfast?" The nurse should give immediate consideration to which of the following?**

1. Has the oxygen cannula been off long enough to cause hypoxia?
2. Is the client's anger related to being hospitalized again?
3. Does the client need a clock in the room to keep track of the time?
4. Is the client accustomed to eating meals at unusual times?

1. *Very good! The need for oxygen is a physiological need. The client's apparent confusion may be a result of decreased oxygen to the brain. The nurse should give immediate consideration to this physiological need. Maslow's Hierarchy of Needs identifies physiological needs as first priorities.*
2. *Wrong. The case scenario tells us that the client is angry, but what he says does not support the idea that he is angry about being hospitalized. Also, this statement indicates a psychological consideration as the explanation for the client's behavior. It must be determined if his behavior is due to a physiological need.*
3. *Wrong. The client appears to be confused about the time because he is asking for his breakfast when it is 5:00 p.m. A clock in his room may help to keep him oriented to the time of day, however, this is not the most immediate concern of the nurse. This option gives a psychological rationale for the client's behavior. This rationale should be explored only after the nurse makes sure that his behavior was not due to a physiological need.*
4. *Wrong. This options gives a psychological rationale for the client's behavior. This reason should be explored only after the nurse makes sure that his behavior was not due to a physiological need. According to Maslow's Hierarchy of Needs, physiological needs receive first priority.*

42. **In treating diabetic ketoacidosis (DKA), the nurse is aware that a goal of treatment is to correct which of the following imbalances?**

1. Hypoglycemia.
2. Dehydration.
3. Hyperkalemia.
4. Respiratory acidosis.

1. *No! Diabetic ketoacidosis (DKA) is caused by an absence or markedly inadequate amount of insulin. This results in a hyperglycemia, with blood glucose levels varying from 300 to 800 mg/dL.*
2. *Correct choice! The hyperglycemia of DKA leads to polyuria and polydipsia with volume depletion. Clients with severe DKA may lose an average of 6.5 liters of water.*
3. *Incorrect. The hyperglycemia of DKA leads to electrolyte loss, especially potassium. Try to recall the pathophysiology of this process and make the correct selection.*
4. *No. In DKA, there is an excess production of ketone bodies because of the lack of insulin that would*

normally prevent this from happening. Ketone bodies are acids, and their accumulation in the circulation leads to metabolic acidosis.

43. **A client, age 65, is receiving doxycycline (Vibramycin) for actinomycosis (fungal infection). The nurse should observe the client for which of the following side effects?**

1. Photosensitivity.
2. Constipation.
3. Ototoxicity.
4. Permanent discoloration of teeth.

1. *Good choice! Photosensitivity is an adverse effect of tetracylines in which the skin reacts abnormally to light, especially ultraviolet radiation or sunlight. The result is an intense sunburn reaction with erythema, macules and gray-blue patches. Prevention involves avoiding direct exposure to sunlight and ultraviolet light and it may help to use a sunscreen with a sun protection factor (SPF) of 15 or greater.*
2. *No, clients on tetracycline therapy often experience GI distress, manifested by anorexia, nausea/vomiting and diarrhea.*
3. *Incorrect. Ototoxicity is a concern when clients are on aminoglycosides or on minocycline (Minocin). It has not been reported as an adverse reaction to Vibramycin.*
4. *No. Although permanent discoloration of the teeth is an adverse reaction, it only affects the neonate in the last half of pregnancy and children under eight years of age. This client is 65 years old.*

44. **To assess for proper placement of a nasogastric tube, the nurse should:**

1. Instill 30 mL of saline into the tube to assess client tolerance.
2. Instill 10 mL of air into the tube and listen for gurgling sounds with a stethoscope over the gastric area.
3. Aspirate stomach contents with a syringe.
4. Place the end of the tube in water to assess for bubbling.

1. *Incorrect and hazardous procedure! This could be dangerous if the tube was in the lungs and not the stomach.*
2. *Incorrect. This method does not provide for a sufficient amount of air to reach the stomach and make any gurgling sounds — at least 30 mL of air is needed. There is a safer and more reliable method among the options given.*
3. *Absolutely correct! Placement should be checked by aspirating gastric contents with a syringe and testing the pH of the aspirate.*
4. *Never, never! This could be dangerous to the client if the tube was incorrectly positioned in the lungs.*

The client could aspirate the water in the glass. Select a safer, more reliable option.

45. While caring for a client receiving fluids using an IV pump plugged into an electrical outlet, the nurse should avoid which action?

1. Palpate the client's IV site while resetting the pump for the next bag of IV solution.
2. Assess the IV site visually and by palpation.
3. Change the tubing according to hospital protocol.
4. Observe the pump for correct operation.

1. *Excellent! You have identified an incorrect action. The client should never be touched at the same time that a piece of electrical equipment is being handled. If there were any electrical current leakage from the pump, it would transfer from the nurse to the client.*
2. *This is a correct nursing action. Assessing an IV site for signs of phlebitis or infection should be done on a regular basis. This question is asking you to identify an incorrect action, however, so this cannot be the correct answer.*
3. *This is a correct nursing action. Whatever protocol the hospital uses should be carefully followed. This question is asking you to identify an incorrect action.*
4. *This is a correct nursing action. The pump should be observed to determine if it is operating correctly. The question is asking you to identify an incorrect action, however, so this cannot be the correct answer.*

46. A client is admitted with end stage cirrhosis of the liver. Which of the following measures would the nurse expect to decrease the serum ammonia level?

1. Administration of vitamin K.
2. Increased fluid intake.
3. Administration of diuretics.
4. Offer low-protein, high-calorie diet.

1. *Incorrect choice. Vitamin K would be given to promote blood clotting and reduce the risk of hemorrhage.*
2. *No. An increased fluid intake would be indicated only to correct any fluid losses from perspiration and fever. This action would not decrease the serum ammonia level.*
3. *Not correct. Diuretics would be ordered to decrease edema and ascites, but would not affect the serum ammonia level.*
4. *Right choice. Ammonia is one of the end products of protein metabolism. A low-protein, high-calorie diet will reduce the source of ammonia and promote adequate carbohydrates for energy requirements while "sparing" protein from breakdown for energy.*

47. A 10-year-old is recovering following an appendectomy. While changing the linens on the client's bed, the nurse notes that drainage from an infected wound has soiled the bed sheet. Which of the following is the best method to use when changing the soiled bed linens?

1. Carefully place the soiled sheet in the cloth linen bag and label it as contaminated.
2. Spray the soiled area with a bleach solution prior to placing it in the linen bag.
3. Carefully place the soiled sheet in a moisture-resistant plastic linen bag designated for soiled articles.
4. Discard the sheet into a plastic trash bag.

1. *No. A cloth linen bag does not protect the laundry employees from exposure to the soiled sheet and organisms that may be present on the sheet.*
2. *Incorrect! Spraying the soiled area of the sheet does not destroy any organisms that may be present on other parts of the sheet but cannot be seen. Spraying the sheet is not practical, since the sheet will be effectively disinfected during laundering. Also, using a cloth linen bag does not protect the laundry employees from exposure to the soiled sheet.*
3. *You are right! Placing the sheet in a moisture-resistant plastic bag protects the laundry employees and others that may come in contact with the bag from exposure to organisms that may be present in the soiled linen.*
4. *Wrong! Discarding linen is neither appropriate or cost-effective. Proper handling by placing the linen in a moisture-resistant bag will protect the nurse and other employees, and the sheet will be effectively disinfected during laundering.*

48. A client is recovering from surgery. He has in place a urinary catheter that needs to be irrigated. The best intervention by the nurse to prevent injury to the mucosa of the bladder is which of the following?

1. Gently compress the ball of the syringe to instill the irrigating solution.
2. Quickly instill the irrigating solution using some pressure to loosen any clots or mucus.
3. After instilling the solution, apply gentle pressure to remove the irrigating solution from the bladder.
4. Place a sterile cap on the end of the drainage tubing to protect it from contamination.

1. *Correct. Gentle instillation creates a flow that helps to dilute and free sediment or debris within the lumen of the catheter.*
2. *No. Using force can injure tissue or cause the solution to leak from the connection. Any suction should be avoided because the mucosa of the bladder is easily injured. Removing the syringe from the catheter will break any suction created by vacuum.*

3. *This is not correct. Using force can injure the mucosa of the bladder.*

4. *A sterile cap can help prevent a potential infection but it does not protect the mucosa of the bladder from injury during irrigation. What was the issue in this question?*

49. **A client is receiving combination chemotherapy for breast cancer. Her most recent complete blood count (CBC) shows the following: Hgb 12.2, Hct 36%, WBC 2.3/cu mm, and platelets 150,000. Which of the following goals should be given priority by the nurse in planning care?**

    1. Prevention of infection.
    2. Maintenance of tissue integrity.
    3. Prevention of injury.
    4. Maintenance of tissue perfusion.

    1. *Excellent! You remembered your normal lab values for a CBC! The low white blood cell count (normal is 4.5-11/cu mm) puts the client at high risk for infection. All other lab values are within normal limits.*

    2. *No, there is no abnormal lab value that would suggest the possibility of skin breakdown.*

    3. *Incorrect. The platelet level is within the normal limits of 150,000-350,000, so the client is not prone to a bleeding tissue injury. There is no evidence of anemia, so the client is not prone to fainting, falls, or mechanical injury.*

    4. *No, the client does not show evidence of anemia. The hemoglobin and hematocrit are both within normal limits, although on the low end of normal—not unusual for a client undergoing chemotherapy.*

50. **Which of the following instructions is appropriate for the nurse to give a client who is to take nitroglycerin (Nitrostat) tablets sublingual for angina pain?**

    1. Take your blood pressure prior to administration of Nitrostat. If the diastolic is less than 80, do not take the pill.
    2. Take the Nitrostat with a full glass of water.
    3. Sit or lie down prior to taking the medication.
    4. Notify the physician immediately if you feel dizzy or get a headache after taking the Nitrostat.

    1. *Wrong. This is not a realistic instruction to give the client. The Nitrostat will decrease blood pressure (as a side effect) but the client with angina is instructed to take the medication at the first sign of chest pain. To take a blood pressure measurement first would delay the prompt treatment needed to dilate the coronary blood vessels.*

    2. *Not appropriate. The sublingual route means that the client puts the pill under the tongue and allows it to dissolve.*

    3. *Yes. The client should be instructed to sit or lie down prior to taking the Nitrostat because of the medication's ability to drop the blood pressure very quickly. This position would also minimize nitroglycerin's side effects of dizziness and weakness.*

    4. *Incorrect. Dizziness and headache are common adverse side effects of nitroglycerin that should decrease with continuing therapy and do not require immediate notification of the physician. The client is instructed to notify the physician if headache is persistent or severe.*

51. **While transferring a client with left-leg weakness from the bed to a wheelchair, the best nursing action is to do which of the following?**

    1. Have the seat of the wheelchair at a right angle to the bed.
    2. Lock the wheels on the bed and the wheelchair.
    3. Allow the client to do as much as possible to increase his sense of independence.
    4. Have the client lock his hands around the nurse's neck to provide the client with a sense of security.

    1. *This is incorrect. This position would require the client to pivot 180 degrees to get into the seat of the wheelchair. The seat of the wheelchair should be parallel with and next to the bed for ease of access for the client.*

    2. *Correct! Locking the wheels of both bed and wheelchair provides for the client's safety by not allowing the equipment to move away from the client, thereby risking an injury from a fall.*

    3. *This is not correct. Although encouraging independence is important, the client's safety is the most important consideration. A client with a weakened lower extremity is at risk for falling.*

    4. *This is wrong! The client can place his hands on the shoulders, but not around the neck, of the nurse. If the client slips, all of the client's weight will be placed on the cervical vertebrae of the nurse, which could cause a spinal cord injury.*

52. **The nurse initiates a diversional activity for a nine-year-old female client who is hospitalized with osteomyelitis. The activity is writing a story about the hospitalization experience. Which statement reflects a positive outcome of this activity?**

    1. The client was actively engaged in writing for one-half hour.
    2. During one-half hour of activity, the client put the light on six times.
    3. The client told her mother she likes her nurse.
    4. Correct grammar was demonstrated when writing the story.

1. *Good! The object a diversional activity is to provide an age appropriate activity that will reduce the stress of hospitalization. This was a good choice of activities because weight bearing is frequently prohibited in treatment of osteomyelitis.*
2. *No, this is not a positive outcome. This statement seems to indicate increased stress and decreased coping.*
3. *No. Nurses want their clients to like them, but that is not the purpose of a diversional activity.*
4. *No. Correct grammar is not the objective of a diversional activity!*

53. **In planning for the care of a 45-year-old woman diagnosed with Addison's disease, which of the following nursing diagnoses would be most appropriate?**

    1. Fluid volume excess related to sodium retention.
    2. Activity intolerance related to muscular weakness and fatigue.
    3. Impaired skin integrity related to pigmentation changes and lesions.
    4. Body image disturbance related to virilization of feminine features.

    1. *Incorrect. The client with Addison's disease has hyponatremia which causes hypovolemia. The correct diagnosis would be fluid volume deficit.*
    2. *Good choice! The client with Addison's disease has a decreased production of adrenal hormones, which include the mineralocorticoids, one of which is aldosterone. Decreased aldosterone causes hyponatremia and hyperkalemia, which cause the muscular weakness and fatigue.*
    3. *No. Even though the client with Addison's disease will have increased pigmentation of the skin giving a "bronze" appearance, there are no lesions or interruption in skin integrity.*
    4. *Incorrect. Recall that Addison's disease is a "hypo" state with decreased production of androgen and estrogen. Virilization for females would be seen in Cushing's syndrome.*

54. **A client is admitted to the hospital with cirrhosis of the liver and possible bleeding esophageal varices. Which of the following symptoms, if observed by the nurse, would help to validate the esophageal varices?**

    1. Swelling in the neck area.
    2. Painless hematemesis.
    3. A dry, hacking cough.
    4. Hemoptysis with chest pain.

    1. *Incorrect. This is not a symptom of bleeding esophageal varices.*
    2. *Correct choice! Bleeding from esophageal varices is frequently abrupt and without pain. Se-*

vere hematemesis and resultant shock may follow, requiring immediate emergency treatment.
3. *No. A client with bleeding esophageal varices will often have a bleeding episode preceded by coughing or sneezing.*
4. *Wrong choice! The bleeding is from the esophagus and not the lungs.*

55. **A 10-year-old client is recovering following an appendectomy. The nurse changes the bed linens and notes that drainage from an infected wound has soiled the bed sheet. A 13-year-old client with a newly applied full leg cast is to share the room. Which of the following best describes the nurse's role in infection control?**

    1. Hand washing.
    2. Using gloves when in contact with blood and body fluids.
    3. Proper disposal of contaminated dressings.
    4. Preventing the onset and spread of infection.

    1. *Wrong. Hand washing is an essential part of the nurse's role in infection control because it helps prevent the transmission of organisms. However, this action is included in another option that is a more comprehensive or global statement of the nurse's role in infection control. Try again.*
    2. *Wrong! Gloves are recommended as part of universal precautions to protect the nurse, however, this action is included in another option that is a more global statement of the nurse's role in infection control. This is not the best option.*
    3. *Wrong. Disposing of contaminated dressings helps prevent the spread of infection to others, however, this action is also included in another option that is a more global statement of the nurse's role in infection control. This is not the best option.*
    4. *Excellent choice! Preventing the onset and spread of infection includes all of the actions presented in the other options. This is the best option because it is a global statement of the nurse's role in infection control.*

56. **A male nurse received a doctor's order to catheterize one of his female clients. The client says, "I'm not going to allow a male nurse to catheterize me." Which of the following statements is most appropriate by the nurse?**

    1. "Your doctor is a male. Would you let him catheterize you?"
    2. "I've done this many times with no problems."
    3. "You can explain to your doctor why the catheter wasn't inserted."
    4. "You appear to be upset. Let me find a female nurse to help with the procedure."

    1. *This response is defensive, focuses on an inappropriate person (the doctor), focuses on an inappro-*

priate issue (whether the client would allow the doctor to catheterize her), and devalues the client's feelings. This response places the client on the defensive and is not therapeutic.

2. *This response is defensive, focuses on an inappropriate person (the nurse), focuses on an inappropriate issue (the nurse's competency), and does not address on the client's feelings or concern. This response is not therapeutic for the client.*

3. *This response is defensive, focuses on an inappropriate person (the doctor), and aggravates the problem. With this response, the nurse will fail to see that the required procedure is performed, which might endanger the client. This response is not professional.*

4. ***Best response! This statement shows empathy, responds to the client's concern, and offers a possible solution to the problem in this situation. The other options are not client-centered, are defensive, and focus on an inappropriate person or issue.***

57. **The client has just returned from the x-ray department after undergoing an upper GI series. Which of the following interventions by the nurse would be appropriate at this time?**

    1. Keep him NPO until the gag reflex returns.
    2. Administer a cleansing enema.
    3. Monitor his vital signs every 15 minutes for one hour or until stable.
    4. Give milk of magnesia 30 mL p.o.

    1. *Incorrect. The client did not need to have his throat anesthetized for this procedure. The gag and cough reflexes remain intact.*

    2. *Not necessary. This protocol would be appropriate after a barium enema.*

    3. *Not needed. Unless the client became symptomatic during the exam, there is no need to monitor his vital signs so closely. The procedure does not interfere with cardiovascular status; the vital signs would be monitored per daily routine.*

    4. ***Correct. The laxative would be essential to facilitate the passage of the barium through the alimentary tract. The stool should be checked for barium color and consistency to determine that all the barium has been evacuated.***

58. **A client is being sent home on isoxsuprine (Vasodilan) for treatment of premature labor. Which of the following actions need to be included in her discharge teaching plan?**

    1. Technique for taking oral temperature.
    2. How to assess her radial pulse.
    3. Procedure to assess her blood sugar.
    4. How to assess fetal heart rate.

    1. *Vasodilan has no effect on body temperature; the client therefore does not need to be taught this technique.*

2. ***Correct. Vasodilan frequently causes tachycardia. Therefore, the client needs to monitor her radial pulse. She is instructed to call her physician if it is 120 bpm or greater.***

3. *Incorrect. Vasodilan does not affect maternal blood sugar like many of the other tocolytic agents; therefore, the mother does not need to be taught this procedure.*

4. *Not correct. Vasodilan can cause maternal tachycardia, so the fetus also is at risk for elevated heart rate. Antepartum clients, however, are instructed to count fetal movements to indicate fetal well-being.*

59. **A male client, admitted with a myocardial infarction (MI) two days ago, develops paroxysmal atrial tachycardia (PAT). The physician orders quinidine sulfate (Quinatime) 300 mg p.o. every three hours until the arrhythmia is terminated. Which baseline data should the nurse obtain prior to starting the quinidine?**

    1. Serum creatinine.
    2. Q-T interval.
    3. Abdominal girth.
    4. Cardiac ejection fraction.

    1. *Incorrect. Quinidine, an antiarrhythmic, is metabolized by the liver with only 10-30% excreted unchanged by the kidneys. This drug has no untoward effect upon the kidneys, although renal function should be periodically monitored during prolonged therapy.*

    2. ***Yes. Quinidine acts to depress automaticity, resulting in prolongation of the Q-T interval (the total time for ventricular depolarization and repolarization). Baseline data documenting the Q-T interval is important.***

    3. *No. This data collection would not be necessary. Quinidine may cause GI symptoms such as diarrhea, nausea, cramping, and anorexia, but does not cause ascites or predispose the client to an intestinal obstruction.*

    4. *Incorrect. Quinidine is an antiarrhythmic that acts to depress automaticity and slow conduction speed, which will decrease the incidence of premature contractions. The cardiac ejection fraction would not be appropriate data to collect at this time because this test gives information about the volume of blood ejected from the left ventricle.*

60. **An 18-year-old hemophiliac is scheduled for wisdom teeth extractions. Which of the following can the nurse anticipate will be given prior to the dental procedure?**

    1. Packed red blood cells.
    2. Prophylactic antibiotics.
    3. Fresh frozen plasma.
    4. Factor VIII concentrate.

1. No, packed red cells would not be necessary, since the underlying problem in hemophilia is deficiency of clotting factors.
2. Incorrect. The concern in this situation is not a potential for infection, but rather a potential for bleeding.
3. No, fresh frozen plasma is not the correct agent. It is preferable to transfuse the client with only the deficient blood factor.
4. **Good choice! Clients are given factor VIII or IX concentrates as a prophylactic measure before dental extractions or surgery, or when actively bleeding. Other blood products are rarely used now.**

61. **When a client is taking nifedipine (Procardia), the nurse must be aware of the potential for:**

1. Hallucinations.
2. Peripheral edema.
3. Hyperglycemia.
4. Photophobia.

1. Incorrect. Hallucinations are not a side effect of Procardia. Dizziness, lightheadedness, giddiness, headache, and nervousness are side effects of Procardia that affect the central nervous system.
2. **Yes! Procardia can cause a non-cardiac dependent peripheral edema, which can be treated with diuretics. The drug should be used cautiously in clients with congestive heart failure or severe hepatic disease.**
3. No. Procardia is a calcium channel blocker and does not have any effect upon the endocrine system. Beta blockers, used as antihypertensives or anti-anginal agents, should be used cautiously in clients with diabetes because they can lower or raise the blood sugar and result in the need for altered insulin dosage requirements. Beta blockers can also mask signs of hypoglycemia.
4. Wrong choice. Photophobia is not a side effect of Procardia therapy—it's a common side effect of atropine administration. Remember that Procardia is a calcium channel blocker, used in the treatment of hypertension and angina pectoris.

62. **The nurse is counseling a parent about the management of her six-year-old child who has chickenpox. Which statement by the parent indicates that the teaching by the nurse has been ineffective?**

1. "I will keep my child's fingernails cut short."
2. "I will keep my child out of school for five days."
3. "If any of the chickenpox become swollen and ooze yellow drainage, I will call the doctor."
4. "I will give my child diphenhydramine (Benadryl) if the itching becomes severe."

1. No, this statement indicates that teaching has been effective. Keeping the child's fingernails short can

help cut down on spread of microorganisms while scratching, if hands are frequently washed. It's important to decrease the risk of a secondary bacterial infection. Excessive scratching can also cause scarring.
2. **This is the correct answer! Chickenpox is contagious from one to two days before the child breaks out with the pox until all the pox have crusted over. This may occur in five days, but may take as long as seven to 10 days. The parent who makes this statement requires more teaching.**
3. No, this statement indicates that teaching has been effective. Chickenpox look like blisters that open and contain drainage. If the pox become very red, swollen, and ooze drainage, there may be a secondary bacterial infection. This requires treatment with antibiotics and the child should be seen by his health care provider.
4. No, this statement indicates that teaching has been effective. Diphenhydramine can be very helpful with severe itching. This will help make the child more comfortable and cut down on scratching, which also decreases the risk of scars and secondary infection.

63. **A four-year-old recently diagnosed with AIDS is due for his preschool immunizations. His immunizations have previously been up to date. Which immunizations would be most appropriate for this client at this time?**

1. MMR and OPV.
2. DTP and Hib.
3. None required.
4. DTP, IPV and MMR.

1. No. Because OPV is a live vaccine, it is contraindicated for the child with AIDS. Even other children in the household should not receive OPV, since the virus can be transmitted (shed) to the immunocompromised child.
2. No. Did you forget that it's too late to give Hib vaccine? If this child is previously up to date, he was immunized at two, four, and six months.
3. This is definitely incorrect! The child who is immunocompromised needs to be protected as much as possible from childhood illness, and schools require evidence for admission.
4. **You correctly identified the need for this child to be immunized against diphtheria, tetanus and pertussis (DTP) and polio (IPV) and measles, mumps, rubella (MMR). IPV should be substituted for OPV to prevent the possibility of causing active polio disease in the immunocompromised client.**

64. **The nurse knows that which of the following is accurate regarding ECT?**

1. Usually requires 10 days to three weeks before depression is noticeably improved.

2. Results in a high incidence of chronic memory problems.
3. Is effective for 60% of persons who receive it.
4. Is used for persons who have not responded to antidepressants.

1. *Incorrect. ECT has a significantly more rapid onset of action than antidepressants and may be used for very severely depressed persons who are also highly suicidal.*
2. *Not a true statement. The side effects of ECT are transient and may include short-term memory loss. It rarely causes chronic memory problems.*
3. *Incorrect statement. ECT is effective treatment for more than 80% of depressed persons who receive it. It does, however, tend to be associated with a high relapse rate.*
4. ***Correct. ECT is not the first choice of treatment for most depressed persons. It is used for individuals who have not responded to antidepressants or who have had adverse reactions to these drugs.***

65. **A 17-year-old client is brought to the emergency room with right lower quadrant pain. He has a low grade fever, nausea, and a WBC of 18,000. The nurse is aware that the client's symptoms are indicative of which of the following conditions?**

1. Hepatitis.
2. Appendicitis.
3. Peritonitis.
4. Gastritis.

1. *Incorrect. Hepatitis would manifest itself with right upper quadrant pain or tenderness over the liver, along with jaundice and anorexia.*
2. ***Correct! The symptoms experienced by the client are the classic signs of appendicitis. If the appendix ruptures, the pain becomes more diffuse; abdominal distention occurs as a result of paralytic ileus, and the client's condition worsens.***
3. *No. The client's symptoms are not severe enough to warrant this diagnosis. Symptoms of peritonitis depend on the location and extent of inflammation. The affected area of the abdomen becomes extremely tender, and the muscles become rigid. Rebound tenderness and ileus may be present, along with the nausea, leukocytosis, and fever seen in this client's situation.*
4. *Incorrect choice. Gastritis is characterized by epigastric pain or tenderness, nausea, and vomiting.*

66. **A 48-year-old male's EKG shows a flattening of the T wave. He was admitted for congestive heart failure. Which of the following laboratory results would the nurse anticipate as most likely to occur with this EKG change?**

1. Hgb of 9.8 gm.
2. Digitalis toxicity.

3. K+ 2.8 mEq/liter.
4. Serum Ca++ 8.0 mg %.

1. *No. The EKG pattern anticipated with a low hemoglobin would be tachycardia.*
2. *Incorrect. Bradycardia, ventricular bigeminy, or ventricular tachycardia are a few of the arrhythmias occurring with toxic digitalis levels.*
3. ***Correct. A flattened T wave or the development of U waves is indicative of a low potassium level.***
4. *No. Hypocalcemia can cause multiple arrhythmias due to the altered cardiac muscle function, but not a flattened T wave.*

67. **A 43-year-old female client has had a total abdominal hysterectomy and bilateral salpingo-oophorectomy for stage III uterine cancer. Which instructions would the nurse anticipate providing?**

1. Estrogen therapy will alleviate the discomfort of surgical menopause.
2. A Papanicolaou smear should be performed every six months.
3. Lubrication can be used to treat vaginal itching and burning.
4. Vaginal intercourse will no longer be possible.

1. *Incorrect. Estrogen therapy is contraindicated in clients with known uterine cancers.*
2. *No. This test is used to detect cancers of the cervix or uterus. In a total abdominal hysterectomy, the uterus and cervix have been removed.*
3. ***Correct! Atrophic vaginal changes occur due to the loss of estrogen postoperatively and may also cause pain during coitus. Lubricants may reduce the symptoms associated with the diminished mucous production.***
4. *No. The client and partner may resume sexual relations after healing of the incision has occurred. The vagina remains following total hysterectomy.*

68. **A client, age 46, is admitted to the hospital with a diagnosis of acute pancreatitis. In assessing the client's condition, the nurse should expect to find an elevation in which of the following serum levels?**

1. Amylase.
2. Bilirubin.
3. Cholesterol.
4. Gastrin.

1. ***Good selection! Serum amylase level is the most important aid in diagnosing acute pancreatitis. Peak levels are reached in 24 hours, with a rapid fall to normal levels within 48 to 72 hours.***
2. *Incorrect. A rise in the serum bilirubin will occur if there is an excessive destruction of red blood cells or if the liver is unable to excrete the normal*

amounts of bilirubin produced due to liver disease.

3. *No. High levels of cholesterol are associated with atherosclerosis and increased risk of coronary artery disease. There is no correlation between cholesterol and pancreatic functioning.*

4. *Incorrect. Gastrin is a hormone secreted by the mucosa of the pylorus of the stomach. Increased gastrin levels are found in stomach cancer, pernicious anemia, and gastric and duodenal ulcers.*

69. **A 32-year-old client is admitted to the emergency room with a respiratory rate of seven per minute. ABG's reveal the following values: pH 7.22; pCO$_2$ 68 mm Hg; HCO$_3$ 28 mEq/L. Which is the proper analysis of this assessment?**

1. Respiratory alkalosis.
2. Metabolic acidosis.
3. Metabolic alkalosis.
4. Respiratory acidosis.

1. *No. The normal arterial pH is 7.35-7.45.*

2. *Incorrect. The normal pCO$_2$ is 35-45 mm Hg. In metabolic acidosis, the pCO$_2$ is kept from rising much above normal.*

3. *That's not correct. Normal values are: pH 7.35-7.45; pCO$_2$ 35-45 mm Hg; HCO$_3$ 23-29 mEq/liter.*

4. *Excellent! When the pH and the pCO$_2$ deviate in opposite directions, it is always a respiratory problem. The normal pH is 7.35-7.45. The pH of 7.22 indicates that the client is acidotic.*

70. **An 83-year-old confused client has wrist restraints for safety reasons. Which of the following nursing interventions is necessary to provide for the client's safety?**

1. Check the pulse, color, and temperature of extremities every shift and report these findings.
2. Make sure the call light is within the client's reach.
3. Notify the client's family of the restraints and explain the rationale for their use.
4. Remove the restraints at night while the client is sleeping.

1. *Wrong! This will not be adequate to protect the client from permanent injury, since the client is at risk of decreased circulation. The extremities should be assessed every two hours.*

2. *Very good! Even though the client is confused, the call light must be available to allow the client to communicate his or her needs. This option is the best choice because it is the only action that provides for the client's immediate safety.*

3. *No. The family should be informed; however, there is another option that is more necessary for the client's immediate safety.*

4. *No. If the client requires restraints because of confusion, the restraints should not be removed at night. This action is incorrect.*

71. **A client, age 83, is admitted to the hospital with complaints of abdominal pain and distention. He has a history of no bowel movement for the past 10 days. After a diagnostic evaluation, it is determined that the client has a fecal impaction. Which of the following treatments can the nurse anticipate will be ordered initially?**

1. Soap suds enemas until clear.
2. Bisacodyl (Dulcolax) suppository.
3. Oil retention enema.
4. Tap water enema.

1. *No, this treatment would not be ordered initially due to the impaction of the stool. The soap suds solution would not be able to bypass the stool to facilitate elimination.*

2. *Incorrect. The suppository would stimulate peristalsis, but would initially be ineffective in moving the impacted stool.*

3. *You are right! The initial administration of an oil retention enema will help to lubricate the impaction so that it can pass more readily through the intestine. The mineral oil enema is given and the client is asked to retain it for 30-60 minutes. This enema is then followed with saline or soap suds enemas until the bowel is clear. At times, a digital extraction of the stool is necessary. Unless adequate lubrication is used, bowel perforation can occur with manual extraction.*

4. *Incorrect choice. Tap water enemas are hypotonic and, therefore, rarely used because they could upset the client's fluid and electrolyte status.*

72. **The nurse is aware that which of the following effects will occur when the client is taking quinidine (Quinatime) and digoxin (Lanoxin) at the same time?**

1. Elevated quinidine levels.
2. Decreased quinidine levels.
3. Elevated digoxin levels.
4. Decreased digoxin levels.

1. *Incorrect. Combining these two antiarrhythmics will not cause an increased quinidine level. Amiodarone (Cordarone), another antiarrhythmic, will increase quinidine levels and the risk of toxicity. Choose again.*

2. *Wrong. Quinidine will not interact with digoxin and cause a decreased quinidine level. Choose another option.*

3. *Absolutely! When the client takes digoxin and quinidine, the drug-drug interaction increases serum digoxin levels and may cause toxicity: dosage reduction is recommended. Quinidine reduces digoxin's renal excretion and displaces digoxin from tissue binding sites. The overall result is an increase in digoxin blood levels.*

4. *Not true. When a client takes these two medications at the same time, the blood digoxin level will not be decreased. Make another selection.*

73. In assessing an adult client with diabetes mellitus, the nurse would expect to observe all of the following characteristics except?

1. Possible increased body weight.
2. Increased urinary output.
3. Periods of polydypsia.
4. Periods of altered pulse rate.

1. *No, the nurse would expect that an adult with diabetes mellitus may have experienced a weight gain. An important difference between the adult and juvenile diabetic is that an adult diabetic gains weight, but a juvenile diabetic loses weight. Since this question has a false response stem, the correct answer will be an UNEXPECTED finding.*
2. *No, increased urinary output is an expected manifestation of adult diabetes. This question has a false response stem, so this is a distractor.*
3. *No, periods of polydipsia is a manifestation of adult diabetes. You are looking for a false statement. This is a distractor.*
4. ***Very good! Periods of altered pulse rate might be characteristic of ketoacidosis, but they are not manifestations of diabetes. The question has a false response stem, so this answer, which is not characteristic of adult diabetes is the correct answer.***

74. A six-year-old male is admitted with a spiral fracture of the humerus and multiple bruises of the forearm. The physician states abuse is suspected. The nurse's initial goal is which of the following?

1. Prevent further abuse of the client.
2. Encourage the client to express his feelings.
3. Determine who is responsible for the abuse.
4. Teach the parents appropriate methods of discipline.

1. ***Correct. Safety first, then interventions that will decrease the chances of further abuse, such as education of parents.***
2. *No. This may sound good, but you've missed the most important nursing responsibility to the client. Maslow's Hierarchy of Needs will help you to select the initial action.*
3. *No, this is not the nurse's main responsibility.*
4. *No, you skipped an important issue and went right for teaching. The issue in this question is child abuse, and the client in the question is the injured child. This cannot be the nurse's initial action in a situation where child abuse is suspected. Look for an option that immediately addresses the safety of the client.*

75. A 25-year-old man was admitted one week ago with a diagnosis of schizophrenia, paranoid type. Since his admission, he has had several verbal outbursts of anger but has not been violent. A staff member tells the nurse that the client is pacing up and down the hall very rapidly and muttering to himself in an angry manner. Which of the following is the best initial nursing action?

1. Prepare an intramuscular injection of haloperidol (Haldol) to give him p.r.n.
2. Observe the client's behavior and approach him in a non-threatening manner.
3. Gather several staff members and approach the client together.
4. Contact the client's psychiatrist and request an order to place him in seclusion.

1. *Wrong! The client may need a p.r.n. dose of an antipsychotic if he is not able to control his behavior, however, this is not the best initial nursing action.*
2. ***Correct. The nurse must first assess the client's condition before deciding on an appropriate intervention. The best initial action is to approach him calmly, in a non-threatening manner, to ask him to verbalize about his problem.***
3. *Although it is important to have sufficient staff available to handle a potentially unsafe situation, there is a better option that more specifically addresses the approach the nurse should take initially.*
4. *This is not correct because the situation does not indicate that this intervention is needed.*

76. A 12-year-old child is being discharged from the hospital with a diagnosis of asthma. She will be maintained on metered dose inhalers at home. The nurse is preparing a care plan on the use of cromolyn sodium (Intal). Which information would the nurse avoid including in the care plan?

1. Intal will decrease the inflammation in your child's bronchioles.
2. Do not rely on Intal for relief of an acute attack.
3. Have your child rinse her mouth after using the puffer.
4. Your child should breathe more easily after a dose of Intal.

1. *Incorrect choice. Intal is a mast cell inhibiter and decreases inflammation in the bronchioles. You are looking for a statement that would NOT be included in the care plan.*
2. *Not the correct choice! Intal has a slow onset and will not relieve an acute asthma attack. A fast acting bronchodilator should be given. This information is correct and should be given to the client.*
3. *Incorrect choice. Intal may cause throat and mouth irritation. Rinsing or gargling after the medication will help relieve the irritation. Remember, this ques-*

tion has a false response stem and is asking for information that should NOT be included in the care plan.

4. *Good! This statement is not true and would not be included in the care plan. Intal is a prophylactic medication and the client will not "feel better" after using it. Expecting otherwise can lead to noncompliance. Clients need to be aware that the Intal is necessary even though its effect is not immediately felt.*

77. **A client, age 20, has been admitted to the hospital after having two tonic-clonic seizures at work. She suddenly gives a short cry and stiffens. What is the initial nursing action?**

1. Make a mental notation of the time after looking at a watch.
2. Place an oral airway in the client's mouth.
3. Loosen the clothing around the neck.
4. Turn her head to the side.

1. *Correct! A major responsibility of the nurse is to observe and record the sequence of symptoms. Duration of each phase of the attack is part of the assessment.*
2. *No. If an aura precedes the seizure, then a padded tongue blade can be inserted between the teeth to reduce the possibility of the tongue or cheek being bitten. The nurse should never attempt to pry open jaws that are clenched in a spasm to insert anything.*
3. *Incorrect. Although this is part of the nursing management, it is not the initial intervention.*
4. *Not the initial action. This is a useful intervention after the seizure to help prevent aspiration. The other appropriate intervention is to protect the head from striking a hard surface during the seizure.*

78. **A 25-year-old client was admitted to the hospital with newly diagnosed diabetes mellitus. She is very concerned about being placed on a calorie-controlled diet, since she has been losing weight even though she has been eating more food. Which of the following statements is the most therapeutic response by the nurse?**

1. "You won't have to worry about weight loss once your sugar is regulated."
2. "The doctor will order enough food for you."
3. "Your body has not been producing the insulin necessary to utilize the calories you were eating. Once you start receiving insulin, you will once again be able to use the calories you eat and a calorie-controlled diet will be recommended to help maintain your weight."
4. "You probably needed to lose some weight to decrease your need for insulin."

1. *Incorrect. This statement fails to address the client's concern regarding her present weight loss and a*

reduced calorie diet. The statement is not an example of the nurse giving information because the statement is not necessarily true.
2. *Wrong! This response does not address the client's concern regarding her present weight loss and a reduced calorie diet. The response also focuses on the doctor, not the client, which is inappropriate.*
3. *Correct. This response briefly explains the relationship between calorie intake and insulin. It is therapeutic because it gives correct information which addresses the client's concern.*

> **STRATEGY ALERT!** Note that the words "calorie-controlled diet" occur in both the case scenario and this option. This is a clue that this might be the correct answer.

4. *Wrong! The nurse does not know that the client needed to lose weight prior to hospitalization. This response also devalues the client's concerns.*

79. **A client has returned to the ambulatory surgery unit after undergoing a bronchoscopy. She complains of a sore throat. Which of the following nursing measures would be most appropriate after the cough reflex returns?**

1. Ice chips.
2. Warm saline gargle.
3. Tepid clear liquids.
4. Viscous Xylocaine mouth swishes p.r.n.

1. *No, Ice chips would have a topical anesthetic effect in the mouth, but would not be as effective in relieving the discomfort of a sore throat.*
2. *Correct! Warm saline gargles are the intervention of choice when a client complains of a sore throat.*
3. *The client may have difficulty drinking clear liquids until the sore throat is relieved. There is an option listed that will help achieve this goal.*
4. *No, this requires a physician's order. You are asked to choose a nursing intervention.*

80. **The nurse's neighbor has a baby who is four weeks old. She tells the nurse that the hospital just called to ask her to bring her baby in to repeat the PKU test done at 24 hours of age. What is the nurse's best response?**

1. "This is quite unusual, I will go with you."
2. "A second specimen is always done to guarantee the child does not have PKU."
3. "Results of early PKU testing are often inconclusive due to inadequate nutritional intake."
4. "I think you should call your pediatrician to be sure he thinks this repeat test is necessary."

1. *Wrong. For an accurate PKU test, the infant needs to ingest sufficient formula or breast milk. Because the hospitalization following delivery is rarely*

longer than 48 hours, adequate ingestion is often not present. Most hospitals complete the PKU testing regardless of the short time span from birth to the sample. Repeat testing is often needed.

2. *Incorrect. Repeat testing is not needed unless the first results are inconclusive.*

3. ***Correct! Many infants need repeat PKU testing because the first test was done prior to adequate intake of formula or breast milk.***

4. *Wrong. This statement suggests that the decision to repeat PKU test should be made by the pediatrician. The testing lab is the correct source to schedule retesting.*

81. **A child, 11 years old, is to receive 400 mL of IV fluid in an eight-hour shift. The IV drip factor is 60. What is the IV rate that will deliver this amount?**

1. 66 mL/hour.
2. 40 mL/hour.
3. 24 mL/hour.
4. 50 mL/hour.

1. *Wrong. 400 mL/8 hours = 50 mL/hour. The drip factor is irrelevant.*

2. *Try this again! 400 mL/8 hours = 50 mL/hour. The drip factor is irrelevant.*

3. *Wrong! 400 mL/8 hours = 50 mL/hour. The drip factor is irrelevant.*

4. ***Correct. 400 mL/8 hours = 50 mL/hour. The drip factor is irrelevant.***

82. **A 55-year-old client has been taking trifluoperazine (Stelazine) for five years to control her paranoid thoughts. When the client's brother comes to visit, he tells the nurse that he strongly believes all psychiatric medications are a form of "chemical mind control." The nurse understands which of the following regarding antipsychotics?**

1. They act directly on specific neurotransmitters in the brain to control the client's psychotic symptoms.

2. They act to sedate the client so she cannot engage in behavior that will cause difficulty for either herself or others.

3. They are a cure for psychotic disorders, like schizophrenic reactions, and are therefore an important part of his sister's treatment plan.

4. They have been in use for close to 30 years and are safe and effective drugs for clients who have problems like his sister's.

1. ***Correct. The specific mechanisms of action are still unknown, but research indicates that antipsychotics act directly on the dopamine receptors in the brain and thereby control many target symptoms of psychosis.***

2. *This is partially correct. Antipsychotic drugs do sedate the client to some degree, but that is not their primary mode of action. Look again at the other options to select one that provides a better rationale.*

3. *This is not correct. There is no known cure for schizophrenic disorders at this time. Many clients with these diagnoses have a chronic illness. Treatment is focused on helping them attain their highest level of functioning using medication and psychosocial therapies.*

4. *Although this is true, it is not the best rationale for the nurse to use in responding to the client's concern.*

83. **A 24-year-old college student is admitted to the emergency room. She is hysterical and states that she was sexually assaulted 20 minutes ago. Which of the following should be the nurse's first priority in this situation?**

1. Remove her clothes carefully, so as not to destroy any evidence.

2. Vaginal exam with lubricant to decrease the pain involved.

3. Place the client in a private room and leave her alone to grieve.

4. Encourage the client to relate what happened and make decisions about the order of examination.

1. *No. Whenever possible, delay the removal of clothes until the client has calmed down and is comfortable with the people providing care to her.*

2. *No. When a vaginal exam is done no lubricant should be used, because it will interfere with specimen collection.*

3. *Wrong, privacy is very important for this client, but it is likely that she is very frightened and upset. A health care provider, preferably a female, should remain with her throughout her emergency room stay.*

4. ***Good choice! Allowing the client to relate her story helps her cope with what has happened to her. Encouraging her to make decisions provides her with a sense of control, which is something she has recently lost.***

84. **A client is addicted to cocaine and is in labor at 35 weeks gestation. She has heard about a drug that will reverse the effects of narcotics, and wants it given to her newborn after delivery. Which of the following statements is the best response by the nurse regarding administration of the naloxone (Narcan)?**

1. "I will notify the neonatologist immediately, so it will be available."

2. "The drug does not reverse the effects of cocaine, so it is not indicated for your baby."

3. "Let's wait and evaluate the condition of your baby before we decide to use this drug."
4. "Giving this drug to your baby will cause immediate withdrawal. It is not indicated."

1. *This is incorrect. Narcan needs to be used very cautiously in drug addicted clients, as well as their newborns, because it can cause rapid withdrawal.*
2. *Incorrect! Narcan would reverse the effects of the cocaine, but rapid withdrawal is not indicated or desired for an addicted neonate.*
3. *Incorrect! This answer suggests that the decision to use Narcan depends on the condition of the neonate. Rapid withdrawal is never indicated in a neonate.*
4. ***Excellent response! This statement reflects the current feelings related to the use of Narcan in treatment of addicted neonates and their mothers.***

85. **In preparing a client for D&C in an outpatient surgery clinic, the nurse must start an intravenous infusion. Each of the following veins is a possible site for the IV. Which would be the best choice initially?**

1. The great saphenous vein on the ankle.
2. The metacarpal vein on the back of the hand.
3. The median basilic vein in the antecubital fossa.
4. The cephalic vein on the forearm.

1. *Veins in the lower extremities should be used for an IV site only as a last resort. This is not the best choice initially.*
2. ***Initially, you should choose the most distal vein on the hand or arm, and then move up the arm for subsequent IV sites.***
3. *An IV site in the antecubital fossa requires immobilization of the elbow. This would not be the best choice initially when other sites are available.*
4. *The key word is "initially." Initially, you should choose the most distal vein on the hand or arm and then move up the arm for subsequent IV sites. When a vein on the hand is available, that should be used before a vein on the forearm.*

86. **Calcium gluconate is being administered to a client with pregnancy induced hypertension. Which of the following actions must the nurse include in the plan of care throughout injection of the drug?**

1. Ventilator assistance.
2. CVP readings.
3. Continuous CPR.
4. EKG tracings.

1. *Incorrect answer. Respiratory arrest is a potential complication of magnesium intoxication. Calcium gluconate should be administered to reverse the effects of the elevated magnesium levels prior to a respiratory arrest, which would necessitate ventilator assistance.*

2. *No. Although many clients receiving intensive care for the treatment of PIH will have a CVP line in place, it is not considered an essential part of care.*
3. *Wrong. Calcium gluconate should be administered prior to the need for CPR.*
4. ***Correct. A potential side effect of calcium gluconate administration is cardiac arrest. Continuous monitoring of cardiac activity through administration of calcium gluconate is an essential part of care.***

87. **The mother of two children tells the nurse during a clinic visit that her older son, age nine, has been acting up since his younger sibling's diagnosis of cerebral palsy. Which of the following would best help the nine-year-old?**

1. Suggest ways that the parents may spend time meeting the needs of the nine-year-old.
2. Explain to the older child that expressions of anger are inappropriate ways of dealing with his emotions.
3. Provide information to the nine-year-old on his sibling's condition as soon as he requests it.
4. Tell the parents that they should not expect their nine-year-old to understand the needs of the disabled child.

1. ***Yes, this is correct. This behavior is probably related to the amount of time and energy that the parents are giving to the child with cerebral palsy. The "well" child also needs his parents' undivided attention at times.***
2. *No, this is unlikely to have a positive result. This is the same as saying, "Your feelings don't count."*
3. *No, facts alone won't improve behavior, and what if the child never asks? The acting up is the child's way of obtaining his parents' attention.*
4. *The nine-year-old does have the cognitive ability to understand simple explanations regarding the care and needs of a child with cerebral palsy; however, this information alone will not improve the behavior of the "well" child.*

88. **Betamethasone (Celestone) is administered at 30 weeks gestation to reduce the risk of RDS in a neonate. The infant is born after two injections are given. As the nurse is planning care for the infant, which of the following should be anticipated as a result of the administration of betamethasone to the mother?**

1. Rapid pulse rate.
2. Sternal retractions.
3. Hypoglycemia.
4. Hypothermia.

1. *Wrong! Betamethasone administration given to the antepartum client does not have an effect on neonatal vital signs. If this neonate has a rapid*

apical pulse, it is related to another cause, most likely his/her prematurity.

2.   *Wrong! It is quite likely that this premature neonate will have some RDS manifested by sternal retractions, but is most likely a result of immature lung development, not related to the administration of betamethasone in any way.*

3.   ***Correct. Betamethasone causes hyperglycemia in the mother, which predisposes the neonate to hypoglycemia in the first hours after delivery.***

4.   *Wrong! Betamethasone does not have any effect on the neonate's ability to maintain body temperature. If hypothermia is present, it is related to another cause, probably immature temperature regulation.*

89.   **Which of the following situations warrant an injection of RHoGAM to an Rh negative woman?**

1.   Vaginal bleeding at 24 weeks and following a voluntary termination of pregnancy at 12 weeks gestation .
2.   An episode of flu at 24 weeks gestation and after surgery for an ectopic pregnancy.
3.   At 28 weeks gestation and after blood transfusions during pregnancy.
4.   While the client is in labor and following the delivery of an Rh positive neonate.

1.   ***Correct, both of these situations indicate an injection of RHoGAM to prevent the formation of Rh negative antibodies. Both of these women have possible exposure to Rh positive blood from the fetus.***

2.   *No, an episode of the flu in an expectant woman is not related to administration of RHoGAM. Following surgery for an ectopic pregnancy is an indicator.*

3.   *RHoGAM would be given prophylactically to all Rh negative mothers with a possible Rh positive fetus at 28 weeks gestation. If an Rh negative mother received a blood transfusion during pregnancy, careful crossmatch would be done using Rh negative blood; therefore, RHoGAM is not indicated.*

4.   *Wrong! RHoGAM is not given to laboring women. It is given to all Rh negative women who deliver a Rh positive neonate and whose blood work indicates there are no already existing Rh antibodies.*

90.   **The client's psychiatrist orders fluphenazine (Prolixin) 10 mg b.i.d. Before the first dose, the client asks the nurse what the medicine is supposed to do. Which response by the nurse would be most therapeutic for a suspicious client?**

1.   "It will help you feel less anxious."
2.   "It is to help make your thinking clearer and decrease your fears."
3.   "This medication will help you maintain self-control."
4.   "This medication will help you get better."

1.   *This is not a true statement. Antipsychotics are often sedating, but that is not their primary mode of action.*

2.   ***Correct. The primary reasons for prescribing antipsychotics for clients with problems like this is to improve their thought processes and control delusional thoughts and hallucinations. This is an accurate and truthful statement, so it is the best response for the nurse to make.***

3.   *This statement is not untrue, but it is not the best response to this client's question.*

4.   *This statement is true, but it does not specifically answer the client's question. It also could be interpreted as patronizing by the client. There is a better option.*

91.   **A nurse on the psychiatric unit poses a question to a client who either does not respond or mumbles incoherently. The nurse will best deal with the client's communication problems by which of the following actions?**

1.   Sitting quietly with the client during their scheduled times without attempting to verbalize until the client indicates a willingness to talk.
2.   Continuing to speak with the client using short, clear statements or open-ended questions about topics that may interest the client.
3.   Continuing to encourage the client to talk by asking direct questions.
4.   Filling silent periods by talking about topics interesting to the nurse.

1.   *The nurse should continue to meet regularly with the client and may also sit quietly without speaking for periods of time. The nurse, however, should not stop verbally communicating with this client because talking with her is the only way to gain her trust.*

2.   ***Correct. The nurse, whose goal is to establish a therapeutic relationship with a client, will have to communicate verbally with the client. Using short, clear statements and open-ended questions are two good ways to go about this, because the client is given the opportunity to respond without feeling pressured to do so.***

3.   *Wrong! Asking direct questions may be perceived by the client as intimidating or not respectful of her privacy.*

4.   *The nurse conveys a lack of interest in the client by rattling on about topics of interest to the nurse. It also conveys that the client is not expected to verbalize.*

92.   **The nurse learns that a depressed client is an expert at crewel embroidery. The nurse buys embroidery materials and asks the client if she will teach crewel work to the nurse. Which of the following is the best rationale for this nursing intervention?**

1. To assess the client's ability to communicate clearly.
2. To distract the client from thinking about her problems.
3. To reinforce the client's identity as a homemaker.
4. To use the client's strengths to build self-esteem.

1. Wrong. Depression may interfere with a person's willingness to communicate, but it is not primarily a communication disorder.

2. Engaging a depressed person in a productive task is one way to interrupt or limit the amount of time spent focusing on negative evaluations of herself but in this case there is a better option.

3. Incorrect. There is no information in the question that indicates the client is a homemaker.

4. Correct. The nurse is attempting to reinforce the client's sense of self-worth by providing an opportunity for the client to succeed at a task that earns positive feedback from the nurse.

93. **The nurse notices a fire in the linen room. Which type of extinguisher should be used?**

1. Dry powder.
2. Water.
3. Dry chemical.
4. Carbon dioxide.

1. Wrong. Dry powder is used for metal fires.

2. Correct! Water may be used on Class A fires, which involve paper, wood or cloth. A soda and acid extinguisher may also be used for this type of fire.

3. Wrong. Dry chemical extinguishers are appropriate for Type C fires, which involve electrical equipment, or Type D fires, which involve combustible metals.

4. Incorrect! A carbon dioxide extinguisher is appropriate for Type B fires, which involve flammable liquids and gases.

94. **The nurse expects that betamethasone (Celestone) would be used with caution in which of the following antepartum clients?**

1. Primigravida with mild PIH.
2. Multigravida with diabetes.
3. Primigravida with AIDS.
4. Multigravida with renal disease.

1. No. Celestone should be used with caution in the client with severe hypertension, but the client with mild PIH does not have severe hypertension.

2. Good! When any client has diabetes, regardless of her gravida, Celestone should be used with caution due to its effect on blood sugar.

3. No. The presence of AIDS has no bearing on the decision to use or not use Celestone on the antepartum client.

4. No. The presence of renal disease is not a contraindication for the use of Celestone in the antepartum client.

95. **A depressed client's progress improves and she now attends group therapy daily. The nurse understands that the most important benefit of group therapy is:**

1. The opportunity to develop social skills.
2. Improving the client's orientation to reality.
3. Gaining support and encouragement from other persons.
4. Developing greater insight into herself and her problems through the feedback provided by the other members.

1. Incorrect choice. Although clients in group therapy do develop better social skills, this is not the primary focus of the treatment.

2. Depressed persons have a negative view of themselves and their situations, and some depressed persons have delusions. Group therapy, however, is not a technique for reality orientation. Try again.

3. Not quite. This is not the most important benefit of group therapy.

4. Correct. Group therapy provides many benefits that occur through the feedback and validation of the other members.

96. **A 17-year-old client is recovering from an appendectomy. When the nurse offers her meperidine (Demerol), she says, "No, I don't want to get hooked." Which of the following is the best initial nursing response?**

1. "You are right. Why take a chance?"
2. "Tell me what you mean by getting hooked."
3. "You will not get addicted for the short amount of time that you will be in the hospital."
4. "The Demerol will make you more comfortable, not make you an addict."

1. Wrong. The client appears to have made an incorrect assumption concerning risks of the medication. This response is not therapeutic because it does not properly address the client's concern about addiction or the issue of the client's physical discomfort. It also blocks communication by using a cliche. ("Why take a chance?")

2. Excellent choice! This response enhances therapeutic communication by asking for clarification. The nurse is addressing the client's concern and asking for important information about the client's knowledge and feelings.

3. Wrong. This statement uses false reassurance and devalues the client's feelings. The nurse should communicate therapeutically by trying to learn more about the client's knowledge and feelings.

4. Wrong. The first part of this response gives the client correct information and addresses the issue of the client's pain. However, the nurse should first ask for clarification of the client's concerns about "getting hooked."

97. In addition to the prophylactic use of nitrates, the nurse can encourage the client to perform which of the following activities, without increasing the risk of an angina attack?

   1. Eating large meals.
   2. Smoking cigarettes.
   3. Walking a treadmill.
   4. Shoveling snow.

   1. *Incorrect. Large meals may precipitate an attack of angina pectoris. Remember that this form of angina is also known as exertional angina.*
   2. *Wrong choice. Clients with angina pectoris should be strongly encouraged to quit smoking, a risk factor that can be corrected like obesity and hypertension.*
   3. ***Absolutely! Clients with a sedentary lifestyle should be encouraged to establish a regular program of aerobic exercise (e.g., walking, jogging, swimming, bicycling).***
   4. *No. Angina pectoris is triggered most often by an increase in physical activity, as well as exposure to cold. Shoveling snow would definitely be contraindicated.*

98. Which of the following lab findings are consistent with a mother to whom the nurse will expect to administer RHoGAM following delivery?

   1. Mother Rh negative with a negative Coombs, father Rh positive, baby Rh negative.
   2. Mother Rh negative with a positive Rh antibody titer, father Rh positive, baby Rh positive.
   3. Mother Rh negative with a negative Coombs, father Rh positive, baby Rh positive.
   4. Mother Rh negative with a positive Coombs, father Rh negative, baby Rh negative.

   1. *Wrong. RHoGAM is not indicated when both mother and baby are RH negative. There is no risk of exposure to Rh positive.*
   2. *Wrong. The Rh positive antibody titer indicates that antibodies are already present. RHoGAM is not effective against already present antibodies.*
   3. ***Correct. This mother should receive RHoGAM because her negative Coombs shows that she has no antibodies in her system (Rh or other). The infant is Rh positive; therefore, the risk of exposure to Rh positive blood cells is present.***
   4. *Wrong choice! This mother and baby are both negative; thus there is no risk of exposure to Rh negative blood cells. Her positive Coombs may be the result of an antibody other than the Rh antibody. Also, two Rh negative parents can only give birth to Rh negative children.*

99. Following a total hip replacement, the nurse takes precautions to ensure that the affected hip is flexed no more than:

   1. 25 degrees.
   2. 60 degrees.
   3. 75 degrees.
   4. 90 degrees.

   1. *No. The client will need to flex the affected hip more than 25 degrees in order to transfer from bed to chair, etc.*
   2. ***Correct. The affected hip is not to be flexed more than 45 to 60 degrees. Limited flexion is maintained during transfers and when sitting, with encouragement to maintain the operative hip in extension.***
   3. *Incorrect. This amount of flexion may jeopardize the positioning of the femoral head component in the acetabular cup. Choose a safer option.*
   4. *Absolutely not! Dislocation may occur with this angle flexion, as it exceeds the limits of the prosthesis.*

100. A 10-year-old girl is admitted with the hospital unit with cystic fibrosis. It is appropriate for the nurse to administer her pancrelipase (Pancrease) at which time?

   1. One hour before meals.
   2. With meals.
   3. One-half hour after meals.
   4. On an empty stomach.

   1. *Wrong! Pancrease is a digestive enzyme. If the medication is given an hour before the meal, the enzyme will not benefit the child.*
   2. ***Right! Pancrease is a digestive enzyme and must be administered with the meal or just before, in order for the food to be properly digested.***
   3. *Incorrect. Pancrease is a digestive enzyme and must be administered with meals. If the medication is administered after the meal, the action will be too late to benefit the child.*
   4. *Incorrect. Pancrease is a digestive enzyme, given to aid in the digestion of food. If given on an empty stomach, it would not be effective.*

NCLEX-RN

Test 8

NCLEX-RN TEST 8

1. A client, 35 years old, has the following laboratory values reported on his chart: Hct 35%, Hgb 13 g/dL, Platelet count 150,000/cu mm, White blood cell count, 6,000. Which of the following laboratory reports would indicate that the client's condition has improved?

   1. Hematocrit 42%.
   2. Hemoglobin 12.8 g/dL.
   3. Platelet count 180,000/cu mm.
   4. White blood cell count 8,000.

2. A postoperative client is ambulatory and wishes to go to the day room. While walking down the hall with the nurse, the client says that she feels faint and starts to fall. Which of the following is the best action for the nurse to take?

   1. Grasp the client around the waist and hold her up so she doesn't fall and injure herself.
   2. Push the client up against the wall to keep her from falling.
   3. Ease the client gently to the floor.
   4. Ask another client to get some help while you support the client to prevent her from falling.

3. While a client is receiving amphotericin B (Fungizone) for her fungal infection, the nurse should constantly monitor for which of the following?

   1. Photosensitivity.
   2. Pale stools.
   3. Dark urine.
   4. Urine output.

4. A six-year-old is newly diagnosed with primary tuberculosis. The nurse is with the physician when he tells the parents the diagnosis. Which of the following is the nurse's immediate priority?

   1. Help the parents plan a nutritionally appropriate diet.
   2. Outline the medication and treatment regime.
   3. Explain hospital policy of isolation of clients with tuberculosis.
   4. Encourage the parents to express their concerns.

5. In addition to routine care, plans by the nurse for the immediate postoperative care of a client who had a laryngectomy will focus on the need for:

   1. Adequate fluid and electrolyte balance.
   2. Prevention of hemorrhage.
   3. Pain control.
   4. A patent airway.

6. A client has just delivered her first infant. He is jaundiced and has an elevated bilirubin. A diagnosis of ABO incompatibility is made. The client asks if she will be given RHoGAM to prevent this problem with future pregnancies. What is the best nursing response?

   1. "We will have to await the results of blood work on you and the baby."
   2. "I will call the physician and see if he wants you to receive RHoGAM."
   3. "RHoGAM is only effective in preventing Rh antibodies."
   4. "Yes, you will get RHoGAM as soon as the lab completes the necessary crossmatch."

7. A 62-year-old male has just been transferred from ICU and is on telemetry. While counting the radial pulse, the nurse notes an irregular rhythm. The progress notes say that the client has had atrial flutter. Which pattern corresponds to this arrhythmia?

   1. Ventricular rate of 82 with an atrial rate of 80.
   2. P waves occurring at .16 sec before each QRS complex.
   3. An atrial rate of 100, with 80 QRS complex/min.
   4. An irregular ventricular rate of 125, with a wide QRS pattern.

8. A 78-year-old client is admitted to the hospital for an exploratory laparotomy. The client's daughter says to the nurse, "I wish I could stay with my father, but I need to go home to see how my children are doing. I really hate to leave my father alone at this time." The best response by the nurse is:

   1. "Your father needs opportunities to be independent. This will help him become self-sufficient."
   2. "Your father is capable of taking care of himself. Try to allow him more independence."
   3. "Stress is not good for your father at this time. Perhaps you could call your children."
   4. "You are feeling concern for both your dad and your children. Let me know when you are leaving, and I'll stay with him."

9. A 55-year-old client is hospitalized following myocardial infarction. He is to be transferred from a cart to a bed in a room in your unit. When transferring the client from a cart to his bed, the priority action is which of the following?

    1. Have the client place his arms on his chest.
    2. Lock the wheels on the cart and the bed.
    3. Have at least four people to help with the transfer.
    4. Use a draw sheet to move the client.

10. A six-month-old male infant with AIDS has a nursing diagnosis of "Altered Growth and Development" on the care plan. Which of the following will most enhance the growth and development of the child?

    1. Encourage the child to eat whatever he wants.
    2. Provide therapy to help the child meet developmental milestones.
    3. Provide nutritional supplements in addition to an adequate diet.
    4. Weigh and measure the infant on a frequent basis.

11. Which statement written by a laryngectomy client preparing for discharge would indicate to the nurse that he needs further teaching?

    1. "I'll remember to buy non-aerosol products for personal grooming."
    2. "I sure will miss taking showers from now on."
    3. "Giving up swimming won't bother me, since I never learned how in the first place."
    4. "I never thought that belching could be transferred into speech, but I'm learning quickly."

12. A three-year-old boy is hospitalized with a broken leg. In assessing the client, the nurse might expect to observe three of the following behaviors about the client. Which behavior would the nurse least expect to observe?

    1. When offered a toy, the client says, "No," but takes the toy and begins to play with it.
    2. When his mother goes for lunch, he plays quietly, but when she goes home at night he cries for her.
    3. He wets the bed at night, even though his mother says he hasn't had an "accident" in six months.
    4. He plays well with boys his age and slightly older, but refuses to play with girls his own age.

13. To monitor a client for the most common complication arising from the administration of total parenteral nutrition, the nurse should do which of the following?

    1. Weigh the client at the same time each day using the same scale.
    2. Keep accurate records of total intake and total output.
    3. Determine the increase or decrease in body weight each day.
    4. Take the client's temperature at least every four hours.

14. A 70-year-old client is admitted to the hospital following a stroke. He has paralysis of the right side and is at risk of developing decubitus ulcers. In caring for this client, which of the following actions by the nurse is appropriate?

    1. Move the client up in bed by sliding him.
    2. Roll the client to his side once a day.
    3. Change the client's position every two hours.
    4. Keep the client in a wheelchair during the morning and afternoon hours.

15. An eight-year-old client was admitted to the hospital with a diagnosis of acute rheumatic fever. Immediately after admission, which of the following assessments by the nurse is most important?

    1. Auscultation of the rate and characteristics of heart sounds.
    2. Determining the location and severity of joint pain.
    3. Identifying the degree of anxiety related to the diagnosis.
    4. Determining the family's emotional and financial needs.

16. Which manifestations can the nurse expect to observe in a client admitted with emphysema?

    1. Dyspnea, bradycardia.
    2. Barrel chest, shallow respirations.
    3. Cyanosis, productive cough.
    4. Asymmetrical chest, dry cough.

17. Many groups of drugs are associated with a life-threatening abstinence syndrome. The nurse understands that which drug group is least likely to present a medical crisis during withdrawal?

    1. Narcotics.
    2. Barbiturates.
    3. Alcohol.
    4. Benzodiazepines.

18. A 20-day-old infant is recovering from surgery for pyloric stenosis. The client's mother asked the nurse, "Now that my son has had this surgery, is it likely that pyloric stenosis will cause trouble later?" Which of the following is the most appropriate response to the client's statement?

1. "Why don't you talk to the doctor about your uncertainties regarding your son's future?"
2. "He might develop obstructive symptoms later. If so, take him immediately to an emergency room."
3. "He will not have symptoms again in childhood, but may have digestive difficulties in his adult life."
4. "Recurrence of the obstruction or repetition of the surgical procedure would be unlikely."

19. **A client is seen in the clinic in the 28th week of gestation. Her blood pressure is 160/100 and she has 2+ protein in her urine. She complains that all her shoes are too tight. Her doctor recommends hospitalization. The admitting nurse must select a bed for the new client. Each room on the unit is a semiprivate room. Which of the following room-mates would be best for the client?**

    1. A 20-year-old primigravida who enjoys loud rock-and-roll music.
    2. A 32-year-old multigravida who enjoys reading romance novels.
    3. A 24-year-old C-section who watches soap operas and game shows on TV.
    4. A 22-year-old primigravida who has many visitors during the afternoon and evening.

20. **The nurse should monitor the client taking ethambutol (Myambutol) for which of the following?**

    1. Urine output.
    2. Jaundice.
    3. Visual acuity.
    4. Arrhythmias.

21. **After one week in an eating disorders program, a client has gained three pounds. She confides to the nurse that she has begun to have the urge to vomit after eating. How can the nurse best handle this?**

    1. Praise the client for having enough trust in the nurse to share this concern.
    2. Establish a contract with the client to seek out a staff member to talk about her feelings after eating including her urge to vomit.
    3. Remove her privileges if she vomits to reinforce that this behavior is not appropriate.
    4. Suggest she share this concern during her next group therapy session.

22. **A 55-year-old client has been taking trifluopera-zine (Stelazine) for five years to control her para-noid thoughts. The client asks her psychiatrist to change her medication to clozapine (Clozaril) be-cause she is worried about developing tardive dyski-nesia. What information should she be given about taking Clozaril drug safely?**

    1. Monthly blood levels have to be taken to monitor the dose.
    2. Drug holidays should be taken periodically.
    3. Weekly white blood counts have to be done.
    4. Monthly AIMS testing is indicated.

23. **A 35-year-old man was in an automobile accident. Initial assessment revealed fractures of the left femur and pelvis and a large contusion on the head. What should be the nurse's priority assessment in order to determine the client's neurological status?**

    1. Pupillary responses.
    2. Verbal responses.
    3. Limb movements.
    4. Level of consciousness.

24. **In planning care for a client prior to delivery, which of the following nursing orders would be most appropriate?**

    1. Assess fluid balance hourly and maintain optimum placental perfusion.
    2. Monitor urine output and assure a brief rest period each shift.
    3. Check the blood pressure before and after each time the client is out of bed.
    4. Observe for amount of edema and provide for di-versionary activities.

25. **Which of the following statements by the nurse indicates the best understanding of the principles of reality orientation?**

    1. "Good morning, Mr. Edwards. Did you sleep well? It's time to get dressed."
    2. "Good morning. This is your second day in Shady Pines and I am your nurse for the day."
    3. "Do you remember who I am? We met yesterday when you were admitted."
    4. "Good morning, how are you? I am your nurse for the day. Is there anything I can do for you right now?"

26. **Twenty-four hours after admission for viral gas-troenteritis, a four-year-old has a temperature of 101° F. What should the nurse do in response to this data?**

    1. Keep the child warm with blankets.
    2. Apply a hypothermia blanket.
    3. Document the temperature.
    4. Call the physician immediately with these find-ings.

27. **A 72-year-old client has a draining pressure sore. The culture of the drainage reveals staphylococci. Which action during the care of this client should be the nurse's highest priority?**

1. Reinforce the pressure dressing with a sterile towel before ambulating the client.
2. Wear gown and gloves when changing the client's bed linen.
3. Use sterile technique when changing the dressing on the pressure sore.
4. Do not allow the client the use of his personal effects until they have been sterilized.

28. **A person in a restaurant puts his hand to his throat. A nurse who sees this happen begins to administer the Heimlich maneuver. After the client falls to the floor the nurse should next:**

1. Check for the pulse.
2. Sweep the mouth.
3. Attempt to ventilate.
4. Administer five abdominal thrusts.

29. **A chronic alcoholic has been hospitalized following a drinking binge. The nurse enters the room and finds the client shouting in a terrified voice, "Get those ants out of my room!" Which of the following statements would be most appropriate at this time?**

1. "Tell me more about the ants that you see in your room."
2. "I'm sure that the ants you see will not harm you."
3. "I don't see any ants, but you seem very frightened."
4. "I do not see anything. This is part of your illness."

30. **The nurse understands that health education is important for persons with stress-related illnesses. After giving a client information about his medications, treatment options, and the role stress plays in his illness, the nurse realizes that the client will most likely follow the treatment plan under which of the following circumstances?**

1. If the nurse refers the client for supportive psychotherapy.
2. If the nurse involves the client in the treatment planning process.
3. If the nurse asks the client if she may speak with his wife.
4. If the nurse recommends that he come in for weekly appointments to review his progress.

31. **Following a CVA, which affected the left side of his brain, a 71-year-old client has his tube feedings discontinued and is ready to begin oral feedings. Which of the following nursing measures ensures client tolerance?**

1. Feed from right side of mouth; upright position; mouth care before feeding.

2. Verbal encouragement; check gag reflex; feed thinned foods and liquids.
3. Check gag reflex; feed on left side of mouth; upright position.
4. Sensory stimulation; verbal encouragement; favorite foods.

32. **A five-year-old client has just returned from cardiac catheterization. The right femoral artery was used for the procedure. What is the first nursing responsibility?**

1. Elevate to high Fowler's position, to improve ventilation.
2. Place the client on the cardiac monitor, to assess for arrhythmias.
3. Assess for dehydration, since the client has been NPO eight hours.
4. Evaluate the catheter insertion site for bleeding.

33. **A client is to begin taking quinidine (Quinatime) 200 mg p.o. every six hours for maintenance treatment of paroxysmal atrial tachycardia (PAT). The nurse will observe for which of the following common side effects associated with quinidine therapy?**

1. Diarrhea.
2. Vertigo.
3. Rashes.
4. Fever.

34. **Soon after being admitted to a rehabilitation unit following a drinking binge, a client says to the nurse, "I don't really need to be here. My wife and family make me drink. My wife spends all my money. My kid just had an accident with his car, which cost me a fortune in repairs." Which of the following is the most appropriate response by the nurse at this time?**

1. "Tell me more about your wife spending all your money."
2. "How did your child's car accident cost you money?"
3. "It sounds like you have financial difficulties."
4. "Tell me more about your concern about being here."

35. **In the pediatric clinic the nurse is working with a family whose three-month-old has been recently diagnosed as having cerebral palsy. Which of the following statements by the mother would indicate that teaching about the disorder has been effective?**

1. "I know that our baby will get worse, because I have seen older children with this disorder."

2. "I am hopeful that the early schooling will increase his ability for self-care."

3. "My husband and I plan to be tested prior to our next baby to predict the possibility of a similar outcome."

4. I am going to ask the doctor to prescribe skeletal muscle relaxants to improve my child's functioning."

36. **A client is admitted to the hospital with an infection of her right arm that requires an incision and drainage. Which of the following nursing actions is most appropriate?**

    1. Wear gloves only when coming in contact with drainage or soiled articles.
    2. Assess the wound to determine what infection control measures are needed to care for the client.
    3. Wear a gown if there is a possibility of the nurse's clothing becoming contaminated by drainage or secretions.
    4. Wash hands before and after care.

37. **Which of the following lab values would the nurse expect is most likely to be found in a client needing calcium gluconate?**

    1. Magnesium level 8 mEq/L.
    2. Calcium level 6 mEq/L.
    3. Magnesium level 2 mEq/L.
    4. Potassium level 3 mEq/L.

38. **In preparing a client to be discharged, the nurse teaches him to position himself for postural drainage. To achieve success in this teaching program, which of the following information about the client is most important?**

    1. The type of bed the client will be using at home for the procedure.
    2. The amount of time required for the client to change positions.
    3. The client's goal concerning his ability to be self-sufficient.
    4. The client's ability to move about without assistance from others.

39. **A 10-year-old boy is in sickle cell crisis. Which of the following nursing actions is contraindicated?**

    1. Administer oxygen via nasal cannula as prescribed.
    2. Encourage the client to increase oral fluid intake.
    3. Administer narcotics only for very severe pain.
    4. Encourage as much exercise as possible during the crisis.

40. **A client is recuperating from gallbladder surgery in which general anesthesia was administered. The nurse should encourage the client to use the incentive spirometry a minimum of how many times per hour?**

    1. Two.
    2. Five to 10.
    3. 10-15.
    4. 20-25.

41. **To reduce the risk of a serious interaction, the nurse would instruct a client taking cefoperazone (Cefobid) to avoid which of the following?**

    1. Wine.
    2. Orange juice.
    3. Food.
    4. Maalox.

42. **A client complains that he is unable to rest because of the noise from the television being used by the other client in the room. The best action by the nurse is which of the following?**

    1. Have the client moved to a private room.
    2. Provide ear phones for the client who is watching television.
    3. Explain that the roommate is hard of hearing, so the television is louder than usual.
    4. Ask the roommate to shut off the television so the client can rest.

43. **In the emergency room a 10-year-old child is admitted with salicylate poisoning. Which is the first step for the nurse to take in the treatment of this client?**

    1. Prevent the absorption of poison.
    2. Determine the number of tablets ingested.
    3. Assess the child.
    4. Pass a Levine tube and prepare for lavage.

44. **While administering a bed bath to a postoperative client, it is important to maintain privacy. Which of the following is the best method for the nurse to use in maintaining the client's privacy?**

    1. Allow the client to wear a gown, and reach under the gown with the washcloth and towel to bathe the client.
    2. Use towels to protect the bed linen.
    3. Cover the client with a bath blanket and expose only the portion of the body that is being bathed.
    4. Use the bed sheet to cover the client during the bath.

45. A 56-year-old male client diagnosed with complete heart block had a demand pacemaker inserted today. The pacer is set for 72 beats/min. Which EKG pattern indicates to the nurse a failure to capture?

    1. QRS complexes occurring at a rate of 73 beats/min and no sharp spikes.
    2. Sharp spikes at 72 per min; QRS complexes at 50 beats/min.
    3. P waves at a rate of 78 per min; QRS complexes at 72 beats/min.
    4. QRS complexes at a rate of 100 beat/min.

46. A 20-year-old college student comes to the campus health service complaining of severe epigastric distress. While doing an assessment, the nurse discovers that she has suffered from severe bulimia since her freshman year. The client tells the nurse, "I know my eating binges and vomiting are not normal, but I cannot do anything about them." What is the most therapeutic nursing response to the client's statement?

    1. "Do you have any idea why you do this?"
    2. "Are you feeling pretty helpless about changing this behavior?"
    3. "Have you noticed any pattern to your eating binges and vomiting?"
    4. "You will stop because you have to. You are destroying your health."

47. A 72-year-old male has just been diagnosed with Parkinson's disease. Which of the following interventions should the nurse avoid?

    1. Plan gait training with physical therapy.
    2. Help wife to assist with dressing.
    3. Order between meal snacks high in fiber.
    4. Ask him to read the newspaper aloud.

48. A nine-year-old female is to be discharged tomorrow. She is being treated for rheumatic fever. Her symptoms are: temperature 100° F, pulse 120/min, and polyarthritis. Which instruction would the nurse anticipate giving to the client's parents?

    1. Administer penicillin as prescribed.
    2. Utilize acetaminophen for joint pain to prevent the possibility of Reye's syndrome.
    3. Allow her to resume normal activities as soon is joint pain is gone.
    4. Teach CPR, because of the possibility of coronary artery sequelae.

49. A client with atelectasis of the left lower lung is to receive intermittent positive pressure breathing (IPPB) four times a day. It would be appropriate for the nurse to instruct the client that:

    1. The treatment will last 45 minutes to an hour each time.
    2. Take short, quick breaths during the treatment to get the maximum benefit from the medication.
    3. The medication used in the treatment may cause nausea, so the physician has prescribed an antiemetic to be given beforehand.
    4. You should notice an increase in productive coughing during and after the treatment. This means that the medication is working.

50. During heroin withdrawal, a client complains continuously to the nursing staff about his discomfort. One day the nurse overhears a nursing assistant say to the client, "You brought on these problems yourself by taking drugs. What did you think would happen when you continued to use heroin?" Which of the following comments to the nursing assistant would be most constructive?

    1. "Your comments were inappropriate. I will have to report this to the supervisor."
    2. "Weren't you a bit hard on this client? He is having a great deal of discomfort."
    3. "This client is getting on all our nerves."
    4. "I overheard you speaking with the client and I thought your comment about his causing his own problems was inappropriate. You have worked well with other addicted clients. What is different about this man?"

51. A chronic alcoholic has been hospitalized following a drinking binge. During a lengthy conversation with the nurse about his long history of alcoholism, the client becomes tense and uncomfortable. Which of the following is the best initial response by the nurse?

    1. "What did I say to make you feel so uncomfortable?"
    2. "Drinking for a long time can make anyone feel uncomfortable."
    3. "At what point did you begin to feel uncomfortable?"
    4. "Talking about your drinking will help you to recover."

52. A client who is 62 years old is scheduled for coronary artery bypass tomorrow. The physician has ordered aspirin 325 mg daily. Which of the following nursing actions would be most appropriate?

1. Explain to the client that aspirin is given because of its anti-inflammatory effects.
2. Tell the client that after surgery he will continue to take aspirin prophylactically.
3. Question the doctor's order, since aspirin could cause postoperative bleeding.
4. Monitor the client's temperature and report elevations to the doctor immediately.

53. **A client, 40 years old, is scheduled to have a bone marrow aspiration to assist with the diagnosis of multiple myeloma. Prior to a bone marrow aspiration, the most important communication from the nurse to the client is which of the following?**

1. The client must be still during the procedure.
2. This test will help to diagnosis multiple myeloma.
3. He will only feel sharp pain for a few minutes.
4. He will receive a sedative, so he will be asleep during the procedure.

54. **While bathing a small child in a tub, the nurse would avoid which of the following?**

1. Check the temperature of the water with a thermometer.
2. Never leave the child unattended.
3. Make sure the temperature in the room is warm.
4. Allow the child to determine if the water temperature is comfortable by placing the child's feet in the water.

55. **The nurse understands that which of the following statements concerning naloxone (Narcan) is accurate?**

1. Narcan is available in two separate strengths, one for adults and one for infants and children.
2. Narcan is available in one strength. Careful calculation for newborns is essential to prevent an overdose.
3. Narcan is available in one strength. It needs to be diluted with normal saline prior to administration to neonates to prevent an overdose.
4. Narcan is available in two strengths, but either can be administered to adults or neonates as long as dosage is calculated using body weight.

56. **A client's mother comes to visit. The client does not acknowledge her greeting and lies down on her bed, curling up into the fetal position while her mother is in the room. After the visit the nurse speaks with the client's mother and returns to the client's room. The client is still lying in a fetal position. What action by the nurse would be most therapeutic at this time?**

1. Ask the client to get up and put away the clothing her mother has brought her.
2. Ask the client why she responded to her mother that way.
3. Sit in a chair next to the bed and ask the client to talk about what happened when her mother visited.
4. Explain unit expectations about how visitors are to be treated.

57. **A 62-year-old female was diagnosed with breast cancer. She has become quiet and thoughtful and says to the nurse, "What do you think people will say about me when I'm gone?" Which of the following responses by the nurse is the most therapeutic?**

1. "You will be remembered as a very nice person."
2. "Do you feel that people will be talking about you after your death?"
3. "At this time, a positive attitude can influence your recovery."
4. "The thought of your breast cancer must seem hopeless."

58. **When making rounds, the nurse notices that a client who is receiving oxygen via nasal cannula has a pack of cigarettes at the bedside. What is the best action by the nurse?**

1. Remove the pack of cigarettes from the bedside.
2. Remind the client not to smoke when oxygen is in use.
3. Ask the client how he obtained the cigarettes.
4. Review the rules of safety with the client's family.

59. **During a home visit by the nurse, the client's wife collapses. There is no pulse or respirations. Which description correctly summarizes the CPR that the nurse would provide?**

1. Five to one ratio of compressions to ventilations, at a rate of 100 beats/min.
2. Fifteen to two ratio of compressions to ventilations, at a rate of 80 beats/min.
3. Fifteen to two ratio of compressions to ventilations, at a rate of 100 beats/min.
4. Five to one ratio of compressions to ventilations, at a rate of 80 beats/min.

60. **The nurse should advise the client that which is the best way to take erythromycin that is not enteric coated?**

1. With meals.
2. With a full glass of water on an empty stomach.
3. With a snack.
4. Crushed and added to food.

61. **The client has not bathed or changed her clothes during the two days she has been on the unit. After suggesting that she take a shower, the client states an emphatic, "No!" and turns her back to the nurse. What is the best action for the nurse to take initially?**

    1. Withdraw and return at a later time.
    2. Question the client about her resistance to showering.
    3. Get another staff member to help get the client into the shower.
    4. Tell her she will be much more acceptable to other people on the unit if she cleans up and changes her clothes.

62. **What information regarding betamethasone (Celestone) is it important for the nurse to know, prior to administration of the drug to the antepartum client?**

    1. When used along with antibiotics, the risk of infection is increased due to the masking effect of antibiotic therapy.
    2. When used for diabetic clients, the risk of hypoglycemia is increased.
    3. When used after 34 weeks gestation, it is most effective in preventing RDS in the neonate.
    4. When used along with tocolytic agents the risk of pulmonary edema is increased.

63. **A two-month-old is having a well baby check-up today. According to the standard immunization schedule, which immunizations would the nurse expect to administer to this child?**

    1. MMR and OPV.
    2. DTP and OPV.
    3. OPV, Hib and DTP.
    4. DTP.

64. **A client has a positive Mantoux skin test following screening for tuberculosis. The nurse interprets this to mean that the client:**

    1. Has active tuberculosis.
    2. Was infectious at one time, but now has inactive tuberculosis.
    3. Will require further evaluation.
    4. Has never been exposed to the tubercle bacillus.

65. **Which statement by the mother indicates that the nurse's teaching about safety for an 18-month-old has been successful?**

    1. "I will give syrup of ipecac immediately if my child swallows a poison."
    2. "I know that once she understands 'no,' she will be safe."

    3. "I watch her every second, so I'm sure she can't get into anything."
    4. "I have locked my medicines up in the medicine cabinet."

66. **As the nurse approaches a schizophrenic, paranoid type client, he looks at her and says, "Back off. Leave me alone." He appears tense and is pacing rapidly. The best nursing response to his remark is which of the following statements?**

    1. "I can't leave you alone when you are this upset. Sit down and try to relax."
    2. "Let's go to your room and you can tell me what is bothering you."
    3. "I will keep my distance as long as you can control yourself. You appear quite angry and I'd like to know more about what is causing you to feel this way."
    4. "I will leave you alone for a few minutes while you try to compose yourself."

67. **A client is to receive cefazolin (Ancef) 500 mg IM every six hours. Which of the following actions taken by the nurse would most effectively decrease irritation at the injection site?**

    1. Use the Z-track method, and inject into the dorsogluteal site.
    2. Do not massage the site after the medication is administered; use gentle pressure only.
    3. Give the medication slowly, over one minute, to allow dispersal time into the muscle.
    4. Use a 1 1/2 inch needle and inject into the ventrogluteal site.

68. **A 24-year-old man is seen in the emergency room following a gunshot wound to the right chest. The triage nurse notes a thick dressing on the right chest, a sucking noise from the wound, BP 100/60, pulse rate 96 and weak, and respiratory rate 40. Which of the following nursing actions would be best initially?**

    1. Remove the dressing to inspect the wound.
    2. Administer oxygen via nasal cannula.
    3. Draw blood for serum chemistries.
    4. Raise the foot of the bed to 90 degrees.

69. **Which of the following statements by the nurse would best describe the action of RHoGAM?**

    1. It destroys Rh antibodies in the Rh negative mother.
    2. It destroys Rh antibodies in the Rh positive newborn.
    3. It prevents the formation of the Rh antibodies in the Rh negative mother.
    4. It prevents the formation of the Rh antibodies in the Rh positive newborn.

70. A client had been brought to the hospital by two coworkers who were also close friends. They reported that, while he had always been a person "on the go", his activity level had increased over the past two weeks to the point that he was working around the clock. They also indicated that he ate and slept very little, and talked almost nonstop. A priority goal of nursing care for this client is to help him do which of the following?

1. Confront the denial of his underlying depression.
2. Participate in group activities.
3. Identify one recreational or leisure activity to pursue.
4. Obtain adequate amounts of rest.

71. The nurse is to instruct parents of young children about poisoning prevention in the home. Which of the following interventions is most important for the parents learn?

1. If the child ingests poison, induce vomiting with syrup of ipecac.
2. If the child ingests poison, the parents should immediately bring the child to the emergency room.
3. Place labels on the parent's telephone, with the Poison Control Center's telephone number, and instructions to call that number after an accidental ingestion.
4. If a poisoning occurs, the nurse will notify social services to investigate the home situation for safety.

72. The physician orders a stool specimen to be collected for ova and parasites. What is the proper procedure for the nurse to use in collection of this specimen?

1. Send entire stool immediately to the lab.
2. Use a sterile container.
3. Take feces from several areas of the bowel movement.
4. Refrigerate specimen until it can be delivered to the lab.

73. A client, 60 years old, is admitted to the hospital with a diagnosis of chest pain. Several days after admission, the client is scheduled for a cardiac catheterization. Client information is obtained by the nurse during an interview prior to the procedure. Which of the following findings should be reported immediately to the physician who will be doing the procedure?

1. The client is allergic to lobster.
2. The client's father smokes heavily.
3. The client's husband died of heart disease.
4. The client is apprehensive about the procedure.

74. Which of the following interventions by the nurse is appropriate to prepare the client for a cholecystography?

1. NPO after midnight.
2. Clear liquid diet the evening before the test.
3. Assess for allergies to iodine or seafood.
4. Special consent form due to the invasive nature of the procedure.

75. A five-year-old child is being seen for a well child visit in a pediatric clinic. The child's father tells the nurse that his wife has recently been diagnosed with tuberculosis. Which of the following statements will guide the nurse in planning the information that will be provided to the parents?

1. It is likely that the child will require medication.
2. Small children do not easily contract TB, if they are otherwise healthy.
3. As long as the child has not exhibited the symptoms of night sweats and/or coughing, there is probably no infection.
4. Direct physical contact must be limited to insure the health of the child.

76. When elderly clients are treated with antidepressant medication, the nurse is guided by which of the following understandings?

1. They will probably require a higher dose of medication than a younger person.
2. Psychotherapy and medication together are usually more effective than either alone in treating elderly depressed clients.
3. Antidepressant medications are usually not well tolerated by elderly clients because of their many side effects.
4. Antidepressants are expensive medications and the potential results may not be worth their cost.

77. A client, age 58, had a hiatal hernia repair three days ago. During this morning's assessment, he tells the nurse that his abdomen "feels swollen," and that he is nauseated, with increased abdominal discomfort. What should be the nurse's initial action?

1. Give the client an antiemetic.
2. Listen for bowel sounds.
3. Insert a nasogastric tube.
4. Measure the client's abdominal girth.

78. After taking erythromycin (Erythrocin) p.o. for seven days, a client develops oral candidiasis. The nurse is aware that this is most likely a result of which type of reaction?

1. Superinfection.
2. Allergic response.
3. Synergistic reaction.
4. Erythromycin toxicity.

79. **A 15-year-old client was just diagnosed with testicular cancer. When the nurse asks the client a question, he angrily spits in the nurse's face. Which of the following responses by the nurse would be best?**

    1. "You are old enough to find a better way to express yourself. The nurses will not want to take care of you if you treat us this way."
    2. "I'm afraid I will have to tell your parents about this. They call every day to talk to the nurses about how you are doing."
    3. "That behavior makes me very angry and I will not tolerate it. I'll be back after I wash my face and we can talk about what's bothering you."
    4. "If you don't want us here right now, we will go. We will come back to change your linens when you are feeling better."

80. **Although most depressed clients do not attempt suicide, an estimated 80% of persons with depression do have suicidal thoughts. Nursing intervention for an elderly widower with agitated depression should be guided by which information, regarding the risk of suicide?**

    1. It is no different than for any other depressed client.
    2. It is lower than that of an elderly man who has never married.
    3. It is quite low.
    4. It is extremely high.

81. **A child with the body-surface area (BSA) of 0.5 square meters is to receive 250 mg of medication. The usual adult dosage is 500 mg/dose. The nurse's safest action is to:**

    1. Give the medication, as the dosage is correct for the child's size.
    2. Give the medication, but request that the dose be reevaluated.
    3. Withhold the medication and notify the prescriber.
    4. Recalculate the dosage and administer a decreased amount.

82. **A client is admitted with bleeding esophageal varices. The physician has opted to use esophageal tamponade with a Sengstaken-Blakemore tube to control the bleeding. Which of the following nursing interventions is appropriate when caring for the client while the Blakemore tube is in place?**

1. Ambulate the client four times a day.
2. Encourage clear liquids.
3. Provide mouth and nares care every two hours.
4. Maintain the manometer pressure of the esophageal balloon at all times to control bleeding.

83. **A 30-year-old single man who works as a computer analyst, is admitted to the hospital with a diagnosis of bipolar mood disorder, acute manic episode. When taking a nursing history which information, if true, would support this diagnosis?**

    1. He describes himself as a "loner" with a history of being withdrawn and aloof in relationships.
    2. His paternal grandfather had mood swings all his life. He died in a mental institution.
    3. He had a similar episode when in college. He dropped out of school without finishing his degree and his friends say he was never the same again.
    4. His parents were divorced when he was a young child.

84. **A 15-year-old client is to have a k-pad, or water system heating device, applied to a pulled muscle. The client tells the nurse that the device does not feel very warm. Which of the following nursing actions is most appropriate?**

    1. Tell the client that these heating devices never feel hot.
    2. Check the temperature setting on the heating unit and feel the pad for warmth.
    3. Call the appropriate repair department and have them fix the unit.
    4. Turn the temperature up on the unit if it doesn't feel warm enough to the client.

85. **Following a motor vehicle accident a 30-year-old male has a $PaCO_2$ of 30 mm Hg on room air. What intervention would be anticipated?**

    1. Rebreathing of expired air.
    2. Encourage deep breathing.
    3. Administration of oxygen.
    4. Treatment with sodium bicarbonate.

86. **A 23-year-old client is seen in the Women's Health Center and is to be treated with erythromycin (Erythromycin Base Filmtab) 250 mg p.o. every six hours for strep throat. With which of the following should the nurse instruct the client to take the drug?**

    1. Milk or an antacid.
    2. Water one hour before or two hours after meals.
    3. Fruit juice.
    4. Food.

87. The nurse observes a depressed client in the day room. She appears to be cold. Which of the following responses by the nurse would be most therapeutic?

    1. "Come with me to your room and we will get a sweater for you."
    2. "Why do you sit here without a sweater when you are cold?"
    3. "What color sweater do you want me to get from your room for you?"
    4. "When you are in the day room, you should dress so that you are not cold."

88. While making rounds at night, the nurse discovers an elderly client in bed and the room filled with smoke. The first action would be which of the following?

    1. Shut the door.
    2. Remove the client from the room.
    3. Call the fire department.
    4. Get a fire extinguisher.

89. While mixing a solution of bleach and water to be used as a disinfectant spray, the nurse discovers that there is more solution than will fit in the spray bottle. The nurse can appropriately deal with the excess in several ways. The least appropriate solution would be to:

    1. Pour the excess solution into an empty container, label the container as to contents, and place it in the cleaning supply closet.
    2. Discard the excess solution.
    3. Use the excess solution for the immediate cleaning job, then discard what is left.
    4. Pour the excess into another cleaning solution container that has only a small amount of an ammonia solution left in the bottom.

90. Postural drainage with percussion is ordered for a client with pneumonia. How would the nurse plan for this procedure?

    1. Perform this procedure before meals.
    2. Cup and clap lightly to avoid causing redness to the client's skin.
    3. Administer bronchodilators after percussion and before postural drainage.
    4. Provide analgesia prior to each treatment.

91. A 68-year-old client is admitted with a broken right arm and contusions to the left wrist following an automobile accident. Which of the following measures would the nurse avoid when feeding the client?

    1. Offer small bites of food.
    2. Order pureed foods.
    3. Have the client use her dentures while eating.
    4. Allow enough time for the client to chew the food well before offering more.

92. A 72-year-old female has fallen, fracturing her left hip. She is admitted in Buck's traction and scheduled for intramedullary nailing tomorrow. The nurse understands that which is the primary rationale for Buck's traction in this client?

    1. To reduce muscle spasm.
    2. To provide for total immobility.
    3. To promote healing of the fracture.
    4. To allow for a 20 pound weight to be applied.

93. A child weighing 1800 gm is admitted to intensive care. The nurse correctly explains to the parents that the infant's weight in pounds is:

    1. 3.9 lbs.
    2. 8.1 lbs.
    3. 18 lbs.
    4. 36 lbs.

94. A client in the intensive care unit is placed on a ventilator. During an electrical storm, the lights go out for a brief period. Some of the lights come back on, but the ventilator is not working. What is the best nursing action?

    1. Remove the client from the ventilator and ventilate with a bag and mask.
    2. Check the electrical outlets to determine if the ventilator is plugged into an emergency power outlet.
    3. Call a code.
    4. Notify the supervisor while ventilating the client with oxygen using positive pressure bag attached to the endotracheal tube.

95. The admitting nurse asks a client what factors, such as a recent change in his life, have contributed to his hospitalization? He replied, "Change...change is money...when you have money you make the change." Which of the following is this statement an example of?

    1. Clanging.
    2. Echolalia.
    3. Perseveration.
    4. Flight of ideas.

96. Clients with Parkinson's disease and myasthenia gravis are both encountered in the neurology clinic. The nursing assistant asks the nurse, "Are these disorders similar?" Which of the following is inaccurate information on which to base a response?

1. Both disorders are characterized by abnormal involuntary movements.
2. Each disorder is managed with specific drug therapy.
3. Crisis states may occur in either disorder due to medication withdrawal.
4. No known cure exists for either disorder.

97. **A woman is admitted to the ICU on a ventilator after attempting suicide. She had been depressed for some time. As the husband is talking with the nurse, he begins to cry. He says, "It's all my fault. I should have been home more often to keep an eye on her." Which of the following statements by the nurse would be most appropriate initially?**

    1. "You seem to regret not being there for your wife. How can you feel that way when you have to earn a living?"
    2. "At this time you need your privacy. I will return later, and we can talk then."
    3. "This is an important issue that you need to bring up at your family therapy session."
    4. "It must have been hard to be away when your wife was so sick."

98. **A 24-year-old female client diagnosed with sciatica is found staring into space with her lunch tray untouched. The client received meperidine (Demerol) 100 mg one hour ago. Which assessment should the nurse make from this scenario?**

    1. The medication dosage is excessive.
    2. The observed behaviors indicate intractable pain.
    3. The client is upset with the care and the food.
    4. The behaviors demonstrate an adjustment to pain.

99. **A client is admitted to the psychiatric unit with a diagnosis of acute depression. After being hospitalized for a few weeks, the client says to the nurse, "I'm a terrible person, and I should be dead." Which of the following responses by the nurse would be appropriate initially?**

    1. "That is why you are here. We are trying to help you with your bad feelings."
    2. "Feeling that way must be awful. What makes you feel so terrible?"
    3. "Feeling like a terrible person is part of your illness. As you get better, those feelings will lessen."
    4. "You are not terrible. You are not a bad person."

100. **The nurse notices a crack in an electrical outlet. The IV pump that is plugged into the outlet appears to be working without any problems. Which of the following is the best nursing action?**

    1. Use another outlet; then call the maintenance department to have the outlet changed.
    2. Since the pump is working, no action is necessary.
    3. Test the outlet by moving the plug a bit in the outlet, and observing if this affects the pump.
    4. Since the outlet works, continue to use it until maintenance can replace it.

NCLEX-RN

Test 8

Questions with Rationales

NCLEX-RN TEST 8 WITH RATIONALES

1. **A client, 35 years old, has the following laboratory values reported on his chart: Hct 35%, Hgb 13 g/dL, Platelet count 150,000/cu mm, White blood cell count, 6,000. Which of the following laboratory reports would indicate that the client's condition has improved?**

   1. Hematocrit 42%.
   2. Hemoglobin 12.8 g/dL.
   3. Platelet count 180,000/cu mm.
   4. White blood cell count 8,000.

   1. *Good choice! A normal hematocrit for a adult male is 42% to 54%. The original laboratory value indicated a low hematocrit. This choice shows a hematocrit within normal limits. This is an indication that the client's condition has improved.*
   2. *A normal hemoglobin for an adult male is 14 to 18. The original laboratory values indicate a low hemoglobin. This option shows a hemoglobin which is still lower. This would not be an indication that the client's condition has improved.*
   3. *Wrong! Normal platelet counts range from 130,000 to 370,000/cu mm. The original laboratory values indicate a platelet count that is within normal limits. This option shows a platelet count that is also within normal limits. This would not be an indication that the client's condition has improved.*
   4. *Wrong! Normal white blood cell counts range from 4,100 to 10,900/cu mm. The original laboratory values indicate a white blood cell count that is within normal limits. This choice shows a white blood cell count that is also within normal limits. This would not be an indication that the client's condition has improved.*

2. **A postoperative client is ambulatory and wishes to go to the day room. While walking down the hall with the nurse, the client says that she feels faint and starts to fall. Which of the following is the best action for the nurse to take?**

   1. Grasp the client around the waist and hold her up so she doesn't fall and injure herself.
   2. Push the client up against the wall to keep her from falling.
   3. Ease the client gently to the floor.
   4. Ask another client to get some help while you support the client to prevent her from falling.

   1. *This is not correct. Preventing injury to the client is the most important action. This option may result in both the client and the nurse falling, putting both individuals at risk for injury.*

   2. *Pushing the client against the wall will not prevent the fall and may cause injury to the client from the impact against the wall.*
   3. ***Right! Easing the client gently to the floor is the best action since it protects both individuals from injury.***
   4. *This is incorrect. Attempting to hold a client who is fainting upright places the nurse at risk for injury. If the client becomes too heavy, then the client may be injured if the nurse becomes fatigued and can no longer support her.*

3. **While a client is receiving amphotericin B (Fungizone) for her fungal infection, the nurse should constantly monitor for which of the following?**

   1. Photosensitivity.
   2. Pale stools.
   3. Dark urine.
   4. Urine output.

   1. *Wrong. Photosensitivity occurs with griseofulvin (Grisactin), not amphotericin B.*
   2. *Wrong. Pale stools occur with ketoconazole (Nizoral), not amphotericin B.*
   3. *Incorrect. Dark urine occurs with ketoconazole (Nizoral), not amphotericin B.*
   4. ***Correct. Amphotericin B causes kidney damage. Impairment of renal function occurs in almost all clients, so it is important to monitor urine output.***

4. **A six-year-old is newly diagnosed with primary tuberculosis. The nurse is with the physician when he tells the parents the diagnosis. Which of the following is the nurse's immediate priority?**

   1. Help the parents plan a nutritionally appropriate diet.
   2. Outline the medication and treatment regime.
   3. Explain hospital policy of isolation of clients with tuberculosis.
   4. Encourage the parents to express their concerns.

   1. *Not the first priority. Nutrition is important, especially the inclusion of high calcium and protein, so that organisms can be walled off in lung tissue. This is particularly important with INH therapy.*
   2. *No, this isn't the first thing to discuss with the parents, although they are both appropriate for discharge planning.*
   3. *Incorrect. This will have to be discussed, but is not the nurse's focus at the time the diagnosis is given.*

Children with primary tuberculosis have minimal pulmonary lesions and therefore are not as infectious as most adults.

4. *Right! This is the priority. You are being questioned here on a major principle of teaching/learning theory. Always allow for the expression of feelings and concerns, before interventions, including teaching.*

5. **In addition to routine care, plans by the nurse for the immediate postoperative care of a client who had a laryngectomy will focus on the need for:**

    1. Adequate fluid and electrolyte balance.
    2. Prevention of hemorrhage.
    3. Pain control.
    4. A patent airway.

    1. *Wrong choice. Although this will be an important postoperative assessment, there is another option that is more critical for the client's safety. The question is asking you to focus on the special needs of a laryngectomy client.*
    2. *Wrong. This is an important postoperative focus for ALL clients. This question asks for specific concerns for a laryngectomy client.*
    3. *No. This is not a priority intervention for a client after neck surgery.*
    4. *Excellent! A patent airway is an immediate priority for a postoperative client, especially after neck surgery.*

6. **A client has just delivered her first infant. He is jaundiced and has an elevated bilirubin. A diagnosis of ABO incompatibility is made. The client asks if she will be given RHoGAM to prevent this problem with future pregnancies. What is the best nursing response?**

    1. "We will have to await the results of blood work on you and the baby."
    2. "I will call the physician and see if he wants you to receive RHoGAM."
    3. "RHoGAM is only effective in preventing Rh antibodies."
    4. "Yes, you will get RHoGAM as soon as the lab completes the necessary crossmatch."

    1. *Wrong choice! RHoGAM has no effect on the prevention of ABO antibodies, only Rh antibodies. Therefore, she will not receive the drug.*
    2. *Incorrect! RHoGAM is never used in the treatment of an ABO incompatibility.*
    3. *Good! You seem to have a good understanding of the indications for the use of RHoGAM in preventing an Rh incompatibility with future pregnancies.*
    4. *Incorrect. RHoGAM is not indicated when an ABO incompatibility is the problem.*

7. **A 62-year-old male has just been transferred from ICU and is on telemetry. While counting the radial pulse, the nurse notes an irregular rhythm. The progress notes say that the client has had atrial flutter. Which pattern corresponds to this arrhythmia?**

    1. Ventricular rate of 82 with an atrial rate of 80.
    2. P waves occurring at .16 sec before each QRS complex.
    3. An atrial rate of 100, with 80 QRS complex/min.
    4. An irregular ventricular rate of 125, with a wide QRS pattern.

    1. *Incorrect. This is ventricular extrasystole.*
    2. *No, this is normal sinus rhythm.*
    3. *Correct. This indicates a lack of conduction between the atria and ventricles, which resulted in additional atrial beats that weren't conducted.*
    4. *No. You selected the life-threatening arrhythmia of ventricular tachycardia.*

8. **A 78-year-old client is admitted to the hospital for an exploratory laparotomy. The client's daughter says to the nurse, "I wish I could stay with my father, but I need to go home to see how my children are doing. I really hate to leave my father alone at this time." The best response by the nurse is:**

    1. "Your father needs opportunities to be independent. This will help him become self-sufficient."
    2. "Your father is capable of taking care of himself. Try to allow him more independence."
    3. "Stress is not good for your father at this time. Perhaps you could call your children."
    4. "You are feeling concern for both your dad and your children. Let me know when you are leaving, and I'll stay with him."

    1. *Wrong! This response is not focused on the client. The client in this question is the daughter, who has shared with the nurse her need to go home to see her children and her reluctance to leave her father. This response is focused on an inappropriate person.*
    2. *Incorrect! This is focused on an inappropriate person and an inappropriate issue. The client in this question is the daughter, who has shared with the nurse her need to go home to see her children and her reluctance to leave her father. This response is focused on the father, not the daughter. It also uses the communication block of giving advice.*
    3. *No! This is focused on an inappropriate person. The client in this question is the daughter, and her need to go home to check on her children is the issue. There is no data to indicate that the father would find it stressful if his daughter went home, or that his condi-*

tion requires the daughter to remain constantly at the hospital. Also, this response uses the communication block of giving advice, and denies the daughter the opportunity to make her own decision and to meet her own needs.

4. *Excellent! This option illustrates the tools of showing empathy and offering self. The client in this question is the daughter. The issue is her need to go home to check on her children. This response recognizes her feelings about both her father and her children. In offering to stay with the father while she is away, the nurse is offering self.*

9. **A 55-year-old client is hospitalized following myocardial infarction. He is to be transferred from a cart to a bed in a room in your unit. When transferring the client from a cart to his bed, the priority action is which of the following?**

   1. Have the client place his arms on his chest.
   2. Lock the wheels on the cart and the bed.
   3. Have at least four people to help with the transfer.
   4. Use a draw sheet to move the client.

   1. *Wrong. Although placing the arms across the chest helps protect the arms from injury, this option is not the priority action which the stem of the question is asking for.*
   2. *Right! Locking the wheels prevents the client from falling to the floor by not allowing the cart or bed to move apart or away from the client. This is the priority action for transferring a client.*
   3. *Four people may or may not be the number needed for a transfer. The number will depend on the size of the client and the size of the persons performing the transfer. The case scenario does not provide enough information for this to be the correct option.*
   4. *Wrong. A draw sheet is often used to transfer clients between two level horizontal surfaces; however, this is neither a requirement or a priority action.*

10. **A six-month-old male infant with AIDS has a nursing diagnosis of "Altered Growth and Development" on the care plan. Which of the following will most enhance the growth and development of the child?**

    1. Encourage the child to eat whatever he wants.
    2. Provide therapy to help the child meet developmental milestones.
    3. Provide nutritional supplements in addition to an adequate diet.
    4. Weigh and measure the infant on a frequent basis.

    1. *No, this is not the best answer.*
    2. *No. Think about Maslow's hierarchy of needs. What need has priority here?*

3. *Yes, that's right. If this child is behind in measurable ways on growth and development, his nutritional needs cannot be met by food alone. He needs extra supplements to help him fight infection and grow.*
4. *No, this doesn't answer the question. These are assessments or means of evaluating responses, but they are not actions to improve or correct the alteration in growth and development.*

11. **Which statement written by a laryngectomy client preparing for discharge would indicate to the nurse that he needs further teaching?**

    1. "I'll remember to buy non-aerosol products for personal grooming."
    2. "I sure will miss taking showers from now on."
    3. "Giving up swimming won't bother me, since I never learned how in the first place."
    4. "I never thought that belching could be transferred into speech, but I'm learning quickly."

    1. *No, the client is correct when he writes this. Clients with a tracheostomy should avoid using aerosol products, which could accidentally be inhaled. He understands his teaching.*
    2. *Yes, this is the inaccurate statement. Clients with a tracheostomy can shower or take a tub bath, as long as care is taken to avoid aspirating water into the opening. The client will need to have his teaching reinforced to include this important fact.*
    3. *No, the client is correct when he writes this. Clients with a tracheostomy should be told to avoid swimming. Remember the risk of aspiration through the opening! This client understands the information given to him.*
    4. *No, this can be an accurate statement made by a tracheostomy client who is learning esophageal speech. Air is swallowed and then moved quickly back up through the esophagus. Clients learn to coordinate lip and tongue movements with the sound produced by the air passing over vibrating folds of the esophagus.*

12. **A three-year-old boy is hospitalized with a broken leg. In assessing the client, the nurse might expect to observe three of the following behaviors about the client. Which behavior would the nurse least expect to observe?**

    1. When offered a toy, the client says, "No," but takes the toy and begins to play with it.
    2. When his mother goes for lunch, he plays quietly, but when she goes home at night he cries for her.
    3. He wets the bed at night, even though his mother says he hasn't had an "accident" in six months.
    4. He plays well with boys his age and slightly older, but refuses to play with girls his own age.

1. *The client's negativism, which results from his growing independence, is typical of behavior the nurse might observe in a three-year-old. This expected behavior is not the answer, because the question has a false response stem.*

2. *Separation anxiety is typical for this age child. This expected behavior is not the answer, because this question has a false response stem. The answer will be something the nurse would NOT expect to observe.*

3. *Regression to previous behaviors and levels of functioning is common when children are hospitalized. Since the question has a false response stem, this option is a distractor and not the answer.*

4. *Correct choice! You would not expect a three-year-old boy to refuse to play with girls of the same age. Three-year-olds do enjoy parallel play and beginning interaction with other children of either sex. (Older children tend to select playmates of the same sex, and then there is little interest in relationships with children of the opposite sex until adolescence.) This unexpected behavior is the correct answer because the question has a false response stem.*

13. **To monitor a client for the most common complication arising from the administration of total parenteral nutrition, the nurse should do which of the following?**

   1. Weigh the client at the same time each day using the same scale.
   2. Keep accurate records of total intake and total output.
   3. Determine the increase or decrease in body weight each day.
   4. Take the client's temperature at least every four hours.

   1. *Try again. The issue in this question is TPN. Weighing the client daily is an appropriate nursing action to assess whether the primary purpose of TPN is being met, but the stem is asking you to select a nursing action that monitors for the most common complication. Poor weight gain can be a problem, but it is not a complication. Note also that the same idea is expressed in Option 3; similar distractors must be wrong and can be eliminated.*

   2. *Wrong. The idea in this option is to record intake and output. This is an appropriate nursing action, but it does not monitor for the most common complication.*

   3. *Weighing the client daily to assess weight and nutritional status is an appropriate nursing action, but it is not the answer to the question. The issue is TPN, and the stem asks you to select a nursing action that monitors for the most common complication. Note that the same idea is expressed in Option 1. Similar distractors must be wrong and can be eliminated.*

4. *Yes, you are correct! Catheter related infections are the most common complication. Taking the client's temperature at least every four hours is the nursing action that monitors for the most common complication.*

> **STRATEGY ALERT!** Note that Options 1 and 3 are very similar to each other—so neither of them can be correct!

14. **A 70-year-old client is admitted to the hospital following a stroke. He has paralysis of the right side and is at risk of developing decubitus ulcers. In caring for this client, which of the following actions by the nurse is appropriate?**

   1. Move the client up in bed by sliding him.
   2. Roll the client to his side once a day.
   3. Change the client's position every two hours.
   4. Keep the client in a wheelchair during the morning and afternoon hours.

   1. *No. Sliding the client causes friction between the sheets and the client, resulting in possible damage to the skin, and possible infection.*

   2. *Try again! The client must be turned to different positions, at least every two hours, to prevent bed sores.*

   3. *Yes! Changing the client's position every two hours helps prevent bed sores.*

   4. *This is an incorrect action, because keeping the client in a wheelchair most of the day can cause bed sores due to lack of circulation to the areas of skin that are in constant contact with the wheelchair.*

15. **An eight-year-old client was admitted to the hospital with a diagnosis of acute rheumatic fever. Immediately after admission, which of the following assessments by the nurse is most important?**

   1. Auscultation of the rate and characteristics of heart sounds.
   2. Determining the location and severity of joint pain.
   3. Identifying the degree of anxiety related to the diagnosis.
   4. Determining the family's emotional and financial needs.

   1. *Excellent! This is the priority assessment because tachycardia and cardiac murmur indicate cardiac involvement. Cardiac involvement may lead to serious and life-threatening complications.*

   2. *Wrong! Pain in one or more joints is characteristic of rheumatic fever. Joint pain is not life-threatening, however, and since there are usually no permanent sequelae, this assessment is not the priority assessment.*

3. *Wrong! Anxiety related to the diagnosis of rheumatic fever and the symptoms and treatment of rheumatic fever is expected. Such anxiety is not life-threatening, however, so during the initial assessment, this would not be the priority.*

4. *No! The length and cost of the treatment needed for rheumatic fever place a burden on the family's emotional and financial resources. However, this would not be the top priority during the initial assessment.*

16. **Which manifestations can the nurse expect to observe in a client admitted with emphysema?**

1. Dyspnea, bradycardia.
2. Barrel chest, shallow respirations.
3. Cyanosis, productive cough.
4. Asymmetrical chest, dry cough.

1. *Wrong. Although dyspnea is seen in clients with emphysema, bradycardia is not. The heart rate will increase as the heart tries to compensate for less oxygen to the tissues.*

2. **Correct assessment! Clients with emphysema lose lung elasticity, the diaphragm becomes permanently flattened by overdistention of the lungs, the muscles of the rib cage become rigid, and the ribs flare outward. This produces the "barrel chest" typical of emphysema clients. Respirations are also shallow because of decreased lung elasticity.**

3. *Incorrect. Clients with emphysema often have skin that is pink in color. Emphysema clients have only a small amount of mucous, unlike the client with bronchitis.*

4. *No, clients with emphysema would not have an asymmetrical (unequal) chest. The chest wall, although altered in shape, is not unequal. Remember that an asymmetrical chest occurs when two or more ribs are fractured, leading to unequal movement of the chest wall on inspiration and expiration. A dry cough may be present, but is not a characteristic sign.*

17. **Many groups of drugs are associated with a life-threatening abstinence syndrome. The nurse understands that which drug group is least likely to present a medical crisis during withdrawal?**

1. Narcotics.
2. Barbiturates.
3. Alcohol.
4. Benzodiazepines.

1. **Correct. The abstinence syndrome following narcotic abuse is uncomfortable, but is not life-threatening.**

2. *This is not correct. The abstinence syndrome associated with barbiturate abuse can involve seizures and lead to death.*

3. *This is not correct. Alcohol withdrawal can involve seizures and lead to death if not medically managed.*

4. *This is not correct. The abstinence syndrome associated with the prolonged use of benzodiazepine anti-anxiety agents can involve seizures and lead to death.*

18. **A 20-day-old infant is recovering from surgery for pyloric stenosis. The client's mother asked the nurse, "Now that my son has had this surgery, is it likely that pyloric stenosis will cause trouble later?" Which of the following is the most appropriate response to the client's statement?**

1. "Why don't you talk to the doctor about your uncertainties regarding your son's future?"
2. "He might develop obstructive symptoms later. If so, take him immediately to an emergency room."
3. "He will not have symptoms again in childhood, but may have digestive difficulties in his adult life."
4. "Recurrence of the obstruction or repetition of the surgical procedure would be unlikely."

1. *Wrong! This is a communication block that places the client's concerns on hold. An answer to the client's question is within the realm of nursing. The nurse should address the issue here and now.*

2. *Wrong! This answer provides incorrect information. A child who has had a surgical repair of pyloric stenosis is not likely to develop obstructive symptoms later. There is no need to evoke fear in the mother by responding in this way.*

3. *The words "will not" make this an absolute statement which is wrong. The primary symptom of pyloric stenosis, projectile vomiting, can be caused by a variety of factors. It is incorrect for the nurse to say that the client will not have this symptom again.*

4. **Good choice! This option is the correct answer because the nurse is providing correct information. Following surgical repair of pyloric stenosis, recurrence of the obstruction or the surgical procedure is not expected.**

19. **A client is seen in the clinic in the 28th week of gestation. Her blood pressure is 160/100 and she has 2+ protein in her urine. She complains that all her shoes are too tight. Her doctor recommends hospitalization. The admitting nurse must select a bed for the new client. Each room on the unit is a semiprivate room. Which of the following roommates would be best for the client?**

1. A 20-year-old primigravida who enjoys loud rock-and-roll music.
2. A 32-year-old multigravida who enjoys reading romance novels.
3. A 24-year-old C-section who watches soap operas and game shows on TV.

4. A 22-year-old primigravida who has many visitors during the afternoon and evening.

1. *Wrong. The client has symptoms of preeclampsia, including hypertension, proteinuria, and ankle edema. Because of the hypertension and danger of seizures, the best environment for her is one that will facilitate rest and relaxation. The roommate in this option will increase the noise in the environment. The same is true of the roommates in Options 3 and 4, and these similar distractors should be eliminated.*

2. *You selected the right answer! The client has symptoms of preeclampsia including hypertension, proteinuria, and ankle edema. Because of the hypertension, there is a danger of seizures. The best environment for her is one that will facilitate rest and relaxation. A roommate who likes quiet activities such as reading will be best.*

> **STRATEGY ALERT!** In each of the other three options, the roommate will increase the noise in the environment. These similar distractors should all be eliminated.

3. *Wrong. The client has symptoms of preeclampsia including hypertension, proteinuria, and ankle edema. Because of the hypertension and danger of seizures, the best environment for her is one that will facilitate rest and relaxation. The roommate in this option will increase the noise in the environment. The same is true of the roommates in Options 1 and 4, and these similar distractors should be eliminated.*

4. *The client has symptoms of preeclampsia including hypertension, proteinuria, and ankle edema. Because of the hypertension and danger of seizures, the best environment for her is one that will facilitate rest and relaxation. The roommate in this option will increase the noise in the environment. The same is true of the roommates in Options 1 and 3, and these similar distractors should be eliminated.*

20. **The nurse should monitor the client taking ethambutol (Myambutol) for which of the following?**

1. Urine output.
2. Jaundice.
3. Visual acuity.
4. Arrhythmias.

1. *Although ethambutol is excreted in the urine, it is not toxic to the kidneys. Try again.*

2. *Ethambutol does not significantly affect the metabolism of the liver. Choose another option.*

3. *Correct! A significant adverse effect of ethambutol is optic neuritis. Baseline vision testing should be performed before use. This drug is not recommended for children under 13 because of the difficulty of assessing visual changes.*

4. *No, Ethambutol is not associated with arrhythmias. Try again.*

21. **After one week in an eating disorders program, a client has gained three pounds. She confides to the nurse that she has begun to have the urge to vomit after eating. How can the nurse best handle this?**

1. Praise the client for having enough trust in the nurse to share this concern.
2. Establish a contract with the client to seek out a staff member to talk about her feelings after eating including her urge to vomit.
3. Remove her privileges if she vomits to reinforce that this behavior is not appropriate.
4. Suggest she share this concern during her next group therapy session.

1. *This response is not incorrect, but it is not the best option.*

2. *Correct. Talking with a staff member will shift her focus from vomiting, to the emotional issues associated with her eating disorder. Seeking out a staff member will also prevent her from following through on her urge to vomit.*

3. *This is not correct. The behavioral program consists of a weight gain protocol with privileges awarded or taken away based on the client's daily weight gain or loss.*

4. *This response is not incorrect, because she would receive helpful feedback from the other members. There is a better option, however, that deals more directly with the problem.*

22. **A 55-year-old client has been taking trifluoperazine (Stelazine) for five years to control her paranoid thoughts. The client asks her psychiatrist to change her medication to clozapine (Clozaril) because she is worried about developing tardive dyskinesia. What information should she be given about taking Clozaril drug safely?**

1. Monthly blood levels have to be taken to monitor the dose.
2. Drug holidays should be taken periodically.
3. Weekly white blood counts have to be done.
4. Monthly AIMS testing is indicated.

1. *Wrong. Blood levels are monitored for clients on lithium to make sure their lithium level is within the therapeutic range. This is done weekly, for the first month, and then every three to six months.*

2. *This is not the best option for this question. Drug holidays are often recommended for clients on antipsychotic drugs to assess for beginning signs of tardive dyskinesia. Clozaril appears less likely to cause TD than other antipsychotic drugs.*

3. *Correct. A particularly severe, life-threatening, form of agranulocytosis is associated with Clozaril. Weekly monitoring of the WBC is essential, even though the occurrence of this adverse effect is quite rare. These blood tests substantially increase the cost of taking this medication.*

4. *Incorrect. AIMS (Abnormal Involuntary Movement Scale) testing monitors clients on antipsychotics for symptoms indicative of tardive dyskinesia. Clozapine is chemically different from other antipsychotics and appears less likely to cause TD.*

23. **A 35-year-old man was in an automobile accident. Initial assessment revealed fractures of the left femur and pelvis and a large contusion on the head. What should be the nurse's priority assessment in order to determine the client's neurological status?**

1. Pupillary responses.
2. Verbal responses.
3. Limb movements.
4. Level of consciousness.

1. *Wrong! The nurse might do this assessment to determine the client's neurological status, but this is not the best answer.*

2. *Wrong! The nurse might do this assessment to determine the client's neurological status, but this is not the best answer.*

3. *Incorrect! The nurse might do this assessment to determine the client's neurological status, but this is not the best answer.*

4. **You are correct! Assessing the client's level of consciousness includes an assessment of verbal responses, limb movements and pupillary responses.**

> **STRATEGY ALERT!** *This is the most inclusive or global response, so this is the best option.*

24. **In planning care for a client prior to delivery, which of the following nursing orders would be most appropriate?**

1. Assess fluid balance hourly and maintain optimum placental perfusion.
2. Monitor urine output and assure a brief rest period each shift.
3. Check the blood pressure before and after each time the client is out of bed.
4. Observe for amount of edema and provide for diversionary activities.

1. **Excellent! Fluid balance has a relationship to blood pressure and should be assessed frequently. Assessment of fluid balance should include recording of intake and output, measurement of**

blood pressure, and observation of amount of edema. To maintain optimum placental perfusion, the nurse should assist the client to turn from side to side, but remain in a lateral position. This is the best choice for a nursing order for a client's plan of care.

2. *No! Monitoring urine output is an important assessment, because oliguria could indicate renal damage in a client with pregnancy induced hypertension. However, output should be monitored more frequently than once a shift. Also, the client should be on bed rest to decrease the need for oxygen by the cells, which will decrease cardiac workload. A brief rest period every shift is not adequate.*

3. *Not the best choice! The blood pressure should be monitored frequently. If the blood pressure is too high, drugs may be used to control it. However, the client should be on bed rest to decrease the need for oxygen by the cells, which will decrease cardiac workload. The client should not be getting out of bed for activities.*

4. *The nurse should observe for the amount of edema and should provide diversionary activities for the client. However, this is not the best answer to this test question. Look for another answer which is broader or more global.*

25. **Which of the following statements by the nurse indicates the best understanding of the principles of reality orientation?**

1. "Good morning, Mr. Edwards. Did you sleep well? It's time to get dressed."
2. "Good morning. This is your second day in Shady Pines and I am your nurse for the day."
3. "Do you remember who I am? We met yesterday when you were admitted."
4. "Good morning, how are you? I am your nurse for the day. Is there anything I can do for you right now?"

1. *This is not correct because it does not orient the client to anything other than his name. Also, the nurse does not wait for the client to answer the initial question before telling him it is time to get dressed. Short statements, made one at a time, should be used with persons who have memory and other cognitive deficits.*

2. **Correct. This statement orients to client to time of day, place and the nurse's identity. It also is a clear statement that does not contain any irrelevant information that could be confusing to the client.**

3. *This is not correct. The client with memory deficits will probably not recognize or remember meeting the nurse the previous day.*

4. *This is not correct. There is a better option.*

26. **Twenty-four hours after admission for viral gastroenteritis, a four-year-old has a temperature of 101° F. What should the nurse do in response to this data?**

    1. Keep the child warm with blankets.
    2. Apply a hypothermia blanket.
    3. Document the temperature.
    4. Call the physician immediately with these findings.

    1. *No, this will further elevate the temperature.*
    2. *No, this fever does not warrant the use of a hypothermia blanket.*
    3. *Yes, that's all that is necessary at this time. Twenty-four hours after admission for a viral illness, this degree of temperature elevation is a common finding.*
    4. *No, not necessary for this degree of temperature in the absence of other data.*

27. **A 72-year-old client has a draining pressure sore. The culture of the drainage reveals staphylococci. Which action during the care of this client should be the nurse's highest priority?**

    1. Reinforce the pressure dressing with a sterile towel before ambulating the client.
    2. Wear gown and gloves when changing the client's bed linen.
    3. Use sterile technique when changing the dressing on the pressure sore.
    4. Do not allow the client the use of his personal effects until they have been sterilized.

    1. *No. Reinforcing the dressing will not prevent the spread of the pathogens.*
    2. *Right! The nurse should always wear a gown and gloves when changing the client's bed linen. The rationale for this is to prevent the spread of pathogens, which may attach to the nurse's clothing during the bed change. When the nurse goes to another client's room, there is no threat of contaminating that client with this client's pathogens. This question is a prioritizing question. Since no physiological need is identified, the priority is safety. By this action, the nurse will provide the safest environment.*
    3. *Sterile technique will help prevent secondary pathogens from infecting the wound, but will not prevent the spread of the pathogens.*
    4. *Sterilizing the client's linen and personal effects will not prevent the spread of the pathogens.*

28. **A person in a restaurant puts his hand to his throat. A nurse who sees this happen begins to administer the Heimlich maneuver. After the client falls to the floor the nurse should next:**

    1. Check for the pulse.
    2. Sweep the mouth.
    3. Attempt to ventilate.
    4. Administer five abdominal thrusts.

    1. *Incorrect. If there is no air moving, it is not appropriate to progress to the pulse check.*
    2. *Correct. The mouth sweep is performed in case the object is high enough in the oral cavity to allow for removal.*
    3. *No. This is not the correct sequence as taught by the American Heart Association or the Red Cross.*
    4. *Not yet. Several steps are missing; rethink this and try again.*

29. **A chronic alcoholic has been hospitalized following a drinking binge. The nurse enters the room and finds the client shouting in a terrified voice, "Get those ants out of my room!" Which of the following statements would be most appropriate at this time?**

    1. "Tell me more about the ants that you see in your room."
    2. "I'm sure that the ants you see will not harm you."
    3. "I don't see any ants, but you seem very frightened."
    4. "I do not see anything. This is part of your illness."

    1. *This option is an inappropriate response because it reinforces the client's hallucination.*
    2. *This option is inappropriate because it reinforces the client's hallucination.*
    3. *Very good! This response presents reality. ("I don't see any ants.") Also, this response illustrates the therapeutic communication tool of showing empathy. By saying, "You seem frightened," the nurse acknowledges the client's feelings.*

    > **STRATEGY ALERT!** Note that the test-taking strategy of looking for similar words in the stem and one of the options would be effective here. The words "frightened" and "terrified" are similar.

    4. *Wrong! In this option the nurse attempts to present reality. ("I do not see anything.") However, the statement of reality should be more specific. ("I don't see any ants.") Also, the response is not empathetic. The nurse should acknowledge the client's feelings.*

30. **The nurse understands that health education is important for persons with stress-related illnesses. After giving a client information about his medications, treatment options, and the role stress plays in his illness, the nurse realizes that the client will most likely follow the treatment plan under which of the following circumstances?**

1. If the nurse refers the client for supportive psychotherapy.
2. If the nurse involves the client in the treatment planning process.
3. If the nurse asks the client if she may speak with his wife.
4. If the nurse recommends that he come in for weekly appointments to review his progress.

1. This is not correct. Some clients may benefit from supportive psychotherapy, but most do not require it unless they have additional mental health problems. A supportive relationship with a health care provider can help the client to cope effectively with the stresses that aggravate the illness.
2. Correct. The client is most likely to follow the treatment plan when he or she has participated in identifying specific problems, setting goals, and choosing the actions needed to work towards those goals.
3. The spouse or other close family members do need information about the client's condition and recommended care, but this is not the best option for this question. Identify the option that will best help the client to comply with his treatment regime.
4. This may be a good approach, but it is not the best option to help the client comply with his treatment regime.

31. Following a CVA, which affected the left side of his brain, a 71-year-old client has his tube feedings discontinued and is ready to begin oral feedings. Which of the following nursing measures ensures client tolerance?

1. Feed from right side of mouth; upright position; mouth care before feeding.
2. Verbal encouragement; check gag reflex; feed thinned foods and liquids.
3. Check gag reflex; feed on left side of mouth; upright position.
4. Sensory stimulation; verbal encouragement; favorite foods.

1. No. This answer suggests feeding on his affected side.
2. Incorrect. Thinned foods and liquids are poorly handled by the client with dysphagia. Thickened liquids and soft foods are best.
3. Excellent reasoning! This includes the important points of: checking to make sure the client will be able to sense the food; approaching it from the unaffected side (with left-brain injury, right-sided involvement would be expected); and feeding in the upright position, which best avoids choking.
4. No. Sensory stimulation may actually be counterproductive. Although none of these actions is completely wrong, they do not answer the question. Select again.

32. A five-year-old client has just returned from cardiac catheterization. The right femoral artery was used for the procedure. What is the first nursing responsibility?

1. Elevate to high Fowler's position, to improve ventilation.
2. Place the client on the cardiac monitor, to assess for arrhythmias.
3. Assess for dehydration, since the client has been NPO eight hours.
4. Evaluate the catheter insertion site for bleeding.

1. No, this is actually contraindicated initially, because this would impede blood flow through the femoral artery.
2. No, this is not a routine for post-catheterization care, unless there were arrhythmias during the procedure.
3. Important, but not the priority. Dehydration is a potential complication and does require assessment of input and output, skin turgor and mucous membranes.
4. Yes, the essential action is to assess the pulse and observe for any evidence of bleeding, either a hematoma or oozing.

33. A client is to begin taking quinidine (Quinatime) 200 mg p.o. every six hours for maintenance treatment of paroxysmal atrial tachycardia (PAT). The nurse will observe for which of the following common side effects associated with quinidine therapy?

1. Diarrhea.
2. Vertigo.
3. Rashes.
4. Fever.

1. Yes. Diarrhea is one of the most frequently occurring side effects of quinidine therapy, a Class IA drug. Other GI symptoms include nausea, cramping, and anorexia. If oral quinidine causes GI upset, the drug may be given with food.
2. Incorrect. Vertigo can occur as a side effect of quinidine therapy, but it is less frequent than another option listed.
3. No. Rashes are not a common side effect of quinidine therapy. Choose another option.
4. Wrong choice. Fever may occur with quinidine therapy, but is not common. Make another selection.

34. Soon after being admitted to a rehabilitation unit following a drinking binge, a client says to the nurse, "I don't really need to be here. My wife and family make me drink. My wife spends all my

money. My kid just had an accident with his car, which cost me a fortune in repairs." Which of the following is the most appropriate response by the nurse at this time?

1. "Tell me more about your wife spending all your money."
2. "How did your child's car accident cost you money?"
3. "It sounds like you have financial difficulties."
4. "Tell me more about your concern about being here."

1. *This response illustrates the non-therapeutic communication block of focusing on inappropriate issues or persons. It is focused on the client's wife, and on money. The issue is the client's alcoholism.*
2. *This response illustrates the non-therapeutic communication block of focusing on inappropriate issues or persons. It is focused on the client's child, and on money. The issue is the client's alcoholism.*
3. *This response illustrates the non-therapeutic communication block of focusing on inappropriate issues. It is focused on the client's financial difficulties. The issue is the client's alcoholism.*
4. ***Correct answer! The client is a chronic alcoholic who is in denial. This response is therapeutic because it focuses on the client's feelings about not needing to be in the hospital.***

> **STRATEGY ALERT!** Note that Options 1, 2 and 3 are similar distractors that focus on financial difficulties.

35. In the pediatric clinic the nurse is working with a family whose three-month-old has been recently diagnosed as having cerebral palsy. Which of the following statements by the mother would indicate that teaching about the disorder has been effective?

1. "I know that our baby will get worse, because I have seen older children with this disorder."
2. "I am hopeful that the early schooling will increase his ability for self-care."
3. "My husband and I plan to be tested prior to our next baby to predict the possibility of a similar outcome."
4. I am going to ask the doctor to prescribe skeletal muscle relaxants to improve my child's functioning."

1. *No. Cerebral palsy is a static neurologic dysfunction. The appearance of deterioration is due to our expectations of increasing gross and fine motor control as a child grows, rather than an actual decrease in function.*
2. ***Correct!! Early intervention programs that include speech and physical therapies provide the best intervention available and the greatest po-***

tential for independence, which is always a goal in chronic conditions.
3. *No. Cerebral palsy is not hereditary. Select another option.*
4. *No, this is too general to be correct. Skeletal muscle relaxants are limited to use with spastic cerebral palsy. Usually they are used only briefly and with older children or adolescents. These drugs do not significantly improve functioning.*

36. A client is admitted to the hospital with an infection of her right arm that requires an incision and drainage. Which of the following nursing actions is most appropriate?

1. Wear gloves only when coming in contact with drainage or soiled articles.
2. Assess the wound to determine what infection control measures are needed to care for the client.
3. Wear a gown if there is a possibility of the nurse's clothing becoming contaminated by drainage or secretions.
4. Wash hands before and after care.

1. *Wrong choice! This action is appropriate to prevent transferring organisms to the nurse or other clients. The other options are also appropriate in caring for this isolation client. This is a prioritizing question. Which of the choices should take priority? Can you identify one which is different from the others?*
2. ***Very good. Assessing the situation should be done before implementing any nursing action. All of the choices are appropriate actions. Which of the choices in this prioritizing question should take priority? In comparing the options, this option is the priority because the nursing process identifies that the nurse should always assess first.***

> **TEST-TAKING TIP:** When you cannot choose the correct option using your nursing knowledge alone, the option that is different from the others may be the correct answer. This option is different because it involves assessing, while the other options involve implementation.

3. *Wrong choice. The nurse should wear a gown in this instance. All of the choices are correct actions. This is a prioritizing question. Which of the options would take priority?*
4. *This is standard nursing protocol for almost any situation. All the options are correct actions, but this option is not the correct choice. This is a prioritizing question. Which of the options would take priority?*

37. Which of the following lab values would the nurse expect is most likely to be found in a client needing calcium gluconate?

1. Magnesium level 8 mEq/L.
2. Calcium level 6 mEq/L.
3. Magnesium level 2 mEq/L.
4. Potassium level 3 mEq/L.

1. *Good choice! A magnesium level of 8 mEq/L is indicative of magnesium toxicity and warrants administration of an antidote such as calcium gluconate.*
2. *Wrong choice! A calcium level of 6 mEq/L is already elevated and administration of calcium gluconate would be dangerous.*
3. *Wrong choice! A magnesium level of 2 mEq/L is considered within a normal range.*
4. *Sorry, try again! A potassium level of 3 mEq/L is considered normal, and even if it was elevated (i.e., above 5 mEq/L) the administration of calcium gluconate would not be used to treat it.*

38. **In preparing a client to be discharged, the nurse teaches him to position himself for postural drainage. To achieve success in this teaching program, which of the following information about the client is most important?**

1. The type of bed the client will be using at home for the procedure.
2. The amount of time required for the client to change positions.
3. The client's goal concerning his ability to be self-sufficient.
4. The client's ability to move about without assistance from others.

1. *Not the best choice! The type of bed the client will be using at home is important information, since a mechanical bed greatly facilitates the procedure. However, postural drainage can be done without a mechanical bed, using things normally found in the home such as pillows and a straight-back chair. The key word in the stem of this question is "most." Which of the priority setting guidelines should be applied in answering this question?*
2. *The amount of time required for the client to change positions is important, but it is not the "most important." Look at the other options. Which of the priority setting guidelines should be applied in answering this question?*
3. *Excellent! The client's motivation and goals are essential for success, and they are a primary concern in any teaching program. Teaching/learning theory tells us that if the client is not motivated or goal directed, the discharge teaching program is unlikely to be effective.*

> **STRATEGY ALERT!** *This option is also more general than any of the other options, which refer to very specific assessments. This is the global response option.*

4. *The client's ability to move about without assistance from others is important, but it is not the "most important" consideration. Which of the priority setting guidelines should be used in answering this question? What is the priority according to those guidelines?*

39. **A 10-year-old boy is in sickle cell crisis. Which of the following nursing actions is contraindicated?**

1. Administer oxygen via nasal cannula as prescribed.
2. Encourage the client to increase oral fluid intake.
3. Administer narcotics only for very severe pain.
4. Encourage as much exercise as possible during the crisis.

1. *Incorrect choice. Hemoglobin S forms a sickled shape in the presence of low oxygen tension, and oxygen is administered to prevent the condition of low oxygen tension. This appropriate action is not the answer to this false response stem.*
2. *Wrong. High fluid intake prevents dehydration, which would encourage aggregation of the cells and vaso-occlusion. This appropriate action is not the answer to this false response stem.*
3. *Wrong choice. Relief of pain is an important goal during a sickle cell crisis. Physical measures, such as application of heat, should be used whenever they are effective. If physical measures are not effective, non-narcotic analgesics should be tried. Narcotics are administered only for severe pain which is not relieved by physical measures and non-narcotic analgesics. Clients with sickle cell anemia are likely to have pain over an extended period of time, and addiction may become a problem.*
4. *Correct, encouraging exercise during a sickle cell crisis would be contraindicated! During a sickle cell crisis, exercise should be kept to a minimum. Clients are usually placed on bed rest to decrease the need for oxygen by the cells. Note that the word "crisis" appears in the stem of the question and in the correct answer.*

40. **A client is recuperating from gallbladder surgery in which general anesthesia was administered. The nurse should encourage the client to use the incentive spirometry a minimum of how many times per hour?**

1. Two.
2. Five to 10.
3. 10-15.
4. 20-25.

1. *Incorrect. Twice an hour would not be an efficient use of incentive spirometry to decrease the risk of atelectasis and/or pneumonia.*
2. *Good choice. Clients should use incentive spirom-*

etry five to 10 times every hour. This device is designed to motivate the client to take deep breaths, and should be included in the postoperative plan of care.

3. *No, this number of times may tire the client and lead to decreased compliance.*

4. *No, this is beyond the reasonable expectation for a postoperative client. Postoperative breathing exercises must be balanced with turning, coughing, and the client's need for rest.*

41. **To reduce the risk of a serious interaction, the nurse would instruct a client taking cefoperazone (Cefobid) to avoid which of the following?**

1. Wine.
2. Orange juice.
3. Food.
4. Maalox.

1. *Correct! When Cefobid is taken with alcohol, acetaldehyde is raised in the blood and produces an Antabuse-like reaction with gastrointestinal symptoms. Avoid the use of alcohol or any over-the-counter medicines that contain alcohol when this medication is involved.*

2. *This is incorrect. Fruit juices are known for their effect when combined with penicillins, not with cefoperazone. Try again.*

3. *Wrong choice! Cephalosporins may be taken with food with no ill effects.*

4. *This is false! Antacids have no effect.*

42. **A client complains that he is unable to rest because of the noise from the television being used by the other client in the room. The best action by the nurse is which of the following?**

1. Have the client moved to a private room.
2. Provide ear phones for the client who is watching television.
3. Explain that the roommate is hard of hearing, so the television is louder than usual.
4. Ask the roommate to shut off the television so the client can rest.

1. *Wrong, moving the client to a private room would eliminate the noisy television. The client, however, would need input to determine if his insurance will cover the cost of a private room, and if not, whether he is willing to pay the difference. This is not the best action by the nurse at this time.*

2. *Correct. Providing ear phones provides both clients with a solution to the problem.*

3. *Wrong! Explaining the action of the roommate indicates to the client that his concerns are not important since nothing is being done to decrease the noise.*

4. *Wrong! Telling the roommate to turn off the television interferes with the roommate's right to watch television.*

43. **In the emergency room a 10-year-old child is admitted with salicylate poisoning. Which is the first step for the nurse to take in the treatment of this client?**

1. Prevent the absorption of poison.
2. Determine the number of tablets ingested.
3. Assess the child.
4. Pass a Levine tube and prepare for lavage.

1. *No, by the time the child is brought to the emergency room there is little chance that absorption can be avoided.*

2. *No, not the first priority.*

3. *Yes, assessment is always the first response, the nurse is initiating the nursing process.*

4. *No, although you may do this procedure, this is not the initial nursing priority. Make an another selection.*

44. **While administering a bed bath to a postoperative client, it is important to maintain privacy. Which of the following is the best method for the nurse to use in maintaining the client's privacy?**

1. Allow the client to wear a gown, and reach under the gown with the washcloth and towel to bathe the client.
2. Use towels to protect the bed linen.
3. Cover the client with a bath blanket and expose only the portion of the body that is being bathed.
4. Use the bed sheet to cover the client during the bath.

1. *This is not correct. The gown should be removed when performing a bed bath. It does not absorb water well and may cause the client to become chilled. The gown is not clean and may be soiled, which would defeat one of the purposes of the bath, which is to cleanse the skin.*

2. *Using towels to protect the bed linen is appropriate during a bed bath; however, the stem of the question asks about maintaining the client's privacy. This option does not address the issue in the question.*

3. *Correct! The nurse should provide privacy by exposing only the portion of the body that is being bathed. A bath blanket should be used because it provides a covering for the client which absorbs water and avoids chilling of the client.*

4. *Wrong choice! While the bed sheet may provide privacy for the client, it does not absorb water well and will result in the client's being chilled.*

45. **A 56-year-old male client diagnosed with complete heart block had a demand pacemaker inserted today. The pacer is set for 72 beats/min. Which EKG pattern indicates to the nurse a failure to capture?**

1. QRS complexes occurring at a rate of 73 beats/min and no sharp spikes.
2. Sharp spikes at 72 per min; QRS complexes at 50 beats/min.
3. P waves at a rate of 78 per min; QRS complexes at 72 beats/min.
4. QRS complexes at a rate of 100 beat/min.

1. *No, this indicates a heart beat above the pacemaker setting. The pacemaker is functioning correctly, sensing the heart beat which is greater than the pacer rate of 72.*
2. **Yes. The pacemaker is firing at the set rate, but the heart is only beating 50 times/min. This may be due to poor positioning of the pacer electrode and is referred to as "lack of capture."**
3. *No. This is a pattern of extra atrial contractions, and does not indicate any pacemaker activity.*
4. *Incorrect. This is the EKG pattern of a tachycardia. Nothing else can be determined from the information provided.*

46. **A 20-year-old college student comes to the campus health service complaining of severe epigastric distress. While doing an assessment, the nurse discovers that she has suffered from severe bulimia since her freshman year. The client tells the nurse, "I know my eating binges and vomiting are not normal, but I cannot do anything about them." What is the most therapeutic nursing response to the client's statement?**

1. "Do you have any idea why you do this?"
2. "Are you feeling pretty helpless about changing this behavior?"
3. "Have you noticed any pattern to your eating binges and vomiting?"
4. "You will stop because you have to. You are destroying your health."

1. *This is not correct. A question that asks "why" is very difficult for the client to answer. There is a better option.*
2. **Correct. The nurse is responding to the feelings the client has expressed. Clarifying feelings is an important first step prior to exploring how to deal with them more effectively.**
3. *This statement is not wrong, but there is a better option.*
4. *This is not correct. The nurse is giving advice in a way that could very well cause the client to feel misunderstood and unwilling to explore her problem further with the nurse.*

47. **A 72-year-old male has just been diagnosed with Parkinson's disease. Which of the following interventions should the nurse avoid?**

1. Plan gait training with physical therapy.
2. Help wife to assist with dressing.
3. Order between meal snacks high in fiber.
4. Ask him to read the newspaper aloud.

1. *Incorrect. This is an appropriate intervention that would be useful to prevent shuffling and propulsive gaits, which puts the client at risk for injury. Look for an INAPPROPRIATE intervention.*
2. **Terrific! This is not the best approach. To maintain ADL's, the client needs extra time without pressure to accomplish the tasks. You must have remembered that in any chronic disorder maintenance of self-care as long as possible is always the objective.**
3. *No, this is appropriate. Constipation and loss of weight are common problems for the client with Parkinson's disease. Look for an INAPPROPRIATE intervention.*
4. *No. Impaired verbal communication may be a result of Parkinson's disease. An intervention to help maintain intonation and articulation is to read aloud. Try to find an INAPPROPRIATE intervention.*

48. **A nine-year-old female is to be discharged tomorrow. She is being treated for rheumatic fever. Her symptoms are: temperature 100° F, pulse 120/min, and polyarthritis. Which instruction would the nurse anticipate giving to the client's parents?**

1. Administer penicillin as prescribed.
2. Utilize acetaminophen for joint pain to prevent the possibility of Reye's syndrome.
3. Allow her to resume normal activities as soon is joint pain is gone.
4. Teach CPR, because of the possibility of coronary artery sequelae.

1. **Yes. Penicillin is the drug of choice. It is given to treat the causative organism and then prophylactically for the rest of her life.**
2. *No, this isn't the most effective treatment for the joint pain. Acetaminophen would only be substituted for the more effective aspirin if there were indications of a viral infection. Prednisone may also be prescribed during the acute phase.*
3. *Only partially correct. The more reliable indicators for recovery are the pulse rate and temperature returning to normal, which indicate that carditis is resolved.*
4. *Coronary artery disease is a complication of Kawasaki disease. The complication of rheumatic fever is mitral and aortic valve stenosis.*

49. A client with atelectasis of the left lower lung is to receive intermittent positive pressure breathing (IPPB) four times a day. It would be appropriate for the nurse to instruct the client that:

    1. The treatment will last 45 minutes to an hour each time.
    2. Take short, quick breaths during the treatment to get the maximum benefit from the medication.
    3. The medication used in the treatment may cause nausea, so the physician has prescribed an antiemetic to be given beforehand.
    4. You should notice an increase in productive coughing during and after the treatment. This means that the medication is working.

    1. *Wrong. IPPB treatments are usually administered for 15 to 20 minutes at a time. This is to prevent tiring of the client and to decrease the risk of side effects from the medications.*
    2. *Wrong. The client is instructed to maintain a slow respiratory rate and to use diaphragmatic breathing during the IPPB treatment.*
    3. *Wrong. The medications used in the IPPB treatment may cause nausea and vomiting if administered too soon after meals. Prevention would mean scheduling the treatments so that they do not take place around mealtime. An antiemetic would therefore be unnecessary.*
    4. *Yes! Coughing is encouraged and indicates that the aerosol medication is liquefying the secretions. IPPB treatments may be followed by chest physiotherapy or postural drainage treatment. The end result is the effective removal of secretions that have accumulated in the lower respiratory tract.*

50. During heroin withdrawal, a client complains continuously to the nursing staff about his discomfort. One day the nurse overhears a nursing assistant say to the client, "You brought on these problems yourself by taking drugs. What did you think would happen when you continued to use heroin?" Which of the following comments to the nursing assistant would be most constructive?

    1. "Your comments were inappropriate. I will have to report this to the supervisor."
    2. "Weren't you a bit hard on this client? He is having a great deal of discomfort."
    3. "This client is getting on all our nerves."
    4. "I overheard you speaking with the client and I thought your comment about his causing his own problems was inappropriate. You have worked well with other addicted clients. What is different about this man?"

    1. *This is not correct. The nurse is responsible for supervising the nursing assistant's work. Therefore, the nurse also is responsible for dealing directly with him on matters that concern the care of*

clients. If the nurse and the nursing assistant are not able to resolve the issue, then approaching the nursing supervisor for consultation may be appropriate.
    2. *This is not the most constructive approach. The nurse's comment will not help the nursing assistant explore his own behavior so that he could deal more constructively with this client in the future.*
    3. *This is not correct. This statement ignores the nursing assistant's inappropriate comment to the client.*
    4. *Correct. The nurse is giving specific feedback about what was observed. The nurse also intervenes to focus the nursing assistant on his behavior in a way that could help him gain insight into his behavior and deal more constructively with this client in the future.*

51. A chronic alcoholic has been hospitalized following a drinking binge. During a lengthy conversation with the nurse about his long history of alcoholism, the client becomes tense and uncomfortable. Which of the following is the best initial response by the nurse?

    1. "What did I say to make you feel so uncomfortable?"
    2. "Drinking for a long time can make anyone feel uncomfortable."
    3. "At what point did you begin to feel uncomfortable?"
    4. "Talking about your drinking will help you to recover."

    1. *Wrong! This response is an illustration of the nontherapeutic communication block of focusing on an inappropriate person. The response is focused on the nurse rather than on the client. The nurse is also accepting responsibility for the client's feelings. Try again.*
    2. *Wrong! This response is an assumption by the nurse. The nurse should seek additional information (do an assessment) before stating the cause of the client's feelings.*
    3. *Right! This response illustrates the therapeutic communication tool of clarification. The nurse needs to gather more information about the client's feelings (do an assessment).*
    4. *Try again! This response illustrates the non-therapeutic communication block of giving advice. It also does not focus on the issue, which is the client's discomfort.*

52. A client who is 62 years old is scheduled for coronary artery bypass tomorrow. The physician has ordered aspirin 325 mg daily. Which of the following nursing actions would be most appropriate?

    1. Explain to the client that aspirin is given because of its anti-inflammatory effects.

2. Tell the client that after surgery he will continue to take aspirin prophylactically.
3. Question the doctor's order, since aspirin could cause postoperative bleeding.
4. Monitor the client's temperature and report elevations to the doctor immediately.

1. *Try again. Although aspirin does have an anti-inflammatory effect, cardiac clients who take 325 mg daily are taking it for its anticoagulation effect. This option is a distractor, because the issue is aspirin and the question is about the use of aspirin preoperatively.*
2. *Although the client might take aspirin prophylactically following surgery to prevent coagulation, he should not take it preoperatively because it may cause bleeding. This option is a distractor.*
3. ***Excellent! Since aspirin interferes with the action of platelets, it may cause bleeding after the surgery. Questioning the doctor's order would be the best action in this case.***
4. *Aspirin is the issue in this question. Aspirin does have an antipyretic effect, but this question is about the use of aspirin preoperatively. Furthermore, the nurse knows that cardiac clients who take 325 mg aspirin daily are taking it for its anticoagulation effect. This option is a distractor. The question contains no data to suggest that the client has a temperature elevation, or that he is at risk for developing a temperature elevation.*

53. **A client, 40 years old, is scheduled to have a bone marrow aspiration to assist with the diagnosis of multiple myeloma. Prior to a bone marrow aspiration, the most important communication from the nurse to the client is which of the following?**

1. The client must be still during the procedure.
2. This test will help to diagnosis multiple myeloma.
3. He will only feel sharp pain for a few minutes.
4. He will receive a sedative, so he will be asleep during the procedure.

1. ***Correct! It is necessary to be still so the physician can accurately insert the needle into the bone marrow of the sternum or iliac crests.***
2. *Incorrect, because the client has not been definitively diagnosed. The nurse's role would not be to cause more fear.*
3. *Incorrect. The area is anesthetized, so the client should only feel momentary discomfort.*
4. *Incorrect! A sedative is not always prescribed, and the dosage would not be enough to cause the client to sleep.*

54. **While bathing a small child in a tub, the nurse would avoid which of the following?**

1. Check the temperature of the water with a thermometer.

2. Never leave the child unattended.
3. Make sure the temperature in the room is warm.
4. Allow the child to determine if the water temperature is comfortable by placing the child's feet in the water.

1. *Wrong choice! The nurse should check the temperature of the water with a thermometer. Water temperature should be between 100° F and 105° F, since the small child's skin is easily burned.*
2. *Wrong choice! A small child may be able to turn the water faucet on and could receive burn injuries. There is also a danger of drowning when a small child is left unattended.*
3. *Wrong choice! The nurse does not want to avoid making sure the temperature of the room is warm. It should be warm to avoid chilling the child.*
4. ***Correct! If the water is too hot, the child may sustain burned feet. Using a thermometer will ensure the correct temperature.***

55. **The nurse understands that which of the following statements concerning naloxone (Narcan) is accurate?**

1. Narcan is available in two separate strengths, one for adults and one for infants and children.
2. Narcan is available in one strength. Careful calculation for newborns is essential to prevent an overdose.
3. Narcan is available in one strength. It needs to be diluted with normal saline prior to administration to neonates to prevent an overdose.
4. Narcan is available in two strengths, but either can be administered to adults or neonates as long as dosage is calculated using body weight.

1. ***Good choice! There are two separate strengths of Narcan. It is critical to check the vial to determine if it is adult or neonatal strength. Failure to do this could result in an overdose or insufficient dosage.***
2. *Wrong choice! There is a dosage for adults as well as one for neonates.*
3. *No. Diluting the adult dose is not needed since there is a neonatal dosage available to provide for safe administration to all ages.*
4. *Incorrect! The adult dosage should be given to adults only, and the neonatal dosage should be used in neonates only.*

56. **A client's mother comes to visit. The client does not acknowledge her greeting and lies down on her bed, curling up into the fetal position while her mother is in the room. After the visit the nurse speaks with the client's mother and returns to the client's room. The client is still lying in a fetal position. What action by the nurse would be most therapeutic at this time?**

1. Ask the client to get up and put away the clothing her mother has brought her.
2. Ask the client why she responded to her mother that way.
3. Sit in a chair next to the bed and ask the client to talk about what happened when her mother visited.
4. Explain unit expectations about how visitors are to be treated.

1. *This is not correct. The nurse is avoiding the client's response to her mother's visit by switching the focus to another task. The nurse is not conveying trustworthiness or an ability to help the client with her recovery, by not dealing with issues as they come up during the day.*
2. *This is a possibility. The nurse is attempting to gather data to do an assessment of what transpired. There is a better option for this question, however, because the client will most likely not be able or willing to respond to a direct question that is phrased in this manner.*
3. **Correct. The nurse is offering self and being available to talk about the situation that just occurred. The nurse is doing this in a way that does not put further pressure on the client. If the client is not able to talk about her mother's visit, the nurse should indicate a willingness to stay with her for a few more minutes and they can sit quietly without talking. This further action will convey that the nurse is willing to accept the client as she is and begin to establish the basis for a therapeutic relationship.**
4. *This is not correct. The nurse is discussing unit rules and not helping the client deal with her feelings about her mother's visit.*

57. **A 62-year-old female was diagnosed with breast cancer. She has become quiet and thoughtful and says to the nurse, "What do you think people will say about me when I'm gone?" Which of the following responses by the nurse is the most therapeutic?**

1. "You will be remembered as a very nice person."
2. "Do you feel that people will be talking about you after your death?"
3. "At this time, a positive attitude can influence your recovery."
4. "The thought of your breast cancer must seem hopeless."

1. *Wrong! This response uses the communication block of false reassurance. There is no indication that the nurse would know what others might say about the client. More importantly, however, this response is not therapeutic because it does not address the client's feelings of hopelessness.*
2. *Not the best choice, because this response does not focus on the appropriate issue. The nurse's re-*

sponse should address the client's feelings of hopelessness.
3. *Wrong! This response blocks communication by giving advice. The nurse's response should encourage the client to explore her feelings.*
4. **Good! This response uses the tool of restatement to focus on the client's feelings of hopelessness. This response is therapeutic because it allows the client to talk about what she has been thinking since she learned of her diagnosis.**

58. **When making rounds, the nurse notices that a client who is receiving oxygen via nasal cannula has a pack of cigarettes at the bedside. What is the best action by the nurse?**

1. Remove the pack of cigarettes from the bedside.
2. Remind the client not to smoke when oxygen is in use.
3. Ask the client how he obtained the cigarettes.
4. Review the rules of safety with the client's family.

1. **This may appear restrictive; however, this is the correct procedure, because the presence of the cigarettes creates a hazard for all the clients in the room and in the vicinity.**
2. *Close, but this is incorrect! This action is appropriate, but it is not sufficient to provide for the safety of the clients in the room.*
3. *Wrong. This would be appropriate if possession of the cigarettes were prohibited. However, this action alone will not provide for the safety of the clients in the room.*
4. *Wrong. This action is appropriate, but it is not sufficient to provide for the safety of the clients in the room.*

59. **During a home visit by the nurse, the client's wife collapses. There is no pulse or respirations. Which description correctly summarizes the CPR that the nurse would provide?**

1. Five to one ratio of compressions to ventilations, at a rate of 100 beats/min.
2. Fifteen to two ratio of compressions to ventilations, at a rate of 80 beats/min.
3. Fifteen to two ratio of compressions to ventilations, at a rate of 100 beats/min.
4. Five to one ratio of compressions to ventilations, at a rate of 80 beats/min.

1. *No, this is incorrect. Go back and reread the question.*
2. *Incorrect. You have selected the correct ratio, but the rate is not fast enough.*
3. **Correct. One-person CPR is performed with 15 compressions and two ventilations. It is necessary to give the compressions at a rate of 100 per minute, since there is a pause after every 15 compressions**

to give the ventilations. This will actually result in approximately 60 compressions per minute to the client.

4. *No, this is not one-person CPR.*

60. The nurse should advise the client that which is the best way to take erythromycin that is not enteric coated?

1. With meals.
2. With a full glass of water on an empty stomach.
3. With a snack.
4. Crushed and added to food.

1. *No. If the client takes a form of erythromycin that is not enteric coated with meals, much of the drug will be lost, because erythromycin can be protein bound.*
2. ***Correct! The best way to take a non-enteric coated erythromycin is with water on an empty stomach. If diarrhea or stomach complications arise, the enteric coated form may be ordered.***
3. *Wrong choice! Mixing with food will bind the drug and make it less available for absorption.*
4. *Wrong choice! The medication should not be crushed; if hard to swallow, a liquid form is available. If it is added to food, less is absorbed.*

61. The client has not bathed or changed her clothes during the two days she has been on the unit. After suggesting that she take a shower, the client states an emphatic, "No!" and turns her back to the nurse. What is the best action for the nurse to take initially?

1. Withdraw and return at a later time.
2. Question the client about her resistance to showering.
3. Get another staff member to help get the client into the shower.
4. Tell her she will be much more acceptable to other people on the unit if she cleans up and changes her clothes.

1. ***Correct. The nurse should withdraw to avoid a power struggle with the client. Later, the nurse can return and offer to help her gather together the things she will need and gently lead her to the shower. This directive approach does not require a decision on the part of the client, so she is more likely to cooperate with the nurse.***
2. *This is not correct. The client's behavior indicates her anxiety level has increased and she probably will not be able to explain her resistance to showering.*
3. *Wrong. If two staff members overpower the client, they will destroy any trust she may have started to develop with the staff as well as further undermine*

her feelings of self-worth. This is not the correct option.

4. *This is not correct. This response would cause harm to the client's self-esteem.*

62. What information regarding betamethasone (Celestone) is it important for the nurse to know, prior to administration of the drug to the antepartum client?

1. When used along with antibiotics, the risk of infection is increased due to the masking effect of antibiotic therapy.
2. When used for diabetic clients, the risk of hypoglycemia is increased.
3. When used after 34 weeks gestation, it is most effective in preventing RDS in the neonate.
4. When used along with tocolytic agents the risk of pulmonary edema is increased.

1. *No. Antibiotics are often given along with Celestone because of the immunosuppressant effects of the drug, which increases the risk of infection.*
2. *Wrong. When given to a diabetic, caution should be used because of the risk of hyperglycemia, not hypoglycemia. However, it is important to remember that when the mother experiences hyperglycemia, the neonate is at high risk for hypoglycemia.*
3. *Incorrect! Betamethasone is rarely used after 34 weeks. It is not felt to have an important effect on fetal lung maturation at this gestational age.*
4. ***Excellent choice! When used along with tocolytic drugs to stop labor, the client needs careful assessment for signs and symptoms of pulmonary edema since the risk is increased.***

63. A two-month-old is having a well baby check-up today. According to the standard immunization schedule, which immunizations would the nurse expect to administer to this child?

1. MMR and OPV.
2. DTP and OPV.
3. OPV, Hib and DTP.
4. DTP.

1. *Incorrect. MMR is not given until the child is 15 months old. Earlier immunization has proven ineffective.*
2. *Partially correct. DTP and OPV are given together at two months, but you are missing something.*
3. ***Yes!! OPV (oral polio), Hib (Haemophilus influenzae type b), and DTP (diphtheria, tetanus, pertussis) reflect the currently recommended schedule for immunization of two-month-old children.***
4. *Incomplete. DTP only protects the child from the diseases of diphtheria, tetanus and pertussis. This does not meet current guidelines.*

64. A client has a positive Mantoux skin test following screening for tuberculosis. The nurse interprets this to mean that the client:

1. Has active tuberculosis.
2. Was infectious at one time, but now has inactive tuberculosis.
3. Will require further evaluation.
4. Has never been exposed to the tubercle bacillus.

1. *No, a positive Mantoux is not diagnostic for active tuberculosis. Remember, the Mantoux is a screening test.*
2. *Incorrect. A positive Mantoux indicates that the body tissues are sensitive to tuberculin, but it does not mean that the client has had the disease.*
3. ***Correct! A positive Mantoux indicates that the person has been exposed to the tubercle bacillus, and further evaluation will be needed through the use of sputum cultures and chest x-rays.***
4. *No. A Mantoux is a screening test for tuberculosis and detects tissue sensitivity to the tubercle bacillus.*

65. Which statement by the mother indicates that the nurse's teaching about safety for an 18-month-old has been successful?

1. "I will give syrup of ipecac immediately if my child swallows a poison."
2. "I know that once she understands 'no,' she will be safe."
3. "I watch her every second, so I'm sure she can't get into anything."
4. "I have locked my medicines up in the medicine cabinet."

1. *Wrong! Syrup of Ipecac is used to induce vomiting. It should only be used after contacting an authority such as Poison Control. If the poison swallowed was a corrosive, vomiting will not be induced as this will burn the esophagus as the poison is vomited.*
2. *Wrong! Toddlers can understand the meaning of the word "no," but are not able to be aware of danger and may proceed anyway if curious. Houseproofing is the way to help keep them more safe.*
3. *Wrong! Even with direct supervision, toddlers still are very vulnerable to falls and other mishaps because of their development. Supervision should be augmented with "childproofing".*
4. ***Correct! Locking up medications and other potential poisons is the only sure way to keep them out of accessibility. Toddlers can climb and can manipulate things with their hands to get what they want. This response ensures the most safety for the child.***

66. As the nurse approaches a schizophrenic, paranoid type client, he looks at her and says, "Back off. Leave me alone." He appears tense and is pacing rapidly. The best nursing response to his remark is which of the following statements?

1. "I can't leave you alone when you are this upset. Sit down and try to relax."
2. "Let's go to your room and you can tell me what is bothering you."
3. "I will keep my distance as long as you can control yourself. You appear quite angry and I'd like to know more about what is causing you to feel this way."
4. "I will leave you alone for a few minutes while you try to compose yourself."

1. *This is not correct. The aggressive person is highly anxious and feeling out of control. He will not be able to sit quietly and relax.*
2. *This is not correct. The nurse cannot discuss the client's concerns until the client first provides assurance that he is able to maintain self-control and not become violent.*
3. ***Correct. The nurse's first concern is to ensure safety. To avoid escalating the client's behavior, the nurse should stay at a comfortable distance and remain calm, while stressing the importance of his maintaining control. Verbal intervention is the least restrictive form of action. If the client does not respond to verbal interventions, then more restrictive measures will have to be used.***
4. *This is not correct. It is not safe to leave a potentially violent client alone.*

67. A client is to receive cefazolin (Ancef) 500 mg IM every six hours. Which of the following actions taken by the nurse would most effectively decrease irritation at the injection site?

1. Use the Z-track method, and inject into the dorsogluteal site.
2. Do not massage the site after the medication is administered; use gentle pressure only.
3. Give the medication slowly, over one minute, to allow dispersal time into the muscle.
4. Use a 1 1/2 inch needle and inject into the ventrogluteal site.

1. ***Excellent! This injection technique is specific for administration of medications known to cause pain or permanent staining of superficial tissues. The dorsogluteal site uses the gluteus medius muscle of the buttocks, a large muscle mass desired in this case.***
2. *Incorrect. Although use of gentle pressure without massage may help to decrease irritation, it is not the most effective technique of the choices given.*
3. *No. This intervention may assist in more even distribution of the medication, but it does not necessarily decrease the risk of irritation.*

4. *Not the best choice. You were correct in choosing the needle length, but the ventrogluteal site, using the gluteus MINIMIS muscle, is not the preferred site. Choose again.*

68. **A 24-year-old man is seen in the emergency room following a gunshot wound to the right chest. The triage nurse notes a thick dressing on the right chest, a sucking noise from the wound, BP 100/60, pulse rate 96 and weak, and respiratory rate 40. Which of the following nursing actions would be best initially?**

    1. Remove the dressing to inspect the wound.
    2. Administer oxygen via nasal cannula.
    3. Draw blood for serum chemistries.
    4. Raise the foot of the bed to 90 degrees.

    1. *This option is incorrect. The dressing should not be removed from a sucking chest wound until chest tube insertion. Removal of the dressing will cause an increase in respiratory difficulty.*
    2. **This is correct. This nursing action is "best initially," because respiratory difficulty is evidenced by the high respiratory rate and the increased heart rate. Administering oxygen will increase the oxygen exchange in the lungs and increase the oxygen available to the tissues. Note that Options 1 and 4 are incorrect, and Option 3 is not a priority.**
    3. *Serum chemistries will be needed, but this nursing action is not the top priority. Immediate intervention is needed for respiratory difficulty as evidenced by the high respiratory rate and the increased heart rate. This option is a distractor. Look for the key words in the question!*
    4. *This option is incorrect. Trendelenburg's position will increase pressure on the heart and lungs, and is contraindicated in a client with an open chest wound.*

69. **Which of the following statements by the nurse would best describe the action of RHoGAM?**

    1. It destroys Rh antibodies in the Rh negative mother.
    2. It destroys Rh antibodies in the Rh positive newborn.
    3. It prevents the formation of the Rh antibodies in the Rh negative mother.
    4. It prevents the formation of the Rh antibodies in the Rh positive newborn.

    1. *Wrong. RHoGAM never destroys antibodies. It prevents them in an Rh negative mother.*
    2. *Wrong. RHoGAM does not destroy antibodies, it prevents formation. Also remember RHoGAM is given to the mother, never the newborn.*
    3. **Correct. Giving RHoGAM to the mother prevents the formation of antibodies in the Rh negative mother.**

4. *Incorrect. RHoGAM is never given to a newborn infant. The only way to prevent Rh antibody formation in the newborn is to prevent them in the mother by administering RHoGAM at appropriate times.*

70. **A client had been brought to the hospital by two coworkers who were also close friends. They reported that, while he had always been a person "on the go", his activity level had increased over the past two weeks to the point that he was working around the clock. They also indicated that he ate and slept very little, and talked almost nonstop. A priority goal of nursing care for this client is to help him do which of the following?**

    1. Confront the denial of his underlying depression.
    2. Participate in group activities.
    3. Identify one recreational or leisure activity to pursue.
    4. Obtain adequate amounts of rest.

    1. *This is not correct. While elated behavior is a mirror image of depression and is thought to represent denial of depressed feelings, it is not a priority goal for his initial nursing care.*
    2. *No! Manic clients are usually social and outgoing and do not require assistance with group participation. Also, group participation is not desirable during the acute stage of illness because the stimulation of group activity will increase the manic client's hyperactivity. This is not the correct option.*
    3. *This is not correct. Manic clients do not usually have difficulty finding activities to pursue.*
    4. **Great job! The manic client who is hyperactive is very much in danger of jeopardizing his physical health because of lack of rest and sleep. Obtaining adequate rest is often a priority nursing goal.**

71. **The nurse is to instruct parents of young children about poisoning prevention in the home. Which of the following interventions is most important for the parents learn?**

    1. If the child ingests poison, induce vomiting with syrup of ipecac.
    2. If the child ingests poison, the parents should immediately bring the child to the emergency room.
    3. Place labels on the parent's telephone, with the Poison Control Center's telephone number, and instructions to call that number after an accidental ingestion.
    4. If a poisoning occurs, the nurse will notify social services to investigate the home situation for safety.

    1. *Wrong. In some poisons, such as lye or petroleum products, vomiting is contraindicated. Identification of the poison is most important before treatment can be initiated.*

2. *No. Immediate measures usually can be instituted by the parents to lessen the severity of the poisoning by preventing or slowing absorption. Depending on the location of the hospital, time may be a factor in the outcome of the situation.*

3. **Correct. The phone number for the Poison Control Center can place the parents in contact with an immediate source of information for initial emergency measures that can be implemented to help decrease the severity of the poisoning prior to transportation to the emergency room.**

4. *Wrong! Accidental poisoning often occurs because of a lack of knowledge on the part of the parents. A social service consult is not necessary unless a pattern of practices indicates an unsafe environment for the children.*

72. **The physician orders a stool specimen to be collected for ova and parasites. What is the proper procedure for the nurse to use in collection of this specimen?**

1. Send entire stool immediately to the lab.
2. Use a sterile container.
3. Take feces from several areas of the bowel movement.
4. Refrigerate specimen until it can be delivered to the lab.

1. **Correct! A stool specimen for ova and parasites should be collected in its entirety, placed in a dry container free of urine, labelled correctly, and sent immediately to the laboratory.**

2. *No, a sterile container is not necessary. The feces should be collected in a dry container free of urine.*

3. *Incorrect procedure. Taking samples from various areas of the stool is done when a stool sample for occult blood is ordered. Choose another option.*

4. *No. Refrigeration will kill the parasites and definitely alter the test results.*

73. **A client, 60 years old, is admitted to the hospital with a diagnosis of chest pain. Several days after admission, the client is scheduled for a cardiac catheterization. Client information is obtained by the nurse during an interview prior to the procedure. Which of the following findings should be reported immediately to the physician who will be doing the procedure?**

1. The client is allergic to lobster.
2. The client's father smokes heavily.
3. The client's husband died of heart disease.
4. The client is apprehensive about the procedure.

1. **Correct. Since lobster and the contrast dye used for a cardiac catheterization both contain iodine,**

the client may have an allergic reaction during the procedure. The doctor who will be doing the procedure needs to know this information immediately to assure the client's safety. Maslow's Hierarchy of Needs indicates that when no physiological need exists, safety needs should get priority attention.

2. *Wrong. The fact that the client's father smokes heavily may be a risk factor for her. However, this is not an immediate threat to her safety.*

3. *Wrong. The client's statement that her husband died of heart disease may be an indication of fear on the part of the client. According to Maslow's Hierarchy of Needs, the need for a sense of security is a higher level need. Priority should be placed on the need for safety.*

4. *Wrong. Apprehension about the procedure indicates a need for security, which is a higher level need according to Maslow's Hierarchy of needs. Priority should be placed on the need for safety.*

74. **Which of the following interventions by the nurse is appropriate to prepare the client for a cholecystography?**

1. NPO after midnight.
2. Clear liquid diet the evening before the test.
3. Assess for allergies to iodine or seafood.
4. Special consent form due to the invasive nature of the procedure.

1. *Incorrect. The client will be NPO from the time the contrast is given, the evening prior to the test, until the examination is completed.*

2. *No. The client is typically given a low fat meal the evening before the x-ray examination, to decrease the stimulation of the gallbladder.*

3. **Correct! An oral iodine contrast substance such as Telepaque or Oragrafin is given, because gallstones are not usually radiopaque. After the administration of the iodinated substance, it takes about 13 hours for it to reach the liver and be excreted into the bile, where it's stored in the gallbladder. It's important to assess for allergies to iodine or seafood.**

4. *Not necessary. Cholecystography is an x-ray examination of the gallbladder, and is not an invasive procedure. A special consent form is not needed.*

75. **A five-year-old child is being seen for a well child visit in a pediatric clinic. The child's father tells the nurse that his wife has recently been diagnosed with tuberculosis. Which of the following statements will guide the nurse in planning the information that will be provided to the parents?**

1. It is likely that the child will require medication.

2. Small children do not easily contract TB, if they are otherwise healthy.
3. As long as the child has not exhibited the symptoms of night sweats and/or coughing, there is probably no infection.
4. Direct physical contact must be limited to insure the health of the child.

1. *Right! The most common source of infection to a child is an adult within the immediate household. Prophylactic medication and or treatment for active disease are a high probability for this child.*
2. *No. Children are at high risk when someone in their household has active tuberculosis. In addition, children in this age group have frequent illness, which makes them a susceptible host.*
3. *No. Symptoms such as coughing are not reliable in small children, so this would be an empty reassurance. Screening with Tine and then PPD would be more appropriate indicators.*
4. *No. How is TB usually transmitted? That's right— droplet. Make another selection.*

76. **When elderly clients are treated with antidepressant medication, the nurse is guided by which of the following understandings?**

1. They will probably require a higher dose of medication than a younger person.
2. Psychotherapy and medication together are usually more effective than either alone in treating elderly depressed clients.
3. Antidepressant medications are usually not well tolerated by elderly clients because of their many side effects.
4. Antidepressants are expensive medications and the potential results may not be worth their cost.

1. *Wrong choice! Elderly persons, and other clients with coexisting medical problems, are treated with lower doses of antidepressants. This cannot be the correct option.*
2. *Correct. Psychotherapy and antidepressant medication usually are more effective in treating elderly clients with clinical depression than either modality used alone.*
3. *Incorrect! Elderly clients are more sensitive to the side effects of antidepressants. Also, the elderly are more likely to be taking other drugs for medical problems which could lead to drug interactions. However, elders can still be effectively treated with antidepressants when their responses to the drug treatment are monitored closely. This is not the correct option.*
4. *This is false! Not all antidepressants are expensive, which is relative in any event. This cannot be the correct option.*

77. **A client, age 58, had a hiatal hernia repair three days ago. During this morning's assessment, he tells the nurse that his abdomen "feels swollen," and that he is nauseated, with increased abdominal discomfort. What should be the nurse's initial action?**

1. Give the client an antiemetic.
2. Listen for bowel sounds.
3. Insert a nasogastric tube.
4. Measure the client's abdominal girth.

1. *Incorrect. Although this action should be taken to prevent vomiting, it is not the initial step in assessing the cause of the client's nausea.*
2. *Absolutely! Paralytic ileus is a complication that may occur after intestinal or abdominal surgery. It's characterized by the absence of bowel sounds, abdominal discomfort, and distention. The nurse would need to complete the assessment before notifying the physician.*
3. *No. Insertion of a nasogastric tube is not an independent nursing action—it requires a physician's order. This intervention may be needed later, but there is an earlier action that is essential.*
4. *Incorrect choice. Unless the nurse had a baseline measurement, this assessment would be of little value at this time. Another action has priority.*

78. **After taking erythromycin (Erythrocin) p.o. for seven days, a client develops oral candidiasis. The nurse is aware that this is most likely a result of which type of reaction?**

1. Superinfection.
2. Allergic response.
3. Synergistic reaction.
4. Erythromycin toxicity.

1. *Correct. Erythromycin, like other antibiotics, may allow overgrowth of nonsusceptible bacteria or fungi—in this case, candida.*
2. *Incorrect choice. Hypersensitivity reactions are characterized by maculopapular rashes, urticaria, wheezing, and diarrhea.*
3. *No, a synergistic response occurs when the effect of two drugs combined is greater than the effect expected if the individual effects of the two drugs acting independently were added together. You only have information about one drug.*
4. *No. Erythromycin toxicity would be manifested by hearing loss (rare) or hepatotoxicity. (Ilosone can damage the liver, causing cholestatic hepatitis— which appears 10-12 days after therapy is started. In most clients, symptoms rapidly disappear when the drug is discontinued.)*

79. **A 15-year-old client was just diagnosed with testicular cancer. When the nurse asks the client a question, he angrily spits in the nurse's face. Which of the following responses by the nurse would be best?**

   1. "You are old enough to find a better way to express yourself. The nurses will not want to take care of you if you treat us this way."
   2. "I'm afraid I will have to tell your parents about this. They call every day to talk to the nurses about how you are doing."
   3. "That behavior makes me very angry and I will not tolerate it. I'll be back after I wash my face and we can talk about what's bothering you."
   4. "If you don't want us here right now, we will go. We will come back to change your linens when you are feeling better."

   1. *Not the best response! This response does not consider that the client's behavior may be severely regressed because of his inability to cope with his diagnosis. It also involves a threat that care will be withheld because of his behavior. This response is not therapeutic because the nurse does not assist the client with expressing his anger or coping with his feelings.*
   2. *No. This response involves a threat to tell the client's parents about his behavior. It is not therapeutic because the nurse does not help the client to express his anger or cope with his feelings. This response also focuses on inappropriate person.*
   3. ***Great choice! This response models behavior for the client, by showing how anger can be expressed appropriately. The response also sets limits, which is appropriate for this age group. This response focuses on the client's feelings.***
   4. *No, this response is not therapeutic. This response focuses on the nurse, rather than on the client in the question. The response also does not acknowledge the client's angry feelings.*

80. **Although most depressed clients do not attempt suicide, an estimated 80% of persons with depression do have suicidal thoughts. Nursing intervention for an elderly widower with agitated depression should be guided by which information, regarding the risk of suicide?**

   1. It is no different than for any other depressed client.
   2. It is lower than that of an elderly man who has never married.
   3. It is quite low.
   4. It is extremely high.

   1. *This statement is inaccurate. An elderly client with agitated depression has a higher risk of suicide than that of most other groups of depressed clients. This is especially true for clients who have persistent insomnia.*

   2. *This statement is inaccurate. Elderly men who have never married have a lower risk of suicide than those who have been widowed, separated, or divorced.*
   3. *This statement is inaccurate. Re-read the question and look for risk factors.*
   4. ***You are right. The elderly widower with an agitated depression is in one of the groups with the highest risk for suicide. The other group with one of the highest rates of suicide is adolescents.***

81. **A child with the body-surface area (BSA) of 0.5 square meters is to receive 250 mg of medication. The usual adult dosage is 500 mg/dose. The nurse's safest action is to:**

   1. Give the medication, as the dosage is correct for the child's size.
   2. Give the medication, but request that the dose be reevaluated.
   3. Withhold the medication and notify the prescriber.
   4. Recalculate the dosage and administer a decreased amount.

   1. *This dose is too high. The correct dose is calculated by dividing the child's BSA by the average adult BSA (1.73) and multiplying by the usual adult dose: 0.5 m² / 1.73 m² x 500 mg = 144.5 mg.*
   2. *Good, you figured out that this dose is incorrect; however, you would never give an incorrect dose. Even if the calculations are reevaluated, the damage has been done. The correct dose is calculated by dividing the child's BSA by the average adult BSA (173 m²) and multiplying by the usual adult dosage: 0.5 m² / 1.73 m² x 500 mg = 144.5 mg.*
   3. ***Correct. The ordered dosage is too high. The correct dose is calculated by dividing the child's BSA by the average adult BSA (1.73 m²) and multiplying by the usual adult dosage: 0.5 m² / 1.73 m² x 500 mg = 144.5 mg.***
   4. *A nurse does not have the authority to override a prescribed dosage. If the nurse knows that the dosage is wrong, the nurse must report the error and request a correct order. The correct dosage is calculated by dividing the child's BSA by the average adult BSA and multiplying by the usual adult dosage: 0.5 m² / 1.73 m² x 500 mg = 144.5 mg.*

82. **A client is admitted with bleeding esophageal varices. The physician has opted to use esophageal tamponade with a Sengstaken-Blakemore tube to control the bleeding. Which of the following nursing interventions is appropriate when caring for the client while the Blakemore tube is in place?**

   1. Ambulate the client four times a day.
   2. Encourage clear liquids.
   3. Provide mouth and nares care every two hours.
   4. Maintain the manometer pressure of the esophageal balloon at all times to control bleeding.

1.   Incorrect. The client must remain on bedrest while the Blakemore tube is in place to prevent accidental dislodgement, which can cause asphyxia. Choose another option.

2.   No. The client will be NPO due to the placement of the tube. Remember that the client will be unable to swallow and may require suctioning of the oral cavity to remove secretions. Make another selection.

*3.   **Correct intervention. If the client is alert, the nurse should provide tissues, and encourage spitting of saliva into a tissue or basin. If the client is not alert, gentle suctioning may be needed.***

4.   Not correct procedure. The esophageal balloon is usually deflated in approximately 12 hours to assess if bleeding has stopped. It can be left inflated for up to 48 hours without tissue damage or severe discomfort. Choose again.

83.   **A 30-year-old single man who works as a computer analyst, is admitted to the hospital with a diagnosis of bipolar mood disorder, acute manic episode. When taking a nursing history which information, if true, would support this diagnosis?**

1.   He describes himself as a "loner" with a history of being withdrawn and aloof in relationships.
2.   His paternal grandfather had mood swings all his life. He died in a mental institution.
3.   He had a similar episode when in college. He dropped out of school without finishing his degree and his friends say he was never the same again.
4.   His parents were divorced when he was a young child.

1.   This is not correct. Most manic clients have had successful relationships and are quite sociable with many acquaintances. In contrast, schizophrenic clients are more likely to be described as aloof and withdrawn.

*2.   **Correct. Most manic clients come from a family where a close relative also suffered from a unipolar or bipolar disorder. The theory that genetic factors are involved in the occurrence of manic-depressive illness results from this observation.***

3.   Ninety percent of manic clients have periods of normal or near normal behavior between manic episodes. Most clients do not experience chronic deterioration after an acute episode of illness.

4.   There is no evidence that a divorce in the family causes manic illness. This is not the correct option.

84.   **A 15-year-old client is to have a k-pad, or water system heating device, applied to a pulled muscle. The client tells the nurse that the device does not feel very warm. Which of the following nursing actions is most appropriate?**

1.   Tell the client that these heating devices never feel hot.
2.   Check the temperature setting on the heating unit and feel the pad for warmth.
3.   Call the appropriate repair department and have them fix the unit.
4.   Turn the temperature up on the unit if it doesn't feel warm enough to the client.

1.   Wrong. Although these heating units do feel warm and not hot, the unit may not be at a therapeutic temperature, and should be assessed to see if it is working properly.

*2.   **Correct! The manufacturer recommends a temperature setting, which should be assessed, as well as whether the pad feels warm.***

3.   Incorrect! The unit may not be malfunctioning, and should be assessed by the nurse before any other action is taken. If the unit is malfunctioning, it should be replaced with another unit, and the malfunctioning unit should be sent to the repair department.

4.   Incorrect! The temperature should not be set above the recommended setting, to avoid causing a burn to the client.

85.   **Following a motor vehicle accident a 30-year-old male has a $PaCO_2$ of 30 mm Hg on room air. What intervention would be anticipated?**

1.   Rebreathing of expired air.
2.   Encourage deep breathing.
3.   Administration of oxygen.
4.   Treatment with sodium bicarbonate.

*1.   **Correct. The report of a $PaCO_2$ below 35 indicates hyperventilation, possibly due to anxiety or pain.***

2.   No, this intervention would be utilized mainly in the presence of increased $PaCO_2$ levels.

3.   Incorrect. PaO_2 levels below 80 mm Hg are treated with oxygen.

4.   Not correct. Sodium bicarbonate is used to treat metabolic acidosis, which would be indicated in abnormal pH, base excess, and HCO_3 readings.

86.   **A 23-year-old client is seen in the Women's Health Center and is to be treated with erythromycin (Erythromycin Base Filmtab) 250 mg p.o. every six hours for strep throat. With which of the following should the nurse instruct the client to take the drug?**

1.   Milk or an antacid.
2.   Water one hour before or two hours after meals.
3.   Fruit juice.
4.   Food.

1. No, erythromycin may bind with the milk or ant-
acid and decrease the amount of drug available for
absorption.

*2. **Correct. Erythromycin base and stearate prepara-***
tions should be given on an empty stomach.

3. Wrong! The acidity of fruit juice may destroy the
drug before it's absorbed.

4. Incorrect choice. Erythromycin base would bind
with the food and make less drug available for
absorption.

87. **The nurse observes a depressed client in the day room. She appears to be cold. Which of the following responses by the nurse would be most therapeutic?**

1. "Come with me to your room and we will get a sweater for you."
2. "Why do you sit here without a sweater when you are cold?"
3. "What color sweater do you want me to get from your room for you?"
4. "When you are in the day room, you should dress so that you are not cold."

*1. **You made the right choice! By volunteering to go***
with the client to get a sweater, the nurse is com-
municating therapeutically by offering self.

2. Wrong! This option uses a "Why" question. This
is an example of the communication block of re-
questing an explanation.

3. Close, since the nurse is offering self by volunteer-
ing to get a sweater for the client. This is not the
best option, because it would be more therapeutic
to assist the client in meeting her own need. Also,
the color of the sweater is not significant, and mak-
ing decisions is often difficult for depressed clients.

4. Wrong! In this option, the nurse is giving advice.
Giving advice is not therapeutic.

88. **While making rounds at night, the nurse discovers an elderly client in bed and the room filled with smoke. The first action would be which of the following?**

1. Shut the door.
2. Remove the client from the room.
3. Call the fire department.
4. Get a fire extinguisher.

1. This is wrong. All the doors on the unit should be
closed to contain the fire. However, since the client
in the room is in immediate danger, this is not the
first nursing action.

*2. **Correct! The client should be removed from im-***
mediate danger before other actions are imple-
mented. The client could be asphyxiated from the
smoke.

3. Wrong. The fire department should be notified once

the client has been removed from the room. Since
the client is in immediate danger of asphyxiation,
this is not the first nursing action.

4. No. Since the room is smoke filled, obtaining a fire
extinguisher before providing for the safety of the
client is not appropriate. The client is in immediate
danger of asphyxiation.

89. **While mixing a solution of bleach and water to be used as a disinfectant spray, the nurse discovers that there is more solution than will fit in the spray bottle. The nurse can appropriately deal with the excess in several ways. The least appropriate solution would be to:**

1. Pour the excess solution into an empty container, label the container as to contents, and place it in the cleaning supply closet.
2. Discard the excess solution.
3. Use the excess solution for the immediate cleaning job, then discard what is left.
4. Pour the excess into another cleaning solution container that has only a small amount of an ammonia solution left in the bottom.

1. No, this is appropriate. All containers should be
labelled with the contents and stored in the appro-
priate area for the contents. Cleaning supplies and
chemicals should not be kept near supplies that are
for oral consumption or other uses where a client
could be injured by someone picking up the wrong
bottle.

2. No, this is appropriate. If there are no available
containers that can be safely used, then discarding
the solution is the best action in order to avoid
poisoning or injury by another person using the
unidentified solution for the wrong purpose.

3. No, this is appropriate. If the solution was pre-
pared because of the need to clean a particular
area, then the person who prepared the solution
can use the excess, and can then discard what is left
after the immediate cleaning task is completed. Any
solution that is not identified has the potential for
being mistakenly misused by another person.

*4. **This is the correct answer, because it is something***
the nurse should not do. Mixing chlorine or
bleach with ammonia produces toxic fumes that
can cause damage to the respiratory tract when
inhaled.

90. **Postural drainage with percussion is ordered for a client with pneumonia. How would the nurse plan for this procedure?**

1. Perform this procedure before meals.
2. Cup and clap lightly to avoid causing redness to the client's skin.
3. Administer bronchodilators after percussion and before postural drainage.

4. Provide analgesia prior to each treatment.

1. *Correct. To facilitate the client's ability to tolerate the procedure, an empty stomach is recommended.*
2. *Incorrect. When performed correctly, percussion causes a slight redness, even though the client's gown or a towel is placed between the percussor's hands and the client's skin.*
3. *No. Bronchodilators would be given approximately 20-30 minutes before the treatment to facilitate the drainage of secretions.*
4. *No, this would be counterproductive. This procedure is not considered painful, and the ability of the client to cough effectively following the treatment may be diminished with analgesia. Make another selection.*

91. **A 68-year-old client is admitted with a broken right arm and contusions to the left wrist following an automobile accident. Which of the following measures would the nurse avoid when feeding the client?**

1. Offer small bites of food.
2. Order pureed foods.
3. Have the client use her dentures while eating.
4. Allow enough time for the client to chew the food well before offering more.

1. *No, this is appropriate. Offering small bites of food helps prevent the client from choking caused by too much food in the mouth.*
2. *That's right, pureed food for this client is inappropriate! A client who is able to chew should receive foods of normal texture. Pureed foods would be used for clients who are not able to chew or do not have teeth.*
3. *No, this is appropriate. Dentures provide the mechanism for the client to chew foods. If dentures are not used, then the client is at risk for choking on unchewed foods that are too large to swallow.*
4. *No, this is very appropriate! Choking can occur if the client does not have time to chew food well. Attempts may be made to swallow large boluses of food, or the mouth may become too full by feeding the client at too fast a pace.*

92. **A 72-year-old female has fallen, fracturing her left hip. She is admitted in Buck's traction and scheduled for intramedullary nailing tomorrow. The nurse understands that which is the primary rationale for Buck's traction in this client?**

1. To reduce muscle spasm.
2. To provide for total immobility.
3. To promote healing of the fracture.
4. To allow for a 20 pound weight to be applied.

1. *This is the correct rationale. Most often Buck's traction is used initially to reduce the severe muscle spasm, which is mainly responsible for the pain associated with a fracture of the femoral head.*
2. *Incorrect. Although the client's mobility is limited by traction, the affected leg is the only part that should be immobilized. The client will be allowed to turn and exercise the unaffected limbs. Be wary of any response that uses absolutes, in this case "total."*
3. *No, not likely. Only persons who are inoperable would have Buck's used for the whole course of treatment. The usual course of treatment includes surgical reduction and pinning.*
4. *Oops, this is incorrect. Buck's is skin traction and the limit for weight is usually five to 10 pounds. If greater weight is needed, skeletal traction must be used.*

93. **A child weighing 1800 gm is admitted to intensive care. The nurse correctly explains to the parents that the infant's weight in pounds is:**

1. 3.9 lbs.
2. 8.1 lbs.
3. 18 lbs.
4. 36 lbs.

1. *Correct. One kilogram is equal to 2.2 pounds. Therefore, the correct weight is calculated by multiplying the weight in kilograms by 2.2. There are 1000 grams in a kilogram. 1.8 kg x 2.2 = 3.96 lbs.*
2. *Incorrect.*
3. *Incorrect.*
4. *Incorrect.*

94. **A client in the intensive care unit is placed on a ventilator. During an electrical storm, the lights go out for a brief period. Some of the lights come back on, but the ventilator is not working. What is the best nursing action?**

1. Remove the client from the ventilator and ventilate with a bag and mask.
2. Check the electrical outlets to determine if the ventilator is plugged into an emergency power outlet.
3. Call a code.
4. Notify the supervisor while ventilating the client with oxygen using positive pressure bag attached to the endotracheal tube.

1. *This is not correct! A client on a ventilator has an endotracheal tube in place. A mask cannot be used since a seal cannot be made.*
2. *Yes! All emergency equipment such as ventilators should be plugged into emergency outlets in case*

of power failure. If the ventilator was not plugged into the appropriate outlet, then the nurse should move the plug to an emergency power outlet.

3. *Wrong choice! It is not necessary to call a code because of equipment malfunction. A code is to be called only if the equipment cannot be readily restored and the client's condition begins to deteriorate.*

4. *Wrong. This option may be necessary if the nurse cannot get the ventilator turned back on. The nurse's first effort, however, should be to restore the functioning of the ventilator.*

95. The admitting nurse asks a client what factors, such as a recent change in his life, have contributed to his hospitalization? He replied, "Change...change is money...when you have money you make the change." Which of the following is this statement an example of?

1. Clanging.
2. Echolalia.
3. Perseveration.
4. Flight of ideas.

1. *Correct. Clanging is speech in which sounds, rather than conceptual relationships, govern word choice. It is most commonly associated with schizophrenia and mania.*

2. *Wrong choice! Echolalia is the repetition or "echoing" of the words or phrases of others. This is not the correct option.*

3. *Wrong. Perseveration is the persistent repetition of words or ideas so that once an individual uses a particular word it recurs. It is most commonly associated with organic mental disorders or schizophrenia.*

4. *Wrong. Flight of ideas refers to a nearly continuous flow of accelerated speech with abrupt changes from topic to topic before the original topic is completed. It is most frequently associated with manic episodes but is also seen in other conditions.*

96. Clients with Parkinson's disease and myasthenia gravis are both encountered in the neurology clinic. The nursing assistant asks the nurse, "Are these disorders similar?" Which of the following is inaccurate information on which to base a response?

1. Both disorders are characterized by abnormal involuntary movements.
2. Each disorder is managed with specific drug therapy.
3. Crisis states may occur in either disorder due to medication withdrawal.
4. No known cure exists for either disorder.

1. *Correct choice. Parkinson's disease clients have a characteristic tremor, while those with myasthenia gravis exhibit muscular weakness.*

2. *No, this is accurate. Levodopa is used with Parkinson's disease, and short acting anticholinesterase medications are used in the treatment of myasthenia gravis.*

3. *Incorrect choice. Crisis states can occur if medication is inadequate or delayed. Both diseases must be recognized and treated immediately.*

4. *No, this statement is accurate. Both diseases are considered degenerative neurologic disorders.*

97. A woman is admitted to the ICU on a ventilator after attempting suicide. She had been depressed for some time. As the husband is talking with the nurse, he begins to cry. He says, "It's all my fault. I should have been home more often to keep an eye on her." Which of the following statements by the nurse would be most appropriate initially?

1. "You seem to regret not being there for your wife. How can you feel that way when you have to earn a living?"
2. "At this time you need your privacy. I will return later, and we can talk then."
3. "This is an important issue that you need to bring up at your family therapy session."
4. "It must have been hard to be away when your wife was so sick."

1. *This response is partly correct, since it begins with the nurse showing empathy for the client. However, the second part of the nurse's response actually rejects the client's feelings and minimizes them, while appearing to show approval for his actions. This response is not therapeutic. When part of an option is a communication block, the option is incorrect.*

2. *Wrong! In this response, the nurse abandons the client when he needs to talk about his feelings, putting his feelings on hold. The client's feelings must be dealt with at this time. Remember, the client in this question is the husband.*

3. *This response puts the client's feelings on hold. The nurse's response should address the client's feelings and encourage him to express them. Remember, the client in this question is the husband.*

4. *Yes! This is the correct answer! This response shows empathy by showing that the nurse understands the husband's feelings. Note that Options 2 and 3 block communication by putting his feelings on hold.*

98. A 24-year-old female client diagnosed with sciatica is found staring into space with her lunch tray untouched. The client received meperidine (Demerol) 100 mg one hour ago. Which assessment should the nurse make from this scenario?

1. The medication dosage is excessive.
2. The observed behaviors indicate intractable pain.
3. The client is upset with the care and the food.
4. The behaviors demonstrate an adjustment to pain.

1. *Incorrect. The assessment does not correlate with an excess of medication. The decrease in appetite could be relevant, but the staring is not. Also, 100 mg of meperidine is an appropriate adult dose of this medication.*
2. ***You are correct! Sciatic pain is severe, which accounts for the anorexia. Lack of interest in the environment would indicate depression, which is indicative of unremitting pain.***
3. *Incorrect. This is not the best choice. Are you reading into the situation?*
4. *No. Coping effectively with pain would be indicated by the client performing activities of daily living rather than being anorectic.*

99. **A client is admitted to the psychiatric unit with a diagnosis of acute depression. After being hospitalized for a few weeks, the client says to the nurse, "I'm a terrible person, and I should be dead." Which of the following responses by the nurse would be appropriate initially?**

1. "That is why you are here. We are trying to help you with your bad feelings."
2. "Feeling that way must be awful. What makes you feel so terrible?"
3. "Feeling like a terrible person is part of your illness. As you get better, those feelings will lessen."
4. "You are not terrible. You are not a bad person."

1. *No. This response appears to support the client's feelings that she is a terrible person. The second part of the response also blocks therapeutic communication by focusing on inappropriate persons — the nurse and others who "are trying to help" the client. This response is not therapeutic.*
2. ***Good choice! This response shows empathy, and then seeks clarification of the client's feelings.***

These two communication tools combine to make a therapeutic response that allows the client to talk about her feelings.
3. *Wrong! This is giving information about the illness. However, at this time, the client's feelings must be addressed before information is given. When a client is distressed and upset, giving an explanation is inappropriate.*
4. *Absolutely not! The nurse's opinion is not important! This response blocks therapeutic communication by putting the nurse in the role of an authority figure, using false reassurance, and devaluing the client's feelings. The nurse's response should encourage the client to explore her feelings with the nurse.*

100. **The nurse notices a crack in an electrical outlet. The IV pump that is plugged into the outlet appears to be working without any problems. Which of the following is the best nursing action?**

1. Use another outlet; then call the maintenance department to have the outlet changed.
2. Since the pump is working, no action is necessary.
3. Test the outlet by moving the plug a bit in the outlet, and observing if this affects the pump.
4. Since the outlet works, continue to use it until maintenance can replace it.

1. ***This is the correct choice! A cracked electrical outlet should never be used and should be replaced, since it has the potential to start an electrical fire or to cause an electrical shock to the person who attempts to insert a plug.***
2. *Wrong choice! Although the electrical outlet is presently working, it could quit working or cause a short and start an electrical fire.*
3. *Try again! Moving the plug in the outlet may cause the outlet to become further damaged and cause an electrical shock or electrical fire.*
4. *Try again! A broken electrical outlet should never be used because of the potential for an electrical fire or short.*

NOTES

NCLEX-RN

Test 9

NCLEX-RN TEST 9

1. **A client is taking both digoxin (Lanoxin) and chlorothiazide (Diuril). The nurse has completed discharge teaching regarding diet. Which of the following menus, if selected by the client, would indicate that she can identify good food sources for potassium?**

   1. Baked chicken, boiled potato, pudding.
   2. Boiled chicken, rice, cranberry juice.
   3. Broiled meat, baked potato, citrus fruit salad.
   4. Beef stew, bread and butter, jello.

2. **While working in a unit where the clients are on cardiac monitors, the nurse hears an alarm and notices that one of the clients has a straight line on the cardiac monitor, indicating a cardiac arrest. Which of the following is the initial nursing action?**

   1. Call a code.
   2. Notify the physician.
   3. Administer cardiopulmonary resuscitation.
   4. Assess the client.

3. **A two-year-old boy with a rectal temperature of 101° F is diagnosed with a viral illness. Which statement by the mother would indicate to the nurse that further teaching is needed?**

   1. "I will give him 1/4 tsp of acetaminophen (Tylenol) for a temperature over 101° F."
   2. "I will give him extra fluids over the next couple of days."
   3. "I will give him two baby aspirin (acetylsalicylic acid) every four hours."
   4. "I will keep him home from day care while he has a fever."

4. **Which of the following findings on assessment would alert the nurse to a possible serious adverse effect of diltiazem (Cardizem) therapy?**

   1. Drowsiness.
   2. Hypertension.
   3. Rhonchi.
   4. Gingival hyperplasia.

5. **A 28-year-old client had a D&C this morning. She has returned to the unit from the recovery room. She says to the nurse, "I am hungry. When can I eat?" In determining when the client can have something by mouth, which of the following nursing actions would demonstrate best judgment?**

   1. Request a diet order from the doctor.
   2. Determine when the next meal will be served.
   3. Use a stethoscope to listen to the client's abdomen.
   4. Check the chart for a diet order.

6. **One morning the nurse asks an elderly client if she had any visitors the day before. She responds that several members of her church choir had been to see her. The nurse knows that only her daughter had visited the day before. A fabrication that is told to mask memory loss is which of the following?**

   1. Delusion.
   2. Illusion.
   3. Confabulation.
   4. Dissociation.

7. **During the resuscitation of a client, the physician orders the client to be defibrillated. The nurse should avoid doing which of the following?**

   1. Moving away from the bed while the client is defibrillated.
   2. Observing the other nurses to be sure they are not in contact with the client or the bed during defibrillation.
   3. Holding the IV pole out of the way while the client is defibrillated.
   4. Making sure the client's chest is dry, except where the electrode paste or pads are applied for placement of the defibrillator paddles.

8. **When approached by a nurse, a very depressed psychiatric client says, "Don't bother me. Find someone else to talk with. I don't have anything worth saying. Go find someone you can help." Which of the following responses by the nurse would be most therapeutic?**

   1. "OK. I'll go now and be back in a half-hour."
   2. "I have the feeling that I upset you. Don't you want to talk to me?"
   3. "I'm assigned to take care of you, and I intend to spend time with you."
   4. "I would like to stay with you for a while."

9. **A 56-year-old client has peripheral vascular disease with intermittent claudication. Which of the following should the nurse avoid including in the plan of care for this client?**

1. Walking in the local shopping mall for a half-hour each day.
2. Wearing elastic support stockings that are rolled at the top.
3. Sitting in a tub of warm water for 15 minutes each day.
4. Elevating the legs above the level of the heart for two minutes.

10. **A postoperative client has an electronic blood pressure machine automatically measuring her blood pressure every 15 minutes. The blood pressure machine is reading the client's blood pressure at more frequent intervals, and the readings are not similar. The nurse checks the machine settings, and observes additional readings, but the problem continues. What is the best nursing action?**

1. Record only those blood pressures that are needed for the 15-minute intervals.
2. Disconnect the machine and measure the blood pressure with a sphygmomanometer and stethoscope.
3. Turn on the machine every 15 minutes to obtain the client's blood pressure.
4. Measure the blood pressure manually in the opposite arm and compare readings obtained by the machine with the readings obtained manually.

11. **A client is admitted to the hospital with a bleeding duodenal ulcer. He is receiving his first unit of blood when he complains of a headache and itching of his skin. Which of the following nursing actions would demonstrate best judgment initially?**

1. Notify the physician.
2. Give Benadryl as ordered.
3. Stop the blood infusion.
4. Send a urine specimen to the lab.

12. **A client was admitted to the hospital with congestive heart failure. The client's history reveals multiple hospitalizations due to chronic obstructive pulmonary disease. Digoxin (Lanoxin) 0.25 mg was ordered daily for the client. The nurse administering digoxin to the client notices that his breakfast is untouched. The client is also complaining of nausea. The nurse checks his vital signs, which are: BP 120/84, P 64, R 22. Which of the following nursing actions would demonstrate best judgment by the nurse?**

1. Ask the dietician to visit the client.
2. Withhold the drug and call the doctor.
3. Remove the breakfast tray from the room.
4. Request an order for an antiemetic.

13. **A client taking alprazolam (Xanax) should be instructed to avoid ingesting certain substances. Which of the following will the nurse be least likely to include in the list of substances to avoid?**

1. Alcohol.
2. Meperidine (Demerol).
3. Flurazepam (Dalmane).
4. Acetaminophen (Tylenol).

14. **A client is 16 weeks pregnant. She asks if she can still ride her bike for exercise now that she is pregnant. The nurse's best response is which of the following statements?**

1. "If you are used to riding, then it is okay."
2. "You probably shouldn't, since you may fall."
3. "How much bike riding do you normally do?"
4. "You should not ride at all during pregnancy."

15. **The doctor has ordered restraints for a very agitated client. When applying restraints to a client, the nurse should avoid which of the following steps?**

1. Using the least restrictive type of restraint that will effectively protect the client from injury.
2. Fastening restraints to the bed frame.
3. Tying the restraint with a knot that cannot be undone easily, in order to prevent the client from untying it.
4. Explaining to the client and family the type of restraint and the reason for applying the restraint.

16. **A client is eight hours postoperative, following a transurethral resection of the prostate gland. Which of the following assessments would be an early indication of a postoperative complication?**

1. Acute pain at the operative site.
2. Pulse rate of 88 and regular.
3. Copious output of bloody urine.
4. Oral temperature of 101.8° F.

17. **A 69-year-old client is admitted to the hospital. She brings all of her medicines, including a bottle with no label. She says this is her cough medicine, which she put in a small bottle so it would fit in her purse. Which of the following nursing actions is best?**

1. Pour the liquid down the drain, since it has no label.
2. Instruct the client concerning safety issues related to this practice and suggest that she have the pharmacy put the medication in smaller containers that will fit in her purse.

3. Send the bottle home with a family member.

4. Tell the client that this is a dangerous practice that could result in the death of one of her small grandchildren.

18. **A client asks the nurse to telephone her husband and ask him if he remembered to pick up his suit at the cleaners. The nurse knows her husband died five years before. The best nursing response is which of the following statements?**

1. "It may seem like your husband is still here, but he did die in 1988."

2. "You miss your husband a lot, don't you? It must seem like he's almost here with you."

3. "You've forgotten that your husband is dead, haven't you?"

4. "Don't worry. Your husband will remember to pick up his cleaning."

19. **A colostomy has been performed on a 48-year-old female diagnosed with colon cancer. Postoperatively, the nurse is preparing to change the dressing. Which of the following would best describe the expected appearance of the stoma within 24 hours of surgery?**

1. Pale, with a mucoid discharge from the ostomy.

2. Bright red, with a few drops of blood appearing from the stoma.

3. Inclusive of a two centimeter area of eschar.

4. Flush with the abdominal wall.

20. **A male client takes a nitroglycerin (Nitrostat) tablet at the onset of anginal pain. His chest pain is relieved, but he complains of a sudden pounding headache. The nurse is aware that the headache represents:**

1. A hypersensitivity reaction.

2. A toxic adverse reaction.

3. An expected adverse reaction.

4. Orthostatic hypotension.

21. **A client diagnosed with emphysema is being prepared for discharge. Which of the following instructions given by the nurse would be most beneficial for improving his gas exchange?**

1. Teaching home oxygen therapy at five liters/minute.

2. Encouraging him to take slow, deep breaths.

3. Demonstrating the proper technique for chest breathing.

4. Teaching him pursed lip breathing.

22. **The physician prescribes cephradine (Velosef) 250 mg p.o. for a client every six hours. Which of the following is best when the nurse administers the drug?**

1. Wait until the client's temperature returns to normal and the WBC count is under 10,000.

2. Wait at least one hour before or two hours after a meal.

3. Give with food or milk.

4. Give only after determining whether the client's prothrombin time is within normal limits.

23. **A client is admitted to a long-term care facility. She requires total care. In providing mouth care to the client, the nurse should do which of the following?**

1. Place the client on her back with a pillow under her head.

2. Use thumb and index finger to keep the client's mouth open.

3. Use a stiff toothbrush to clean the client's teeth.

4. Place the client on her side before starting mouth care.

24. **A client in an extended care facility is in the dining room, having dinner with the other clients. The client has stopped eating, is grasping his throat with his hands, and cannot talk. The first and most effective action by the nurse is which of the following?**

1. Call a code and obtain assistance, before taking further action.

2. Perform the Heimlich maneuver.

3. Place the client on the floor and begin mouth-to-mouth resuscitation.

4. Slap the client on the back several times.

25. **A premature infant weighed only three pounds seven ounces at birth. Following a lengthy stay in the hospital, her weight has increased to five pounds. She will be discharged soon. Which of the following statements by the mother would indicate to the nurse that additional teaching is needed prior to discharge?**

1. "My baby is so fragile that I will need to be very careful about everything that I do for her."

2. "I know that my baby will need to see the doctor regularly for awhile, and I have the appointments on my calendar."

3. "My mother is going to stay with me for several weeks to help me with my older children."

4. "I have the nursery, clothing, bottles and diapers all ready for the day we bring our baby home."

26. **A 32-year-old client has second and third degree burns over 36% of his body. He is receiving IV fluids at the rate of 450 mL per hour. Serial CVP readings during the first five hours following admission are 3.5, 4.5, 5.0, 6.0 and 8.0. Which of the following is the best interpretation of this data?**

1. Changes in readings may indicate poor technique in measuring CVP.
2. Fluid therapy should continue until CVP is within normal limits.
3. Rapid infusion of fluids has resulted in serious circulatory overload.
4. The consistent rise in CVP is an expected response to fluid therapy.

27. **An 84-year-old married man is admitted from his home to a skilled nursing facility with a diagnosis of Alzheimer's disease. While speaking with the admitting nurse, his wife begins to cry and says, "I never thought it would come to this. I feel so guilty bringing him here." Which nursing response is best?**

1. "You have done all you could. We will take good care of him here."
2. "This has been a difficult time for you. Let's find a quiet place where we can talk."
3. "Admitting your husband was the right decision. He requires more care then you can provide at home."
4. "What are you feeling guilty about?"

28. **A client, 45 years old, had a left pneumonectomy for squamous cell carcinoma. The nurse is assessing her respiratory status on the second post-operative day, using auscultation. Which of the following descriptions of breath sounds is expected?**

1. Breath sounds absent on the left side.
2. Rales heard bilaterally in the bases.
3. Rhonchi heard over the large airways.
4. Crackling sounds heard symmetrically on inspiration.

29. **A client is receiving an intravenous infusion. The nurse should observe the client for signs of infiltration of the IV solution, which would include all of the following except:**

1. The infusion rate slows or stops while the tubing is not kinked.
2. The area around the injection site feels warm to the touch.
3. Swelling, hardness or pain located around the needle site.
4. Blood fails to return in the tubing when the bottle is lowered.

30. **A client is admitted to the hospital following a spontaneous abortion that occurred in her home. The nurse has done an assessment and has determined that the client's condition is stable at this**

time. The client is crying and says to the nurse, "I am so upset. My husband and I wanted a baby so much. Now what will we do?" Which of the following responses by the nurse would be best initially?

1. "Are you feeling overwhelmed?"
2. "You can have another baby soon."
3. "At this time, your husband's support is really important."
4. "There are many options that may be helpful to you, such as genetic counseling."

31. **Before administering the first dose of ceftriaxone (Rocephin) IV to a client, the nurse takes a drug history. The nurse would be especially concerned about any previous reactions to which of the following drugs?**

1. Aminoglycosides.
2. Macrolides.
3. Penicillins.
4. Sulfonamides.

32. **A two-year-old is hospitalized with bacterial pneumonia. The nurse will monitor her respiratory status closely. Which of the following signs/symptoms would the nurse expect to observe as the earliest indication of difficulty?**

1. Respiratory rate of 40 to 48.
2. Blood pressure of 80/60.
3. Cyanosis of mucous membranes.
4. Circumoral/periorbital pallor.

33. **A client with angina pectoris is to take nadolol (Corgard) 40 mg p.o. daily. Which of the following conditions in the client's health history would cause the nurse to question the order for Corgard?**

1. Asthma.
2. Hypothyroidism.
3. Hypertension.
4. Renal insufficiency.

34. **The nurse understands that, physiologically, the difference between angina and myocardial infarction is which of the following?**

1. With angina, arterial perfusion is briefly inadequate. With myocardial infarction, arterial perfusion is cut off permanently.
2. With angina, the enzymes SGOT, LDH, and CPK are elevated. With myocardial infarction, they are not elevated.
3. With angina, adrenocorticosteroids are released to reduce the inflammatory reaction. With myocardial infarction, these hormones are absent.

4. With angina, hypertension and congestive heart failure are absent. With myocardial infarction, hypertension and congestive heart failure are present.

35. **A client is admitted to the abuse treatment unit for a heroin addiction. On the client's third day in the hospital, a friend visits in the evening. The nurse notices that the client seems much more relaxed after his friend leaves. The client tells the nurse that the worst of his withdrawal symptoms from heroin seem to be over. What action by the nurse would be best?**

    1. Obtain a urine specimen to send for a drug screen.
    2. Congratulate him for staying with the program.
    3. Ask about his relationship with his friend to evaluate whether the friend could be a good source of emotional support.
    4. Continue to assess his withdrawal symptoms.

36. **A client who gave birth two days ago is in the bathroom after taking a shower. The nurse hears a loud thud and, after opening the bathroom door, sees the client on the floor and a hair dryer in the sink with the basin full of water. The first action would be which of the following?**

    1. Assess the client to determine if she is breathing.
    2. Assess the client for a heart rate.
    3. Unplug the hair dryer, while taking care not to touch the client or any water or wet surface.
    4. Perform a neurological assessment.

37. **In caring for a 16-year-old client with ulcerative colitis, the nurse understands that an important difference between ulcerative colitis and a conversion disorder is that in ulcerative colitis:**

    1. The physical symptoms are consciously selected by the person.
    2. The physical symptoms are relieved when the mental conflict is resolved.
    3. The physical symptoms may be fatal to the person if left untreated.
    4. The person characteristically has an attitude of indifference toward the physical symptoms.

38. **A 47-year-old school teacher, was admitted to the Coronary Care Unit with a diagnosis of myocardial infarction. After her condition was stabilized, she says to the nurse, "All this equipment is making me nervous. Am I so sick that I need all of this?" Which of the following responses by the nurse would be best initially?**

    1. "All of this equipment can be frightening."
    2. "You won't need the equipment very long."
    3. "Why does the equipment bother you?"
    4. "Let me tell you about what each machine does."

39. **In teaching a 42-year-old client with a history of urolithiasis with uric acid stones, which of the following suggestions would the nurse avoid?**

    1. Drink plenty of fluids, but only early in the day.
    2. Plan for moderate exercise several times a week.
    3. Limit intake of foods high in protein and purine.
    4. Avoid dehydration caused by excessive perspiration.

40. **Prior to delivery, a client is treated with magnesium sulfate. It is noted that her respiratory rate is 12 and deep tendon reflexes are O. Which of the following nursing interventions would be most appropriate?**

    1. Turn off the magnesium sulfate and prepare to give calcium gluconate if ordered by the doctor.
    2. Notify the doctor and the operating room staff to prepare for an immediate C-section.
    3. Monitor blood pressure, urine output and the change in amount of sacral edema.
    4. Put the client in Trendelenburg position and bring the emergency cart into her room.

41. **Which of the following lab values should be monitored by the nurse while the client is taking procainimide (Procan SR) for maintenance therapy after an episode of atrial flutter?**

    1. Potassium.
    2. Platelet count.
    3. Blood urea nitrogen (BUN).
    4. T-3, T-4.

42. **A client is admitted to the psychiatric unit for depression. The nurse observes an improvement in the client's grooming when the client comes to breakfast freshly bathed wearing clean clothes and with her hair combed. Which of the following responses by the nurse would be the most therapeutic?**

    1. "You must be getting better—you look great."
    2. "Let's go put some make-up on to make you look even better."
    3. "Why did you get all dressed up today? Is it a special occasion?"
    4. "You look very nice in your clean dress after your bath and shampoo."

43. **A physician prescribes procainimide (Pronestyl)**

500 mg p.o. every six hours as maintenance therapy after a client's ventricular arrhythmia is corrected. The nurse is aware that which of the following adverse reactions is particularly associated with use of this drug?

1. Hyperglycemia.
2. Hypokalemia.
3. Thrombocytopenia.
4. Hypertension.

44. The preprinted care plan states that the client in Buck's traction has a nursing diagnosis of "high risk for alteration in skin integrity." Which is the best plan to monitor skin integrity?

1. Instruct the client to describe any pain experienced under the boot.
2. Remove the traction and boot to examine the skin each shift.
3. Paint the skin with betadine, which will toughen the skin to breakdown.
4. Observe for any drainage through the boot and report to the physician immediately.

45. The nurse is to administer a blood transfusion to a nine-year-old male hospitalized in sickle cell crisis. Which of the following interventions would most enhance the client's coping ability?

1. Explain the procedure in full detail, so that he will have a complete understanding of what is being done.
2. Have the client role play the fears and frustrations he is experiencing.
3. Encourage the client to write a story about his hospitalization experiences.
4. Allow the client to choose the arm in which he wants the transfusion to be given.

46. An elderly client is going to be discharged to a long-term care facility. What nursing action is best for promoting her continued recovery?

1. Reviewing her nursing care plan with her daughter.
2. Discussing her nursing care needs with her physician.
3. Telephoning the charge nurse at the long-term care facility to explain her nursing care needs.
4. Sending a written summary of her nursing care plan to the long-term care facility.

47. A client is to have a perineal examination, which requires the dorsal recumbent position. Which of the following procedures by the nurse provides the client with the most privacy?

1. Place a bath blanket on the client with one corner

at the chest, two corners wrapped around the feet and legs, and the fourth corner draped between the client's legs.
2. Drape a draw sheet over the client's knees covering the abdomen and legs.
3. Place a bath blanket on the client, with the top at the chest and the bottom draped over the knees to cover the legs and feet.
4. Close the examination room door.

48. After a depressed client is discharged, her husband stops attending family counseling sessions. A nurse from the counseling center makes a follow-up phone call, and the husband says that he doesn't have time for "all that talking." Which of the following responses by the nurse would be most therapeutic?

1. "Because your wife's condition is improving, you will be less involved in family therapy."
2. "You should continue attending the counseling sessions until the therapist tells you to stop."
3. "It must be difficult for you to talk about these family problems"
4. "Continuing counseling is necessary if your wife is to continue making progress."

49. A gastric washing is to be performed on a 15-year-old with possible tuberculosis. When should the nurse anticipate performing this procedure for the best result?

1. Any time when a parent is available to support the client emotionally.
2. Upon awakening in the morning, before breakfast.
3. After the client finishes consuming the contrast media.
4. Following the administration of a mild sedation.

50. Calcium gluconate should be administered with great caution to clients with certain health conditions. The nurse understands that all of the following are health problems that warrant caution when administering calcium gluconate except:

1. Renal transplant.
2. Class II cardiac disease.
3. Epilepsy.
4. Lanoxin therapy.

51. The nurse enters the anorexic client's room and finds her doing vigorous push-ups on the floor. What is the most therapeutic nursing action?

1. Remind her that if her weight decreases she will lose a privilege.
2. Leave the room, permitting her to exercise in pri-

vate.

3. Ask her to stop doing the push-ups and suggest she pursue a less strenuous activity.
4. Wait for her to finish exercising and ask her why she feels the need to exercise.

52. **A client is given IV ritodrine (Yutopar) to postpone labor. Which of the following statements by the client indicates to the nurse that further education is needed?**

1. "If my weight increases several pounds in a day, I need to call my physician."
2. "If my pulse rate is greater than 120, I should call my doctor immediately."
3. "If I get symptoms of a cold, I should get plenty of rest and force fluids."
4. "If I can palpate uterine contractions, I should call my doctor immediately."

53. **A client is to have a urine specimen obtained for routine analysis and culture sensitivity. While collecting the specimen for the lab, the nurse decreases the possibility of transferring microorganisms to others by which of the following actions?**

1. Wearing gloves when handling the specimen container.
2. Applying a label with the client's name and hospital number to the specimen container.
3. Checking the client's identification bracelet.
4. Having the client bring the specimen to the nurses' station when she obtains it.

54. **A client is given procainimide (Pronestyl) 100 mg slow IV push after developing paroxysmal atrial tachycardia. If Pronestyl is given too rapidly, the nurse is aware that the client may develop**

1. AV block.
2. Hypotension.
3. Seizures.
4. Severe throbbing headache.

55. **The nurse discovers a fire in the hospital. Which of the following actions would place the client at risk?**

1. Sound the nearest fire alarm.
2. Move clients who are in the immediate area of the fire.
3. Turn off any oxygen or electrical equipment.
4. Open the doors and windows to let the smoke out.

56. **A client had a myocardial infarction. The nurse visits him at home one week following his discharge. He is taking chlorothiazide (Diuril) 500 mg daily and digoxin (Lanoxin) 0.25 mg daily. The nurse should give top priority to assessing the client's knowledge related to which of the following?**

1. Sources of potassium.
2. Sources of sodium.
3. Activity restrictions.
4. Signs of a heart attack.

57. **A nine-year-old child is discharged following acute rheumatic fever and endocarditis. Which statement by the parents indicates to the nurse that the parents have the best understanding of rheumatic heart disease?**

1. "We will keep low cholesterol foods in our diet."
2. "We may need to move to a warmer climate."
3. "Our son should not participate in sports."
4. "This therapy includes long-term medications."

58. **The nurse is monitoring a client who is on penicillin G potassium IV therapy. Which of the following lab values would be of immediate concern to the nurse when monitoring a client while on this penicillin therapy?**

1. Sodium: 150 mEq/L.
2. Potassium: 5.2 mEq/L.
3. WBC: 13,000/cu mm.
4. Hgb: 14.2 g/dl.

59. **A young client is paralyzed from the waist down. He has a TV, radio, video tape player, stereo, and video game unit, all of which are turned on most of the day. The nurse notices that there are not enough electrical outlets, and that extension cords with multiple outlets are in use to accommodate this equipment. The best nursing action would be to:**

1. Have the client's family take some of the equipment home.
2. Inform the client that an overloaded circuit can cause an electrical fire, and, therefore, the extension cords are not allowed.
3. Tell the client that only single-outlet cords can be used, and that the staff will check often to see if he wants to use anything not currently connected.
4. Call the maintenance department and have more wall outlets installed in the client's room.

60. A client was admitted to the psychiatric unit for obsessive compulsive disorder. The nurse notes that the client's ritualistic behavior of handwashing has increased at bedtime. Which of the following responses by the nurse would be most therapeutic?

   1. "So that you can get to bed on time, you need to start getting ready earlier than the other clients."
   2. "You have one hour to get ready for bed. Then we will talk for a half-hour before you go to sleep."
   3. "I understand you need to reduce your anxiety by washing your hands, so go to bed when you feel tired."
   4. "If you don't stop washing you hands so much, I will have to notify your doctor."

61. In caring for a client immediately following a cardiac catheterization procedure, which of the following nursing actions is appropriate?

   1. Apply warm compresses to the puncture site.
   2. Assist with passive range of motion exercises.
   3. Monitor the client for cardiac arrhythmias.
   4. Assist the client into high Fowler's position.

62. An anorexic client is preparing for discharge from the hospital. Her weight has stabilized and she has agreed to attend outpatient therapy. The nurse would avoid including which of the following provisions in her discharge plans?

   1. Referral to a local eating disorders support group.
   2. Continued family therapy.
   3. Medication management.
   4. Primary health care.

63. The nurse is working in a pediatric clinic. Which of the following clients would be least likely to test HIV positive?

   1. A two-month-old whose mother has been an IV drug addict for two years.
   2. A 15-year-old who has been on treatment for hemophilia since infancy.
   3. An eight-year-old whose best friend is HIV positive.
   4. A 16-year-old who is sexually active.

64. The nurse is taking vital signs and notices an irregularity in the heart rate. Which of the following nursing actions would be most appropriate?

   1. Request the assistance of another staff member and take an apical/radial pulse.
   2. Count the apical pulse rate for one full minute and describe the irregularity in the chart.
   3. Call the doctor and request an order for a Holter monitor recording for the next day.
   4. Take the pulse at each peripheral site and count the rate for 30 seconds.

65. The nurse understands that which of the following statements regarding the administration of RHoGAM is accurate?

   1. It must be given IV, soon after delivery to the mother.
   2. It must be given IM to the mother, within three days after delivery.
   3. It must be given IM, to both the mother and neonate, within 72 hours after delivery.
   4. It must be given to the mother during labor to prevent the formation of antibodies.

66. When administering RHoGAM, the nurse should be aware of the potential adverse reactions in the client. Which of the following clinical findings could be anticipated by the nurse to result from RHoGAM administration?

   1. Rapid pulse rate.
   2. Elevated temperature.
   3. Hot, reddened area around injection site.
   4. Low blood sugar.

67. A disruptive 10-year-old child is having difficulty interacting with other children on the unit. Which of the following nursing actions would be best initially?

   1. Have a unit conference with other staff members and discuss strategies to solve the problem.
   2. Talk to the child about the behavior that is causing the problem and identify possible solutions.
   3. Tell the other children to stop teasing the client and observe for changes in the client's behavior.
   4. Tell the client's mother that she needs to talk to her son about his disruptive behavior.

68. Which of the following approaches is best when the nurse is taking the blood pressure of a client with hypertension?

   1. Measure the blood pressure under the same conditions each time.
   2. Take the blood pressure with the client sitting on the side of the bed.
   3. Place the blood pressure cuff on the right arm above the elbow.
   4. Measure the blood pressure with the client in supine position.

69. **Because a client is taking atenolol (Tenormin), which of the following interventions is most critical for the nurse to include in the plan of care?**

    1. Monitor intake and output.
    2. Do not give Tenormin if apical pulse is less than 50 beats per minute.
    3. Administer Tenormin one hour before or two hours after meals.
    4. Instruct client to change position slowly, especially lying to standing.

70. **A client, age 63, is being treated for Legionnaires' disease with erythromycin estolate (Ilosone). Which of the following conditions, if given in his medical history, would the nurse understand to be a contraindication the use of this drug?**

    1. Pyelonephritis.
    2. Cirrhosis.
    3. Coronary artery disease.
    4. Emphysema.

71. **A client has undergone a transurethral resection of the prostate to correct benign prostatic hypertrophy. He has returned from the recovery room with an indwelling urinary catheter. For several hours the urinary output has been adequate. However, the nurse notes that the catheter has drained no urine during the last hour. What should the nurse do first?**

    1. Offer the client 100 mL of oral fluids each hour.
    2. Irrigate the catheter according to the postoperative orders.
    3. Call the physician and request an increase in IV fluid rate.
    4. Monitor the vital signs every 15 minutes for one hour.

72. **The nurse finds an elderly client standing in a puddle of water in the hallway of the unit. The nurse does not know this client. Which of the following actions should the nurse take initially?**

    1. Ask the client for her name and room number.
    2. Wipe up the water until the floor is completely dry.
    3. Call the supervisor for assistance in identifying the client.
    4. Have the client wait in the lounge until security arrives.

73. **In which of the following client situations does the nurse understand that the administration of betamethasone (Celestone) is both advisable and safe?**

    1. Gestational age 30 weeks, insulin dependent diabetic mother, no tocolysis given.

    2. Gestational age 28 weeks, mother with mild PIH, no tocolysis given.
    3. Gestational age 35 weeks, no tocolysis given.
    4. Gestational age 30 weeks, chronic hypertensive mother, tocolysis given.

74. **Which of the following activities would be appropriate for the nurse to suggest to a manic client?**

    1. A daily walk on the hospital grounds.
    2. Playing a computer game with another client.
    3. Participation in a basketball game with other male clients.
    4. Reading quietly in his room.

75. **Following a normal vaginal delivery, a client is given an IV containing oxytocin (Pitocin). To evaluate the effectiveness of this drug, the nurse needs to assess which of the following?**

    1. Pulse rate.
    2. Blood pressure.
    3. Urinary output.
    4. Fundal consistency.

76. **The nurse assists an angry, confused client with a displaced oxygen cannula and raises the head of the bed to high Fowler's position. The nurse places his dinner on the overbed table and prepares the dinner by cutting the meat and spreading the bread according to the client's preference. It is essential for the nurse to carry out which of the following nursing actions before leaving the room?**

    1. Ask the client if he needs further assistance with his meals.
    2. Assist the client with menu selections for the following day.
    3. Tell the client when the nurse will return to his room.
    4. Place the call bell where the client can easily reach it.

77. **A 10-week-old male is admitted to the pediatric unit with a diagnosis of inorganic failure to thrive. He is the first child of a 16-year-old mother and a 17-year-old father. Which of the following would the nurse select as the priority nursing diagnosis?**

    1. Altered nutrition: less than body requirements related to physical abuse.
    2. Sensory/perceptual alterations (gustatory) related to infant deprivation.
    3. Altered growth and development related to poor suck.
    4. Altered parenting related to knowledge deficit.

78. **Because of hyperactivity and difficulty sleeping, the most therapeutic room arrangement that the nurse can make for a manic client is which of the following?**

    1. A private bedroom.
    2. A semi-private room with a roommate who has a similar problem.
    3. Either a private or semi-private room.
    4. Direct admission to the seclusion room until his activity level becomes more subdued.

79. **A diabetic client, age 75, is prescribed ampicillin (Omnipen) by his physician. The nurse should give highest priority to asking the client which of the following questions, before he leaves the clinic?**

    1. Which method do you use to monitor your glucose level?
    2. Do you have any food allergies?
    3. Do you have any difficulty swallowing capsules?
    4. Do you have a history of liver disease?

80. **A 38-year-old is admitted to the hospital for a severe episode of gastrointestinal bleeding secondary to a peptic ulcer. He is scheduled for an upper GI series. In preparing the client for this diagnostic procedure, which of the following should the nurse include in teaching for the client?**

    1. An upper GI series will take five or six hours to complete. Since you will be waiting much of this time, you should take something to read with you.
    2. This is a series of x-rays in which the entire GI tract is delineated. A liquid suspension of barium sulfate taken orally is the contrast medium.
    3. The client should not eat or drink anything after midnight on the evening before the test. However, following the first x-rays, full liquids are allowed.
    4. A laxative is administered the day before the test. On the morning of the test, soap suds enemas are given until the returns are clear.

81. **A manic client tells the nurse that his latest computer project is "revolutionizing the industry." He also states, "IBM and Apple are both going under because their products cannot compete with mine." In choosing how to respond, the nurse is best guided by the knowledge that:**

    1. This statement is grandiose and does not require a response.
    2. This statement represents the client's inability to deal with inner feelings of inadequacy and vulnerability.
    3. Manic clients are prone to exaggerate the facts of a situation.
    4. This is a delusional statement that should be confronted to correct the client's perception of reality.

82. **A client who is 43 years old has a long history of peptic ulcer. She is admitted now for treatment of pyloric obstruction. An order has been written for a nasogastric tube. The nurse understands that the best rationale for the use of the nasogastric tube is:**

    1. Collection of laboratory specimens.
    2. Supplying nutrients via tube feedings.
    3. Decompression of the stomach.
    4. Administration of medications.

83. **A client was admitted to the psychiatric unit with a diagnosis of bipolar mood disorder. At 3:00 a.m., the client ran to the nurses station demanding that she see her therapist immediately. Which of these responses by the nurse would be best initially?**

    1. "Calm down, go back to your room, and I'll try to get in touch with your therapist right away."
    2. "Regulations state that I can't call the therapist in the middle of the night except in an emergency."
    3. "You must be very upset about something to want to see your therapist in the middle of the night."
    4. "You are being unreasonable and I will not call your therapist at 3:00 in the morning."

84. **The nurse understands that the effective use of limit-setting with hyperactive clients requires all of the following except:**

    1. Providing a consistent, structured environment so the client knows what is expected of him or her.
    2. The specific limits to be used must be understood and agreed upon by all staff members on all shifts.
    3. The client's requests for greater freedom should be granted to evaluate the progress that has been made.
    4. Consequences should be direct results of behavior and perceived by the client as negative outcomes.

85. **In addition to nitrate therapy, a client is to begin nifedipine (Procardia) 10 mg p.o. every six hours. When giving this medication along with nitrates, the nurse will observe for:**

    1. Tremor.
    2. Tetany.
    3. Hypotension.
    4. Hyperkalemia.

86. **A 22-year-old sustained a fracture of the tibia and fibula while playing football. A long leg cast was applied, and the client was admitted to the orthopedic unit. Following four weeks of bed rest, the nurse notes decreased breath sounds in the lower lobes of both lungs. What is the best explanation for this change in breath sounds?**

1. The client did not take deep breaths while the nurse examined his lower lobes.
2. Because of improper positioning, the client has developed pulmonary edema.
3. Atelectasis, caused by immobility, has resulted in the decreased breath sounds.
4. The client's resistance is down, and he has caught a cold from someone else.

87. **A 36-year-old client has hypertension and is treated with chlorothiazide (Diuril). Which of the following should the nurse include in the teaching plan?**

1. Dietary sodium should be restricted to one gram daily.
2. Avoid using Diuril with other antihypertensives.
3. Orthostatic hypotension may be a side effect.
4. It is unnecessary to increase dietary potassium.

88. **The nurse understands that, in comparing skeletal traction to skin traction, which statement is correct?**

1. Skeletal traction can be utilized longer than skin traction.
2. Clients in skin traction have more pain than those in skeletal traction.
3. Skin traction is more likely to be complicated by osteomyelitis.
4. The risk of skin breakdown is greater with skeletal traction.

89. **A client is hospitalized with schizophrenia. During a conversation with a female nurse, the client seemed relaxed initially, but then became restless and began wringing his hands. The nurse stated to the client that he seemed tense, and he agreed. Which of these responses by the nurse would demonstrate the best understanding at this time?**

1. "Do you often feel tense when you are talking to a woman?"
2. "What were we discussing when you began to feel uncomfortable?"
3. "Did I say something wrong that made you feel tense?"
4. "I sometimes feel tense, too, when I am talking to a stranger."

90. **What information about diet should the nurse give all clients taking lithium?**

1. Sodium intake should be restricted to 1200 mg per day.
2. Fluid intake should not exceed 1000 mL per day.
3. An adequate daily intake of sodium and fluids should be maintained.
4. Sodium and fluid intake should be increased.

91. **A client, 23 years old, has a fractured right femur. She is placed in skeletal traction with a Thomas splint and Pearson attachment. Which of the following interventions for positioning this client is appropriate?**

1. Position the client's right foot on the bed in direct line with the femur.
2. Use trochanter rolls to prevent abduction of the right leg.
3. Allow the client to turn slightly from side to side above the waist.
4. Maintain the client flat with only brief periods with her head elevated.

92. **The nurse observes that in the first few days of hospitalization, an 18-month-old client sits quietly sucking her thumb in the corner of her crib. When the nurse approaches the crib, the client shyly turns her head away from the nurse. Which interpretation of her behavior is most justifiable?**

1. The behavior is indicative of pathological reaction to hospitalization.
2. The relationship between parents and child needs to be evaluated.
3. The behavior demonstrates an anxiety reaction to the stress of hospitalization.
4. The negative behavior is a beginning attempt at autonomy.

93. **A eight-year-old client is admitted with a diagnosis of acute rheumatic fever. During the first few days after admission, the nurse would demonstrate best judgment by suggesting which of the following activities for the client?**

1. Playing computer games in the game room.
2. Visiting with several school friends.
3. Completing school assignments.
4. Listening to favorite cassette tapes.

1. No. The client should be on bedrest during the acute phase of rheumatic fever. Rest is very important because it decreases the cardiac workload. The nurse should promote rest.

2. No. Visiting with several school friends does not promote rest during the acute phase.

3. No. Completing school assignments does not promote rest during the acute phase.

4. Yes! This is the best answer! The client should be on bedrest during the acute phase of rheumatic fever. Rest is very important because it decreases the cardiac workload. The nurse should promote rest.

94. **A 65-year-old male is admitted to the emergency department with unequal grips and aphasia. The goal of initial treatment for this client is best achieved by which of the following actions?**

    1. Preparing to begin an IV infusion.
    2. Raising the HOB to 30 degrees.
    3. Monitoring BP.
    4. Explaining MRI to the client and family.

95. **After four weeks of hospitalization, the client says to the nurse, "My son called and told me that my boss has hired someone to take my place." Which of the following is the most therapeutic response by the nurse?**

    1. "I don't understand why your son would tell you that now."
    2. "You must feel very concerned about your boss not holding your job."
    3. "There isn't anything you can do about that until you go home."
    4. "Why don't you call your wife and see if she can change his mind?"

96. **A 40-year-old client is returning from surgery with a radium implant for the treatment of endometrial cancer. Which nursing diagnosis would be most helpful in planning this client's care?**

    1. Alteration in nutrition related to anorexia.
    2. Body image disturbance related to alopecia.
    3. Alteration in mobility related to bedrest.
    4. Potential for injury related to radiation.

97. **The nurse understands that a client with primary degenerative dementia experiences:**

    1. Memory loss gradually progressing to disorientation.
    3. Personality traits develop that are opposite of original traits.

    4. Increased auditory and visual acuity offset other losses.

98. **A 38-year-old is admitted to the hospital with recurrence of the symptoms of leukemia. The client says to the nurse, "The doctor told me that my blood condition is too severe to be treated successfully. I guess I don't have long to live." Which of these responses by the nurse would be best?**

    1. "Tell me exactly what your doctor meant when he said that your condition was too severe."
    2. "Do you think that having a good mental outlook can help you at this time?"
    3. "Your condition is very serious."
    4. "How long do feel that you have left to live?"

99. **A 39-year-old female has had a right radical mastectomy. Which activity would the nurse anticipate being the most difficult for this client four days postoperatively?**

    1. Brushing her hair with her right hand.
    2. Eating with her right hand.
    3. Active-assisted range of motion of the right hand.
    4. Washing her hands in a basin.

100. **The physician prescribes verapamil (Calan) 100 mg p.o. three times a day for a client with angina pectoris. The client states: "My brother takes Calan for high blood pressure. Do you think the doctor made a mistake?" The nurse's most therapeutic response would be:**

    1. "I'll check with the physician to verify the order."
    2. "Calan is effective in two ways: to treat angina and to manage high blood pressure."
    3. "Are you concerned that you might have high blood pressure?"
    4. "No, the physician has prescribed Calan so that you will not develop high blood pressure."

NCLEX-RN

Test 9

Questions with Rationales

NCLEX-RN TEST 9 WITH RATIONALES

1. **A client is taking both digoxin (Lanoxin) and chlorothiazide (Diuril). The nurse has completed discharge teaching regarding diet. Which of the following menus, if selected by the client, would indicate that she can identify good food sources for potassium?**

   1. Baked chicken, boiled potato, pudding.
   2. Boiled chicken, rice, cranberry juice.
   3. Broiled meat, baked potato, citrus fruit salad.
   4. Beef stew, bread and butter, jello.

   1. *Wrong choice! Chicken and potato are both good sources of potassium, but since the potato is boiled it has lost significant amounts of potassium. Milk products contain some potassium but are not considered a good source.*
   2. *Wrong choice! Chicken is a good source of potassium, but since it is boiled it has lost significant amounts of potassium. Rice and cranberry juice contain only small amounts of potassium.*
   3. ***Very good! Broiled meat, baked potato and citrus fruit salad are all good sources of potassium and the cooking methods have not depleted this nutrient.***
   4. *Wrong choice! Beef is a good source of potassium, but bread, butter and jello are not.*

2. **While working in a unit where the clients are on cardiac monitors, the nurse hears an alarm and notices that one of the clients has a straight line on the cardiac monitor, indicating a cardiac arrest. Which of the following is the initial nursing action?**

   1. Call a code.
   2. Notify the physician.
   3. Administer cardiopulmonary resuscitation.
   4. Assess the client.

   1. *Since machines used to monitor clients can malfunction, calling a code is not the initial nursing action.*
   2. *This action may be necessary, but it is not the initial nursing response. The physician may not have to be notified if the client did not have a cardiac arrest. A lead may have come loose or the monitor may be malfunctioning.*
   3. *This action may be necessary, but it is not the initial nursing response. The nurse needs more information.*
   4. ***Correct! Assessing the client will provide the nurse with knowledge to make an appropriate decision. If the client is able to be aroused or a pulse is***

palpated, then the client did not have a cardiac arrest, and there is a problem with the monitoring equipment.

3. **A two-year-old boy with a rectal temperature of 101° F is diagnosed with a viral illness. Which statement by the mother would indicate to the nurse that further teaching is needed?**

   1. "I will give him 1/4 tsp of acetaminophen (Tylenol) for a temperature over 101° F."
   2. "I will give him extra fluids over the next couple of days."
   3. "I will give him two baby aspirin (acetylsalicylic acid) every four hours."
   4. "I will keep him home from day care while he has a fever."

   1. *No, Acetaminophen is an antipyretic that is appropriate for use in children. This statement does not indicate a need for further teaching, which is the focus of this false response stem question.*
   2. *Wrong choice! Giving the child extra fluids will maintain hydration by replacing fluid lost in the fever. This statement does not indicate a need for further teaching.*
   3. ***This is the correct choice! Aspirin is contraindicated in viral illness because it has been associated with Reyes syndrome, a potentially fatal illness. This mother definitely needs further teaching.***
   4. *Wrong choice! If he is kept at home while ill, the child will not place other children at risk, or be exposed to additional illnesses. This statement does not indicate a need for further teaching.*

4. **Which of the following findings on assessment would alert the nurse to a possible serious adverse effect of diltiazem (Cardizem) therapy?**

   1. Drowsiness.
   2. Hypertension.
   3. Rhonchi.
   4. Gingival hyperplasia.

   1. *No. Drowsiness is a side effect, but is not common (like fatigue) nor is it serious or life-threatening.*
   2. *Incorrect. Cardizem is a calcium channel blocker used alone or in combination with other agents in the management of hypertension. A common side effect of Cardizem is hypotension.*
   3. ***Correct choice. Edema is a frequently occurring***

side effect of Cardizem therapy. Clients should be assessed for signs of congestive heart failure such as peripheral edema, rales/crackles, dyspnea, and/or weight gain.

4. *Wrong. Cardizem may occasionally cause gingival hyperplasia, but it's not life-threatening. The client is advised to maintain good oral hygiene and have regular dental examinations and cleaning to prevent gingival tenderness, bleeding, and enlargement.*

5. **A 28-year-old client had a D&C this morning. She has returned to the unit from the recovery room. She says to the nurse, "I am hungry. When can I eat?" In determining when the client can have something by mouth, which of the following nursing actions would demonstrate best judgment?**

1. Request a diet order from the doctor.
2. Determine when the next meal will be served.
3. Use a stethoscope to listen to the client's abdomen.
4. Check the chart for a diet order.

1. *Before the client can have anything by mouth, bowel activity must return to normal. Further assessment is needed before requesting a diet order from the doctor. Note that Options 1 and 4 are similar because they both focus on the diet order, and similar distractors can be eliminated.*

2. *The time of the next meal is not relevant. After a client has been NPO for surgery, the first thing given by mouth is usually ice chips or ice water, which are available anytime.*

3. ***This is the correct answer! Before giving the client anything by mouth, assess bowel function by listening to the abdomen with a stethoscope.***

> **STRATEGY ALERT!** Note that Options 1 and 4 both focus on the diet order. These two similar distractors can be eliminated.

4. *Before the client can have anything by mouth, bowel activity must return to normal. Further assessment is needed before looking for a diet order. Note that Options 1 and 4 are similar because they both focus on the diet order, and similar distractors can be eliminated.*

6. **One morning the nurse asks an elderly client if she had any visitors the day before. She responds that several members of her church choir had been to see her. The nurse knows that only her daughter had visited the day before. A fabrication that is told to mask memory loss is which of the following?**

1. Delusion.
2. Illusion.
3. Confabulation.
4. Dissociation.

1. *This is not correct. A delusion is a false, fixed belief. Delusional thinking is most often associated with schizophrenia and other psychotic disorders.*

2. *This is not correct. An illusion is a sensory misperception and not a thinking problem.*

3. ***Correct. Confabulation is making up responses that are inaccurate but sound appropriate. It is done to avoid the embarrassment about memory loss.***

4. *This is not correct. Dissociation is the defense mechanism of separating aspects of memory or emotions from the rest of one's conscious awareness or identity.*

7. **During the resuscitation of a client, the physician orders the client to be defibrillated. The nurse should avoid doing which of the following?**

1. Moving away from the bed while the client is defibrillated.
2. Observing the other nurses to be sure they are not in contact with the client or the bed during defibrillation.
3. Holding the IV pole out of the way while the client is defibrillated.
4. Making sure the client's chest is dry, except where the electrode paste or pads are applied for placement of the defibrillator paddles.

1. *The nurse does not want to avoid moving away while the client is defibrillated! Touching the bed or the client may result in the nurse receiving an electrical shock, since the electricity the client receives can be conducted to anything with which the client is in contact.*

2. *This is a correct action, and, therefore, not the correct answer to this question. The nurse should observe for other nurses who may be so involved in performing a particular task, such as starting an intravenous, that the physician's order may not be heard. Observing their actions and alerting them may protect them from an electrical injury.*

3. ***That's right! The nurse should avoid touching the IV pole because the pole may conduct electricity by way of the IV fluid that the client is receiving. Touching it could result in an electrical shock to the nurse.***

4. *This is a correct action, and, therefore, not the correct answer to this question. Moisture is an excellent conductor of electricity. During defibrillation, the electricity will follow the path of least resistance, which could be any moisture on the chest, and which could result in burns to the chest area where the moisture is present.*

8. When approached by a nurse, a very depressed psychiatric client says, "Don't bother me. Find someone else to talk with. I don't have anything worth saying. Go find someone you can help." Which of the following responses by the nurse would be most therapeutic?

    1. "OK. I'll go now and be back in a half-hour."
    2. "I have the feeling that I upset you. Don't you want to talk to me?"
    3. "I'm assigned to take care of you, and I intend to spend time with you."
    4. "I would like to stay with you for a while."

    1. *This is not correct. The client is a very depressed person. The appropriate nursing action for a very depressed client is to stay with the client. This option does not allow the nurse to remain with the client, and the client's safety may therefore be jeopardized.*
    2. *This response is focused on the nurse. Focusing on the nurse is not therapeutic for the client and cannot be the correct answer in a communication question.*
    3. *Wrong! This answer is focused on the needs of the nurse rather than on the needs of the client. Focusing on the nurse is not therapeutic for the client and is not the correct answer for a communication question.*
    4. ***Excellent! The client is a very depressed client. The appropriate nursing action for a very depressed client is to stay with the client. This response allows the nurse to remain with the client. At the same time, the nurse communicates caring.***

9. A 56-year-old client has peripheral vascular disease with intermittent claudication. Which of the following should the nurse avoid including in the plan of care for this client?

    1. Walking in the local shopping mall for a half-hour each day.
    2. Wearing elastic support stockings that are rolled at the top.
    3. Sitting in a tub of warm water for 15 minutes each day.
    4. Elevating the legs above the level of the heart for two minutes.

    1. *Walking, particularly on a level surface such as in a shopping mall, is an effective exercise that will enhance arterial blood supply and decrease venous congestion in the lower extremities. This question has a false response stem, which means you need to choose an option that represents something the client should NOT do.*
    2. ***Correct answer! This is something the client should not do. Wearing elastic stockings that are rolled at the top may act as a tourniquet and produce stasis, rather than decrease venous congestion.***

    3. *Although a hot bath would be contraindicated, a warm bath is good therapy. A hot bath will increase the metabolism of the cells in the tissues, which will increase the circulatory demand. A bath that is warm, but not hot, will stimulate circulation. This question has a false response stem, so you need to choose an option that is something the client should NOT do.*
    4. *Elevating the legs above the level of the heart for a short period of time will use gravity to drain venous congestion. Look for the option that describes something the client should NOT do.*

10. A postoperative client has an electronic blood pressure machine automatically measuring her blood pressure every 15 minutes. The blood pressure machine is reading the client's blood pressure at more frequent intervals, and the readings are not similar. The nurse checks the machine settings, and observes additional readings, but the problem continues. What is the best nursing action?

    1. Record only those blood pressures that are needed for the 15-minute intervals.
    2. Disconnect the machine and measure the blood pressure with a sphygmomanometer and stethoscope.
    3. Turn on the machine every 15 minutes to obtain the client's blood pressure.
    4. Measure the blood pressure manually in the opposite arm and compare readings obtained by the machine with the readings obtained manually.

    1. *This is incorrect. Although blood pressure readings are being obtained, the fact that the machine is taking the blood pressure more frequently and the measurements obtained are not similar suggests that the machine is malfunctioning and is in need of repair.*
    2. ***Very good. If there is a question concerning the reliability of the monitoring equipment, a manual check should be made, so that a client does not receive medical treatment because of an erroneous measurement.***
    3. *No. Since the measurements and the operation of the machine appear to be questionable, the machine should be taken out of service and repaired.*
    4. *Although this option appears to provide a means of checking the machine, the fact that it is not operating correctly suggests that it should not be used until it has been checked by a biomedical technician.*

11. A client is admitted to the hospital with a bleeding duodenal ulcer. He is receiving his first unit of blood when he complains of a headache and itching of his skin. Which of the following nursing actions would demonstrate best judgment initially?

1. Notify the physician.
2. Give Benadryl as ordered.
3. Stop the blood infusion.
4. Send a urine specimen to the lab.

1. *Incorrect. Headaches and itching skin are symptoms of a blood transfusion reaction, which is a medical emergency. The physician should be notified, but this should not be the initial action.*

2. *No! Headaches and itching skin are symptoms of a blood transfusion reaction, which is a medical emergency. Benadryl may be ordered to treat itching, but this should not be the initial action.*

3. ***Very good! Headaches and itching skin are symptoms of a blood transfusion reaction, which can be life-threatening. The nurse assesses the symptoms and makes a diagnosis that this is a medical emergency. The nurse must stop the transfusion immediately to prevent a more severe reaction. Maslow's Hierarchy of Needs indicates that physiological and safety needs receive priority. There is a possibility of anaphylactic shock, which is a life-threatening complication.***

4. *Wrong choice! Headache and itching skin are symptoms of a blood transfusion reaction, which is a medical emergency. A urine specimen may be sent to the lab to determine the presence of hematuria, but this should not be the initial action.*

12. **A client was admitted to the hospital with congestive heart failure. The client's history reveals multiple hospitalizations due to chronic obstructive pulmonary disease. Digoxin (Lanoxin) 0.25 mg was ordered daily for the client. The nurse administering digoxin to the client notices that his breakfast is untouched. The client is also complaining of nausea. The nurse checks his vital signs, which are: BP 120/84, P 64, R 22. Which of the following nursing actions would demonstrate best judgment by the nurse?**

1. Ask the dietician to visit the client.
2. Withhold the drug and call the doctor.
3. Remove the breakfast tray from the room.
4. Request an order for an antiemetic.

1. *Wrong! It is likely that the client is not eating because he is nauseated secondary to digoxin toxicity. The dietitian may be able to identify and provide foods that are the client's preferences, but it is likely that he still will not eat because of the nausea. In addition, if the digoxin toxicity is not treated, it may lead to serious complications such as cardiac arrhythmias.*

2. ***Excellent! It is likely that the client is not eating because he is nauseated secondary to digoxin toxicity. Another symptom of digoxin toxicity is bradycardia. The client's pulse rate is not 60 or less, but at 64, it is borderline. Because of the***

serious nature of complications that may develop if digoxin toxicity is not treated (cardiac arrhythmias), the nurse should withhold the drug and call the doctor.

3. *Wrong! It would be appropriate for the nurse to remove the breakfast tray from the room. Clients who are nauseated do not want to see or smell food. However, this action is not the most appropriate action. It is likely that the client's nausea is secondary to digoxin toxicity. Because of the serious nature of complications that may develop if digoxin toxicity is not treated (cardiac arrhythmias), the nurse should withhold the drug and call the doctor.*

4. *Wrong! It is likely that the client's nausea is secondary to digoxin toxicity. Because of the serious nature of the complications that may develop if digoxin toxicity is not treated (cardiac arrhythmias), the nurse should withhold the drug and call the doctor.*

13. **A client taking alprazolam (Xanax) should be instructed to avoid ingesting certain substances. Which of the following will the nurse be least likely to include in the list of substances to avoid?**

1. Alcohol.
2. Meperidine (Demerol).
3. Flurazepam (Dalmane).
4. Acetaminophen (Tylenol).

1. *Wrong! A client taking Xanax should be instructed to avoid the use of alcohol because their central nervous system depressant effects will be potentiated and could lead to accidental overdose and death. This is a negative response stem and so the correct answer is an option that does not have to be avoided by the client taking Xanax.*

2. *Try again. Clients on Xanax should avoid the use of other CNS depressants, such as Dalmane, because of their potentiation effects. This is a negative response question, so the correct answer is an option that does not have to be avoided by the client taking Xanax.*

3. *Incorrect choice. Clients on Xanax should avoid other benzodiazepine drugs, such as Dalmane, because of the potentiation effects. This is a negative response question, so the correct answer is an option that does not have to be avoided by the client taking Xanax.*

4. ***Correct! This client could safely take acetaminophen. Since this question has a negative response stem, the correct answer is an option that does not have to be avoided by the client taking Xanax.***

14. **A client is 16 weeks pregnant. She asks if she can still ride her bike for exercise now that she is pregnant. The nurse's best response is which of the following statements?**

1. "If you are used to riding, then it is okay."
2. "You probably shouldn't, since you may fall."
3. "How much bike riding do you normally do?"
4. "You should not ride at all during pregnancy."

1. *This statement may be appropriate, depending on how much exercise the client is talking about. The nurse does not have sufficient information at this point to select this as the correct response. Which of the priority setting guidelines should be used in answering this question?*
2. *This statement may be appropriate during the latter part of pregnancy, when balance can present a problem, however, in this question the client is only 16 weeks pregnant. If the client rides regularly, it is not necessary to prohibit a moderate amount of bike riding because of balance alone at this stage of pregnancy. Does the nurse have enough information at this point to answer the client's question? Which of the priority setting guidelines should be used in answering this test question?*
3. *Correct. The nurse doesn't have enough information to answer the client's question. The nurse must first assess what she usually does for exercise. This question uses the nursing process as a priority setting guideline. The nursing process tells us to always assess first.*

> **STRATEGY ALERT!** Note that the other three options are all implementations. Also, Options 2 and 4 both tell the client that it is inadvisable for her to ride, so neither of these can be correct.

4. *No. Exercise during pregnancy is important. In most cases, a pregnant client can continue with the type of exercise she does when she is not pregnant. Does the nurse have enough information to answer this client's question about bicycle riding?*

15. **The doctor has ordered restraints for a very agitated client. When applying restraints to a client, the nurse should avoid which of the following steps?**

1. Using the least restrictive type of restraint that will effectively protect the client from injury.
2. Fastening restraints to the bed frame.
3. Tying the restraint with a knot that cannot be undone easily, in order to prevent the client from untying it.
4. Explaining to the client and family the type of restraint and the reason for applying the restraint.

1. *No, the nurse wants to use the least restrictive type of restraint since over-restraining a client can intensify the problems caused by immobility. The question asks you to identify an action that the nurse should AVOID.*
2. *The nurse does not want to avoid fastening the restraints to the bed frame. The bed frame rather than the side rails should be used to attach the restraints because the bed frame is more stable.*

Lowering side rails that have restraints attached can result in injury to the client. The question asks you to identify an incorrect action.
3. *Very good! This is something that the nurse should avoid. Restraints should be tied with knots that can be undone easily, in case the client's well being necessitates removal of the restraints. To protect the client from releasing the restraints, the knot should be placed where the client cannot reach it.*
4. *Incorrect choice. Restraints can increase the client's confusion and cause anger and hostility in the client and family. An explanation concerning the client's safety can help to promote understanding and cooperation. This is not the correct answer, however, because the question asks you to identify something the nurse should AVOID.*

16. **A client is eight hours postoperative, following a transurethral resection of the prostate gland. Which of the following assessments would be an early indication of a postoperative complication?**

1. Acute pain at the operative site.
2. Pulse rate of 88 and regular.
3. Copious output of bloody urine.
4. Oral temperature of 101.8° F.

1. *Incorrect. Acute pain in the operative site is expected following surgery. It should be treated with medication as ordered, to keep the client as comfortable as possible and to allow the client to participate in care by coughing, deep breathing, and ambulating as ordered.*
2. *Wrong. A regular pulse rate of 88 is within normal limits and would not indicate an early postoperative complication.*
3. *Wrong. Copious output of bloody urine is expected following a transurethral resection of the prostate gland. Plenty of fluids are provided to this client initially through an IV to stimulate output of large amounts of urine. The increased urine output serves to flush the bloody clot from the bladder following the operation.*
4. *Correct. An oral temperature of 101.8° F represents a slight temperature elevation. This is an important assessment. A temperature elevation postoperatively could suggest either an infection or atelectasis of the lungs. In either case, this would be considered a postoperative complication.*

17. **A 69-year-old client is admitted to the hospital. She brings all of her medicines, including a bottle with no label. She says this is her cough medicine, which she put in a small bottle so it would fit in her purse. Which of the following nursing actions is best?**

1. Pour the liquid down the drain, since it has no label.
2. Instruct the client concerning safety issues related to this practice and suggest that she have the pharmacy put the medication in smaller containers that will fit in her purse.
3. Send the bottle home with a family member.
4. Tell the client that this is a dangerous practice that could result in the death of one of her small grandchildren.

1. *Wrong. The medication belongs to the client and may be expensive. Although placing medication in an unlabelled container is not a safe practice, the client should be informed of the hazard and be told of safer alternatives.*
2. **Yes, best choice! Instructing the client regarding safety issues and discussing alternatives allows the client to participate in health care decisions, which results in a higher rate of compliance.**
3. *No. The bottle can be sent home with a family member; however, this is a safety issue which should be discussed with the client.*
4. *No. Using fear as an approach is not appropriate, and this response by the nurse is not therapeutic. In addition, labelling the bottle will not prevent small children from ingesting the contents if given access to the medication. All medications must be kept out of the reach of children.*

18. **A client asks the nurse to telephone her husband and ask him if he remembered to pick up his suit at the cleaners. The nurse knows her husband died five years before. The best nursing response is which of the following statements?**

1. "It may seem like your husband is still here, but he did die in 1988."
2. "You miss your husband a lot, don't you? It must seem like he's almost here with you."
3. "You've forgotten that your husband is dead, haven't you?"
4. "Don't worry. Your husband will remember to pick up his cleaning."

1. *This response is an attempt to orient the client to reality. It is not incorrect, but it is not the best response.*
2. **Correct. This nursing response validates the client's feelings and acknowledges her experience. This is the best option because the nurse is responding to the feelings underlying the client's comment, instead of the disordered content.**
3. *This is not correct because the nurse is responding only to the content in the client's statement. The response indicates no empathy for how the client is feeling.*
4. *This is not correct because it validates a reality that does not exist.*

19. **A colostomy has been performed on a 48-year-old female diagnosed with colon cancer. Postoperatively, the nurse is preparing to change the dressing. Which of the following would best describe the expected appearance of the stoma within 24 hours of surgery?**

1. Pale, with a mucoid discharge from the ostomy.
2. Bright red, with a few drops of blood appearing from the stoma.
3. Inclusive of a two centimeter area of eschar.
4. Flush with the abdominal wall.

1. *No. This would indicate a reduced blood supply. The mucous may be present, but it does not indicate a functioning or healthy stoma.*
2. **Great! A small amount of blood from the stoma would be acceptable and indicates a healthy bowel with a good blood supply.**
3. *No, this indicates tissue death either from a burn or gangrene. This stoma is not healthy.*
4. *Not likely. As the stoma matures it will shrink, but immediately after surgery, the stoma is usually edematous. A stoma flush with the abdomen is not desirable, since it will be difficult to ensure maintenance of skin integrity.*

20. **A male client takes a nitroglycerin (Nitrostat) tablet at the onset of anginal pain. His chest pain is relieved, but he complains of a sudden pounding headache. The nurse is aware that the headache represents:**

1. A hypersensitivity reaction.
2. A toxic adverse reaction.
3. An expected adverse reaction.
4. Orthostatic hypotension.

1. *Incorrect. A hypersensitivity (allergic) reaction to Nitrostat would not be evidenced by a headache.*
2. *No, a headache after use of Nitrostat does not indicate a toxic adverse reaction. Remember that nitroglycerin is a potent vasodilator.*
3. **Yes! Adverse reactions commonly associated with nitrates include a headache, sometimes with throbbing, due to vasodilation of cerebral blood vessels. This side effect should decrease with continuing therapy. The client should notify the physician if the headache is persistent or severe. Sometimes aspirin or acetaminophen may be ordered to treat headache: it may or may not be effective.**
4. *Wrong choice. Orthostatic hypotension is manifested by dizziness or lightheadedness when changing position from lying to standing (due to sudden drop in blood pressure). Make another selection.*

21. A client diagnosed with emphysema is being pre-pared for discharge. Which of the following in-structions given by the nurse would be most ben-eficial for improving his gas exchange?

    1. Teaching home oxygen therapy at five liters/minute.
    2. Encouraging him to take slow, deep breaths.
    3. Demonstrating the proper technique for chest breathing.
    4. Teaching him pursed lip breathing.

    1. *Incorrect! Remember that low concentrations of oxygen (one to two liters/minute) are indicated for clients with COPD.*
    2. *No. Although this is an expected outcome, the nurse must teach the client how to achieve this effect.*
    3. *No! The client with COPD should be taught dia-phragmatic breathing, which helps to reduce the respiratory rate and increases alveolar ventila-tion.*
    4. ***Good choice! Pursed lip breathing slows expira-tion, prevents collapse of lung units, and helps the client to control the rate and depth of respira-tions.***

22. The physician prescribes cephradine (Velosef) 250 mg p.o. for a client every six hours. Which of the following is best when the nurse administers the drug?

    1. Wait until the client's temperature returns to nor-mal and the WBC count is under 10,000.
    2. Wait at least one hour before or two hours after a meal.
    3. Give with food or milk.
    4. Give only after determining whether the client's prothrombin time is within normal limits.

    1. *Incorrect. A cardinal rule of antibiotic therapy is that the client is always instructed to take the medi-cation exactly as prescribed, at evenly spaced in-tervals, for the full length of time prescribed or until all the drug is gone. Absence of signs of infec-tion is no indication to discontinue treatment.*
    2. *Taking cephalosporins on an empty stomach may exacerbate the GI distress often associated with these medications.*
    3. ***Good choice! Velosef is well absorbed orally and can be taken with food or milk if gastric irritation develops.***
    4. *No. Velosef does not affect the client's clotting times. NOTE: Certain cephalosporins (Cefobid, Cefotan, Moxam) may cause hypoprothrombinemia; there-fore, bleeding time and PT should be monitored when these drugs are given.*

23. A client is admitted to a long-term care facility. She requires total care. In providing mouth care to the client, the nurse should do which of the following?

    1. Place the client on her back with a pillow under her head.
    2. Use thumb and index finger to keep the client's mouth open.
    3. Use a stiff toothbrush to clean the client's teeth.
    4. Place the client on her side before starting mouth care.

    1. *Wrong. Placing the client on her back during mouth care could result in aspiration of fluid into the lungs.*
    2. *Wrong. A padded tongue blade — not a thumb or an index finger — should be used to keep the client's mouth open.*
    3. *No. A soft toothbrush should be used, not a stiff one.*
    4. ***This is correct, because placing the client on her side encourages fluids to run out of her mouth.***

24. A client in an extended care facility is in the din-ing room, having dinner with the other clients. The client has stopped eating, is grasping his throat with his hands, and cannot talk. The first and most effective action by the nurse is which of the following?

    1. Call a code and obtain assistance, before taking further action.
    2. Perform the Heimlich maneuver.
    3. Place the client on the floor and begin mouth-to-mouth resuscitation.
    4. Slap the client on the back several times.

    1. *It is not necessary to call a code at this time. Also, choking requires immediate intervention. Waiting for help places the client at further risk.*
    2. ***Excellent choice! The Heimlich maneuver is the most effective method to clear an obstructed air-way of a choking person.***
    3. *This action is inappropriate and might cause fur-ther danger to the client. Mouth-to-mouth resusci-tation is indicated after the airway has been cleared, for a client who has ceased breathing. Mouth-to-mouth resuscitation performed on a choking client could lodge the food even further into the airway.*
    4. *Wrong. The client is choking. Slapping a person on the back is not the best intervention for choking.*

25. A premature infant weighed only three pounds seven ounces at birth. Following a lengthy stay in the hospital, her weight has increased to five pounds. She will be discharged soon. Which of the following statements by the mother would in-dicate to the nurse that additional teaching is needed prior to discharge?

1. "My baby is so fragile that I will need to be very careful about everything that I do for her."
2. "I know that my baby will need to see the doctor regularly for awhile, and I have the appointments on my calendar."
3. "My mother is going to stay with me for several weeks to help me with my older children."
4. "I have the nursery, clothing, bottles and diapers all ready for the day we bring our baby home."

1. *Caring for a premature infant at home should not be any different from caring for a full term baby. This statement does reflect a need for further instruction.*
2. *Wrong! Regular doctor appointments are especially important for premature infants because there is a greater risk for anemia and failure to thrive. This correct statement is not the answer, however, because this question has a false response stem. You are looking for a statement by the mother that is not correct.*
3. *Extra help with household chores and older children is additional support that is helpful when mother and baby are adjusting to a new schedule. This correct statement is not the answer to this question, which has a false response stem.*
4. *This comment indicates that the mother is prepared to provide care for the baby at home. This is not the answer to this question, which has a false response stem.*

26. **A 32-year-old client has second and third degree burns over 36% of his body. He is receiving IV fluids at the rate of 450 mL per hour. Serial CVP readings during the first five hours following admission are 3.5, 4.5, 5.0, 6.0 and 8.0. Which of the following is the best interpretation of this data?**

1. Changes in readings may indicate poor technique in measuring CVP.
2. Fluid therapy should continue until CVP is within normal limits.
3. Rapid infusion of fluids has resulted in serious circulatory overload.
4. The consistent rise in CVP is an expected response to fluid therapy.

1. *Wrong. Fluctuations in CVP readings may result from poor technique. However, the stem asks you to select the best interpretation, and the gradual increase in these readings does not suggest poor technique.*
2. *While it is true that fluid therapy should continue in order to maintain adequate hydration, the data indicate that CVP is already within normal limits. You are looking for the best interpretation.*
3. *Wrong choice! There is no data to suggest circulatory overload. The CVP is within normal limits.*

4. *Correct choice! Rapid infusion of fluids in this burn client is meant to achieve and maintain adequate hydration. The CVP readings are now within normal limits. This is the best interpretation of the data.*

27. **An 84-year-old married man is admitted from his home to a skilled nursing facility with a diagnosis of Alzheimer's disease. While speaking with the admitting nurse, his wife begins to cry and says, "I never thought it would come to this. I feel so guilty bringing him here." Which nursing response is best?**

1. "You have done all you could. We will take good care of him here."
2. "This has been a difficult time for you. Let's find a quiet place where we can talk."
3. "Admitting your husband was the right decision. He requires more care then you can provide at home."
4. "What are you feeling guilty about?"

1. *This statement is not the best nursing response because it is a form of false reassurance. The nurse is assuming the wife did all she could. The nurse can not know this without further assessment.*
2. *Correct. The nurse is acknowledging the wife's feelings and is offering self to assist her with them. The nursing goal is to help the wife deal with her feelings so she will be able to support her husband with his adjustment to the nursing home.*
3. *This is not the best option. The nurse is giving advice instead of helping the wife to deal constructively with her feelings.*
4. *This is not correct. The wife has told the nurse that she feels guilty about admitting her husband to the long-term care facility. Asking this question indicates that the nurse either has not listened or is not sensitive to the wife's feelings.*

28. **A client, 45 years old, had a left pneumonectomy for squamous cell carcinoma. The nurse is assessing her respiratory status on the second postoperative day, using auscultation. Which of the following descriptions of breath sounds is expected?**

1. Breath sounds absent on the left side.
2. Rales heard bilaterally in the bases.
3. Rhonchi heard over the large airways.
4. Crackling sounds heard symmetrically on inspiration.

1. *Correct. Since pneumonectomy involves the removal of a lung, no breath sounds should be heard on the operative side.*
2. *Rales, which are produced by moisture in the tracheobronchial tree, would not be heard on the operative side after a pneumonectomy. The word*

"bilaterally" makes this option a false statement, and not the answer.

3. *Incorrect. Normal vesicular breath sounds would not be heard on the operative side after a pneumonectomy.*

4. *Following a pneumonectomy, the operative side should have no breath sounds. The word "symmetrically" makes this an inaccurate statement and a distractor, since this question has a true response stem.*

29. **A client is receiving an intravenous infusion. The nurse should observe the client for signs of infiltration of the IV solution, which would include all of the following except:**

    1. The infusion rate slows or stops while the tubing is not kinked.
    2. The area around the injection site feels warm to the touch.
    3. Swelling, hardness or pain located around the needle site.
    4. Blood fails to return in the tubing when the bottle is lowered.

    1. *Wrong! One sign of infiltration is that the infusion rate slows or stops while the tubing is not kinked. Since this question has a false response stem, you are looking something that would NOT be present when an IV is infiltrated.*
    2. ***Very good! The area around the injection site would not feel warm to the touch when the IV is infiltrated. Since the IV fluid is at room temperature, it is cooler than body temperature. The area around the injection site will feel cool to the touch when the IV is infiltrated. If the area around the injection site feels warm to the touch, it may indicate infection or phlebitis.***
    3. *Wrong choice. One sign of infiltration is swelling, hardness, or pain located around the needle site. Since this question has a false response stem, you are looking for something that would NOT be present when an IV is infiltrated.*
    4. *Not the correct choice! One sign of infiltration is that the blood fails to return in the tubing when the bottle is lowered. Since this question has a false response stem, you are looking for something that would NOT be present when an IV is infiltrated.*

30. **A client is admitted to the hospital following a spontaneous abortion that occurred in her home. The nurse has done an assessment and has determined that the client's condition is stable at this time. The client is crying and says to the nurse, "I am so upset. My husband and I wanted a baby so much. Now what will we do?" Which of the following responses by the nurse would be best initially?**

    1. "Are you feeling overwhelmed?"
    2. "You can have another baby soon."
    3. "At this time, your husband's support is really important."
    4. "There are many options that may be helpful to you, such as genetic counseling."

    1. ***Yes! You are correct! In this option, the nurse is using the tools of showing empathy and restatement to acknowledge the client's feelings and encourage the client to express her concerns.***

    > **PRIORITY ALERT!** *Communication theory indicates that the priority is to deal with the client's feelings.*

    2. *In this option the nurse's response gives false reassurance, and demeans the client's feelings. This response is not therapeutic and cannot be the answer.*
    3. *This option is focused on an inappropriate person and an inappropriate issue. This response blocks communication because it does not recognize the client's feelings.*
    4. *In this response the nurse is giving information, but it is not a therapeutic response because the client is very upset and the response fails to recognize her feelings. The client might even interpret this response as demeaning. Also, we do not have any information to indicate that the problem is genetic. The nurse's response should first address the client's feelings.*

31. **Before administering the first dose of ceftriaxone (Rocephin) IV to a client, the nurse takes a drug history. The nurse would be especially concerned about any previous reactions to which of the following drugs?**

    1. Aminoglycosides.
    2. Macrolides.
    3. Penicillins.
    4. Sulfonamides.

    1. *Incorrect. There is no evidence of cross-sensitivity between cephalosporins and aminoglycosides.*
    2. *No. Macrolides are often prescribed for clients who are allergic to penicillin.*
    3. ***Correct. Cephalosporins and penicillins may have cross-sensitivity (5-10% risk) due to similarities in their chemical structures. Physicians may prescribe cephalosporins even for clients allergic to penicillins; however, if the client reports a serious reaction or anaphylaxis to penicillin, cephalosporins should not be used.***
    4. *Incorrect. There is no evidence of cross-sensitivity between cephalosporins and sulfonamides.*

32. **A two-year-old is hospitalized with bacterial pneumonia. The nurse will monitor her respiratory status closely. Which of the following signs/symptoms would the nurse expect to observe as the earliest indication of difficulty?**

    1. Respiratory rate of 40 to 48.
    2. Blood pressure of 80/60.
    3. Cyanosis of mucous membranes.
    4. Circumoral/periorbital pallor.

    1. *Correct. One early indication of respiratory difficulty is an increased respiratory rate. A respiratory rate of 40 to 48 is rapid for a two-year-old.*
    2. *Blood pressure of 80/60 is within normal limits for a two-year-ole and does not indicate increased respiratory difficulty.*
    3. *Cyanosis of mucous membranes is certainly a sign of respiratory difficulty. However, this is a late sign. The nurse should be alert for early signs so that appropriate intervention can begin.*
    4. *Wrong! Circumoral/periorbital pallor is certainly a sign of respiratory difficulty. However, this is a late sign. The nurse should be alert for early signs so that appropriate intervention can begin.*

33. **A client with angina pectoris is to take nadolol (Corgard) 40 mg p.o. daily. Which of the following conditions in the client's health history would cause the nurse to question the order for Corgard?**

    1. Asthma.
    2. Hypothyroidism.
    3. Hypertension.
    4. Renal insufficiency.

    1. *Correct. Corgard is a beta-adrenergic blocker. This means that the drug works by blocking the sympathetic response at the receptor site. Blocking the sympathetic response in the bronchioles can cause bronchospasms in clients with obstructive pulmonary disease (e.g., asthma, emphysema).*
    2. *No. Nadolol can mask signs of hyperthyroidism (and also hypoglycemia). The client's thyroid studies and blood glucose levels will need to be monitored regularly.*
    3. *Wrong choice. Recall that nadolol is a beta-adrenergic blocker, used in the management of angina pectoris AND also used alone or in combination with other agents in the treatment of hypertension. A side effect of nadolol is hypotension—not hypertension.*
    4. *Incorrect choice. Nadolol should be used cautiously in clients with renal impairment because 70% of the drug is excreted unchanged by the kidneys; however, renal insufficiency is not a contraindication.*

34. **The nurse understands that, physiologically, the difference between angina and myocardial infarction is which of the following?**

    1. With angina, arterial perfusion is briefly inadequate. With myocardial infarction, arterial perfusion is cut off permanently.
    2. With angina, the enzymes SGOT, LDH, and CPK are elevated. With myocardial infarction, they are not elevated.
    3. With angina, adrenocorticosteroids are released to reduce the inflammatory reaction. With myocardial infarction, these hormones are absent.
    4. With angina, hypertension and congestive heart failure are absent. With myocardial infarction, hypertension and congestive heart failure are present.

    1. *Correct. The arterial supply is inadequate in angina but permanently blocked in a myocardial infarction. This is the best answer!*
    2. *Wrong! In fact, the opposite is true: after an infarction, the enzymes are elevated. Since there is no muscle or tissue damage in angina, the enzymes are not elevated. This is a distractor. Try again!*
    3. *This is a good distractor; but it is incorrect. There is no inflammatory reaction in a myocardial infarction. Were you confused by this option? When you are deciding between two options, always choose what you know for sure!*
    4. *This option looks like a possibility. The statement is false, however, because these are complications that may be associated with either angina or a myocardial infarction. They are not characteristic of just one of these conditions. This option is a distractor. Try again!*

    > **STUDY TIP:** *You may wish to select the other options to see why they are incorrect.*

35. **A client is admitted to the abuse treatment unit for a heroin addiction. On the client's third day in the hospital, a friend visits in the evening. The nurse notices that the client seems much more relaxed after his friend leaves. The client tells the nurse that the worst of his withdrawal symptoms from heroin seem to be over. What action by the nurse would be best?**

    1. Obtain a urine specimen to send for a drug screen.
    2. Congratulate him for staying with the program.
    3. Ask about his relationship with his friend to evaluate whether the friend could be a good source of emotional support.
    4. Continue to assess his withdrawal symptoms.

    1. *Correct. A drug screen should be done when the nurse observes that the client's withdrawal symp-*

toms dramatically improve, especially when the withdrawal syndrome has not run its full course. In the case of opioids, including heroin, this is seven to 10 days.

2. *This is not correct. The nursing priority is to assess the reason for this client's improvement.*

3. *The issue in this question is the sudden improvement in withdrawal symptoms. The nurse needs to accurately assess the reason for this client's improvement, since the withdrawal syndrome has not run its full course.*

4. *The issue in this question is the sudden improvement in withdrawal symptoms. The nurse needs to accurately assess the reason for this client's improvement, since the withdrawal syndrome has not run its full course.*

36. **A client who gave birth two days ago is in the bathroom after taking a shower. The nurse hears a loud thud and, after opening the bathroom door, sees the client on the floor and a hair dryer in the sink with the basin full of water. The first action would be which of the following?**

1. Assess the client to determine if she is breathing.
2. Assess the client for a heart rate.
3. Unplug the hair dryer, while taking care not to touch the client or any water or wet surface.
4. Perform a neurological assessment.

1. *Wrong. While this is important and should be done, it is not the first action, since the safety of the nurse may also be at stake in this situation.*

2. *Wrong. Assessing the heart rate is not the first nursing action during an emergency.*

3. **Correct. The hair dryer in a basin of water appears to be the cause of this client's problem. The dryer still poses a serious electrical hazard and should be carefully unplugged, so that the nurse does not also become injured and unable to help the client.**

4. *No. While this is an appropriate measure, the safety of the nurse may be at stake in this situation. This option is not the first action to initiate.*

37. **In caring for a 16-year-old client with ulcerative colitis, the nurse understands that an important difference between ulcerative colitis and a conversion disorder is that in ulcerative colitis:**

1. The physical symptoms are consciously selected by the person.
2. The physical symptoms are relieved when the mental conflict is resolved.
3. The physical symptoms may be fatal to the person if left untreated.
4. The person characteristically has an attitude of indifference toward the physical symptoms.

1. *No. The physical symptoms are not consciously selected in either illness.*

2. *Not correct! Ulcerative colitis is a psychosomatic disorder. The symptoms decrease as the mental conflict is relieved in both psychosomatic and conversion disorders. The stem asks you to identify a characteristic of ulcerative colitis but not conversion disorders. This is a good distractor!*

3. **This is correct! The potential for loss of life is a major difference between these two illnesses. The client with ulcerative colitis (a psychosomatic disorder) may die from his illness if there is no medical intervention. The client with a conversion disorder (for example, hysterical blindness) will not die from his physical symptoms. In this question, the nurse understands that the client with ulcerative colitis may die without medical intervention.**

4. *This is a false statement, because it represents a characteristic of a conversion disorder. The client with ulcerative colitis is very concerned about his medical problem, since it is life-threatening.*

38. **A 47-year-old school teacher, was admitted to the Coronary Care Unit with a diagnosis of myocardial infarction. After her condition was stabilized, she says to the nurse, "All this equipment is making me nervous. Am I so sick that I need all of this?" Which of the following responses by the nurse would be best initially?**

1. "All of this equipment can be frightening."
2. "You won't need the equipment very long."
3. "Why does the equipment bother you?"
4. "Let me tell you about what each machine does."

1. **Best choice! The nurse's first response should recognize the client's feelings. Communication theory indicates that the client's feelings should receive priority.**

2. *Incorrect. This response may be false reassurance, and it doesn't address the client's feelings. This response is not therapeutic.*

3. *Wrong. This response is an intimidating "why" question. Questions that begin with who, what, when, where and how are less intimidating and more therapeutic. What is the priority in communication theory?*

4. *Incorrect! This response indicates that the nurse is going to teach the client about the function of each piece of equipment. Giving information is a communication tool, but it is not the priority in communication theory. To be therapeutic, the nurse should first address the client's feelings.*

39. **In teaching a 42-year-old client with a history of urolithiasis with uric acid stones, which of the following suggestions would the nurse avoid?**

1. Drink plenty of fluids, but only early in the day.
2. Plan for moderate exercise several times a week.
3. Limit intake of foods high in protein and purine.
4. Avoid dehydration caused by excessive perspiration.

1. *Correct! This option is the inappropriate. Stones form more readily in concentrated urine, and high fluid intake throughout the day assures dilute urine. This option includes limiting intake of fluids to early in the day, which may cause concentrated urine during the night.*
2. *Incorrect choice. Immobility may lead to slowing of drainage from the kidneys, which would encourage the formation of stones. Moderate exercise is appropriate.*
3. *Metabolic breakdown of protein foods high in purine yields uric acid. Limiting the intake of these foods is appropriate because it will decrease the amount of uric acid available for stone formation. This correct statement is not the answer to this false response stem.*
4. *Stones form more readily in concentrated urine, and dehydration leads to concentrated urine. High fluid intake throughout the day will assure dilute urine and is appropriate. This correct statement is not the answer to this false response stem.*

40. **Prior to delivery, a client is treated with magnesium sulfate. It is noted that her respiratory rate is 12 and deep tendon reflexes are O. Which of the following nursing interventions would be most appropriate?**

1. Turn off the magnesium sulfate and prepare to give calcium gluconate if ordered by the doctor.
2. Notify the doctor and the operating room staff to prepare for an immediate C-section.
3. Monitor blood pressure, urine output and the change in amount of sacral edema.
4. Put the client in Trendelenburg position and bring the emergency cart into her room.

1. *Very good! Magnesium sulfate has caused central nervous system depression. The antidote for magnesium sulfate is calcium gluconate. The nurse should recognize the symptoms and prepare for the treatment as ordered by the doctor.*
2. *Wrong! Magnesium sulfate has caused central nervous system depression. The best course of action is to treat the cause of the problem before serious damage is done to the mother and/or baby. A C-section is not indicated.*
3. *Wrong! Monitoring blood pressure, urine output and sacral edema are appropriate nursing actions for a client with pregnancy induced hypertension. However, in this case the client also has central nervous system depression secondary to adminis-*

tration of magnesium sulfate. The best course of action is to treat the cause of the problem before serious damage is done to the mother and/or the baby. The nurse should recognize these symptoms and prepare for the treatment as ordered by the doctor.
4. *No! Trendelenburg position is used for clients in shock when the blood pressure drops. This position is not indicated for this client. The client has central nervous system depression secondary to administration of magnesium sulfate. The nurse should recognize these symptoms and prepare for the treatment as ordered by the doctor. The best course of action is to treat the cause of the problem before serious damage is done to the mother and/or the baby.*

41. **Which of the following lab values should be monitored by the nurse while the client is taking procainimide (Procan SR) for maintenance therapy after an episode of atrial flutter?**

1. Potassium.
2. Platelet count.
3. Blood urea nitrogen (BUN).
4. T-3, T-4.

1. *Wrong choice. Procan SR will not affect the potassium level. This lab value should be monitored closely when the client is taking diuretics, especially furosemide (Lasix) or one of the thiazides.*
2. *Absolutely! The complete blood count (CBC) should be monitored weekly during the first three months of therapy because procainimide can decrease platelet counts due to quinidine-platelet complexes, which cause platelet destruction.*
3. *Incorrect. The blood urea nitrogen (BUN) is not affected by procainimide therapy. The drug, however, may cause an increase in AST, ALT, LDH, and bilirubin levels.*
4. *No, procainimide does not affect the thyroid gland; therefore, the T-3 and T-4 levels would not change.*

42. **A client is admitted to the psychiatric unit for depression. The nurse observes an improvement in the client's grooming when the client comes to breakfast freshly bathed wearing clean clothes and with her hair combed. Which of the following responses by the nurse would be the most therapeutic?**

1. "You must be getting better—you look great."
2. "Let's go put some make-up on to make you look even better."
3. "Why did you get all dressed up today? Is it a special occasion?"
4. "You look very nice in your clean dress after your bath and shampoo."

1. *Wrong. The first part of the option is an example of false reassurance. The fact that the client looks good does not assure that she is getting better. Sometimes depressed clients appear improved after having made a suicide decision. This response is not therapeutic.*
2. *Wrong. This option devalues the client's behavior because it implies that what she did isn't good enough.*
3. *Wrong. This option requests an explanation. "Why" questions block therapeutic communication.*
4. ***Very good! This option acknowledges and affirms the client's behavior.***

43. **A physician prescribes procainimide (Pronestyl) 500 mg p.o. every six hours as maintenance therapy after a client's ventricular arrhythmia is corrected. The nurse is aware that which of the following adverse reactions is particularly associated with use of this drug?**

    1. Hyperglycemia.
    2. Hypokalemia.
    3. Thrombocytopenia.
    4. Hypertension.

    1. *Incorrect. The endocrine system is not affected by Pronestyl, which is an antiarrhythmic agent. Make another selection.*
    2. *Wrong. Hypokalemia is seen in clients who take diuretics for hypertension control. Pronestyl has no apparent effect upon electrolyte levels.*
    3. ***Good choice! Pronestyl can cause leukopenia and thrombocytopenia. The client is advised to notify the physician immediately if signs of thrombocytopenia (unusual bleeding or bruising) or leukopenia (sore throat, mouth, or gums) occur. The medication may be discontinued if these problems occur.***
    4. *Not true. Hypotension is an expected side effect of Pronestyl therapy. Parameters for pulse and blood pressure should be monitored periodically during oral administration of this antiarrhythmic.*

44. **The preprinted care plan states that the client in Buck's traction has a nursing diagnosis of "high risk for alteration in skin integrity." Which is the best plan to monitor skin integrity?**

    1. Instruct the client to describe any pain experienced under the boot.
    2. Remove the traction and boot to examine the skin each shift.
    3. Paint the skin with betadine, which will toughen the skin to breakdown.
    4. Observe for any drainage through the boot and report to the physician immediately.

    1. *Incorrect. The client can be instructed to report*

pain, but this is not the best method to assess skin integrity.
2. ***This is correct. The best method of assessment is a visual inspection to pick up early signs of skin changes.***
3. *You're not answering the question. This is an intervention, not an assessment or monitoring function.*
4. *No. By the time that drainage has occurred there is a serious interruption in the skin integrity. This is not the best way to determine alterations in skin integrity.*

45. **The nurse is to administer a blood transfusion to a nine-year-old male hospitalized in sickle cell crisis. Which of the following interventions would most enhance the client's coping ability?**

    1. Explain the procedure in full detail, so that he will have a complete understanding of what is being done.
    2. Have the client role play the fears and frustrations he is experiencing.
    3. Encourage the client to write a story about his hospitalization experiences.
    4. Allow the client to choose the arm in which he wants the transfusion to be given.

    1. *No, a full explanation isn't appropriate. He is very ill. This response is not age appropriate.*
    2. *No, a role play would take too long before doing the procedure. This might be something to do when the treatment is complete and his condition is stable, to allow expression of his fears.*
    3. *Incorrect. This might be appropriate for later, however, the stem states that this child is in sickle cell crisis. This indicates acute illness, and he is too sick to write stories.*
    4. ***This is an appropriate measure, which allows the child some control over the situation but does not delay the necessary care.***

46. **An elderly client is going to be discharged to a long-term care facility. What nursing action is best for promoting her continued recovery?**

    1. Reviewing her nursing care plan with her daughter.
    2. Discussing her nursing care needs with her physician.
    3. Telephoning the charge nurse at the long-term care facility to explain her nursing care needs.
    4. Sending a written summary of her nursing care plan to the long-term care facility.

    1. *This is not the best action. The family should know about the client's needs for care, but there is a better way to promote continuity of care.*
    2. *This is not the best action even for clients who will*

continue to use the same physician. Select the option that would better promote the continuity of her nursing care.

3. *This is a possibility, but there is a better option.*

4. *Correct. A written summary of her nursing care plan is the best way of conveying the client's nursing care needs to the nurses who will actually work with her in the long-term care facility.*

47. **A client is to have a perineal examination, which requires the dorsal recumbent position. Which of the following procedures by the nurse provides the client with the most privacy?**

1. Place a bath blanket on the client with one corner at the chest, two corners wrapped around the feet and legs, and the fourth corner draped between the client's legs.

2. Drape a draw sheet over the client's knees covering the abdomen and legs.

3. Place a bath blanket on the client, with the top at the chest and the bottom draped over the knees to cover the legs and feet.

4. Close the examination room door.

1. *Correct! This option provides the most privacy for the client by keeping the client completely covered until the examination is performed. The examiner can lift the corner of the blanket that is between the client's legs and expose only the perineal area.*

2. *This option does not provide much privacy since the legs are not wrapped and the sheet must be pushed up to expose the perineum, which exposes the legs and thighs.*

3. *This is not correct. Since the blanket must be pushed up to examine the perineum, the client's legs and thighs are completely exposed.*

4. *Draping the client properly provides more privacy, since anyone can open the examination room door.*

48. **After a depressed client is discharged, her husband stops attending family counseling sessions. A nurse from the counseling center makes a follow-up phone call, and the husband says that he doesn't have time for "all that talking." Which of the following responses by the nurse would be most therapeutic?**

1. "Because your wife's condition is improving, you will be less involved in family therapy."

2. "You should continue attending the counseling sessions until the therapist tells you to stop."

3. "It must be difficult for you to talk about these family problems"

4. "Continuing counseling is necessary if your wife is to continue making progress."

1. *Wrong! This option is an example of false reassur-*

ance. An improvement in the client's condition does not mean that therapy can be discontinued. Also, this response is inappropriate because it is the therapist's role to determine the length of family therapy, not the nurse's.

2. *Wrong! This option is an example of the nurse giving advice. This is a communication block. It is unlikely that the client will return to counseling sessions as a result of this response.*

3. *Good choice! This option is an example of the nurse showing empathy. The husband's comment to the nurse states that he is having difficulty with "talking" sessions, and the nurse is showing an understanding of his feelings. The nurse is also helping the client focus on what it is about the counseling that bothers him. Helping the client explore his feelings at this time is pivotal to the family's continuing therapy and for the long-term benefit of his wife.*

4. *Wrong. The husband is the client in this question, and his feelings about the family therapy are the issue. This response focuses on an inappropriate person (his wife), and an inappropriate concern (his wife's progress). This response also blocks communication by giving advice. To be therapeutic, the nurse's response must deal with the client's feelings about the family therapy.*

49. **A gastric washing is to be performed on a 15-year-old with possible tuberculosis. When should the nurse anticipate performing this procedure for the best result?**

1. Any time when a parent is available to support the client emotionally.

2. Upon awakening in the morning, before breakfast.

3. After the client finishes consuming the contrast media.

4. Following the administration of a mild sedation.

1. *No, but this is a good distractor! "Any time" makes this incorrect. Furthermore, not all adolescents even want the parent present during procedures, although this should be offered.*

2. *Correct! To obtain the best possible specimen the client should not eat or get up before the Levine tube is inserted and the specimen obtained. The object is to collect a specimen with the greatest possible concentration of tubercle bacilli that have been swallowed during the night.*

3. *No. Contrast media is not used; this is not a radiographic study.*

4. *Incorrect. This is not a painful procedure. With an appropriate explanation, the nurse should anticipate cooperation from this client.*

50. **Calcium gluconate should be administered with great caution to clients with certain health condi-**

tions. The nurse understands that all of the following are health problems that warrant caution when administering calcium gluconate except:

1. Renal transplant.
2. Class II cardiac disease.
3. Epilepsy.
4. Lanoxin therapy.

1. *Incorrect answer. Clients who have renal disease should not receive calcium gluconate unless great caution is used.*
2. *Wrong answer. Many of the adverse reactions to calcium gluconate are related to cardiac activity. It should be used with great caution in the client with pre-existing cardiac disease.*
3. **Correct. The presence of epilepsy has no effect on the decision to use calcium gluconate and the subsequent need for monitoring the client.**
4. *Wrong. Great caution needs to be exercised when administering calcium gluconate to a digitalized client.*

51. **The nurse enters the anorexic client's room and finds her doing vigorous push-ups on the floor. What is the most therapeutic nursing action?**

1. Remind her that if her weight decreases she will lose a privilege.
2. Leave the room, permitting her to exercise in private.
3. Ask her to stop doing the push-ups and suggest she pursue a less strenuous activity.
4. Wait for her to finish exercising and ask her why she feels the need to exercise.

1. *This is not correct. Vigorous physical exercise is a compulsive behavior in anorexic clients, and the threat of losing privileges will not deter the client from this activity.*
2. *This is not correct. Active intervention is required to prevent the client from continuing to lose weight.*
3. **Correct. The nurse has to actively intervene to interrupt undesirable behaviors, such as vigorous exercise. The goal of treatment is to promote weight gain through behavior modification.**
4. *This is not correct. Active intervention on the part of the nurse is needed to prevent further weight loss by burning calories. Discussing feelings indicates that the nurse does not understand the compulsive nature of some of the client's behaviors.*

52. **A client is given IV ritodrine (Yutopar) to postpone labor. Which of the following statements by the client indicates to the nurse that further education is needed?**

1. "If my weight increases several pounds in a day, I need to call my physician."

2. "If my pulse rate is greater than 120, I should call my doctor immediately."
3. "If I get symptoms of a cold, I should get plenty of rest and force fluids."
4. "If I can palpate uterine contractions, I should call my doctor immediately."

1. *Wrong choice! A frequent complication of ritodrine therapy is pulmonary edema. An early warning sign is a rapid weight gain.*
2. *Wrong choice! Tachycardia is a common side effect of ritodrine therapy. Clients are taught to report pulse rates greater than 120.*
3. **Good choice! The symptoms of a cold might be the early signs of pulmonary edema and the client needs to be seen immediately.**
4. *Wrong choice! Clients receiving tocolysis should palpate the uterus several times throughout the day to assess for mild contractions. Aggressive treatment of early labor is the best way to prevent preterm labor.*

53. **A client is to have a urine specimen obtained for routine analysis and culture sensitivity. While collecting the specimen for the lab, the nurse decreases the possibility of transferring microorganisms to others by which of the following actions?**

1. Wearing gloves when handling the specimen container.
2. Applying a label with the client's name and hospital number to the specimen container.
3. Checking the client's identification bracelet.
4. Having the client bring the specimen to the nurses' station when she obtains it.

1. **Best choice! Universal precautions include the wearing of gloves when touching anything that may be contaminated with body fluids.**
2. *Wrong! Identifying the specimen container is an appropriate intervention but it does not decrease the possibility of transferring microorganisms to others.*
3. *Wrong choice! The client's identification bracelet should be checked to determine the origin of the specimen but doing so does not decrease the possibility of transferring microorganisms to others.*
4. *Wrong choice! Having the client bring a urine specimen to the nursing station is not an appropriate nursing action, since the possibility of the patient contaminating a clean surface is present. The nurse should tell the client to let the staff know when the specimen is ready and collect it from the client's room.*

54. **A client is given procainimide (Pronestyl) 100**

mg slow IV push after developing paroxysmal atrial tachycardia. If Pronestyl is given too rapidly, the nurse is aware that the client may develop

1.   AV block.
2.   Hypotension.
3.   Seizures.
4.   Severe throbbing headache.

1.   *Incorrect. AV block (heart block) can occur when the client receives verapamil (Calan), a calcium channel blocker. Heart block is an uncommon side effect of Pronestyl therapy.*
2.   **Yes. Blood pressure should be monitored continuously throughout IV administration. If the blood pressure drops more than 15 mm. Hg., IV administration is usually discontinued. The client should remain supine to minimize hypotension.**
3.   *Wrong choice. Seizures are an adverse life-threatening side effect seen more often in clients receiving lidocaine. Choose again.*
4.   *No. Recall that a headache is a common side effect of nitroglycerin therapy. The central nervous side effects seen with Pronestyl use are confusion and dizziness.*

55. **The nurse discovers a fire in the hospital. Which of the following actions would put the client at risk?**

1.   Sound the nearest fire alarm.
2.   Move clients who are in the immediate area of the fire.
3.   Turn off any oxygen or electrical equipment.
4.   Open the doors and windows to let the smoke out.

1.   *This is an appropriate action in case of fire. This question has a negative response stem, and is looking for an action that is UNSAFE.*
2.   *This is an appropriate action in case of fire. The stem of this question is looking for an option that is NOT safe.*
3.   *This is an appropriate action in case of fire. This question has a false response stem, and is asking for an option that is UNSAFE.*
4.   **Correct option! Opening doors and windows makes the fire worse by providing more oxygen. Doors and windows should be shut.**

56. **A client had a myocardial infarction. The nurse visits him at home one week following his discharge. He is taking chlorothiazide (Diuril) 500 mg daily and digoxin (Lanoxin) 0.25 mg daily. The nurse should give top priority to assessing the client's knowledge related to which of the following?**

1.   Sources of potassium.
2.   Sources of sodium.
3.   Activity restrictions.
4.   Signs of a heart attack.

1.   **Very good! Because the client is taking both Diuril and digoxin, the nurse should focus on his knowledge related to sources of potassium. Diuril depletes potassium. If the potassium level is too low, digoxin toxicity may lead to serious cardiac arrhythmias. This is the top priority because lack of understanding may be life-threatening very quickly.**
2.   *No! The client is probably on a sodium restricted diet. Too much sodium will increase the cardiac workload. The nurse should assess the client's knowledge of sources of sodium, but based on the information provided in the case scenario this is not the top priority.*
3.   *Wrong! The client will increase his activity gradually as he recuperates from the myocardial infarction. The nurse should assess the client's knowledge of activity restrictions, but based on the information provided in the case scenario this is not the top priority.*
4.   *Wrong choice! The nurse should assess the client's knowledge of the signs of another heart attack, but based on the information provided in the case scenario this is not the top priority.*

57. **A nine-year-old child is discharged following acute rheumatic fever and endocarditis. Which statement by the parents indicates to the nurse that the parents have the best understanding of rheumatic heart disease?**

1.   "We will keep low cholesterol foods in our diet."
2.   "We may need to move to a warmer climate."
3.   "Our son should not participate in sports."
4.   "This therapy includes long-term medications."

1.   *This is incorrect! Using low cholesterol foods is a good idea; however, it is not a specific need for the child recovering from endocarditis.*
2.   *Although rheumatic fever is more common in cool, humid climates, moving to a warmer climate will not alleviate any symptoms or decrease that child's chance of recurrence significantly.*
3.   *Wrong! There is a long period of convalescence following endocarditis, in which the child's activity must be restricted. Many of these children, however, recover and pursue sports and strenuous physical exercise.*
4.   **Correct! Because children who have had rheumatic fever are more susceptible to repeated attacks, they are advised to be on continuous prophylactic doses of antibiotics, usually penicillin.**

58. The nurse is monitoring a client who is on penicillin G potassium IV therapy. Which of the following lab values would be of immediate concern to the nurse when monitoring a client while on this penicillin therapy?

    1. Sodium: 150 mEq/L.
    2. Potassium: 5.2 mEq/L.
    3. WBC: 13,000/cu mm.
    4. Hgb: 14.2 g/dL.

    1. *Incorrect. Although this value represents slight hypernatremia, penicillin G potassium does not contain sodium salts and therefore will not upset that electrolyte balance.*
    2. **Right! Hyperkalemia, potentially fatal, can result from IV administration of penicillins that contain potassium, especially in the presence of renal insufficiency.**
    3. *An elevated WBC is an indication for giving IV antibiotics (indicative of an infectious process). It is not an unexpected lab finding in this situation.*
    4. *No. There is no reason to report a NORMAL hemoglobin value. Please review your normal lab values!*

59. A young client is paralyzed from the waist down. He has a TV, radio, video tape player, stereo, and video game unit, all of which are turned on most of the day. The nurse notices that there are not enough electrical outlets, and that extension cords with multiple outlets are in use to accommodate this equipment. The best nursing action would be to:

    1. Have the client's family take some of the equipment home.
    2. Inform the client that an overloaded circuit can cause an electrical fire, and, therefore, the extension cords are not allowed.
    3. Tell the client that only single-outlet cords can be used, and that the staff will check often to see if he wants to use anything not currently connected.
    4. Call the maintenance department and have more wall outlets installed in the client's room.

    1. *The client should not be deprived of activities that he finds entertaining. This option does not solve the problem at hand, either, since an electrical fire could occur while waiting for the family to take the equipment home.*
    2. *Although this is a true statement, it does not provide any alternatives for consideration of the client.*
    3. **Good choice. This option allows the client the continued use of his electrical devices, and pro-** *vides for safety by decreasing the possibility of an electrical fire.*
    4. *Revamping the physical structure of a building is an administrative decision. Adding electrical outlets is expensive, and may not comply with fire or electrical codes. Also, this option does not solve the problem at hand, since an electrical fire could occur while waiting for the electrical work to be done.*

60. A client was admitted to the psychiatric unit for obsessive compulsive disorder. The nurse notes that the client's ritualistic behavior of handwashing has increased at bedtime. Which of the following responses by the nurse would be most therapeutic?

    1. "So that you can get to bed on time, you need to start getting ready earlier than the other clients."
    2. "You have one hour to get ready for bed. Then we will talk for a half-hour before you go to sleep."
    3. "I understand you need to reduce your anxiety by washing your hands, so go to bed when you feel tired."
    4. "If you don't stop washing you hands so much, I will have to notify your doctor."

    1. *Wrong. The issue in this question is the need for controlling the client's handwashing behavior at bedtime. This option focuses on getting to bed on time, but does not address the need for setting limits on the handwashing behavior.*
    2. **Good choice! The issue in this question is the need for controlling the client's handwashing behavior at bedtime. This option sets limits by allowing a specific amount of time for getting ready for bed. This option also is an example of the nurse offering self, because the nurse offers to talk for a half-hour before the client sleeps.**
    3. *The issue in this question is the need for controlling the client's handwashing behavior at bedtime. This option does not set limits, but allows the client to wash her hands indefinitely. Her need for sleep may be compromised with this option.*
    4. *The issue in this question is the need for controlling the client's handwashing behavior at bedtime. Instead of setting limits, this option uses the inappropriate threat of notifying the doctor of the client's behavior. The client's need for sleep may be compromised, since this response permits the client to wash her hands indefinitely and puts her needs on hold until the doctor is available. This response is not therapeutic for the client.*

61. In caring for a client immediately following a cardiac catheterization procedure, which of the following nursing actions is appropriate?

1. Apply warm compresses to the puncture site.
2. Assist with passive range of motion exercises.
3. Monitor the client for cardiac arrhythmias.
4. Assist the client into high Fowler's position.

1. This is incorrect. Since bleeding is a major complication following a cardiac catheterization, heat is never applied.

2. This is incorrect. Since bleeding is a major complication following a cardiac catheterization, movement is limited in the involved extremity.

3. This is correct. The heart muscle may be irritable following this procedure, and serious arrhythmias may occur.

> **STRATEGY ALERT!** This is the only correct option in this question. Note also that the word "cardiac" in the stem of the question is repeated in this option — and that the issue is cardiac catheterization. In this question, these similar words are a good clue!

4. This is incorrect. This position could obstruct arterial blood flow and lead to formation of a thrombus. The involved extremity must be properly aligned and immobilized immediately after the procedure.

62. An anorexic client is preparing for discharge from the hospital. Her weight has stabilized and she has agreed to attend outpatient therapy. The nurse would avoid including which of the following provisions in her discharge plans?

1. Referral to a local eating disorders support group.
2. Continued family therapy.
3. Medication management.
4. Primary health care.

1. This cannot be the correct option. Support groups are very important for eating disorder clients, to help them deal more effectively with the developmental issues of adolescence while maintaining a healthy attitude toward eating and body weight.

2. This cannot be the correct option. Family therapy will continue to help the client and the family members to relate more effectively with each other.

3. Correct. Medication is not commonly used in the treatment of clients with eating disorders. Therefore, the nurse would not expect to include this information in the client's discharge plans.

4. This cannot be the correct option. Primary health care, through a pediatrician, nurse practitioner, or family physician, is important to monitor her general physical health and treat any medical problems that may develop in the future.

63. The nurse is working in a pediatric clinic. Which of the following clients would be least likely to test HIV positive?

1. A two-month-old whose mother has been an IV drug addict for two years.
2. A 15-year-old who has been on treatment for hemophilia since infancy.
3. An eight-year-old whose best friend is HIV positive.
4. An 16-year-old who is sexually active.

1. Incorrect option. This history would place the infant at high risk for HIV, since infection in utero through the placenta is a means of communicating the virus. Many IV drug abusers are HIV positive.

2. No. This child is at risk, since the blood supply was not consistently tested until the late 1980s.

3. Very good! You recognized this is a "casual social contact," which would be considered a low risk for transmission.

4. No, this adolescent is at risk. It may be that a condom is being used, but only abstinence offers complete protection from this form of transmission.

64. The nurse is taking vital signs and notices an irregularity in the heart rate. Which of the following nursing actions would be most appropriate?

1. Request the assistance of another staff member and take an apical/radial pulse.
2. Count the apical pulse rate for one full minute and describe the irregularity in the chart.
3. Call the doctor and request an order for a Holter monitor recording for the next day.
4. Take the pulse at each peripheral site and count the rate for 30 seconds.

1. Wrong. An apical/radial pulse is used to identify a deficit between the apical and radial rates. It is not used to assess irregularity in the pulse, which is the issue in this question. This option doesn't describe the most appropriate nursing action when assessing a cardiac irregularity.

2. Correct. When the pulse is regular, it may be counted for 15 seconds and multiplied by four, or counted for 30 seconds and multiplied by two. However, if the pulse is irregular, it must be counted for a full minute to obtain an accurate rate. The irregularity should be described in the chart.

> **STRATEGY ALERT!** Note that the word "irregularity" appears in the stem of the question and in this option.

3. Wrong! An irregular pulse rate should be followed up immediately, generally by continuously monitoring the cardiac rhythm by telemetry. A Holter monitor recording the next day may be too late!

4. Incorrect. Assessment of all peripheral pulses is appropriate for a client with a cardiovascular problem. That assessment, however, is related to adequacy of circulation to each extremity rather than to regularity of the heart rate. Consequently, this option does not address the issue in this question. The stem asks you to select the most appropriate nursing action when assessing a cardiac irregularity.

65. The nurse understands that which of the following statements regarding the administration of RHoGAM is accurate?

1. It must be given IV, soon after delivery to the mother.
2. It must be given IM to the mother, within three days after delivery.
3. It must be given IM, to both the mother and neonate, within 72 hours after delivery.
4. It must be given to the mother during labor to prevent the formation of antibodies.

1. No. RHoGAM is never administered IV. Before administration, blood laboratory evaluation needs to be done on the blood sample of both mother and newborn.
2. **Correct! It is important that RHoGAM is given to the mother prior to discharge from the hospital, which is rarely longer than three days. If an omission of the drug is discovered after this time, it is felt best to administer RHoGAM since no harm could result. It is unclear how long it takes for the formation of Rh antibodies to occur.**
3. Incorrect. RHoGAM is never administered to the neonate.
4. No, assessment of the blood of the mother and newborn must be completed prior to the administration of RHoGAM. It is, however, given prophylactically at 28 weeks gestation.

66. When administering RHoGAM, the nurse should be aware of the potential adverse reactions in the client. Which of the following clinical findings could be anticipated by the nurse to result from RHoGAM administration?

1. Rapid pulse rate.
2. Elevated temperature.
3. Hot, reddened area around injection site.
4. Low blood sugar.

1. No. RHoGAM has no documented effect on maternal pulse rate.
2. **Correct! Fever is a common response to RHoGAM. The client should still be evaluated carefully for an infection. It cannot be assumed the fever is the result of RHoGAM until other causes are eliminated.**

3. Wrong choice! Soreness at the injection site is commonly seen, but a hot reddened area is cause for concern. It could indicate an infection in the injection site.
4. No. The administration of RHoGAM has no documented effect on the maternal blood sugar.

67. A disruptive 10-year-old child is having difficulty interacting with other children on the unit. Which of the following nursing actions would be best initially?

1. Have a unit conference with other staff members and discuss strategies to solve the problem.
2. Talk to the child about the behavior that is causing the problem and identify possible solutions.
3. Tell the other children to stop teasing the client and observe for changes in the client's behavior.
4. Tell the client's mother that she needs to talk to her son about his disruptive behavior.

1. No. The client in this question is the child, and the issue is disruptive behavior. This option is only indirectly related to the client. This is not the best option.
2. **You are correct. Since the child is the client in this question, the correct answer must be related to him. This option deals directly with the issue of the client's behavior.**
3. The client in this question is the child, not the other children on the unit. The answer should be related to the client. Also, "telling" the other children what to do about the problem is characteristic of an authority figure and is not therapeutic in the nurse-client relationship. The nurse's response must be therapeutic for the client.
4. Wrong. This option focuses on inappropriate person, the client's mother. Also, "telling" the client's mother what she "needs" to do is characteristic of an authority figure and is not therapeutic in the nurse-client relationship.

68. Which of the following approaches is best when the nurse is taking the blood pressure of a client with hypertension?

1. Measure the blood pressure under the same conditions each time.
2. Take the blood pressure with the client sitting on the side of the bed.
3. Place the blood pressure cuff on the right arm above the elbow.
4. Measure the blood pressure with the client in supine position.

1. **Congratulations! This is the correct answer. The nurse should record the client's position in the chart so that the next reading may be done with the client in the same position.**

> **STRATEGY ALERT!** *The other three options are similar to each other in that they each describe a specific position or method. This is a broader or more global response.*

2. *This is not the answer. The client may be sitting, lying or standing when blood pressure is measured. The nurse should record the client's position in the chart so that the reading may be done with the client in the same position each time.*

3. *This is not the answer. The blood pressure cuff may be placed above the elbow on either the right or left arm.*

4. *This is not the answer. The client may be sitting, lying or standing when blood pressure is measured. The nurse should record the client's position in the chart so that the reading may be done with the client in the same position each time.*

69. **Because a client is taking atenolol (Tenormin), which of the following interventions is most critical for the nurse to include in the plan of care?**

1. Monitor intake and output.
2. Do not give Tenormin if apical pulse is less than 50 beats per minute.
3. Administer Tenormin one hour before or two hours after meals.
4. Instruct client to change position slowly, especially lying to standing.

1. *Wrong choice. This is not the most critical intervention, although it is important to monitor for the life-threatening side effects of congestive heart failure and pulmonary edema. Daily weights would be the most valuable assessment tool in this case.*

2. *Correct. Because atenolol is a beta-blocker, one of the major side effects (which is also life-threatening) is bradycardia. The nurse must take the apical pulse prior to administration. If the rate is less than 50 beats per minute, the medication should be withheld and the physician notified.*

3. *Incorrect option. Atenolol may be administered without regards to meals. Tablets may be crushed or mixed with fluids if the client has difficulty swallowing.*

4. *No, although this is an appropriate instruction to give the client to decrease the incidence of orthostatic hypotension, it is not the most critical intervention. Orthostatic hypotension is not typically a life-threatening condition and is preventable: the client is taught to make position changes slowly, especially lying to standing.*

70. **A client, age 63, is being treated for Legionnaires' disease with erythromycin estolate (Ilosone). Which of the following conditions, if given in his medical history, would the nurse understand to be a contraindication the use of this drug?**

1. Pyelonephritis.
2. Cirrhosis.
3. Coronary artery disease.
4. Emphysema.

1. *Incorrect. Ninety-five percent of the excretion of erythromycin is via the liver and bile; only five percent is in urine. There is no significant effect upon renal function.*

2. *Good answer! Erythromycin estolate is contraindicated in clients with hepatic disease because the drug may be hepatotoxic, causing cholestatic jaundice. The risk of liver damage is increased if erythromycin is given concurrently with other hepatotoxic agents, e.g., estrogens, piperacillin, and sulfonamides.*

3. *Wrong! There is no known contraindication for the use of erythromycin in clients with a history of coronary artery disease. Make another choice.*

4. *No, there is no known contraindication for the use of erythromycin in clients with COPD. Erythromycin may be ordered for COPD clients who develop respiratory tract infections caused by group A beta-hemolytic streptococci or other bacteria.*

71. **A client has undergone a transurethral resection of the prostate to correct benign prostatic hypertrophy. He has returned from the recovery room with an indwelling urinary catheter. For several hours the urinary output has been adequate. However, the nurse notes that the catheter has drained no urine during the last hour. What should the nurse do first?**

1. Offer the client 100 mL of oral fluids each hour.
2. Irrigate the catheter according to the postoperative orders.
3. Call the physician and request an increase in IV fluid rate.
4. Monitor the vital signs every 15 minutes for one hour.

1. *Wrong. A sudden stop in urine output from the catheter following prostate surgery is probably a result of an occluded catheter. Increasing oral fluids without removing the obstruction in the catheter will just cause the client to be uncomfortable.*

2. *You are correct! A sudden stop in urine output from the catheter following prostate surgery is probably a result of an occluded catheter. Irrigation will remove a clot from the catheter. Note that the word "catheter" appears in the stem of the question and in the correct answer.*

3. *A sudden stop in urine output from the catheter following prostate surgery is probably a result of an occluded catheter. Increasing IV fluids without removing the obstruction in the catheter will just cause the client to be uncomfortable.*

4. *Wrong. Monitoring the vital signs is not relevant because there is no indication in the case scenario that the vital signs are not stable.*

72. **The nurse finds an elderly client standing in a puddle of water in the hallway of the unit. The nurse does not know this client. Which of the following actions should the nurse take initially?**

    1. Ask the client for her name and room number.
    2. Wipe up the water until the floor is completely dry.
    3. Call the supervisor for assistance in identifying the client.
    4. Have the client wait in the lounge until security arrives.

    1. *Wrong. The issue in this question is the puddle of water on the floor. The water on the floor threatens the safety of the client and others on the unit. After the nurse assures safety, she can identify the client and assist with getting her back to where she belongs.*
    2. *Very good! The issue in this question is the puddle of water on the floor. The water on the floor threatens the safety of the client and others on the unit. The nurse's first action should be to alleviate the safety hazard by wiping up the water.*

    > **PRIORITY ALERT!** *Maslow's Hierurchy of Needs Indicates that when no physiological need exists, safety needs should receive priority. Note: the word "water" in the question is repeated in this option. The test-taking strategy of looking for similar words in the question would identify this option as a possible answer.*

    3. *Wrong! The issue in this question is the puddle of water on the floor. The water on the floor threatens the safety of the client and others on the unit. After the nurse assures safety, she can identify the client and assist with getting her back to where she belongs.*
    4. *The issue in this question is the puddle of water on the floor. The water on the floor threatens the safety of the client and others on the unit. Asking the client to wait in the lounge until security arrives does not assure safety. Someone may still slip on the puddle of water and injure themselves.*

73. **In which of the following client situations does the nurse understand that the administration of betamethasone (Celestone) is both advisable and safe?**

    1. Gestational age 30 weeks, insulin dependent diabetic mother, no tocolysis given.
    2. Gestational age 28 weeks, mother with mild PIH, no tocolysis given.
    3. Gestational age 35 weeks, no tocolysis given.
    4. Gestational age 30 weeks, chronic hypertensive mother, tocolysis given.

    1. *No, use of betamethasone in a diabetic client needs to be carefully considered because of the resulting*

hyperglycemia. *Some sources list diabetes as a contraindication, while others suggest using it with caution.*
    2. *Yes, this client is an excellent candidate for betamethasone therapy. Her hypertension related to PIH is not severe at this point, and the stress of the PIH on the fetus, as well as the administration of betamethasone, will accelerate fetal lung maturation in this very premature infant. The fact that she has not received tocolysis is another positive aspect.*
    3. *No. Betamethasone is not given after 34 weeks because the risk of neonatal RDS after that gestational age is low.*
    4. *No, the use of betamethasone in clients with hypertension needs to be considered carefully. In addition, this client is receiving tocolysis, which increases the risk of pulmonary edema. The effects of the chronic hypertension on the fetus might be enough to accelerate fetal lung maturity.*

74. **Which of the following activities would be appropriate for the nurse to suggest to a manic client?**

    1. A daily walk on the hospital grounds.
    2. Playing a computer game with another client.
    3. Participation in a basketball game with other male clients.
    4. Reading quietly in his room.

    1. *Correct. Physical exercise involving large motor skills is an appropriate way for him to work off excess energy and emotional tension.*
    2. *This is not correct. Competitive games will tend to increase his anxiety and tension and therefore escalate his hyperactivity.*
    3. *Incorrect response! Basketball games tend to be competitive and overly stimulating. This activity would escalate his behavior, so it is not the correct option.*
    4. *This is not correct. Because mania is associated with a short attention span and high level of distractibility, the client is usually not able to sit and read quietly by himself.*

75. **Following a normal vaginal delivery, a client is given an IV containing oxytocin (Pitocin). To evaluate the effectiveness of this drug, the nurse needs to assess which of the following?**

    1. Pulse rate.
    2. Blood pressure.
    3. Urinary output.
    4. Fundal consistency.

    1. *Wrong. Tachycardia is a side effect of Pitocin, but it does not confirm the effectiveness of the drug.*
    2. *Wrong. Hypotension is a side effect of Pitocin, but does not confirm the effectiveness of the drug.*

3. *Wrong. A decrease in urinary output is a side effect, but does not confirm the effectiveness of the drug.*

4. ***Correct. Pitocin is given to prevent or treat uterine atony. If Pitocin is effective, the fundus will be firm on palpation.***

76. **The nurse assists an angry, confused client with a displaced oxygen cannula and raises the head of the bed to high Fowler's position. The nurse places his dinner on the overbed table and prepares the dinner by cutting the meat and spreading the bread according to the client's preference. It is essential for the nurse to carry out which of the following nursing actions before leaving the room?**

1. Ask the client if he needs further assistance with his meals.
2. Assist the client with menu selections for the following day.
3. Tell the client when the nurse will return to his room.
4. Place the call bell where the client can easily reach it.

1. *While this option is an appropriate nursing action, it might not be a priority. Look to see whether any of the other options identify a physiological need or a safety need (Maslow's Hierarchy of Needs).*

2. *Although this option is an appropriate nursing action, it might not be a priority. What is the issue in this question? Does this option focus on a priority in any of the four guidelines? Look to see whether any of the other options identify a physiological need or a safety need (Maslow's Hierarchy of Needs).*

3. *This option is an inappropriate nursing action! Because the client is confused and hypoxic, his condition warrants frequent checks. Look to see whether any of the other options identify a physiological need or a safety need (Maslow's Hierarchy of Needs).*

4. ***Yes! This is the correct answer! This option focuses on the client's need for a safe environment. Because of his confused behavior, providing a safe environment in which the client has access to a call bell is a priority.***

> **PRIORITY ALERT!** *Maslow's Hierarchy of Needs is used as a guideline in this question. If none of the options identifies a physiological need, then the option that identifies a safety need receives priority.*

77. **A 10-week-old male is admitted to the pediatric unit with a diagnosis of inorganic failure to thrive. He is the first child of a 16-year-old mother and a 17-year-old father. Which of the following would the nurse select as the priority nursing diagnosis?**

1. Altered nutrition: less than body requirements related to physical abuse.
2. Sensory/perceptual alterations (gustatory) related to infant deprivation.
3. Altered growth and development related to poor suck.
4. Altered parenting related to knowledge deficit.

1. *No, this is not the priority, because you have no assessment data to back this up. You would need information regarding the type and amount of nutrition offered.*

2. *No. The definition of inorganic failure to thrive is that there is no physiologic reason for the failure to gain weight, so that makes the initial part of the statement incorrect.*

3. *Did you read the "related to"? This infant does exhibit altered growth patterns, since this, by definition, is failure to thrive, but not because of a poor suck.*

4. ***Correct! The rationale for this choice is that adolescent parents have few parenting skills. This nursing diagnosis would be the most helpful in designing interventions to improve the infant's prognosis. These parents need modeling of nurturing and infant stimulation behaviors.***

78. **Because of hyperactivity and difficulty sleeping, the most therapeutic room arrangement that the nurse can make for a manic client is which of the following?**

1. A private bedroom.
2. A semi-private room with a roommate who has a similar problem.
3. Either a private or semi-private room.
4. Direct admission to the seclusion room until his activity level becomes more subdued.

1. ***Very good. A private room is ideal for a manic client who easily becomes over-stimulated by the number of persons and activities in the environment of an inpatient unit. A private room can be used to take "time-outs" during the day and to settle down to sleep at night.***

2. *This is not correct. The client should not be given a roommate who is also hyperactive because the situation would be too stimulating for either of them.*

3. *This is not the correct option.*

4. *This is not the correct option. Legal and ethical guidelines require treatment in the least restrictive setting. Seclusion is only used when there is a specific need to do so and this need is documented in writing by the staff. Also, a psychiatrist's order has to be obtained before a person can be placed in seclusion.*

79. **A diabetic client, age 75, is prescribed ampicillin (Omnipen) by his physician. The nurse should give highest priority to asking the client which of the following questions, before he leaves the clinic?**

    1. Which method do you use to monitor your glucose level?
    2. Do you have any food allergies?
    3. Do you have any difficulty swallowing capsules?
    4. Do you have a history of liver disease?

    1. *Excellent focus! You recall that clients with diabetes who use copper sulfate urine glucose tests (Clinitest) may have false-positive results when taking ampicillin. It's important for the nurse to assess which glucose testing method (urine, blood) the client uses, in order to determine if he/she should use an alternate method, such as Tes-Tape or Clinistix.*
    2. *Incorrect choice. Asking the client about food allergies will not help the nurse determine if there is an allergy to penicillin.*
    3. *Not the best choice. This question, although relevant to determine if the client may need a liquid suspension, does not have priority over another action that addresses the ongoing assessment of the client's health status. Try to find that option.*
    4. *Not correct. Penicillins (except Nafcillin) are excreted mostly unchanged in urine. Nafcillin is extensively metabolized in the liver. Hepatic function is not a major concern with most penicillins. Make another choice.*

80. **A 38-year-old is admitted to the hospital for a severe episode of gastrointestinal bleeding secondary to a peptic ulcer. He is scheduled for an upper GI series. In preparing the client for this diagnostic procedure, which of the following should the nurse include in teaching for the client?**

    1. An upper GI series will take five or six hours to complete. Since you will be waiting much of this time, you should take something to read with you.
    2. This is a series of x-rays in which the entire GI tract is delineated. A liquid suspension of barium sulfate taken orally is the contrast medium.
    3. The client should not eat or drink anything after midnight on the evening before the test. However, following the first x-rays, full liquids are allowed.
    4. A laxative is administered the day before the test. On the morning of the test, soap suds enemas are given until the returns are clear.

    1. *Good choice! An upper GI series is a series of x-rays that delineates the upper portion of the GI tract. It takes five or six hours to complete because the series of x-rays follows the progress of the con-*
    trast medium through the GI tract. The client waits during much of this time, and reading material helps to pass the time. Note that the test-taking strategy of looking for similar words would be a clue in answering this question, because the phrase "upper GI Series" appears in both this option and in the stem.*
    2. *The absolute word "entire" makes this option wrong. An upper GI Series delineates only the upper portion of the GI tract.*
    3. *This is incorrect. The client should be NPO after midnight and should continue fasting until the test is over.*
    4. *This is incorrect. Laxatives and enemas are contraindicated prior to an upper GI.*

81. **A manic client tells the nurse that his latest computer project is "revolutionizing the industry." He also states, "IBM and Apple are both going under because their products cannot compete with mine." In choosing how to respond, the nurse is best guided by the knowledge that:**

    1. This statement is grandiose and does not require a response.
    2. This statement represents the client's inability to deal with inner feelings of inadequacy and vulnerability.
    3. Manic clients are prone to exaggerate the facts of a situation.
    4. This is a delusional statement that should be confronted to correct the client's perception of reality.

    1. *This statement is an example of grandiosity, but the client's statement should not be ignored because he might misinterpret the nurse's response as agreement. There is a better option.*
    2. *Correct. The elated mood and grandiose statements of manic clients often reflect their inner feelings of inadequacy and vulnerability. The nurse's response should focus on underlying themes and feelings instead of the content of the client's statements.*
    3. *This is an accurate statement, but there is a better option.*
    4. *The client's comment is a grandiose delusion but reality testing is not appropriate. There is a better option.*

82. **A client who is 43 years old has a long history of peptic ulcer. She is admitted now for treatment of pyloric obstruction. An order has been written for a nasogastric tube. The nurse understands that the best rationale for the use of the nasogastric tube is:**

    1. Collection of laboratory specimens.
    2. Supplying nutrients via tube feedings.
    3. Decompression of the stomach.
    4. Administration of medications.

1. A nasogastric tube is sometimes used for collection of laboratory specimens, but no data is given in this question that would make this the correct answer or the best rationale. Be careful not to "read into" the question!

2. A nasogastric tube is sometimes used for feeding, but this option is a distractor. Read the question again carefully! Because of the obstruction, tube feeding is contraindicated.

3. *Excellent! Removal of gastric secretions and gas from the stomach is needed because of the obstruction. Good choice!*

4. While a nasogastric tube may be used for administration of medications, no data is given in this question to support this choice as the correct answer. Be careful not to "read into" the question!

83. **A client was admitted to the psychiatric unit with a diagnosis of bipolar mood disorder. At 3:00 a.m., the client ran to the nurses station demanding that she see her therapist immediately. Which of these responses by the nurse would be best initially?**

    1. "Calm down, go back to your room, and I'll try to get in touch with your therapist right away."
    2. "Regulations state that I can't call the therapist in the middle of the night except in an emergency."
    3. "You must be very upset about something to want to see your therapist in the middle of the night."
    4. "You are being unreasonable and I will not call your therapist at 3:00 in the morning."

    1. Wrong! It is difficult for an agitated client to follow complex directives, and this option gives several directives at one time. Also, this response is not therapeutic because it does not address the client's feelings.
    2. Wrong! This option focuses on regulations, which is an inappropriate issue, and it does not address the client's feelings. This response is not therapeutic.
    3. *Good choice! This option is an example of the nurse showing empathy. This response addresses the client's feelings and offers an opportunity for the client to clarify the situation.*
    4. Wrong! The nurse is showing disapproval. This is a communication block.

84. **The nurse understands that the effective use of limit-setting with hyperactive clients requires all of the following except:**

    1. Providing a consistent, structured environment so the client knows what is expected of him or her.
    2. The specific limits to be used must be understood and agreed upon by all staff members on all shifts.
    3. The client's requests for greater freedom should be

granted to evaluate the progress that has been made.
    4. Consequences should be direct results of behavior and perceived by the client as negative outcomes.

    1. Wrong choice! The key to effective limit-setting is to provide a structure that is consistently enforced.
    2. This is an effective measure, so it cannot be the correct option.
    3. *Correct! The need for limits should be reevaluated at regular intervals. The decision to relax specific restrictions should be based on the client's ability to demonstrate more responsible and controlled behavior and not on specific requests alone. This is the correct option because it is a false statement.*
    4. This is an effective measure, so it cannot be the correct option. Limits should be simple and applied at the time the problem behavior occurs. Also, limits are most effective when the client perceives them as undesirable and therefore receives no secondary gains from their use.

85. **In addition to nitrate therapy, a client is to begin nifedipine (Procardia) 10 mg p.o. every six hours. When giving this medication along with nitrates, the nurse will observe for:**

    1. Tremor.
    2. Tetany.
    3. Hypotension.
    4. Hyperkalemia.

    1. Incorrect. Tremor is not a side effect of nifedipine therapy. The only musculoskeletal side effect is muscle cramps.
    2. No. Tetany is not seen in clients who take Procardia. The only musculoskeletal side effect is muscle cramps. Make another selection.
    3. *Yes. Procardia, as a calcium channel blocker, reduces peripheral vascular resistance. With concurrent use of nitrates (which are potent vasodilators), Procardia can cause hypotension with initial administration.*
    4. Wrong. Procardia, a calcium channel blocker, and nitrates (vasodilators) do not affect the potassium level. Recall that electrolyte levels, especially potassium, are important to monitor in clients taking cardiac glycosides and diuretics.

86. **A 22-year-old sustained a fracture of the tibia and fibula while playing football. A long leg cast was applied, and the client was admitted to the orthopedic unit. Following four weeks of bed rest, the nurse notes decreased breath sounds in the lower lobes of both lungs. What is the best explanation for this change in breath sounds?**

    1. The client did not take deep breaths while the nurse examined his lower lobes.
    2. Because of improper positioning, the client has developed pulmonary edema.

3. Atelectasis, caused by immobility, has resulted in the decreased breath sounds.
4. The client's resistance is down, and he has caught a cold from someone else.

1. *Wrong! Breath sounds may be decreased if the client does not take deep breaths. However, there is no data in the case scenario to support the idea that this occurred. Do not "read into" the question!*
2. *Wrong choice! Pulmonary edema is not a likely reason for the decreased breath sounds. Pulmonary edema is usually a complication of heart failure, not a complication of immobility. There is also no information in the case scenario that would indicate improper positioning.*
3. ***Congratulations! Immobility can cause atelectasis, which results in decreased breath sounds. This is the most plausible reason for the decreased breath sounds. Note that all the other options involve "reading into" the question.***

> **STRATEGY ALERT!** *The phrase "decreased breath sounds" in the stem is repeated in Option 3, which is a clue that this option may be the answer.*

4. *Wrong! There is no data in this question to support the idea that the client has a cold.*

87. **A 36-year-old client has hypertension and is treated with chlorothiazide (Diuril). Which of the following should the nurse include in the teaching plan?**

1. Dietary sodium should be restricted to one gram daily.
2. Avoid using Diuril with other antihypertensives.
3. Orthostatic hypotension may be a side effect.
4. It is unnecessary to increase dietary potassium.

1. *Wrong choice! Diuril is a thiazide diuretic that causes sodium loss in the urine. Sodium restriction is not indicated. This statement is false.*
2. *Diuril is sometimes used with other antihypertensive medications to counteract the effect of sodium retention. This statement is false.*
3. ***Yes. Thiazide diuretics such as Diuril may cause orthostatic hypotension. This information should be included in the teaching plan.***
4. *Diuril, a thiazide diuretic, causes potassium loss in the urine. Increased dietary intake or potassium supplements are indicated. This statement is false.*

88. **The nurse understands that, in comparing skeletal traction to skin traction, which statement is correct?**

1. Skeletal traction can be utilized longer than skin traction.

2. Clients in skin traction have more pain than those in skeletal traction.
3. Skin traction is more likely to be complicated by osteomyelitis.
4. The risk of skin breakdown is greater with skeletal traction.

1. ***Very good. The rationale for the use of skeletal traction is that a greater weight can be applied, and the traction can be utilized longer.***
2. *No. This is too general to be true. The client's injury and pain tolerance are two variables that would have to be assessed.*
3. *Incorrect. The opposite is true; skeletal traction puts the client at greater risk, since the wire or pin is placed through the skin into the bone, where osteomyelitis would occur.*
4. *Too general. The client's nutritional level, hydration, and type of fracture all need to be evaluated to assess the potential for skin breakdown. All persons in traction are at high risk for skin breakdown due to limited positioning and mobility.*

89. **A client is hospitalized with schizophrenia. During a conversation with a female nurse, the client seemed relaxed initially, but then became restless and began wringing his hands. The nurse stated to the client that he seemed tense, and he agreed. Which of these responses by the nurse would demonstrate the best understanding at this time?**

1. "Do you often feel tense when you are talking to a woman?"
2. "What were we discussing when you began to feel uncomfortable?"
3. "Did I say something wrong that made you feel tense?"
4. "I sometimes feel tense, too, when I am talking to a stranger."

1. *Wrong! This option is an assumption that the client is feeling tense because he is talking to a woman.*
2. ***This is the correct answer! This answer seeks clarification by asking for information about when the client became tense.***
3. *Wrong! This option is focused on the nurse and is not therapeutic for the client.*
4. *Incorrect! This response may appear to be the nurse showing empathy, but in fact it is focused on the nurse. The response should be focused on the client's feelings. This option is not therapeutic for the client.*

90. **What information about diet should the nurse give all clients taking lithium?**

1. Sodium intake should be restricted to 1200 mg per day.

2. Fluid intake should not exceed 1000 mL per day.
3. An adequate daily intake of sodium and fluids should be maintained.
4. Sodium and fluid intake should be increased.

1. *No. Restricting sodium intake could lead to a rise in lithium levels with potential toxicity. Also, conditions that cause the loss of sodium from the body, such as vomiting and diarrhea, can lead to lithium toxicity as well.*
2. *No. Clients taking lithium should drink six to eight glasses of water a day to maintain a normal state of hydration.*
3. *Correct. Consistent intake of sodium and fluids is needed to avoid lithium toxicity. Clients should be advised to contact their psychiatrist to report any medical conditions that cause them to lose sodium, such as vomiting, diarrhea, or profuse sweating. The psychiatrist will advise them on what to do to avert lithium toxicity.*
4. *No. A normal intake of sodium and fluids should be maintained so that the serum lithium level will remain within the therapeutic range. Increasing sodium intake would lead to the excretion of lithium, thereby lowering its serum level and increasing the risk of another manic episode.*

91. **A client, 23 years old, has a fractured femur. She is placed in skeletal traction with a Thomas splint and Pearson attachment. Which of the following interventions for positioning this client is appropriate?**

1. Position the client's right foot on the bed in direct line with the femur.
2. Use trochanter rolls to prevent abduction of the right leg.
3. Allow the client to turn slightly from side to side above the waist.
4. Maintain the client flat with only brief periods with her head elevated.

1. *No, incorrect. The foot should be off the bed at all times to prevent decubitus ulcers from forming.*
2. *No, not correct. The right leg is already stabilized by virtue of the traction and weights.*
3. *Correct. The client may change position without disturbing the line of traction because the counterforce is provided with counterweights, rather than by using the client's weight.*
4. *Wrong. With the Thomas splint and Pearson attachment the hips should be in a 20-degree flexed position to maintain the correct pull.*

92. **The nurse observes that in the first few days of hospitalization, an 18-month-old client sits quietly sucking her thumb in the corner of her crib. When the nurse approaches the crib, the client shyly turns her head away from the nurse. Which interpretation of her behavior is most justifiable?**

1. The behavior is indicative of pathological reaction to hospitalization.
2. The relationship between parents and child needs to be evaluated.
3. The behavior demonstrates an anxiety reaction to the stress of hospitalization.
4. The negative behavior is a beginning attempt at autonomy.

1. *At 18 months, the client is able to identify the nurse as a stranger. Her behavior is appropriate. There is no evidence of pathology.*
2. *No data about the relationship between the client and her parents is provided. The conclusion that the relationship between parents and child need to be evaluated is an assumption. As a general rule, you should not make assumptions when answering NCLEX/CAT-RN questions.*
3. *Correct. Hospitalization is stressful, regardless of the age of the hospitalized client. However, for an 18-month-old, separation from her parents adds to that stress. The client's behavior is demonstrating an anxiety reaction to the stress of hospitalization.*
4. *Erikson's development theory identifies the developmental conflict for children age one to three as autonomy versus shame and doubt. An 18-month-old may be beginning to develop autonomy. However, since the client is hospitalized, her behavior has most likely regressed to the developmental conflict of trust versus mistrust.*

93. **A eight-year-old client is admitted with a diagnosis of acute rheumatic fever. During the first few days after admission, the nurse would demonstrate best judgment by suggesting which of the following activities for the client?**

1. Playing computer games in the game room.
2. Visiting with several school friends.
3. Completing school assignments.
4. Listening to favorite cassette tapes.

1. *No. The client should be on bedrest during the acute phase of rheumatic fever. Rest is very important because it decreases the cardiac workload. The nurse should promote rest.*
2. *No. Visiting with several school friends does not promote rest during the acute phase.*
3. *No. Completing school assignments does not promote rest during the acute phase.*
4. *Yes! This is the best answer! The client should be on bedrest during the acute phase of rheumatic fever. Rest is very important because it decreases the cardiac workload. The nurse should promote rest.*

94. **A 65-year-old male is admitted to the emergency department with unequal grips and aphasia. The goal of initial treatment for this client is best achieved by which of the following actions?**

1. Preparing to begin an IV infusion.
2. Raising the HOB to 30 degrees.
3. Monitoring BP.
4. Explaining MRI to the client and family.

1. *No, this is not the first measure.*
2. *Right! This limits the area of damage by reducing the intracranial pressure. This is a secondary prevention intervention.*
3. *No, the key words in the question are "goal of initial treatment." Although monitoring of BP is an important assessment, it is not treatment.*
4. *Incorrect. Diagnosis is not the first measure; you've skipped an important intervention.*

95. **After four weeks of hospitalization, the client says to the nurse, "My son called and told me that my boss has hired someone to take my place." Which of the following is the most therapeutic response by the nurse?**

1. "I don't understand why your son would tell you that now."
2. "You must feel very concerned about your boss not holding your job."
3. "There isn't anything you can do about that until you go home."
4. "Why don't you call your wife and see if she can change his mind?"

1. *Wrong. The son is not the client in this question. Focusing on an inappropriate person is a communication block. This response is not therapeutic.*
2. *Good choice! This option is an example of the nurse showing empathy by showing an understanding of the client's feelings.*
3. *This response fails to address the client's feelings and also blocks communication by giving advice. This response is not therapeutic.*
4. *This option blocks communication by focusing on an inappropriate person—the client's wife. The response should be focused on the client. The nurse is also blocking communication by giving advice.*

96. **A 40-year-old client is returning from surgery with a radium implant for the treatment of endometrial cancer. Which nursing diagnosis would be most helpful in planning this client's care?**

1. Alteration in nutrition related to anorexia.
2. Body image disturbance related to alopecia.
3. Alteration in mobility related to bedrest.
4. Potential for injury related to radiation.

1. *Not at this time. Intake and output must be monitored, but implants do not carry a high risk of causing anorexia.*
2. *Incorrect. Alopecia is not a side effect of implanted radium.*

3. *Correct. This is the most global choice. Interventions that would be planned include: isometric exercise, skin care, and monitoring of elimination, which may be altered since the client must remain on her back during the treatment with radium.*
4. *No. Generally, potential nursing diagnoses are not the priority of care.*

97. **The nurse understands that a client with primary degenerative dementia experiences:**

1. Memory loss gradually progressing to disorientation.
3. Personality traits develop that are opposite of original traits.
4. Increased auditory and visual acuity offset other losses.

1. *This is incorrect. Short-term memory loss is typically an initial symptom.*
2. *Correct! A gradual progression of symptoms is typical of primary degenerative dementia.*

> **STRATEGY ALERT!** Note that this option is also more global than any of the other options.

3. *Incorrect. An exaggeration of previous traits is typical.*
4. *Incorrect. Perceptual disturbances may require eyeglasses, a hearing aid, and an increased attention to safety in the environment.*

98. **A 38-year-old is admitted to the hospital with recurrence of the symptoms of leukemia. The client says to the nurse, "The doctor told me that my blood condition is too severe to be treated successfully. I guess I don't have long to live." Which of these responses by the nurse would be best?**

1. "Tell me exactly what your doctor meant when he said that your condition was too severe."
2. "Do you think that having a good mental outlook can help you at this time?"
3. "Your condition is very serious."
4. "How long do feel that you have left to live?"

1. *This response focuses on the wrong issue. What the doctor told the client is not the issue here. The issue is the client's feelings about having a severe, life-threatening disease.*
2. *Wrong! The nurse acknowledges the tenseness of the situation but also gives advice by asking this question. To be therapeutic for the client, the nurse's response should show empathy. At this time, it is inappropriate for the nurse to give the client information about the importance of a positive outlook. The nurse must first address the client's feelings.*

3. *This is the best answer! This option recognizes the seriousness of the situation and allows the client to talk about her feelings.*

4. *The issue in this question is the client's feelings about having a severe, life-threatening disease. The nurse's response in this option focuses on an inappropriate concern. This response is not therapeutic.*

99. **A 39-year-old female has had a right radical mastectomy. Which activity would the nurse anticipate being the most difficult for this client four days postoperatively?**

   1. Brushing her hair with her right hand.
   2. Eating with her right hand.
   3. Active-assisted range of motion of the right hand.
   4. Washing her hands in a basin.

   1. *Good reasoning. Abduction of the arm away from the body would be the most difficult, and usually would be the last type of movement to be regained by the post-mastectomy client.*

   2. *No, this isn't too difficult. The arm motion necessary for eating mainly involves the hand, wrist, and elbow.*

   3. *Incorrect. This is an early postoperative activity because active-assisted means that the client does what she is able with the nurse assisting.*

   4. *No, this isn't too difficult. The affected arm can be held low, and only the fingers and wrist moved.*

100. **The physician prescribes verapamil (Calan) 100 mg p.o. three times a day for a client with angina pectoris. The client states: "My brother takes Calan for high blood pressure. Do you think the doctor made a mistake?" The nurse's most therapeutic response would be:**

   1. "I'll check with the physician to verify the order."
   2. "Calan is effective in two ways: to treat angina and to manage high blood pressure."
   3. "Are you concerned that you might have high blood pressure?"
   4. "No, the physician has prescribed Calan so that you will not develop high blood pressure."

   1. *Wrong selection. A nurse making this response does not understand the actions of Calan!*

   2. *Correct. Calan does have more than one action as described above. This can be confusing for clients who have known Calan as an antihypertensive medication.*

   3. *No. This answer does not address the client's concerns nor does it reflect the nurse's understanding of the actions of Calan.*

   4. *Incorrect choice. The physician has prescribed Calan to control the angina attacks. Recall that Calan has many uses: anti-anginal, antihypertensive, antiarrhythmic and coronary vasodilator.*

NCLEX-RN

Test 10
Pharmacology

NCLEX-RN TEST 10

1. A client has been given instructions about taking enteric-coated erythromycin. Which of the following statements made by the client indicates to the nurse the need for further teaching?

   1. "I can take these pills with my meals."
   2. "The medicine has been coated so that it dissolves in my intestine, not my stomach."
   3. "It's okay to crush a tablet as long as I make sure it dissolves completely in water before swallowing it."
   4. "It's important that I finish the entire prescription, even if I don't feel sick anymore."

2. Benzodiazepine anti-anxiety drugs are used primarily to treat anxiety and stress-related conditions. The nurse should know that individual drugs in this family have other uses as well. All of the following conditions are treated with one or more of these drugs except:

   1. Insomnia.
   2. Status epilepticus.
   3. Skeletal muscle injuries.
   4. Chronic pain syndrome.

3. A two-year-old admitted with seizures is receiving phenytoin (Dilantin) in suspension form. What should the nurse do before administering each dose?

   1. Be sure the client has not eaten within the hour.
   2. Shake the container vigorously.
   3. Perform mouth care.
   4. Warm the solution before administering.

4. A chronic alcoholic client is experiencing alcohol withdrawal. Which of the following medications might the nurse expect to be prescribed to medically manage her alcohol withdrawal?

   1. Buspirone (BuSpar).
   2. Propranolol (Inderal).
   3. Hydroxyzine (Atarax).
   4. Chlordiazepoxide (Librium).

5. A 19-year-old client is in crisis and is admitted to the hospital. Her medical record indicates a history of drug abuse. Which of the following types of medications would the nurse expect to be prescribed in limited amounts, if at all, for this client?

   1. Antipsychotics.
   2. Antiparkinsonian agents.
   3. Tricyclic antidepressants.
   4. MAO inhibitor antidepressants.

6. A client is being treated with cefoxitin (Mefoxin) for a staphylococcus wound infection. When instructing the client about this drug, the nurse should tell him about which of the following adverse reactions?

   1. Headaches.
   2. Anorexia.
   3. Glossitis.
   4. Diarrhea.

7. The nurse is administering penicillin G potassium IV to a 70-year-old retired teacher. Which of the following is it important for the nurse to monitor when administering penicillin to this client?

   1. Potassium level.
   2. Seizures.
   3. Platelet count.
   4. Hematocrit and hemoglobin.

8. The antihistamine hydroxyzine (Vistaril) is frequently used for preoperative medication. Which of the following actions would the nurse least expect Vistaril to effectively produce?

   1. Controlling emesis.
   2. Diminishing anxiety.
   3. Reducing the amount of narcotics needed for pain relief.
   4. Skeletal muscle relaxation.

9. In preparing to begin an aminophylline infusion, which of the following approaches by the nurse would be best?

   1. Prepare a solution containing enough drug to last 24 hours.
   2. Obtain an infusion pump to regulate the flow of the drug.
   3. Insert a large IV catheter to assure adequate dilution.
   4. Initiate measurement of I&O to monitor for fluid retention.

10. Which of the following signs/symptoms should the nurse instruct a client to report immediately to the physician when beginning a course of penicillin therapy?

   1. Indigestion, nausea.
   2. Hives, itching.
   3. Ringing in the ears, dizziness.
   4. Headaches, drowsiness.

11. A 63-year-old client is receiving large doses of IV vancomycin (Vancocin). Which of the following precautions should the nurse take while administering this drug?

   1. Assess for loss of hearing.
   2. Assess for changes in vision.
   3. Keep the client on bed rest during medication administration.
   4. Provide a laxative during treatment.

12. The nurse knows that, for a chronically ill psychiatric client with a history of drug abuse, which of the following is a disadvantage of buspirone (BuSpar)?

   1. The two to three week lag time before it effectively reduces anxiety.
   2. Its abuse potential.
   3. Its potent sedative properties.
   4. Its relatively long half-life.

13. A client is receiving a thiazide diuretic. The nurse observes that the client demonstrates an understanding of his diet by selecting which of the following foods?

   1. Apricots.
   2. Milk.
   3. Beef.
   4. Pork.

14. A client is a newly diagnosed hypertensive. She is taking clonidine (Catapres) in the transdermal form. What statement by the client indicates to the nurse a need for further teaching?

   1. "I have trimmed the patch to make it fit better under my blouse."
   2. "I am reapplying the patch every seven days."
   3. "I understand that I can shower as usual."
   4. "I will notify my doctor if I get a rash."

15. The nurse understands that ferrous sulfate absorption will be increased if given with which of the following?

   1. Milk.
   2. Water.
   3. Orange juice.
   4. Meals.

16. The psychiatrist has prescribed diazepam (Valium) for an outpatient. Which of the following should the nurse caution the client to avoid ingesting?

   1. Diuretics.
   2. Cheddar cheese.
   3. Coffee.
   4. Alcoholic beverages.

17. The nurse knows that which of the following statements is inaccurate regarding benzodiazepine anti-anxiety drugs?

   1. They may cause rebound insomnia if discontinued rapidly.
   2. They are safer and more effective for insomnia than barbiturates.
   3. They can be taken safely for one to two weeks.
   4. They are used to treat sleep apnea.

18. A client is receiving cyclophosphamide (Cytoxan) for treatment of her leukemia. The nurse has noticed that she vomited after each of her previous doses. To prevent vomiting, what should the nurse do?

   1. Contact the physician for an antiemetic order prior to treatment.
   2. Withhold fluids prior to and during treatments.
   3. Suggest to the client that she eat before receiving her treatment.
   4. Explain that vomiting cannot be prevented and provide the client with an emesis basin during treatments.

19. The nurse knows that abrupt withdrawal of which of the following medications could be life-threatening?

   1. Amitriptyline (Elavil).
   2. Flurazepam (Dalmane).
   3. Fluoxetine (Prozac).
   4. Fluphenazine (Prolixin).

20. A client has just returned to the unit after having major surgery and is complaining of pain. The physician has ordered morphine sulfate to control her pain. Before administering the medication, what should the nurse do first?

1. Discuss the side effects with the client.
2. Take the client's vital signs.
3. Provide mouth care.
4. Have the client turn, cough and deep breathe.

21. **The doctor has ordered ergonovine (Ergotrate) for a client. Which of the following conditions, if present, would warrant the nurse to use caution when administering the ergonovine?**

    1. Diabetes.
    2. Pre-eclampsia.
    3. Uterine atony.
    4. Anemia.

22. **The nurse knows that which of the following medications is often prescribed for treating the extrapyramidal side effects associated with antipsychotics?**

    1. Phenelzine (Nardil).
    2. Bupropion (Wellbutrin).
    3. Amantadine (Symmetrel).
    4. Hydroxyzine (Atarax).

23. **A client, 83, is a widow with Alzheimer's disease. She has begun to strike out at staff members when they try to assist her to bed at night. In addition, the staff members report she is awake and restless most of the night. After further assessment, the nurse decides to contact the physician for a medication order. The nurse anticipates the physician will most likely order:**

    1. Diazepam (Valium) 10 mg p.r.n.
    2. Hydroxyzine (Vistaril) 50 mg b.i.d.
    3. Chlorpromazine (Thorazine) 10 mg t.i.d.
    4. Haloperidol (Haldol) 2 mg hs.

24. **Ampicillin (Omnipen) is dispensed in a preparation of 125 mg/5 mL. The orders are 100 mg/kg/day to be given every four hours. The client weighs 33 pounds. How many mL should the nurse administer for the 9:00 a.m. dose?**

    1. 15 mL.
    2. 10 mL.
    3. 2 mL.
    4. 22 mL.

25. **The nurse understands that naloxone (Narcan) is given to achieve which of the following actions?**

    1. To accentuate the effects of narcotics in a laboring woman.
    2. To depress the activity of the central nervous system (CNS) in the woman who received narcotics in labor.

3. To block the effects of narcotics on the CNS in a woman in labor.
4. To withdraw narcotics from the body of a laboring woman.

26. **The client is diabetic and has been prescribed cefonicid (Monocid). He regularly tests his urine for glucose. Which of the following instructions would be most appropriate for the nurse to give to a client before he starts the Monocid?**

    1. Use a second-voided urine specimen when testing for glucose using the Clinitest method.
    2. Have your physician adjust your insulin dosage to reflect the need for increased insulin during cephalosporin therapy.
    3. Use an alternate method of urine testing (Clinistix or Tes-Tape) while taking Monocid.
    4. Have the diabetic clinician teach you the use of a glucometer to test for capillary blood sugar while taking Monocid.

27. **A client, age 34, is admitted to the psychiatric unit with a diagnosis of generalized anxiety disorder. He tells the admitting nurse that he is a recovering alcoholic who has not had a drink in two years. He also requests that the nurse telephone his physician to ask for a "tranquilizer" because he is so restless and on edge. Which of the following will the psychiatrist most likely order?**

    1. Chlordiazepoxide (Librium).
    2. Lorazepam (Ativan).
    3. Hydroxyzine (Vistaril).
    4. Oxazepam (Serax).

28. **A client is to receive intravenous antibiotics. Which of the following is the priority nursing action when preparing to administer this medication?**

    1. Determine if the client has any allergies.
    2. Determine the route of administration.
    3. Check the client's name band.
    4. Check the dosage against the physician's order.

29. **The nurse is caring for a diabetic client, who is currently taking cephalexin (Keflex). The nurse should advise the client of which of the following?**

    1. Clinitest or copper sulfate urine glucose tests give false positive results.
    2. Blood sugar may drop without warning.
    3. A source of sugar should always be carried with the client.
    4. A medic alert bracelet should always be worn.

30. A client is highly allergic to penicillin, but in need of a therapeutic plan of care. In carrying out the therapeutic plan of care for a client, the nurse is aware that which of the following antibiotics would be safe to administer?

    1. Ampicillin (Omnipen).
    2. Cefazolin (Ancef).
    3. Erythromycin ethylsuccinate (E.E.S.).
    4. Moxalactam (Moxam).

31. It is the beginning of summer, and a 14-year-old client is taking minocycline (Minocin) for her acne. What advice should the nurse give the client?

    1. Take the medication on an empty stomach with a glass of water.
    2. Minocin makes the skin photosensitive, so shield your skin from the sun and use a sun screen.
    3. Stay inside, as this medication will react with the sun.
    4. Take this drug at night before bedtime.

32. A six-month-old client has been prescribed erythromycin ethylsuccinate (Pediamycin) for an infection. Of what instruction should the nurse remind the client's mother before she gives this medication?

    1. Mix the medication in the client's formula.
    2. Be sure to keep the medication refrigerated and to shake it well before giving to the client.
    3. Keep the medication near the client's bed as a reminder to give it to him around the clock.
    4. This medication should be mixed in the client's baby food and given at each meal.

33. In order to monitor for toxicity of aminoglycosides, what test does the nurse expect might be done to measure the drug level in the blood?

    1. Blood urea nitrogen (BUN) and creatinine clearance.
    2. Peak and trough drug levels.
    3. Hematocrit and hemoglobin levels.
    4. Liver function studies.

34. While on warfarin (Coumadin), the nurse will expect that the client will be monitored by which blood test?

    1. APTT (activated partial thromboplastin time).
    2. Lee White clotting time.
    3. Platelet counts.
    4. PT (prothrombin time).

35. It is expected that the client will be on narcotics for four to five days after surgery. What precautions should the nurse take with the client to prevent complications?

    1. Provide bed rest for the first two to three days.
    2. Put the side rails up and items the client is likely to need, such as the client's water and cigarettes, close to her bed and within her reach.
    3. Encourage the client to call for help to ambulate.
    4. Suggest that the client limit the use of her medications, as addiction may result.

36. The nurse is caring for a client with a myocardial infarction who is taking chlorothiazide (Diuril) and digoxin (Lanoxin). Which diet would be most appropriate to be included in the nursing care?

    1. Diet low in sodium and saturated fats, high in potassium.
    2. Diet low in unsaturated fats, sodium and potassium.
    3. Diet high in potassium, Vitamin C and protein.
    4. Diet low in sodium and saturated and unsaturated fats.

37. A client, age 22, is admitted with a diagnosis of acute psychotic reaction, r/o schizophrenia. Because the client is very agitated, he is started on chlorpromazine (Thorazine) 100 mg, t.i.d. After three days, he is much calmer and his nurse begins to teach him about his medication. Which one of the following statements about his medication is most accurate?

    1. "This medication is a sedative to calm you down."
    2. "This medication acts on the chemical regulators in your brain to help control your symptoms."
    3. "This medication will cure your disorder."
    4. "We do not know how this medication works, but we do know it will help you control your behavior."

38. A new diabetic client requires daily injections of insulin. Which of the following would indicate to the nurse that the client may have an inaccurate understanding concerning the administration of his injections?

    1. The client states that he will change injection sites.
    2. The client tells the nurse that he needs to buy some alcohol.
    3. The client tells the nurse that his brother also is a diabetic and that he will be able to share all of the supplies with him.
    4. The client tells the nurse that his wife will be giving him the injections.

39. A newly diagnosed diabetic who also has adult primary open-angle glaucoma is admitted for regulation of his blood sugars. The client receives pilocarpine (Pilocar) 2% one drop q.i.d. to the OD. Instillation of this drug requires which of the following actions by the nurse?

    1. Asking the client to look straight ahead.
    2. Pressing on the lacrimal sac for one minute after instillation.
    3. Instructing the client to squeeze his eye shut after instillation.
    4. Cleansing the eye first, then wiping from the outer to the inner canthus.

40. Which of the following diagnostic studies can the nurse anticipate will be completed regularly for a client taking isoniazid (INH)?

    1. AST, ALT.
    2. WBC count.
    3. Bone marrow aspirations.
    4. Creatinine & BUN.

41. The client is an infant who weighs 8.6 kilograms. The caloric requirement for this client is 120 cal/kg/24 hours. The formula prescribed has 20 calories in two ounces. How many mL of formula does the nurse understand that the infant needs in a 24-hour period?

    1. 1032 mL.
    2. 3096 mL.
    3. 103 mL.
    4. 1548 mL.

42. A client has been receiving ritodrine therapy for the last 24 hours to stop her premature labor. The attempts are unsuccessful and she delivers an infant at 31 weeks gestation. In assessing the neonate, which of the following should the nurse anticipate as a result of the ritodrine (Yutopar) therapy?

    1. Hypoglycemia.
    2. Hypothermia.
    3. Respiratory distress.
    4. Hypertension.

43. A 42-year-old client is being treated for congestive heart failure. Included in his orders is a prescription for furosemide (Lasix) 20 mg p.o. daily. The nurse administering this drug should be alert for which of the following complications?

    1. Fluid and electrolyte imbalances.
    2. Decreased potassium excretion.

    3. Increased serum calcium level.
    4. Shift of fluid into the cells.

44. A woman is in ICU following a cesarean section, complicated with severe PIH and magnesium intoxication, as a result of prolonged magnesium sulfate therapy. She received an IV bolus of calcium gluconate to treat the hypermagnesemia. The nurse should understand that the side effects of calcium gluconate include which of the following?

    1. Hypertension.
    2. Tachycardia.
    3. Arrhythmia.
    4. Pulmonary edema.

45. Which of the following are major side effects that the nurse might anticipate observing in the client receiving antiparkinsonian drugs?

    1. Blurred vision, mental confusion, dry mouth and constipation.
    2. Orthostatic hypotension, palpitations and tremors.
    3. Insomnia, sedation and constipation.
    4. Occipital headache, neck stiffness, nausea and vomiting.

46. The nurse understands that all of the following would be included in the care of a client with an aspirin overdose except:

    1. Gastric lavage or emesis.
    2. Administration of activated charcoal.
    3. Increasing the acidity of the urine.
    4. Hemodialysis or peritoneal dialysis.

47. A pregnant client has a severe iron deficiency anemia. The physician orders an injection of iron dextran (Imferon) IM. How should the nurse plan to administer the injection?

    1. Use a size 23-25 gauge needle and administer it in the deltoid muscle.
    2. Use a size 20 or 22 gauge needle and administer it deep in the thigh.
    3. Select a 19-20 gauge needle and administer using the Z track method.
    4. Select an 18 gauge needle and give deep in the buttocks.

48. The nurse should advise a client taking rifampin (Rifadin) for treatment of TB to avoid which of the following?

1. Antacids containing magnesium.
2. Aspirin products.
3. OTC cold products.
4. Alcoholic beverages.

49. A client is being treated for gastrointestinal bleeding. The client tells the nurse that he slept very well after taking temazepam (Restoril) and asks if he can continue to take Restoril at home because he suffers from chronic insomnia. Which of the following considerations are important for the nurse to make the best response?

    1. He may not need a sleep medication after his gastrointestinal bleeding is treated in the hospital.
    2. He would benefit more by seeking other methods of relieving his chronic insomnia.
    3. It is too soon to be concerned with his discharge plans.
    4. This could be a good plan for the client's insomnia, since he responded well to the Restoril while in the hospital.

50. A client, age 54, is hospitalized for gastrointestinal bleeding. He is given temazepam (Restoril) at bedtime to help him sleep. What nursing action is indicted immediately following his dose?

    1. Raise the side rails on his bed and tell him to use his call light to summon the nurse if he has to get up during the night.
    2. Keep a padded tongue blade at the bedside and observe for seizures.
    3. Monitor his blood pressure and respirations.
    4. Observe and record his sleep patterns.

51. A client receives haloperidol (Haldol) 5 mg t.i.d. Several days into treatment, the nurse notices that the client is walking stiffly with a shuffling gait. What nursing action is indicated at this time?

    1. Take her blood pressure before her next dose.
    2. Withhold the Haldol until the symptom disappears.
    3. Chart her observations on the client's record.
    4. Obtain an order for an antiparkinsonian drug.

52. The physician has changed a client's antihypertensive medication from hydralazine (Apresoline) to metoprolol (Lopressor). The nurse understands that this change would mean the client is less likely to experience:

    1. Reflex tachycardia.
    2. Hypotension.
    3. Sodium retention.
    4. Dizziness.

53. The nurse must correctly calculate the daily dosage of a new medication for a child weighing 69 pounds. The physician has ordered 10 mcg/kg/day in three divided doses. The nurse has on hand 0.1 mg tablets. What is the daily dosage in milligrams?

    1. 10.45 mg.
    2. 0.69 mg.
    3. 3.1 mg.
    4. 0.31 mg.

54. A client is hospitalized for gastrointestinal bleeding and is being treated with temazepam (Restoril). After the client's physician examined him, the nurse noted the physician had written an order for the client to begin taking amitriptyline (Elavil). Which of the following actions would be best initially by the nurse?

    1. Revise his medication schedule so that Elavil is administered during the day and the Restoril hs.
    2. Monitor the client's vital signs closely.
    3. Question the physician about administering both Elavil and Ativan to the client.
    4. Assess the client for signs and symptoms of depression.

55. A client is seen in the antepartum testing unit for a contraction stress test. Which of the following oxytocic drugs will be used to complete this test?

    1. Ergotamine (Ergomar).
    2. Methylergonovine (Methergine).
    3. Ergonovine (Ergotrate).
    4. Oxytocin (Pitocin).

56. A client is receiving methotrexate (Mexate) for his lung cancer. When he returns to the clinic he reports that his gums are beginning to bleed. What action should the nurse take?

    1. Tell the client that bleeding gums is perfectly normal.
    2. Tell the client not to brush his teeth for a few days.
    3. Consult with his doctor and have the lab draw blood work, especially platelets.
    4. Have the client call his dentist.

57. A blood transfusion using packed cells (250 mL) is ordered to be infused in four hours. The blood set delivers 10 gtt/mL. The nurse calculates the proper drip rate of the unit of packed cells as:

    1. 42 gtts/min.
    2. 63 gtts/min.
    3. 10 gtts/min.
    4. 16 gtts/min.

3. Edema of feet and hands.
4. Red-orange discoloration to all body fluids.

58. A client has been taking isoniazid (INH) and rifampin (Rifadin) for three weeks after being diagnosed with TB. He calls the Health Clinic and tells the nurse that he has noted a reddish-orange color to his urine. Which of the following statements by the nurse would be the most accurate response?

1. "I'll make an appointment for you to see the doctor this afternoon. You may have developed a bleeding problem, which is not uncommon with these drugs."
2. "The reddish color is a side effect of the INH. Stop taking it for two to three days and the discoloration should go away. The doctor may want to change your drug therapy."
3. "The discoloration is due to rifampin. It may turn all body fluids orange-red. This is a harmless side effect."
4. "You should increase your fluid intake while on these medications. They are known to cause bladder irritation when taken together."

59. A two-year-old client has been receiving bleomycin (Blenoxane) IV for treatment of his Wilm's tumor. The next dose is due at 2:00 pm. What must the nurse do before hanging the medication?

1. Change the client's diaper.
2. Be sure the IV is patent.
3. Talk to the client's mother about all the possible side effects of the drug.
4. Be sure the client has had his lunch.

60. A physician prescribes para-aminosalicylic acid (PAS) for a client who has been diagnosed with tuberculosis. To decrease the GI symptoms of nausea/vomiting associated with PAS, the nurse should instruct the client to do which of the following?

1. Take the medication at bedtime.
2. Have the physician prescribe an antiemetic to be taken 30 minutes before the PAS.
3. Take the medication with food or an antacid.
4. Crush the tablets and dissolve them completely in water before swallowing.

61. A client is diagnosed with active tuberculosis and is started on a treatment regimen of isoniazid (INH) and ethambutol (Myambutol). Which of the following signs/symptoms reported by the client would necessitate the discontinuation of ethambutol?

1. Anorexia, nausea/vomiting.
2. Loss of color discrimination.

62. A hospitalized six-month-old, whose mother brings in expressed breast milk, took two ounces of breast milk at 8:00 a.m., three ounces at 11:00 a.m. and two and one-half ounces at 1:00 p.m. What should the nurse record on this client's intake record for the shift?

1. 150 mL.
2. 225 mL.
3. 240 mL.
4. 375 mL.

63. A client is taking erythromycin delayed-release capsules (Eryc) for a urinary tract infection. By the fourth day of a 10-day treatment, he tells the nurse he's fine now and will keep the remainder of his medicine for another infection. Which of the following is the most therapeutic response by the nurse?

1. "Good idea, you will save lots of money that way."
2. "You should always take the full course of antibiotics because it is still possible for many of the bacteria to be in your urinary tract."
3. "Take at least one more day of medication."
4. "That would really be a stupid thing to do."

64. A client is receiving magnesium sulfate as treatment for pregnancy induced hypertension. Which of the following assessments would warrant turning off the magnesium sulfate IV drip?

1. Respirations 16/minute.
2. Urinary output 100 mL in five hours.
3. Reflexes depressed +1.
4. Fetal heart rate 158, decreased variability.

65. The nurse understands that which of the following are common side effects of benzodiazepine anti-anxiety medications?

1. Insomnia.
2. Headache.
3. Confusion.
4. Dizziness.

66. On the third day of amoxicillin (Amoxil) therapy, a client develops diarrhea. The nurse should instruct the client to do which of the following?

1. Stop taking the drug as this is an indication of toxicity.
2. Contact her physician about treatment of the diarrhea.

3. Drink extra liquids to compensate for the fluid lost in the diarrhea.
4. Take an over-the-counter antidiarrheal agent according to package directions.

67. **The client is receiving propranolol (Inderal) for anxiety. In reviewing the client's discharge plans, the nurse needs to emphasize which of the following?**

1. Inderal should be discontinued by gradually tapering it off over time.
2. Inderal should not be taken during pregnancy.
3. Inderal is contraindicated for clients with asthma.
4. Inderal is a safe medication with no known adverse effects.

68. **The nurse knows that peripheral neuropathy, a side effect from the use of isoniazid (INH), is treated by administering which of the following at the same time INH is given?**

1. Vitamin C.
2. Vitamin B6 (Pyridoxine).
3. Steroids.
4. Combinations of vitamins and steroids.

69. **The nurse caring for a person whose anxiety is being treated with hydroxyzine (Vistaril) should know that this person is likely to complain of:**

1. Dry mouth and nasal stuffiness.
2. Headaches.
3. Nausea and vomiting.
4. Diarrhea.

70. **A woman receives naloxone (Narcan) just prior to her rapid vaginal delivery. In planning for her postpartum care, the nurse needs to be aware that the Narcan could cause which of the following?**

1. Respiratory depression.
2. Supine hypotension.
3. Increased lochia.
4. Urticaria.

71. **A mother at 34 weeks gestation is receiving magnesium sulfate to treat severe PIH. Twenty-six hours after the medication is started, the woman delivers by cesarean section. Which of the following clinical findings should the nurse caring for the newborn anticipate as a result of the magnesium sulfate therapy?**

1. Hypoglycemia.
2. Hypothermia.
3. Respiratory depression.
4. Hyperreflexia.

72. **Chlorothiazide (Diuril) is ordered b.i.d. for a infant weighing 6.5 kg. It is supplied in elixir form 100 mg/tsp. The recommended dosage for Diuril is 25 mg/kg/day. How many mL should the nurse give to the child for each dose?**

1. 6.15 mL.
2. 8.13 mL.
3. 4.06 mL.
4. 0.81 mL.

73. **A client is being treated with cisplatin (Platinol) for his cancer. After several treatments he begins to complain of fatigue and wants to sleep all day. Which of the following nursing actions is most appropriate?**

1. Advise the client about the dangers of immobility.
2. Check lab values of RBCs, hematocrit and hemoglobin, as he is likely to be anemic.
3. Call in the family for counseling, since the client is depressed and may become suicidal.
4. Set up an exercise plan.

74. **A client, age 82, is admitted to the psychiatric unit for a diagnostic work-up because she had become increasingly forgetful and disoriented at home. She has been taking lorazepam (Ativan) 0.5 mg p.r.n. to control her restlessness. The Ativan is not an indication for the nurse's plan of care to include close observation of the client for which of the following?**

1. Orthostatic hypotension.
2. Increased anxiety.
3. Hyperexcitation.
4. Hallucinations.

75. **A client is given a six dose series of ergonovine (Ergotrate) following a vaginal delivery. Which of the following assessments must be completed on this client while she is receiving the ergonovine?**

1. Urinary output.
2. Apical pulse.
3. Blood pressure.
4. Oral temperature.

76. **Before beginning a client's rifampin (Rifadin) therapy, the nurse should warn him that this medication can cause which adverse side effect?**

1. Turn urine, sweat, tears and saliva to a red-orange color.
2. Cause stools to turn black.
3. Stain his teeth.
4. Cause constipation.

77. **Which of the following statements made by a client would indicate to the nurse that the client has an accurate understanding of oral cloxacillin (Tegopen) administration?**

    1. "I'll take the medicine with milk or an antacid so that my stomach won't get upset."
    2. "I'll take the Tegopen with a large glass of fruit juice so that I get extra Vitamin C for wound healing."
    3. "I'll take the medicine either one hour before or two hours after meals so that it will work better."
    4. "I'll take the Tegopen at the same time as my blood pressure and heart pills so that I don't forget to take it."

78. **A medication is ordered t.i.d. for a child weighing 16 lbs 12 oz. The recommended dosage is 0.03 mg/kg/day. How many milligrams should the nurse administer to the child per dose?**

    1. 0.06 mg.
    2. 0.22 mg.
    3. 0.08 mg.
    4. 0.16 mg.

79. **An elderly client is disoriented, confused and agitated and is receiving lorazepam (Ativan). Because the client is receiving Ativan, which of the following nursing actions is a priority?**

    1. Observing the client for beginning signs of tardive dyskinesia.
    2. Warning the client not to drive her automobile or engage in activities that require alertness.
    3. Check the client's serum level of medication frequently.
    4. Monitor the client closely when she ambulates.

80. **A psychiatric client becomes very agitated. His psychiatrist prescribes chlorpromazine (Thorazine) 50 mg by intramuscular injection, p.r.n. What instructions should the nurse give the client when administering the injection?**

    1. "You will need to lie down when I give this injection and should remain in this position for at least 30 minutes."
    2. "You have to hold your arm still when I give you the injection so the medication goes in properly."
    3. "This medication can only be given by injection."
    4. "I have to give you an injection because you need a larger dose than I can safely give you by mouth."

81. **The nurse is planning care for a client receiving nifedipine (Adalat) for treatment of preterm labor. Which of the following maternal assessment must be included?**

    1. Temperature.
    2. Blood sugar.
    3. Blood pressure.
    4. Pedal pulses.

82. **A client is being treated with large doses of IV vancomycin (Vancocin). He complains that his arm is sore. Which of the following nursing actions is most appropriate at this time?**

    1. Immediately assess placement of the needle in the vein, as this drug can cause tissue damage if allowed to infiltrate.
    2. Assure the client that this drug burns a little as it infuses, but there is nothing to worry about.
    3. Alert emergency surgery, as infiltration of Vancocin may necessitate surgery.
    4. Apply cold compresses to the site after the medication has infused.

83. **Two days after a psychiatric inpatient begins taking fluphenazine (Prolixin), she comes to the nursing station. The nurse observes she is very frightened, her head is twisted to one side, her back is arched and her eyes are rolled up. The best action for the nurse to take, initially, after reassuring the client that the nurse knows what is wrong and can help, is to do which of the following?**

    1. Check her for cogwheeling.
    2. Telephone her physician to report the client's condition.
    3. Give her a p.r.n. dose of haloperidol (Haldol) to relax her.
    4. Give her a p.r.n. dose of benztropine mesylate (Cogentin) IM.

84. **Before starting a tricyclic antidepressant, a complete medical history and physical exam should be done. The nurse knows that which of the following tests are an essential part of this pre-treatment screening?**

    1. An electrocardiogram (EKG).
    2. A thyroid scan.
    3. Liver function tests.
    4. A creatinine clearance test.

85. **The nurse knows that the chief reason for using para-aminosalicylic acid (PAS) in the treatment of tuberculosis is which of the following?**

1. It is a substitute for ethambutol (Myambutol) in TB regimes for pediatric clients.
2. It is prophylactic for tuberculosis.
3. It treats severe disseminated tuberculosis.
4. It treats extrapulmonary tuberculosis.

86. **The doctor orders D5 1/2 NS with KCl 10 mEq/liter at 30 mL/hr. The nurse is going to hang a 500 mL bag. KCl is supplied 20 mEq/10 mL. How many mL of KCl will be added to the IV solution?**

    1. 1.5 mL.
    2. 2.5 mL.
    3. 5 mL.
    4. 10 mL.

87. **A psychiatrist informs the nurse that a client with an obsessive-compulsive disorder is to start on psychotropic medication. Which of the following medications, specifically indicated for the treatment of obsessive-compulsive disorder, does the nurse anticipate the psychiatrist will order?**

    1. Clomipramine (Anafranil) or fluoxetine (Prozac).
    2. Amitriptyline (Elavil) or trazodone (Desyrel).
    3. Alprazolam (Xanax) or diazepam (Valium).
    4. Haloperidol (Haldol) or fluphenazine (Prolixin).

88. **Which of the following disease conditions would the nurse expect to contraindicate the use of rifampin (Rifadin) in a client with tuberculosis?**

    1. Active hepatitis.
    2. Hypertension.
    3. Pyelonephritis.
    4. Parkinsonism.

89. **A client is receiving oxytocin (Pitocin) for induction of labor. Which of the following conditions would warrant the nurse discontinuing the intravenous infusion of Pitocin?**

    1. Fetal heart rate baseline 140-160 bpm.
    2. Contractions every one and one-half minutes, each lasting 70-80 seconds.
    3. Maternal temperature 101.2° F.
    4. Early decelerations in the fetal heart rate.

90. **The nurse notices that a two-year-old client who is receiving bleomycin (Blenoxane) IV is not voiding adequately, what action should be taken initially?**

    1. Stop the drug immediately.
    2. Assess intake and output, be sure that the client is adequately hydrated.

3. Give a diuretic.
4. Do nothing; a decrease in urine is an expected side effect.

91. **The physician ordered gr 3/4; on hand are 15 mg tablets. How many tablet(s) should the nurse give?**

    1. Three tablets.
    2. One tablet.
    3. Two tablets.
    4. One and a half tablets.

92. **If a client with thrombophlebitis is started on IV antibiotics, how should the nurse plan to administer the IV antibiotics?**

    1. Consult with the physician because another IV line will be needed since heparin is not compatible with most other IV medications.
    2. Plan to piggyback the additional medications into the heparin line.
    3. Refuse to give the additional medications as it would be unsafe practice.
    4. Tell the client to watch for additional side effects, as heparin and other medications usually do not mix.

93. **A client diagnosed with TB has been taking isoniazid (INH) 300 mg p.o. daily for six weeks. He now complains of numbness and tingling in his hands and feet. Which of the following medications will most likely be ordered by the physician to decrease these symptoms?**

    1. Isoxsuprine (Vasodilan).
    2. Dipyridamole (Persantine).
    3. Pyridoxine (Vitamin B6).
    4. Cyclandelate (Cyclospasmol).

94. **A 33-year-old client is in counseling for generalized anxiety disorder. The psychiatrist prescribes buspirone (BuSpar) to control her extreme restlessness and irritability. The nurse knows that which of the following side effects is most common when taking buspirone?**

    1. Drowsiness.
    2. Sedation.
    3. Ataxia.
    4. Headaches.

95. **A client is receiving magnesium sulfate for treatment of severe pregnancy induced hypertension (PIH). She begins to show symptoms of magnesium intoxication and the decision is made to administer calcium gluconate. Which of the following best describes the procedure the nurse should use for injection of calcium gluconate?**

1. Rapid IV administration via IV push.
2. Slow IV administration via piggyback IV drip.
3. Slow IV administration via IV push.
4. IM injection to provide for slow absorption.

96. **A client is receiving ritodrine (Yutopar) for treatment of premature labor. Which clinical finding would warrant further assessments to evaluate this client?**

    1. Maternal heart rate 124/minute for 10 minutes.
    2. Fetal heart rate 174 bpm.
    3. Blood pressure drop from 120/68 to 110/60.
    4. Respiratory rate 34/minute for 10 minutes.

97. **Ampicillin/sulbactam (Unasyn) 250 mg is diluted in 50 mL of D5W. The antibiotic is to be delivered in 20 minutes though a soluset (set delivers 60 gtt per mL). Which is the correct rate for the nurse to set in order to deliver the medication in 20 minutes?**

    1. 50 microgtt/min.
    2. 17 microgtt/min.
    3. 150 microgtt/min.
    4. 38 microgtt/min.

98. **Four days after admission, a client who is taking haloperidol (Haldol) is pacing up and down the hallway. The nurse observes him and assesses further by asking the client how he feels. He replies that he is very restless and can't seem to sit still. The nurse diagnoses the problem as the extrapyramidal side effect termed:**

    1. Dystonia.
    2. Parkinsonism.
    3. Tardive dyskinesia.
    4. Akathisia.

99. **A client is being given an aminoglycoside for his bacterial infection. The nurse can aid in minimizing the risk of aminoglycoside toxicity through which of the following actions?**

    1. Weighing the client daily.
    2. Encouraging the client to drink at least 2000 mL of fluid daily.
    3. Monitoring blood pressure prior to drug administration.
    4. Instructing the client to take the medicine with food.

100. **Which of the following clinical findings would indicate to the nurse that an antepartum client is experiencing an adverse reaction to betamethasone (Celestone)?**

    1. Blood pressure 90/52.
    2. Blood sugar 64.
    3. Muscle weakness or cramping.
    4. Temperature 103° F.

NOTES

NCLEX-RN

Test 10

Pharmacology Questions with Rationales

NCLEX-RN TEST 10 WITH RATIONALES

1.   A client has been given instructions about taking enteric-coated erythromycin. Which of the following statements made by the client indicates to the nurse the need for further teaching?

  1.   "I can take these pills with my meals."
  2.   "The medicine has been coated so that it dissolves in my intestine, not my stomach."
  3.   "It's okay to crush a tablet as long as I make sure it dissolves completely in water before swallowing it."
  4.   "It's important that I finish the entire prescription, even if I don't feel sick anymore."

  1.   *Incorrect choice. This statement indicates that the client knows that enteric-coated tablets may be taken with meals. The client does understand the drug therapy.*
  2.   *No. The client does understand the drug therapy. Enteric-coated means that the medication is protected from the acid media of the stomach and can thus pass safely into the duodenum, where it is absorbed.*
  3.   *Correct! You remembered that enteric-coated tablets cannot be crushed. Another drug form that should not be crushed is the sustained release form, often identified with key suffixes attached to the drug's name: Dur (as in duration), SR (sustained release), CR (controlled release), SA (sustained action), and Contin (continuous). Trade names may also imply sustained release: spansules, extentabs, extencaps.*
  4.   *Wrong choice! This client does understand a key principle in antibiotic therapy: take the medication for as long as prescribed, usually seven to 10 days, even if beginning to feel better. You are asked to find an area where the client requires further instruction.*

2.   Benzodiazepine anti-anxiety drugs are used primarily to treat anxiety and stress-related conditions. The nurse should know that individual drugs in this family have other uses as well. All of the following conditions are treated with one or more of these drugs except:

  1.   Insomnia.
  2.   Status epilepticus.
  3.   Skeletal muscle injuries.
  4.   Chronic pain syndrome.

  1.   *Benzodiazepine anti-anxiety drugs are used as hypnotics to induce sleep in persons who suffer from a short-term sleep disorder. This is not the correct option because the stem is asking for a false response.*
  2.   *Incorrect choice. Valium is used to treat certain seizure disorders, such as status epilepticus. This cannot be the answer because the question has a false response stem.*
  3.   *Benzodiazepine anti-anxiety medications have muscle relaxant properties and are used to treat various conditions that cause muscle spasm, such as whiplash injuries.*
  4.   *Correct. Chronic pain syndrome is treated with antidepressants, not anti-anxiety drugs.*

3.   A two-year-old admitted with seizures is receiving phenytoin (Dilantin) in suspension form. What should the nurse do before administering each dose?

  1.   Be sure the client has not eaten within the hour.
  2.   Shake the container vigorously.
  3.   Perform mouth care.
  4.   Warm the solution before administering.

  1.   *This is incorrect. Phenytoin should be given with meals to decrease gastric problems.*
  2.   *Correct! It is important for the nurse to shake the container, as clients can be under-medicated if the medication is not evenly distributed.*
  3.   *This is incorrect. Although mouth and dental care are needed, and clients do need to consult their dentist, mouth care is not needed before each dose.*
  4.   *This action is not necessary; the diluent for oral use will hasten dissolution if warmed.*

4.   A chronic alcoholic client is experiencing alcohol withdrawal. Which of the following medications might the nurse expect to be prescribed to medically manage her alcohol withdrawal?

  1.   Buspirone (BuSpar).
  2.   Propranolol (Inderal).
  3.   Hydroxyzine (Atarax).
  4.   Chlordiazepoxide (Librium).

  1.   *This is not the correct medication. BuSpar has no CNS depressant properties, so it cannot be used in withdrawing clients from alcohol.*
  2.   *This is not the correct medication. Inderal is a beta-blocker used to treat clients with anxiety. It is not used in alcohol withdrawal because it is not a CNS depressant.*

3. *This is not the correct medication. Atarax is an antihistamine that can be used as a mild sedative-hypnotic agent. It is not used in alcohol withdrawal because it is not a CNS depressant.*

4. *Correct. Librium is a relatively long acting CNS depressant that is used to treat alcohol withdrawal. It is substituted for alcohol during the detoxification process to prevent the occurrence of delirium tremens.*

5. **A 19-year-old client is in crisis and is admitted to the hospital. Her medical record indicates a history of drug abuse. Which of the following types of medications would the nurse expect to be prescribed in limited amounts, if at all, for this client?**

   1. Antipsychotics.
   2. Antiparkinsonian agents.
   3. Tricyclic antidepressants.
   4. MAO inhibitor antidepressants.

   1. *This is not correct. Antipsychotics do not have abusive properties.*
   2. *Correct. Antiparkinsonian agents, used to treat the extrapyramidal side effects of antipsychotics, can produce a state of euphoria and therefore have the potential for abuse.*
   3. *This is not correct. Antidepressants do not have properties that could lead to abuse.*
   4. *This is not the correct answer. MAOIs are not associated with any abuse potential.*

6. **A client is being treated with cefoxitin (Mefoxin) for a staphylococcus wound infection. When instructing the client about this drug, the nurse should tell him about which of the following adverse reactions?**

   1. Headaches.
   2. Anorexia.
   3. Glossitis.
   4. Diarrhea.

   1. *Incorrect choice. Although headaches may result when clients take certain cephalosporins with alcohol, they are not a common reaction to Mefoxin administration.*
   2. *No, anorexia is not a common side effect of Mefoxin administration.*
   3. *Incorrect. Glossitis (inflammation of the tongue) is not commonly seen in clients taking Mefoxin.*
   4. *Correct! Diarrhea, maculopapular rash, urticaria, hemolytic anemia and pseudomembranous colitis are common adverse reactions to Mefoxin.*

7. **The nurse is administering penicillin G potassium IV to a 70-year-old retired teacher. Which of the following is it important for the nurse to monitor when administering penicillin to this client?**

   1. Potassium level.
   2. Seizures.
   3. Platelet count.
   4. Hematocrit and hemoglobin.

   1. *You are correct! Deaths have resulted from the toxic effects of potassium in the presence of renal insufficiency.*
   2. *This is incorrect. Neurological deficits, including seizures, are not side effects of penicillin.*
   3. *This is not correct. Penicillin has no effect on platelets.*
   4. *This is incorrect. Penicillin does not effect the production of red blood cells, so the hematocrit and hemoglobin would not be affected.*

8. **The antihistamine hydroxyzine (Vistaril) is frequently used for preoperative medication. Which of the following actions would the nurse least expect Vistaril to effectively produce?**

   1. Controlling emesis.
   2. Diminishing anxiety.
   3. Reducing the amount of narcotics needed for pain relief.
   4. Skeletal muscle relaxation.

   1. *Wrong choice! Vistaril is an effective antiemetic and is used to control nausea and vomiting in pre- and postoperative clients. This cannot be the correct option because the stem is asking for an action not expected with Vistaril.*
   2. *Wrong! Vistaril is used to diminish anxiety in surgical clients as well as in persons with moderate anxiety states.*
   3. *Wrong. When Vistaril is used for surgical clients, narcotic requirements may be significantly reduced.*
   4. *Correct. The benzodiazepines produce skeletal muscle relaxation; Vistaril does not.*

9. **In preparing to begin an aminophylline infusion, which of the following approaches by the nurse would be best?**

   1. Prepare a solution containing enough drug to last 24 hours.
   2. Obtain an infusion pump to regulate the flow of the drug.
   3. Insert a large IV catheter to assure adequate dilution.
   4. Initiate measurement of I&O to monitor for fluid retention.

1. *This is incorrect. Since aminophylline can be very toxic if infused too quickly, the total daily dose should be divided into several IV containers. If the infusion rate increases, a limited amount of drug will be infused.*

2. **Correct. Since aminophylline can be very toxic if infused too quickly, a pump should be used to regulate the flow of this drug. Note that the word "infusion" appears in the stem of the question and in the correct answer.**

3. *The size of the IV catheter is not relevant to dilution of the drug. The drug is diluted in the IV solution, not in the vein.*

4. *I&O should be monitored, but the nurse will be looking for dehydration rather than fluid retention, since aminophylline acts as a diuretic.*

10. **Which of the following signs/symptoms should the nurse instruct a client to report immediately to the physician when beginning a course of penicillin therapy?**

    1. Indigestion, nausea.
    2. Hives, itching.
    3. Ringing in the ears, dizziness.
    4. Headaches, drowsiness.

    1. *Incorrect. These two symptoms of GI distress are often experienced by clients on antibiotic therapy. Although problematic, they do not constitute an immediate threat to the client's life.*

    2. **Good choice. The development of hives, itching, and/or wheezing are indicative of a possible hypersensitivity reaction, which could progress to anaphylactic shock. Even if a client has previously taken penicillin without problems, there is still a chance of a subsequent reaction with future doses. Clients should always be instructed to report these symptoms to the physician immediately.**

    3. *No. These two symptoms are not indicative of potential adverse reactions to penicillin.*

    4. *Sorry, this is not correct! These two symptoms are not indicative of adverse reactions to penicillin therapy.*

11. **A 63-year-old client is receiving large doses of IV vancomycin (Vancocin). Which of the following precautions should the nurse take while administering this drug?**

    1. Assess for loss of hearing.
    2. Assess for changes in vision.
    3. Keep the client on bed rest during medication administration.
    4. Provide a laxative during treatment.

    1. **Correct, this medication does impair hearing, especially in elderly individuals.**

2. *No. This medication does not impair vision. Its main toxicities involve hearing, and liver and kidney function.*

3. *Wrong. Keeping a 63-year-old on bedrest for the period of time of IV administration would lead to complications of immobility and would not be a safe nursing practice.*

4. *Wrong choice! Providing a laxative is not necessary, as constipation is not a side effect of Vancocin.*

12. **The nurse knows that, for a chronically ill psychiatric client with a history of drug abuse, which of the following is a disadvantage of buspirone (BuSpar)?**

    1. The two to three week lag time before it effectively reduces anxiety.
    2. Its abuse potential.
    3. Its potent sedative properties.
    4. Its relatively long half-life.

    1. **Correct. BuSpar is an effective nonbenzodiazepine anti-anxiety drug used for persons with anxiety disorders. It would not be a drug of choice for a client with acute anxiety, such as a person in crisis, because of its two to three week lag time.**

    2. *No. BuSpar does not have an abuse potential because of its long lag time.*

    3. *Incorrect. Unlike the benzodiazepines, BuSpar has no sedative-hypnotic properties and no abuse potential.*

    4. *Wrong! BuSpar's half life is only two to five hours, one of the shortest of the anti-anxiety medications.*

13. **A client is receiving a thiazide diuretic. The nurse observes that the client demonstrates an understanding of his diet by selecting which of the following foods?**

    1. Apricots.
    2. Milk.
    3. Beef.
    4. Pork.

    1. **Good choice! Of all the foods listed, apricots have the most potassium. Since the client is receiving a thiazide diuretic, potassium needs to be replaced.**

    2. *Wrong! Milk is higher in sodium than in potassium and because the client is receiving a thiazide diuretic, his potassium needs to be replaced.*

    3. *This choice is incorrect. Because the client is receiving a thiazide diuretic, his potassium needs to be replaced. Of the four foods listed, which is the highest in potassium?*

    4. *This choice is incorrect. Because the client is receiving a thiazide diuretic, his potassium needs to be replaced. Of the four foods listed, which is the highest in potassium?*

14. A client is a newly diagnosed hypertensive. She is taking clonidine (Catapres) in the transdermal form. What statement by the client indicates to the nurse a need for further teaching?

1. "I have trimmed the patch to make it fit better under my blouse."
2. "I am reapplying the patch every seven days."
3. "I understand that I can shower as usual."
4. "I will notify my doctor if I get a rash."

1. Good! If the patch is trimmed, part of the medication will be removed, thus reducing the dose.
2. The client is following the proper routine for Catapres patches by reapplying the patch every seven days.
3. No misunderstanding here! The client is correct in understanding that she can shower or bathe as usual.
4. Not misunderstood! A rash may indicate hypersensitivity, and the client is quite right to report one. Remember, this question asks for an option that indicates that the client did NOT understand the teaching.

15. The nurse understands that ferrous sulfate absorption will be increased if given with which of the following?

1. Milk.
2. Water.
3. Orange juice.
4. Meals.

1. Milk or dairy products cause a decrease in iron absorption. Try again.
2. No. Water does not facilitate absorption.
3. Correct. Vitamin C will potentiate the absorption of iron.
4. Iron is highly protein bound, so meals, especially of eggs, beans, or cereals will inhibit absorption. When iron is taken with food, absorption may be decreased by 1/3 to 1/2.

16. The psychiatrist has prescribed diazepam (Valium) for an outpatient. Which of the following should the nurse caution the client to avoid ingesting?

1. Diuretics.
2. Cheddar cheese.
3. Coffee.
4. Alcoholic beverages.

1. Wrong. This is not the correct substance. Diuretics are contraindicated for clients on lithium because they could potentially deplete their normal sodium level and increase the risk of toxicity. Look again at the other options to select the one specifically contraindicated for clients on Valium.

2. Wrong. This is not the correct substance. Cheddar cheese is contraindicated for clients on MAO inhibitors because it could cause a hypertensive crisis.
3. This is a possibility. Coffee would tend to increase the discomfort of an anxious client taking Valium, but it is not the best option. Read the other options to identify the one that is particularly unsafe for a person on Valium.
4. Correct. Drinking alcoholic beverages would potentiate the CNS depressant effects of Valium. This could produce extreme sedation and potentially lead to a lethal overdose.

17. The nurse knows that which of the following statements is inaccurate regarding benzodiazepine anti-anxiety drugs?

1. They may cause rebound insomnia if discontinued rapidly.
2. They are safer and more effective for insomnia than barbiturates.
3. They can be taken safely for one to two weeks.
4. They are used to treat sleep apnea.

1. No, a significant side effect of the benzodiazepines is the rebound insomnia that develops when the medication is withdrawn. Persons who have been taking these medications over several weeks should taper off their dose slowly. This is not the correct option because the stem is asking for an INACCURATE completion.
2. No. Benzodiazepines are safer and more effective than barbiturates, so this cannot be the correct option.
3. No. Benzodiazepines are effective in improving sleep for several weeks before tolerance develops, so this cannot be the correct option.
4. Yes, this is the inaccurate statement. Benzodiazepines are contraindicated in the treatment of sleep apnea, as they would further aggravate the central nervous system depression that exists in sleep apnea.

18. A client is receiving cyclophosphamide (Cytoxan) for treatment of her leukemia. The nurse has noticed that she vomited after each of her previous doses. To prevent vomiting, what should the nurse do?

1. Contact the physician for an antiemetic order prior to treatment.
2. Withhold fluids prior to and during treatments.
3. Suggest to the client that she eat before receiving her treatment.
4. Explain that vomiting cannot be prevented and provide the client with an emesis basin during treatments.

1. An excellent response. The nurse may be able to prevent nausea and vomiting with an antiemetic prior to treatments.

2. No. Fluids should not be withheld prior to or during treatments. It is important that clients stay well hydrated to prevent kidney damage.

3. Wrong. Eating before treatments would not solve the problem of vomiting. The client could possibly even aspirate on her vomitus.

4. Wrong choice! While the client may indeed need the emesis basin, the nurse may prevent vomiting by administering an antiemetic before administration of the medication.

19. The nurse knows that abrupt withdrawal of which of the following medications could be life-threatening?

1. Amitriptyline (Elavil).
2. Flurazepam (Dalmane).
3. Fluoxetine (Prozac).
4. Fluphenazine (Prolixin).

1. No, although tricyclic antidepressants, like Elavil, should be tapered off gradually over several weeks to avoid mild withdrawal symptoms and rebound depression. Abrupt withdrawal is not life-threatening.

*2. **Correct. Dalmane is a commonly used sedative-hypnotic in the benzodiazepine family. Abrupt withdrawal after long-term use leads to an abstinence syndrome with seizures. It can be life-threatening.***

3. Prozac is a non-tricyclic antidepressant. It should be tapered off gradually to avoid headache and other mild withdrawal symptoms but abrupt withdrawal is not life-threatening.

4. Prolixin is an antipsychotic drug. Abrupt withdrawal could lead to a return of psychotic symptoms but no other withdrawal syndrome.

20. A client has just returned to the unit after having major surgery and is complaining of pain. The physician has ordered morphine sulfate to control her pain. Before administering the medication, what should the nurse do first?

1. Discuss the side effects with the client.
2. Take the client's vital signs.
3. Provide mouth care.
4. Have the client turn, cough and deep breathe.

1. Clients do need to be informed of possible side effects; but the nurse should save teaching until the client is more alert.

*2. **Correct! Vital signs should be taken before administering morphine to provide a baseline for measuring respiratory depression, which can occur afterwards.***

3. Wrong. Mouth care will be needed postoperatively but it is not needed prior to morphine administration.

4. This is not the best choice! The client will be better able to cooperate when she has less pain, after the medication is administered.

21. The doctor has ordered ergonovine (Ergotrate) for a client. Which of the following conditions, if present, would warrant the nurse to use caution when administering the ergonovine?

1. Diabetes.
2. Pre-eclampsia.
3. Uterine atony.
4. Anemia.

1. Wrong. Ergotrate can be used without concern in the client with diabetes.

*2. **Yes, excellent choice! Ergotrate should be used with caution in the client with pre-eclampsia because of the high risk of increased blood pressure in an already hypertensive client.***

3. Wrong choice! Ergotrate is used to treat uterine atony, which is relaxation of the uterus following delivery.

4. Incorrect. Whether or not the client has anemia has no bearing on the administration of ergotrate.

22. The nurse knows that which of the following medications is often prescribed for treating the extrapyramidal side effects associated with antipsychotics?

1. Phenelzine (Nardil).
2. Bupropion (Wellbutrin).
3. Amantadine (Symmetrel).
4. Hydroxyzine (Atarax).

1. No, this medication is not correct. Nardil is an MAO inhibitor antidepressant. Read the other options to identify the medication used to treat EPS.

2. Not correct. Wellbutrin is one of the newer drugs for treating depression.

*3. **Correct. Amantadine (Symmetrel) is an antiparkinsonian drug used to treat extrapyramidal side effects.***

4. This option is not correct. Atarax is an antihistamine used to treat mild to moderate anxiety states.

23. A client, 83, is a widow with Alzheimer's disease. She has begun to strike out at staff members when they try to assist her to bed at night. In addition, the staff members report she is awake and restless most of the night. After further assessment, the nurse decides to contact the physician for a medication order. The nurse anticipates the physician will most likely order:

1. Diazepam (Valium) 10 mg p.r.n.
2. Hydroxyzine (Vistaril) 50 mg b.i.d.
3. Chlorpromazine (Thorazine) 10 mg t.i.d.
4. Haloperidol (Haldol) 2 mg hs.

1. *This is not a good choice. Valium is a long-acting anti-anxiety drug. It is not recommended for elderly clients, who may experience paradoxical responses, such as excitement and delirium. The elderly are also particularly sensitive to its side effects.*

2. *This is not a good choice. Vistaril, an antihistamine, is sometimes used as a mild anti-anxiety agent or sedative-hypnotic. It is not effective for agitated or combative behavior.*

3. *This is a possibility. Thorazine is a low potency antipsychotic that has highly sedative and anticholinergic properties. It would not be a good choice for an elderly lady with an organic mental disorder because of its side effects.*

4. ***Correct. Haldol is frequently prescribed, in low doses, for elderly clients to help control agitation and promote sleep.***

24. **Ampicillin (Omnipen) is dispensed in a preparation of 125 mg/5 mL. The orders are 100 mg/kg/day to be given every four hours. The client weighs 33 pounds. How many mL should the nurse administer for the 9:00 a.m. dose?**

    1. 15 mL.
    2. 10 mL.
    3. 2 mL.
    4. 22 mL.

    1. *No, this isn't right. Use four instead of six when dividing, after finding the total number of milligrams the client should receive in a 24-hour period. Remember, "every four hours" means the client will receive the drug six times each day.*

    2. ***Correct. This is how we did this problem: 33 lbs ÷ 2.2 kg/lb = 15 kg. Plug this into the equation 100 mg/15 kg/day, and you get 1500 mg/day. Then divide by the number of doses per day, which is 6: 1500 ÷ 6 = 250 mg/dose. Now D/H x Volume is 250 mg/125 mg x 5 mL = 10 mL.***

    3. *No! Did you remember to multiply by 5 mL at the very end?*

    4. *No, this isn't correct. Did you remember to convert to kilograms?*

25. **The nurse understands that naloxone (Narcan) is given to achieve which of the following actions?**

    1. To accentuate the effects of narcotics in a laboring woman.
    2. To depress the activity of the central nervous system (CNS) in the woman who received narcotics in labor.
    3. To block the effects of narcotics on the CNS in a woman in labor.

    4. To withdraw narcotics from the body of a laboring woman.

    1. *Incorrect. Narcan does not accentuate anything, it blocks the effects of narcotics.*

    2. *This is incorrect, since Narcan blocks the depressing effects of narcotics on the CNS, rather than depressing the CNS system itself.*

    3. ***Correct. By blocking the effects of narcotics on the CNS, it prevents CNS and respiratory depression in the neonate following delivery.***

    4. *This is a false statement. The word "withdraw" makes this answer incorrect. There is no way to remove narcotics from the body following administration. Narcan blocks the effects of narcotics.*

26. **The client is diabetic and has been prescribed cefonicid (Monocid). He regularly tests his urine for glucose. Which of the following instructions would be most appropriate for the nurse to give to a client before he starts the Monocid?**

    1. Use a second-voided urine specimen when testing for glucose using the Clinitest method.
    2. Have your physician adjust your insulin dosage to reflect the need for increased insulin during cephalosporin therapy.
    3. Use an alternate method of urine testing (Clinistix or Tes-Tape) while taking Monocid.
    4. Have the diabetic clinician teach you the use of a glucometer to test for capillary blood sugar while taking Monocid.

    1. *Incorrect. Recall that cephalosporins and penicillins may cause false positive reactions with copper sulfate urine glucose tests. A second-voided specimen will not alter this effect.*

    2. *Wrong. There should be no need for adjustment in insulin requirements while taking cephalosporins.*

    3. ***Excellent! Glucose enzymatic tests such as these two methods will not give false positive results to urine testing. Using an alternate urine testing method will require minimal adjustment on the client's part vs. learning to test capillary blood glucose levels.***

    4. *Not the best option. It's not necessary to have a client learn a new route/technique of glucose testing when he is already familiar with urine testing. The antibiotic therapy is not a permanent change.*

27. **A client, age 34, is admitted to the psychiatric unit with a diagnosis of generalized anxiety disorder. He tells the admitting nurse that he is a recovering alcoholic who has not had a drink in two years. He also requests that the nurse telephone his physician to ask for a "tranquilizer" because he is so restless and on edge. Which of the following will the psychiatrist most likely order?**

1. Chlordiazepoxide (Librium).
2. Lorazepam (Ativan).
3. Hydroxyzine (Vistaril).
4. Oxazepam (Serax).

1. *This is not correct. Librium is a benzodiazepine anti-anxiety agent. It is used to medically withdraw persons from alcohol because it is a central nervous system depressant that is cross-tolerant with alcohol. Because Librium is associated with both tolerance and physical dependence, it is not an appropriate medication for the client.*
2. *Wrong. Ativan is a benzodiazepine anti-anxiety agent that is associated with tolerance and physical dependence. It is not the correct option for a person with a history of substance abuse.*
3. **Correct. Vistaril is an antihistamine that is used as an anti-anxiety agent. It is an appropriate choice for someone with a history of substance abuse because it is less likely than other classes of anti-anxiety agents to lead to tolerance and physical dependence.**
4. *Serax is a benzodiazepine anti-anxiety agent that is associated with tolerance and physical dependence. It is not the best option for a person with a history of substance abuse.*

28. **A client is to receive intravenous antibiotics. Which of the following is the priority nursing action when preparing to administer this medication?**

1. Determine if the client has any allergies.
2. Determine the route of administration.
3. Check the client's name band.
4. Check the dosage against the physician's order.

1. **Excellent choice! An allergy to an antibiotic can cause serious side effects. This is the priority nursing action, since the safety of the client is the issue. This option assesses before implementing.**
2. *The physician or pharmacist determines the route of administration, while the nurse implements the order. If there is a question about the route, the nurse needs to clarify the order.*
3. *The client's name band should be checked before administering any medication. However, the priority nursing action is to note any allergies before administering any medication, especially antibiotics. If the client has an allergy that contraindicates giving the antibiotic, the nurse will not be administering the medication.*
4. *Determining that the dose is correct is a nursing standard for medication preparation. However, if the client is allergic to the medication, the nurse need not prepare it. Notifying the physician of this fact is the next step and the priority nursing action.*

29. **The nurse is caring for a diabetic client, who is currently taking cephalexin (Keflex). The nurse should advise the client of which of the following?**

1. Clinitest or copper sulfate urine glucose tests give false positive results.
2. Blood sugar may drop without warning.
3. A source of sugar should always be carried with the client.
4. A medic alert bracelet should always be worn.

1. **This statement is correct! Clients should use glucometers, or glucose enzymatic tests like Clinistix, which are much more reliable tests than Clinitest or copper sulfate urine glucose tests.**
2. *This is not correct. This reaction is not caused by antibiotics.*
3. *This is not the answer. This statement is true for all diabetics, regardless of being on medications. The correct answer will relate specifically to the effect of cephalexin on diabetics.*
4. *All diabetics should wear a medic alert bracelet. However, this does not address the client's need for advice on how cephalexin will affect him.*

30. **A client is highly allergic to penicillin, but in need of a therapeutic plan of care. In carrying out the therapeutic plan of care for a client, the nurse is aware that which of the following antibiotics would be safe to administer?**

1. Ampicillin (Omnipen).
2. Cefazolin (Ancef).
3. Erythromycin ethylsuccinate (E.E.S.).
4. Moxalactam (Moxam).

1. *Incorrect. This drug belongs to the penicillin family and would be contraindicated for a client with known hypersensitivity. NOTE: The generic names of all penicillins end in "-cillin."*
2. *No, recall that cefazolin belongs to the cephalosporin family and that there is a possibility of cross-sensitivity (cephalosporins are chemical modifications of the penicillin structure).*
3. **Good choice! You remembered that macrolides are prescribed for clients who are allergic to penicillin. The most important antimicrobial agent in that group is erythromycin.**
4. *Not correct. Moxam is a member of the cephalosporin family and should not be used (or should be used with caution) for penicillin-sensitive clients since cross-sensitivity may occur.*

31. **It is the beginning of summer, and a 14-year-old client is taking minocycline (Minocin) for her acne. What advice should the nurse give the client?**

1. Take the medication on an empty stomach with a glass of water.

2.   Minocin makes the skin photosensitive, so shield your skin from the sun and use a sun screen.
3.   Stay inside, as this medication will react with the sun.
4.   Take this drug at night before bedtime.

1.   While this is true of almost all of the tetracyclines, Minocin was developed to be taken with meals.

2.   You chose the correct answer! All the tetracyclines cause photosensitivity and Minocin is no exception. Clients should stay out of the sun or at least use a sun screen. Good answer!

3.   Wrong! It would be inadvisable to suggest that a 14-year-old stay inside during the summer. Look for a better option.

4.   Wrong! The drug must be taken at intervals around the clock to be effective.

32. **A six-month-old client has been prescribed erythromycin ethylsuccinate (Pediamycin) for an infection. Of what instruction should the nurse remind the client's mother before she gives this medication?**

1.   Mix the medication in the client's formula.
2.   Be sure to keep the medication refrigerated and to shake it well before giving to the client.
3.   Keep the medication near the client's bed as a reminder to give it to him around the clock.
4.   This medication should be mixed in the client's baby food and given at each meal.

1.   Mixing medications in formula is not advisable and is not good practice. If the client does not take his entire bottle, much of the medication will be wasted. Also, this question does not indicate whether the client is bottle fed or breast fed.

2.   Correct, you remembered that this medication comes in a suspension that needs to be refrigerated and shaken well before administration.

3.   Keeping medication near the baby's bed is not a safe practice for any medication. This drug must be refrigerated.

4.   No, mixing medication in food would decrease its absorption. It is also not good practice to mix medications with food.

33. **In order to monitor for toxicity of aminoglycosides, what test does the nurse expect might be done to measure the drug level in the blood?**

1.   Blood urea nitrogen (BUN) and creatinine clearance.
2.   Peak and trough drug levels.
3.   Hematocrit and hemoglobin levels.
4.   Liver function studies.

1.   No. BUN and creatinine clearance monitor the renal function. They can tell if renal function is

getting too low, which would prevent elimination of the drugs from the body.

2.   Correct. The peak and trough tell the highest and lowest concentrations of the drug in the body. The trough is very sensitive—if the lowest concentration of the drug in the body is at a high level, then the drug will become toxic and cause damage.

3.   Wrong. Hematocrit and hemoglobin levels are useful to know, but they do not monitor the blood level of an aminoglycoside.

4.   Liver function studies will monitor the level of liver enzymes, not the level of an aminoglycoside in the body.

34. **While on warfarin (Coumadin), the nurse will expect that the client will be monitored by which blood test?**

1.   APTT (activated partial thromboplastin time).
2.   Lee White clotting time.
3.   Platelet counts.
4.   PT (prothrombin time).

1.   No, this lab test monitors the action of heparin.

2.   No, this is an older screening test used to check on many clotting factors.

3.   Incorrect. Coumadin does not affect the platelets.

4.   Correct. PT time is the correct test for monitoring coumadin use.

35. **It is expected that the client will be on narcotics for four to five days after surgery. What precautions should the nurse take with the client to prevent complications?**

1.   Provide bed rest for the first two to three days.
2.   Put the side rails up and items the client is likely to need, such as the client's water and cigarettes, close to her bed and within her reach.
3.   Encourage the client to call for help to ambulate.
4.   Suggest that the client limit the use of her medications, as addiction may result.

1.   This is incorrect. This is much too long to be on bed rest.

2.   Wrong! The client should not be smoking at all; if allowed, someone should be with her, since she is using narcotics.

3.   Correct! Hypotension can occur, and she should have help with ambulating to prevent falling.

4.   This is incorrect. Fewer than one percent of clients become addicted to narcotics used after surgery for pain.

36. **The nurse is caring for a client with a myocardial infarction who is taking chlorothiazide (Diuril) and digoxin (Lanoxin). Which diet would be most appropriate to be included in the nursing care?**

1. Diet low in sodium and saturated fats, high in potassium.
2. Diet low in unsaturated fats, sodium and potassium.
3. Diet high in potassium, Vitamin C and protein.
4. Diet low in sodium and saturated and unsaturated fats.

1. *Good choice! Sodium would be restricted to decrease the circulating blood volume and reduce the cardiac workload. Saturated fats would be decreased to prevent further atherosclerotic heart disease. Potassium should be increased in his diet because Diuril causes the excretion of potassium in the urine. It is vital to keep potassium within the normal limits because a low potassium level may lead to arrhythmias in a client who is taking digoxin.*
2. *Incorrect! Both saturated and unsaturated fats are restricted in a weight reduction diet. However, we have no information that this client needed to be placed on a weight reduction diet. Also, due to the drugs, loss of potassium can present a problem. Supplements of potassium are needed to prevent cardiac arrhythmias.*
3. *Incorrect. A diet high in potassium is needed because of the loss of potassium due to digoxin and Diuril. There is no reason for increasing Vitamin C or protein.*
4. *Both saturated and unsaturated fats are restricted in a weight reduction diet. However, we have no information that this client needed to be placed on a weight reduction diet. Also, due to the drugs, loss of potassium can present a problem. Supplements of potassium are needed to prevent cardiac arrhythmias. Note that Option 2 also includes low unsaturated fats — both of these options are incorrect.*

37. **A client, age 22, is admitted with a diagnosis of acute psychotic reaction, r/o schizophrenia. Because the client is very agitated, he is started on chlorpromazine (Thorazine) 100 mg, t.i.d. After three days, he is much calmer and his nurse begins to teach him about his medication. Which one of the following statements about his medication is most accurate?**

1. "This medication is a sedative to calm you down."
2. "This medication acts on the chemical regulators in your brain to help control your symptoms."
3. "This medication will cure your disorder."
4. "We do not know how this medication works, but we do know it will help you control your behavior."

1. *Wrong. Antipsychotic medications, like Thorazine, may calm an agitated client, but they are not sedatives. They also control other symptoms of psychosis, such as delusions and other thought disturbances.*

2. *Excellent! Antipsychotic medications are thought to act directly on the dopamine receptors in the brain to prevent the re-uptake of dopamine and thereby control psychotic symptoms.*
3. *No, antipsychotics control symptoms but do not cure the psychotic disorder.*
4. *This is not completely accurate. We do not know the exact mechanisms of action, but research has provided some information about how these drugs work. Antipsychotics block dopamine receptors in the brain, thereby controlling the target symptoms of psychosis.*

38. **A new diabetic client requires daily injections of insulin. Which of the following would indicate to the nurse that the client may have an inaccurate understanding concerning the administration of his injections?**

1. The client states that he will change injection sites.
2. The client tells the nurse that he needs to buy some alcohol.
3. The client tells the nurse that his brother also is a diabetic and that he will be able to share all of the supplies with him.
4. The client tells the nurse that his wife will be giving him the injections.

1. *Wrong choice, because daily injections will require rotation of the sites to insure absorption and prevent complications that can result from overuse of an injection site.*
2. *This statement indicates that the client understands that alcohol is needed for disinfection.*
3. *Correct choice! This option indicates that the nurse needs further clarification to be sure that the client is not planning to share needles with his brother. Needles are disposable and not to be reused by anyone. This evaluation question has a false response stem. This statement by the client does not indicate an understanding by the client of how to care for his health problem.*
4. *Although this should be a concern for the nurse, it does not address the issue in the question, which concerns the client's understanding of injection technique.*

39. **A newly diagnosed diabetic who also has adult primary open-angle glaucoma is admitted for regulation of his blood sugars. The client receives pilocarpine (Pilocar) 2% one drop q.i.d. to the OD. Instillation of this drug requires which of the following actions by the nurse?**

1. Asking the client to look straight ahead.
2. Pressing on the lacrimal sac for one minute after instillation.
3. Instructing the client to squeeze his eye shut after instillation.

4. Cleansing the eye first, then wiping from the outer to the inner canthus.

1. *Incorrect. When instilling eye drops, the client is instructed to look upward since they are less likely to blink in this position.*
2. **Correct. This prevents the medication from running out of the eye and down the duct.**
3. *Incorrect. Squeezing can injure the eye and push out the medication. The client should be instructed to close the eyelids but not to squeeze them shut.*
4. *Incorrect. The eye should be wiped from the inner to the outer canthus cleaning toward the inner canthus. Wiping from the outer to the inner canthus would cause contamination of the lacrimal duct and possibly the other eye.*

40. **Which of the following diagnostic studies can the nurse anticipate will be completed regularly for a client taking isoniazid (INH)?**

    1. AST, ALT.
    2. WBC count.
    3. Bone marrow aspirations.
    4. Creatinine & BUN.

    1. **Good choice!! AST (SGOT) and ALT (SGPT) are studies of liver function. These enzymes are used to monitor the effects of INH that might be toxic to the liver and should be monitored before drug therapy is started and at least monthly during the course of therapy.**
    2. *No. The WBC would not be monitored separately to assess for complications from INH therapy.*
    3. *Incorrect. Although aplastic anemia can result from INH therapy, it is not common. A complete blood count would be a more effective screening tool than invasive (and painful) bone marrow aspirations.*
    4. *Not a correct option. INH is not considered to be a nephrotoxic agent; therefore, kidney function studies would not be indicated.*

41. **The client is an infant who weighs 8.6 kilograms. The caloric requirement for this client is 120 cal/kg/24 hours. The formula prescribed has 20 calories in two ounces. How many mL of formula does the nurse understand that the infant needs in a 24-hour period?**

    1. 1032 mL.
    2. 3096 mL.
    3. 103 mL.
    4. 1548 mL.

    1. *Incorrect.*
    2. *Terrific! You did all the steps: 120 cal x 8.6 kg = 1032 cal/day, then D/H x Volume is expressed 1032/20 x 60 mL = 3096 mL.*
    3. *Incorrect. Remember to convert the two ounces to mL.*

4. *Wrong. Did you use the two ounces at the end of the calculation, or did you guess?*

42. **A client has been receiving ritodrine therapy for the last 24 hours to stop her premature labor. The attempts are unsuccessful and she delivers an infant at 31 weeks gestation. In assessing the neonate, which of the following should the nurse anticipate as a result of the ritodrine (Yutopar) therapy?**

    1. Hypoglycemia.
    2. Hypothermia.
    3. Respiratory distress.
    4. Hypertension.

    1. **Correct. Ritodrine causes maternal hyperglycemia when the mother has high blood sugar just prior to delivery. The neonate is at high risk for hypoglycemia.**
    2. *Wrong! Ritodrine has no effect on newborn body temperature.*
    3. *Wrong. It has been suggested that ritodrine therapy may decrease neonate respiratory distress rather than increase the risk. Any stress stimulates surfactant production, thus reducing the risk of RDS. Ritodrine therapy may be a stressor.*
    4. *Wrong. Ritodrine therapy may be related to newborn hypotension but not hypertension.*

43. **A 42-year-old client is being treated for congestive heart failure. Included in his orders is a prescription for furosemide (Lasix) 20 mg p.o. daily. The nurse administering this drug should be alert for which of the following complications?**

    1. Fluid and electrolyte imbalances.
    2. Decreased potassium excretion.
    3. Increased serum calcium level.
    4. Shift of fluid into the cells.

    1. **Yes! You are correct! Lasix is a potent loop diuretic that can cause rapid changes in fluid and electrolyte balances. Note that this option is also more global and the others are more specific.**
    2. *This is incorrect. With Lasix, potassium excretion is increased and may lead to hypokalemia. Increased intake of potassium in the diet is required to maintain potassium balance.*
    3. *This is incorrect. Lasix causes increased calcium excretion, which may lead to a decreased serum calcium level.*
    4. *This is incorrect. Lasix is a potent loop diuretic that will cause a loss of fluid in the urine and eventually may cause dehydration, not a shift of fluid into the cells.*

44. A woman is in ICU following a cesarean section, complicated with severe PIH and magnesium intoxication, as a result of prolonged magnesium sulfate therapy. She received an IV bolus of calcium gluconate to treat the hypermagnesemia. The nurse should understand that the side effects of calcium gluconate include which of the following?

1. Hypertension.
2. Tachycardia.
3. Arrhythmia.
4. Pulmonary edema.

1. No, hypotension, rather than hypertension, is a side effect of calcium gluconate.
2. No, bradycardia, not tachycardia, is a side effect of calcium gluconate.
3. That's right! Arrhythmias are a side effect of calcium gluconate. Therefore, careful monitoring of the EKG needs to be done for a client who receives calcium gluconate.
4. No, pulmonary edema is not an expected side effect of calcium gluconate administration.

45. All of the following are major side effects that the nurse might anticipate observing in the client receiving antiparkinsonian drugs except:

1. Blurred vision, mental confusion, dry mouth and constipation.
2. Orthostatic hypotension, palpitations and tremors.
3. Insomnia, sedation and constipation.
4. Occipital headache, neck stiffness, nausea and vomiting.

1. Correct. The side effects of antiparkinsonian drugs result from their anticholinergic properties. Antidepressants and antipsychotics also have these side effects, in addition to others.
2. Incorrect. These are the side effects commonly seen with tricyclic antidepressants. Read the options to identify the side effects for antiparkinsonian drugs.
3. These are the side effects of MAO inhibitor antidepressants, so this cannot be the answer.
4. No, try again. These are symptoms of hypertensive crisis, a serious adverse effect of MAOIs.

46. The nurse understands that which of the following would not be included in the care of a client with an aspirin overdose?

1. Gastric lavage or emesis.
2. Administration of activated charcoal.
3. Increasing the acidity of the urine.
4. Hemodialysis or peritoneal dialysis.

1. No, emesis or lavage is recommended. The question is looking for an inappropriate action.

2. Not the correct answer. Charcoal will absorb the aspirin. This question has a false response stem and it is looking for an inappropriate action.
3. Good! This is the inappropriate action. Aspirin is excreted more rapidly by the kidney in an alkaline medium. This is achieved by giving acetazolamide (Diamox) and an alkaline IV solution containing sodium bicarbonate.
4. No, either hemodialysis or peritoneal dialysis may be necessary in a severe overdose. This question has a false response stem and is looking for an inappropriate action.

47. A pregnant client has a severe iron deficiency anemia. The physician orders an injection of iron dextran (Imferon) IM. How should the nurse plan to administer the injection?

1. Use a size 23-25 gauge needle and administer it in the deltoid muscle.
2. Use a size 20 or 22 gauge needle and administer it deep in the thigh.
3. Select a 19-20 gauge needle and administer using the Z track method.
4. Select an 18 gauge needle and give deep in the buttocks.

1. Wrong. Review your needle sizes. A 23-25 gauge is very small, and would not be suitable for iron, as iron is thicker than this gauge allows. Remember, too, that iron must be given deep into the muscle, and a 23-25 gauge needle is short. In addition, iron is never given in the deltoid, only the buttocks, as this is a larger muscle mass.
2. Wrong choice. Please review your needle sizes; a 20-22 gauge is too small for iron injections. Iron must be given in the buttocks—not the thigh.
3. Correct. Iron must be given in the Z track method to prevent staining of tissue. A 19-20 gauge needle is the correct size. It should be at least two inches long.
4. Incorrect. An 18 gauge needle is not the correct size—this is too large. You also need to remember that iron has to be given by the Z track method into the buttocks.

48. The nurse should advise a client taking rifampin (Rifadin) for treatment of TB to avoid which of the following?

1. Antacids containing magnesium.
2. Aspirin products.
3. OTC cold products.
4. Alcoholic beverages.

1. Incorrect. Rifadin should be taken on an empty stomach, but if GI irritation occurs, the client may need to take the drug with food or an antacid.
2. No. There is no contraindication for taking aspirin products while the client is on Rifadin.

3.   *Incorrect choice. Clients may take OTC cold prepa-rations if necessary.*

4.   *Good choice!! Clients should be advised to avoid alcoholic beverages while taking Rifadin because alcohol may increase the risk of hepatotoxicity and increase the rate of Rifadin metabolism. Dosage adjustment may be necessary.*

49.   **A client is being treated for gastrointestinal bleed-ing. The client tells the nurse that he slept very well after taking temazepam (Restoril) and asks if he can continue to take Restoril at home be-cause he suffers from chronic insomnia. Which of the following considerations are important for the nurse to make the best response?**

1.   He may not need a sleep medication after his gas-trointestinal bleeding is treated in the hospital.
2.   He would benefit more by seeking other methods of relieving his chronic insomnia.
3.   It is too soon to be concerned with his discharge plans.
4.   This could be a good plan for the client's insomnia, since he responded well to the Restoril while in the hospital.

1.   *Wrong. The client reported that he suffered from chronic insomnia, so this cannot be the correct option because his sleep problems are apparently unrelated to his gastrointestinal bleeding.*

2.   *Correct. The nurse should instruct the client that Restoril, and other benzodiazepines, can only be taken for short periods of time because prolonged use leads to tolerance and dependency. An assess-ment should be done to identify the cause of the client's insomnia and other approaches to its man-agement recommended.*

3.   *This is not correct. The nurse should capitalize on every opportunity to provide client education. Also, discharge planning is an ongoing process for ev-ery hospitalized client.*

4.   *This is not correct. Prolonged use of benzodiaz-epines, such as Restoril, for problems sleeping can lead to tolerance and physical dependency.*

50.   **A client, age 54, is hospitalized for gastrointesti-nal bleeding. He is given temazepam (Restoril) at bedtime to help him sleep. What nursing action is indicted immediately following his dose?**

1.   Raise the side rails on his bed and tell him to use his call light to summon the nurse if he has to get up during the night.
2.   Keep a padded tongue blade at the bedside and observe for seizures.
3.   Monitor his blood pressure and respirations.
4.   Observe and record his sleep patterns.

1.   *Correct. Restoril is a benzodiazepine that is often prescribed to induce sleep. Ataxia and dizziness are common side effects. The bed rails of a hospi-talized client should be raised and instructions given to call for assistance before getting up dur-ing the night to prevent falling and the risk of injuries.*

2.   *This is not correct. Seizures are associated with withdrawal from prolonged use of high doses of benzodiazepines. They are not a side effect of Restoril when taken for nighttime sedation on a short-term basis.*

3.   *This is not correct. Depressed blood pressure and respirations are associated with intravenous ad-ministration of benzodiazepines, such as Valium, which may be given IV to manage delirium tre-mens (Dts).*

4.   *This is not correct. The nurse should observe and record his sleep patterns, but this is not an immedi-ate action.*

51.   **A client receives haloperidol (Haldol) 5 mg t.i.d. Several days into treatment, the nurse notices that the client is walking stiffly with a shuffling gait. What nursing action is indicated at this time?**

1.   Take her blood pressure before her next dose.
2.   Withhold the Haldol until the symptom disappears.
3.   Chart her observations on the client's record.
4.   Obtain an order for an antiparkinsonian drug.

1.   *This would be correct if the client were experiencing postural hypotension. It is not the correct option for the symptom of a shuffling gait.*

2.   *This option would only be appropriate for unusu-ally severe extrapyramidal side effects. There is a better option.*

3.   *The nurse should chart the observations, but this action would not help the client who is experiencing extrapyramidal side effects.*

4.   *Correct. The client is experiencing parkinsonian side effects to the Haldol. The nurse should ob-tain an order from the psychiatrist for an antiparkinsonian drug to counter these side ef-fects.*

52.   **The physician has changed a client's antihyper-tensive medication from hydralazine (Apresoline) to metoprolol (Lopressor). The nurse understands that this change would mean the client is less likely to experience:**

1.   Reflex tachycardia.
2.   Hypotension.
3.   Sodium retention.
4.   Dizziness.

1. *Correct choice! Apresoline can trigger reflex stimulation of the heart, thereby causing cardiac work and myocardial oxygen demand to increase. Reflex tachycardia can be prevented with a beta-blocker such as metoprolol (Lopressor).*

2. *Wrong. Metoprolol, a beta-adrenergic blocker, will decrease the blood pressure as an expected side effect of the drug's action. Recall that this drug can be used alone or in combination with other agents in the treatment of hypertension and angina pectoris.*

3. *Incorrect. Edema is just as much a concern when the client takes Lopressor as when the client takes Apresoline. Clients should be assessed routinely for evidence of congestive heart failure: peripheral edema, dyspnea, rales/crackles, fatigue, weight gain, and jugular venous distention.*

4. *No. Dizziness is a side effect of both medications. The client should be cautioned to avoid sudden changes in position to minimize orthostatic hypotension, which can cause dizziness and lightheadedness.*

53. **The nurse must correctly calculate the daily dosage of a new medication for a child weighing 69 pounds. The physician has ordered 10 mcg/kg/day in three divided doses. The nurse has on hand 0.1 mg tablets. What is the daily dosage in milligrams?**

    1. 10.45 mg.
    2. 0.69 mg.
    3. 3.1 mg.
    4. 0.31 mg.

    1. *Incorrect. Were you distracted by the "three divided doses?" Go back and look at the question again.*
    2. *Incorrect. Did you convert the pounds to kilograms?*
    3. *Wrong placement of the decimal. Did you forget how many micrograms in a milligram? Try to correct your answer.*
    4. *Correct. Convert pounds to kilograms: 69 lbs ÷ 2.2 lb/ kg = 31.363 kg. Plug this into the equation: 10 mcg/31.363 kg/day = 313.63 mcg/day. To convert mcg to mg, divide by 1000: 313.63 mcg ÷ 1000 mcg/mg = .31 mg.*

54. **A client is hospitalized for gastrointestinal bleeding and is being treated with temazepam (Restoril). After the client's physician examined him, the nurse noted the physician had written an order for the client to begin taking amitriptyline (Elavil). Which of the following actions would be best initially by the nurse?**

    1. Revise his medication schedule so that Elavil is administered during the day and the Restoril hs.

    2. Monitor the client's vital signs closely.
    3. Question the physician about administering both Elavil and Ativan to the client.
    4. Assess the client for signs and symptoms of depression.

    1. *This is not correct. Elavil is a tricyclic anti-depressant that is very sedating. It is often chosen for depressed clients who also have difficulty sleeping. There is a better option.*
    2. *This is not the best option. The client's vital signs should be monitored when he is placed on Elavil because it may cause orthostatic hypotension. Review the choices to select a better one.*
    3. *Correct. Benzodiazepines, such as Restoril, potentiate the effects of other central nervous system depressants, such as the tricyclic, Elavil. The nurse should contact the physician to question the safety of administering these two medications to the client.*
    4. *This is an appropriate nursing action, but it is not the best initial action.*

55. **A client is seen in the antepartum testing unit for a contraction stress test. Which of the following oxytocic drugs will be used to complete this test?**

    1. Ergotamine (Ergomar).
    2. Methylergonovine (Methergine).
    3. Ergonovine (Ergotrate).
    4. Oxytocin (Pitocin).

    1. *No, look again! Ergotamine is a drug to treat migraine headaches and has no effect on uterine activity.*
    2. *No! Remember Methergine is never given to an antepartum client.*
    3. *No! Ergotrate, like Methergine, is never administered to a client prior to the 4th stage of labor.*
    4. *Excellent choice! Pitocin is the only oxytocic drug that may be safely administered to an antepartum woman.*

56. **A client is receiving methotrexate (Mexate) for his lung cancer. When he returns to the clinic he reports that his gums are beginning to bleed. What action should the nurse take?**

    1. Tell the client that bleeding gums is perfectly normal.
    2. Tell the client not to brush his teeth for a few days.
    3. Consult with his doctor and have the lab draw blood work, especially platelets.
    4. Have the client call his dentist.

    1. *Not the best choice! It would be unwise to tell the client not to worry. Bleeding is a side effect of methotrexate.*

2. *Wrong, having the client avoid brushing will not solve the problem of his bleeding gums.*

3. *Correct. You remembered that antineoplastic medications suppress the bone marrow and can decrease platelets.*

4. *Wrong! While he may need to see his dentist on a regular basis, the bleeding is due to the side effect of the medication and needs to be evaluated by the oncologist or the doctor treating the cancer.*

57. **A blood transfusion using packed cells (250 mL) is ordered to be infused in four hours. The blood set delivers 10 gtt/mL. The nurse calculates the proper drip rate of the unit of packed cells as:**

1. 42 gtts/min.
2. 63 gtts/min.
3. 10 gtts/min.
4. 16 gtts/min.

1. *Wrong choice. Hint—the blood is to take four hours to infuse.*

2. *Not right. Reread the question and try this calculation again, setting it up with total drops divided by total minutes.*

3. *Great! Here's how the math works: 250 mL x 10 gtt/min divided by 4 hr x 60 min = 2500 total drops divided by 240 total minutes = 10 gtts/min.*

4. *No, look at the information given in the stem: 10 drops = 1 mL.*

58. **A client has been taking isoniazid (INH) and rifampin (Rifadin) for three weeks after being diagnosed with TB. He calls the Health Clinic and tells the nurse that he has noted a reddish-orange color to his urine. Which of the following statements by the nurse would be the most accurate response?**

1. "I'll make an appointment for you to see the doctor this afternoon. You may have developed a bleeding problem, which is not uncommon with these drugs."

2. "The reddish color is a side effect of the INH. Stop taking it for two to three days and the discoloration should go away. The doctor may want to change your drug therapy."

3. "The discoloration is due to rifampin. It may turn all body fluids orange-red. This is a harmless side effect."

4. "You should increase your fluid intake while on these medications. They are known to cause bladder irritation when taken together."

1. *Not correct. Although thrombocytopenia may occur when taking these medications, it is not a common adverse reaction.*

2. *No, the reddish discoloration is not due to INH. Clients should never be instructed to periodically stop taking their medications.*

3. *Good choice. Rifampin will turn body fluids such as tears, sweat, saliva and urine an orange-red color. Advise the client of possible permanent stains on clothes and soft contact lenses.*

4. *No, these drugs are not considered to be bladder irritants. They are, however, potentially hepatotoxic agents.*

59. **A two-year-old client has been receiving bleomycin (Blenoxane) IV for treatment of his Wilm's tumor. The next dose is due at 2:00 pm. What must the nurse do before hanging the medication?**

1. Change the client's diaper.
2. Be sure the IV is patent.
3. Talk to the client's mother about all the possible side effects of the drug.
4. Be sure the client has had his lunch.

1. *Wrong. The nurse may need to change the diaper, but this is not a priority action before hanging a toxic antineoplastic agent. The nurse does need to keep track of intake and output, but can do so at intervals during the day.*

2. *Correct. Being sure the needle is in the vein is a must before hanging this medication, since tissue damage will occur if the medication gets into the tissues.*

3. *Wrong. The client's mother should have had some instruction about the medication before the course of treatment. She may need reminders, but it should not be necessary for her to know all the possible side effects before each dose.*

4. *Incorrect. Nausea and vomiting are common side effects of bleomycin. It would be more appropriate to administer an antiemetic before administration, not lunch.*

60. **A physician prescribes para-aminosalicylic acid (PAS) for a client who has been diagnosed with tuberculosis. To decrease the GI symptoms of nausea/vomiting associated with PAS, the nurse should instruct the client to do which of the following?**

1. Take the medication at bedtime.
2. Have the physician prescribe an antiemetic to be taken 30 minutes before the PAS.
3. Take the medication with food or an antacid.
4. Crush the tablets and dissolve them completely in water before swallowing.

1. *Incorrect. The normal dosage of PAS is 10-12 grams daily in three or four doses. It could not be taken all at one time.*

2. *Wrong. There should not be a need for this intervention. If the nausea/vomiting is that severe, a change in medication therapy would be indicated.*

There is another option that would help decrease the side effects without the use of additional drugs.

3. *Correct! Nearly all clients taking PAS report GI irritation of one form or another. Taking the drug with food or an antacid prevents some but not all of the irritation produced by the drug therapy.*

4. *No. This intervention, although perfectly acceptable, will not decrease the GI symptoms. PAS is not well tolerated by most clients, but there is an intervention that will help decrease the severity of the nausea/vomiting.*

61. **A client is diagnosed with active tuberculosis and is started on a treatment regimen of isoniazid (INH) and ethambutol (Myambutol). Which of the following signs/symptoms reported by the client would necessitate the discontinuation of ethambutol?**

    1. Anorexia, nausea/vomiting.
    2. Loss of color discrimination.
    3. Edema of feet and hands.
    4. Red-orange discoloration to all body fluids.

    1. *Incorrect. These side effects are not common when a client is taking ethambutol, which is well absorbed from the GI tract in either the presence or absence of food.*

    2. *Correct!! The most commonly reported toxic reaction to normal therapeutic doses of ethambutol is indeed visual disturbance. Examples include changes of color vision (especially red and green) and loss of visual acuity. These signs are cause to terminate ethambutol use.*

    3. *No, this side effect is not related to ethambutol therapy.*

    4. *This is not related to ethambutol therapy. Recall that discoloration of body fluids is a side effect of rifampin and is harmless.*

62. **A hospitalized six-month-old, whose mother brings in expressed breast milk, took two ounces of breast milk at 8:00 a.m., three ounces at 11:00 a.m. and two and one-half ounces at 1:00 p.m. What should the nurse record on this client's intake record for the shift?**

    1. 150 mL.
    2. 225 mL.
    3. 240 mL.
    4. 375 mL.

    1. *No, that's not right. Check your work.*
    2. *Right, this was an easy one for you! Multiply the total ounces by 30 mL per oz: 7.5 x 30 = 225 mL.*
    3. *No, you made an error. Try this again.*
    4. *Incorrect, try the math again.*

63. **A client is taking erythromycin delayed-release capsules (Eryc) for a urinary tract infection. By the fourth day of a 10-day treatment, he tells the nurse he's fine now and will keep the remainder of his medicine for another infection. Which of the following is the most therapeutic response by the nurse?**

    1. "Good idea, you will save lots of money that way."
    2. "You should always take the full course of antibiotics because it is still possible for many of the bacteria to be in your urinary tract."
    3. "Take at least one more day of medication."
    4. "That would really be a stupid thing to do."

    1. *Although saving money is of interest, if the client only takes a few days of the medication, the bacteria that are left only become sensitized to the antibiotic and may become resistant. When the bacteria start to grow again, the client will need more potent and expensive medications to treat his infection.*

    2. *This is the correct response. It is important to take the full course of medications unless there are untoward effects like severe diarrhea, or sensitivity reactions. Medications should not be shared or saved.*

    3. *Wrong! Taking the medication for one more day would still cause bacterial resistance to develop and would not be beneficial.*

    4. *No! This would not be a professional statement.*

64. **A client is receiving magnesium sulfate as treatment for pregnancy induced hypertension. Which of the following assessments would warrant turning off the magnesium sulfate IV drip?**

    1. Respirations 16/minute.
    2. Urinary output 100 mL in five hours.
    3. Reflexes depressed +1.
    4. Fetal heart rate 158, decreased variability.

    1. *No! This is an expected respiratory rate for a client receiving magnesium sulfate. Some references suggest allowing respirations to go as low as 14/minute but all references agree that 16 or above is acceptable for the client with magnesium sulfate.*

    2. *Correct. Urinary output is critical to the excretion of magnesium from the system. References suggest discontinuing the magnesium sulfate when the hourly output is less than 25-30 mL per hour. 100 mL in five hours is only 20 mL per hour; therefore, the magnesium sulfate IV should be discontinued immediately.*

    3. *Not correct! Reflexes are normally +2. In a client receiving magnesium sulfate it is expected that there will be hyporeflexia. It is acceptable to continue the medication.*

    4. *No! A fetal heart rate of 158 is within normal range and the decrease in variability is an expected response to the magnesium sulfate.*

65. **The nurse understands that which of the following are common side effects of benzodiazepine anti-anxiety medications?**

   1. Insomnia.
   2. Headache.
   3. Confusion.
   4. Dizziness.

   1. *Insomnia is a paradoxical reaction to these drugs, not a common side effect. Other symptoms of paradoxical excitement are increased anxiety, racing thoughts, increased energy and impulsiveness.*
   2. *Headache is a rare side effect. It is usually treated with a mild analgesic.*
   3. *Confusion is a rare side effect. It is usually treated by lowering the dose of the medication.*
   4. **Correct. *Dizziness is a common side effect. Other common side effects are drowsiness and sedation.***

66. **On the third day of amoxicillin (Amoxil) therapy, a client develops diarrhea. The nurse should instruct the client to do which of the following?**

   1. Stop taking the drug as this is an indication of toxicity.
   2. Contact her physician about treatment of the diarrhea.
   3. Drink extra liquids to compensate for the fluid lost in the diarrhea.
   4. Take an over-the-counter antidiarrheal agent according to package directions.

   1. *Incorrect choice. Diarrhea is an adverse reaction to Amoxil and not a toxic reaction. It's not an indication to stop taking the medication.*
   2. **Correct. *Diarrhea is often an adverse GI reaction to amoxicillin therapy. It is advisable to contact the physician before adding any new drug to a treatment regimen, including over-the-counter (OTC) antidiarrheal agents.***
   3. *Although drinking extra fluids is appropriate to prevent fluid volume deficit, the client needs intervention to control diarrhea and to prevent electrolyte depletion (especially potassium).*
   4. *This is not sound judgment on the nurse's part. Clients should be cautioned about taking over-the-counter (OTC) drugs without notifying their primary care giver. NOTE: Only OTC drugs with kaolin or attapulgite should be used to control the diarrhea.*

67. **The client is receiving propranolol (Inderal) for anxiety. In reviewing the client's discharge plans, the nurse needs to emphasize which of the following?**

   1. Inderal should be discontinued by gradually tapering it off over time.

2. Inderal should not be taken during pregnancy.
3. Inderal is contraindicated for clients with asthma.
4. Inderal is a safe medication with no known adverse effects.

   1. **Correct. *Rapid withdrawal from Inderal (in cardiac clients) has been associated with cardiac arrhythmias and sudden death. As a general rule, it is discontinued by gradually tapering it off over time to avoid any adverse responses.***
   2. *This is not correct. All medications should be avoided during pregnancy. However, Inderal is unlikely to cause any problems in the baby.*
   3. *This is an accurate statement, but it is not the best response to this question. The client's physical health was evaluated prior to starting Inderal to rule out any contraindications. There is a more important point for the nurse to emphasize prior to her discharge.*
   4. *Inderal is a relatively safe medication, but it does have adverse effects. This is not the correct option.*

68. **The nurse knows that peripheral neuropathy, a side effect from the use of isoniazid (INH), is treated by administering which of the following at the same time INH is given?**

   1. Vitamin C.
   2. Vitamin B6 (Pyridoxine).
   3. Steroids.
   4. Combinations of vitamins and steroids.

   1. *No! Vitamin C does not alter neuritis.*
   2. **Good choice! *Peripheral neuritis results from a deficiency in pyridoxine (B6), which is caused when INH forms a complex with the vitamin. Oral administration of the vitamin increases its availability and eliminates neuritis.***
   3. *Steroids are not used for this condition.*
   4. *Vitamins in general are not useful with peripheral neuritis.*

69. **The nurse caring for a person whose anxiety is being treated with hydroxyzine (Vistaril) should know that this person is likely to complain of:**

   1. Dry mouth and nasal stuffiness.
   2. Headaches.
   3. Nausea and vomiting.
   4. Diarrhea.

   1. **Correct. *Like Vistaril, all antihistamines have anticholinergic properties. Dry mouth and nasal stuffiness are possible side effects.***
   2. *This is not correct. Headaches are not a common side effect of the antihistamines used to control anxiety.*
   3. *Wrong. Antihistamines have antiemetic properties and therefore reduce the occurrence of nausea and vomiting. This is not the correct option.*

4. *This is not correct. Because antihistamines have anticholinergic properties, they do not cause diarrhea. In fact, they are sometimes associated with constipation.*

70. **A woman receives naloxone (Narcan) just prior to her rapid vaginal delivery. In planning for her postpartum care, the nurse needs to be aware that the Narcan could cause which of the following?**

1. Respiratory depression.
2. Supine hypotension.
3. Increased lochia.
4. Urticaria.

1. *Wrong! Narcan is used to treat respiratory depression. It does not cause it.*
2. *Wrong. Supine hypotension is not seen in clients receiving Narcan. Side effects are rare with recommended doses, since Narcan has no pharmacologic activity of its own.*
3. ***Yes, you are correct! Increased PTT has been documented with clients receiving Narcan. Therefore, vaginal bleeding needs to be assessed frequently after administration.***
4. *Wrong. Urticaria is not related to the administration of Narcan.*

71. **A mother at 34 weeks gestation is receiving magnesium sulfate to treat severe PIH. Twenty-six hours after the medication is started, the woman delivers by cesarean section. Which of the following clinical findings should the nurse caring for the newborn anticipate as a result of the magnesium sulfate therapy?**

1. Hypoglycemia.
2. Hypothermia.
3. Respiratory depression.
4. Hyperreflexia.

1. *Wrong. Magnesium sulfate has no effect on the mother's blood sugar and, therefore, no effect on the fetal/neonatal blood sugar. This premature infant may experience hypoglycemia, but it is related to prematurity.*
2. *Wrong. This premature infant will very likely experience hypothermia, but it is not related to the magnesium sulfate. It would be related to his immature temperature control mechanisms.*
3. ***Yes, you are correct! Magnesium sulfate will cause CNS depression in the neonate. Therefore, this infant needs to be monitored carefully for signs of respiratory depression.***
4. *No! The magnesium sulfate is likely to cause hyporeflexia rather than hyperreflexia in this neonate.*

72. **Chlorothiazide (Diuril) is ordered b.i.d. for a infant weighing 6.5 kg. It is supplied in elixir form 100 mg/tsp. The recommended dosage for Diuril is 25 mg/kg/day. How many mL should the nurse give to the child for each dose?**

1. 6.15 mL.
2. 8.13 mL.
3. 4.06 mL.
4. 0.81 mL.

1. *Wrong. Go back and look at your equation. You may have inverted the information.*
2. *No. Did you forget the equivalent number of mL in one teaspoon?*
3. ***Right! 25 mg x 6.5 kg = 162.5 mg/day. Divide this by 2, because the drug is ordered b.i.d. (162.5/ 2 = 81.25). Then D/H x Volume expressed as 81.25 mg/100 mg x 5 mL (5 mL = 1 tsp) = 4.06 mL.***
4. *No. You may not have converted the tsp to mL.*

73. **A client is being treated with cisplatin (Platinol) for his cancer. After several treatments he begins to complain of fatigue and wants to sleep all day. Which of the following nursing actions is most appropriate?**

1. Advise the client about the dangers of immobility.
2. Check lab values of RBCs, hematocrit and hemoglobin, as he is likely to be anemic.
3. Call in the family for counseling, since the client is depressed and may become suicidal.
4. Set up an exercise plan.

1. *Incorrect. Although there are dangers of immobility, this action does not address the cause of the problem.*
2. ***Great work! If the RBCs are low, treatment may need to be delayed until the blood counts are higher.***
3. *Wrong choice. A family session may be needed later. However, physical causes, which are more easily corrected, will be assessed first.*
4. *Wrong. A consult of this type may be needed to help the client and family, but physical causes must be ruled out first.*

74. **A client, age 82, is admitted to the psychiatric unit for a diagnostic work-up because she had become increasingly forgetful and disoriented at home. She has been taking lorazepam (Ativan) 0.5 mg p.r.n. to control her restlessness. The Ativan is not an indication for the nurse's plan of care to include close observation of the client for which of the following?**

1. Orthostatic hypotension.
2. Increased anxiety.
3. Hyperexcitation.
4. Hallucinations.

1. Excellent choice! Orthostatic hypotension is a side effect of antipsychotics and tricyclic antidepressants. It is not a side effect of the benzodiazepines, like Ativan. This is the correct option because the stem is asking for a false response.

2. *Wrong. Increased anxiety is one of the symptoms of paradoxical excitement that can occur in elderly persons, like the client. This cannot be the correct option because the stem is asking for a false response.*

3. *Wrong choice! Hyperexcitation is one of the symptoms of paradoxical excitement that can occur in elderly clients. This cannot be the correct option because the stem is asking for the symptom that does not occur with Ativan.*

4. *Wrong choice! Hallucinations are one of the symptoms of paradoxical excitement that can occur in elderly clients. It is not the correct option.*

75. **A client is given a six dose series of ergonovine (Ergotrate) following a vaginal delivery. Which of the following assessments must be completed on this client while she is receiving the ergonovine?**

1. Urinary output.
2. Apical pulse.
3. Blood pressure.
4. Oral temperature.

1. *No! Although urinary output is an important assessment for the client receiving Pitocin, Ergotrate has no known effect on urinary output.*

2. *No! Changes in pulse rate are not associated with the administration of Ergotrate.*

3. Good thinking! Ergotrate may cause a rise in blood pressure. Therefore, careful monitoring should be done while the client is receiving the drug.

4. *No! Body temperature is not affected by ergotrate.*

76. **Before beginning a client's rifampin (Rifadin) therapy, the nurse should warn him that this medication can cause which adverse side effect?**

1. Turn urine, sweat, tears and saliva to a red-orange color.
2. Cause stools to turn black.
3. Stain his teeth.
4. Cause constipation.

1. Very good! Rifampin frequently causes secretions to have a red-orange color.

2. *It is iron that causes stools to turn black, not rifampin.*

3. *Teeth are stained from taking liquid iron preparations, not from taking rifampin.*

4. *Although rifampin can cause gastric complaints, constipation is not one of them. Nausea is more likely.*

77. **Which of the following statements made by a client would indicate to the nurse that the client has an accurate understanding of oral cloxacillin (Tegopen) administration?**

1. "I'll take the medicine with milk or an antacid so that my stomach won't get upset."
2. "I'll take the Tegopen with a large glass of fruit juice so that I get extra Vitamin C for wound healing."
3. "I'll take the medicine either one hour before or two hours after meals so that it will work better."
4. "I'll take the Tegopen at the same time as my blood pressure and heart pills so that I don't forget to take it."

1. *No. The client should not need milk or antacids. If abdominal cramping, diarrhea and weight loss occur, pseudomembranous colitis should be suspected.*

2. *Incorrect. Penicillins should not be taken with acidic fruit juices or carbonated beverages since both may facilitate decomposition of penicillins.*

3. Correct! You remembered that most oral penicillins are bound to food and are poorly absorbed in acid media. They should be taken on an empty stomach to minimize bonding. NOTE: Amoxicillin is one penicillin that is well absorbed orally and may be given with meals.

4. *Not a wise choice. The client may take his other medications with meals or at different time intervals than suggested for antibiotics. Most antibiotics should be given at evenly-spaced intervals, usually every four to six hours to maintain proper serum concentrations, not on a q.i.d. or b.i.d. regimen.*

78. **A medication is ordered t.i.d. for a child weighing 16 lbs 12 oz. The recommended dosage is 0.03 mg/kg/day. How many milligrams should the nurse administer to the child per dose?**

1. 0.06 mg.
2. 0.22 mg.
3. 0.08 mg.
4. 0.16 mg.

1. *No, this isn't it. Remember to convert the 12 ounces to a decimal and don't round off prematurely.*

2. *No. Make sure to solve for the information requested in the question.*

3. That's right! Divide 12 ounces by 16 to convert the ounces to a decimal (.75) so that you know the child weighs 16.75 lbs. Divide by 2.2 to convert to kilograms: 16.75 ÷ 2.2 = 7.613 kg. Multiply the weight in kg times the dose per kg per day: 7.613 x .03 mg = .228 mg/day. The last step is to divide by three (you are asked to solve for each dose, and the drug is ordered t.i.d.): .228 ÷ 3 = .076. Then round off to .08 mg.

4. *No. Check your work and make sure you converted pounds to kilograms.*

79. **An elderly client is disoriented, confused and agitated and is receiving lorazepam (Ativan). Because the client is receiving Ativan, which of the following nursing actions is a priority?**

1. Observing the client for beginning signs of tardive dyskinesia.
2. Warning the client not to drive her automobile or engage in activities that require alertness.
3. Check the client's serum level of medication frequently.
4. Monitor the client closely when she ambulates.

1. *Wrong. Tardive dyskinesia is an adverse effect of antipsychotics. This is not the correct option.*
2. *This is accurate, but it is not a priority for the client while she is hospitalized.*
3. *Serum levels are checked frequently when elderly client's are taking the tricyclic antidepressants and lithium. This is not correct for Ativan.*
4. *Correct. Elderly clients may become dizzy or ataxic when taking benzodiazepines, like Ativan. They should be monitored closely when they are out of bed and ambulatory to prevent falls and possible injuries.*

80. **A psychiatric client becomes very agitated. His psychiatrist prescribes chlorpromazine (Thorazine) 50 mg by intramuscular injection, p.r.n. What instructions should the nurse give the client when administering the injection?**

1. "You will need to lie down when I give this injection and should remain in this position for at least 30 minutes."
2. "You have to hold your arm still when I give you the injection so the medication goes in properly."
3. "This medication can only be given by injection."
4. "I have to give you an injection because you need a larger dose than I can safely give you by mouth."

1. *Correct. Antipsychotic medications like Thorazine cause postural hypotension, which is most intense when the drug is given by the intramuscular route. The client should lie down for the IM injection and remain in this position for at least 30 minutes to permit his blood pressure to stabi-*

lize. If he should get up sooner, he may become dizzy and could fall and sustain an injury.
2. *This is, in general, a true statement, but it is not the best option. Read the options to identify the instruction that specifically relates to a property of Thorazine.*
3. *Not an accurate statement. Thorazine can be given orally, in tablet or liquid forms, as well as by injection.*
4. *No, injectable antipsychotics are four to 10 times more potent than their p.o. counterparts, so lower doses are used.*

81. **The nurse is planning care for a client receiving nifedipine (Adalat) for treatment of preterm labor. Which of the following maternal assessment must be included?**

1. Temperature.
2. Blood sugar.
3. Blood pressure.
4. Pedal pulses.

1. *Wrong! Adalat has no known effect on maternal body temperature.*
2. *Wrong! Adalat has no effect on maternal blood sugar.*
3. *Right! Hypotension is an adverse reaction to Adalat. Therefore, careful assessment of maternal blood pressure needs to be included in the plan of care.*
4. *Wrong! The presence, absence, or quality of pedal pulse is not related to the administration of Adalat to a client.*

82. **A client is being treated with large doses of IV vancomycin (Vancocin). He complains that his arm is sore. Which of the following nursing actions is most appropriate at this time?**

1. Immediately assess placement of the needle in the vein, as this drug can cause tissue damage if allowed to infiltrate.
2. Assure the client that this drug burns a little as it infuses, but there is nothing to worry about.
3. Alert emergency surgery, as infiltration of Vancocin may necessitate surgery.
4. Apply cold compresses to the site after the medication has infused.

1. *Best decision. Vancomycin (Vancocin) is irritating to tissues and can cause damage if allowed to infiltrate.*
2. *No, this would not be an appropriate action. The drug should be infusing through a large vein and should not be allowed to infiltrate.*
3. *This action is not necessary and would be an overreaction.*

4. *Placing cold compresses on the site after the medication has already infused into the tissues would not be wise. The medication should not be allowed to infuse into the tissue.*

83. **Two days after a psychiatric inpatient begins taking fluphenazine (Prolixin), she comes to the nursing station. The nurse observes she is very frightened, her head is twisted to one side, her back is arched and her eyes are rolled up. The best action for the nurse to take, initially, after reassuring the client that the nurse knows what is wrong and can help, is to do which of the following?**

    1. Check her for cogwheeling.
    2. Telephone her physician to report the client's condition.
    3. Give her a p.r.n. dose of haloperidol (Haldol) to relax her.
    4. Give her a p.r.n. dose of benztropine mesylate (Cogentin) IM.

    1. *This is not the best initial action. Cogwheeling is a term describing muscle rigidity in the arms of clients with parkinsonism, a type of extrapyramidal side effect. Read the other options to identify the best nursing action for the EPS the client is experiencing.*
    2. *This is not the best initial action. Acute dystonic reactions are extremely frightening for clients and require an emergency response by the nurse. Telephoning the physician takes time away from intervening to directly resolve the crisis.*
    3. *This action is incorrect. Haldol is a high potency antipsychotic, as is Prolixin. Both these drugs are associated with a high incidence of extrapyramidal side effects, such as acute dystonic reactions. Giving Haldol will not improve the client's condition and might make it worse.*
    4. **Correct! This is an emergency situation for the client because it is so frightening. If dystonic reactions are not treated promptly, they could lead to respiratory collapse. The correct nursing action is to give an intramuscular injection of an antiparkinsonian drug, such as Cogentin, as promptly as possible. Oral medication can be given for less severe reactions.**

84. **Before starting a tricyclic antidepressant, a complete medical history and physical exam should be done. The nurse knows that which of the following tests are an essential part of this pre-treatment screening?**

    1. An electrocardiogram (EKG).
    2. A thyroid scan.
    3. Liver function tests.
    4. A creatinine clearance test.

1. **Correct. An EKG should be done to rule out any pre-existing cardiac conduction problems. This is important because tricyclic antidepressants are known to cause tachycardia and cardiac irregularities in some clients, especially in those who are over the age of 40.**
2. *This is not correct. A pre-treatment thyroid scan does not have to be done. Clients on thyroid hormone can also take antidepressants, but they should be monitored closely.*
3. *This is not correct. Some clients experience liver toxicity within the first eight weeks of antidepressant treatment. This is a rare hypersensitivity to the medication, not the result of liver disease.*
4. *This is not correct. Kidney function does not have to be tested to begin treatment with antidepressants. It does have to be tested before beginning lithium.*

85. **The nurse knows that the chief reason for using para-aminosalicylic acid (PAS) in the treatment of tuberculosis is which of the following?**

    1. It is a substitute for ethambutol (Myambutol) in TB regimes for pediatric clients.
    2. It is prophylactic for tuberculosis.
    3. It treats severe disseminated tuberculosis.
    4. It treats extrapulmonary tuberculosis.

    1. **Good choice! PAS is substituted for ethambutol in children because there are no optic effects.**
    2. *Isoniazid (INH), not para-aminosalicylic acid, is used as a prophylaxis for TB.*
    3. *This is not correct. A combination of TB drugs will be employed if dissemination occurs in order to bring the disease under control.*
    4. *This is incorrect. If tuberculosis is extrapulmonary, then it is disseminated; and several drugs would need to be used for treatment.*

86. **The doctor orders D5 1/2 NS with KCl 10 mEq/liter at 30 mL/hr. The nurse is going to hang a 500 mL bag. KCl is supplied 20 mEq/10 mL. How many mL of KCl will be added to the IV solution?**

    1. 1.5 mL.
    2. 2.5 mL.
    3. 5 mL.
    4. 10 mL.

    1. *No, not enough KCl. This dose would under-medicate the client.*
    2. **Yes, that's right. First, 5 mEq of KCl is desired, because only a 500 mL bag of solution is being medicated, instead of a liter. D/H x Volume = 5 mEq/20 mEq x 10 mL = 2.5 mL.**
    3. *No, some information in the case scenario was disregarded.*
    4. *Incorrect. This amount would result in overmedicating the client. Remember to check your work and ask if this is a logical answer.*

87. A psychiatrist informs the nurse that a client with an obsessive-compulsive disorder is to start on psychotropic medication. Which of the following medications, specifically indicated for the treatment of obsessive-compulsive disorder, does the nurse anticipate the psychiatrist will order?

1. Clomipramine (Anafranil) or fluoxetine (Prozac).
2. Amitriptyline (Elavil) or trazodone (Desyrel).
3. Alprazolam (Xanax) or diazepam (Valium).
4. Haloperidol (Haldol) or fluphenazine (Prolixin).

1. *Correct. Anafranil and Prozac are two antidepressants that specifically act on the neurotransmitter, serotonin. They are used to treat obsessive-compulsive disorder.*
2. *This is not correct. These drugs are used to treat depression and have no effect on obsessive-compulsive disorder.*
3. *This is not correct. These drugs are anti-anxiety agents but have not demonstrated any therapeutic effects with obsessive-compulsive disorder. They also can lead to physiological dependency.*
4. *This is not correct. Haldol and Prolixin are antipsychotic drugs and have not demonstrated any therapeutic effects with obsessive-compulsive disorder.*

88. Which of the following disease conditions would the nurse expect to contraindicate the use of rifampin (Rifadin) in a client with tuberculosis?

1. Active hepatitis.
2. Hypertension.
3. Pyelonephritis.
4. Parkinsonism.

1. *Correct!! Clients with impaired hepatic function should not receive rifampin unless absolutely essential, because of the common adverse reaction of hepatotoxicity.*
2. *Incorrect. This disease condition is not a contraindication for use of rifampin.*
3. *No, a kidney infection is not a contraindication for the use of rifampin. The drug and its metabolites are excreted primarily in bile.*
4. *Parkinson's disease is not a contraindication for taking Rifadin.*

89. A client is receiving oxytocin (Pitocin) for induction of labor. Which of the following conditions would warrant the nurse discontinuing the intravenous infusion of Pitocin?

1. Fetal heart rate baseline 140-160 bpm.
2. Contractions every one and one-half minutes, each lasting 70-80 seconds.
3. Maternal temperature 101.2° F.
4. Early decelerations in the fetal heart rate.

1. *This fetal heart rate is within the normal range and a good prognostic sign.*
2. *Correct! This contraction pattern is indicative of hyperstimulation of the uterus, and could result in injury to the mother and fetus if not corrected.*
3. *This temperature is definitely abnormal, but Pitocin is not related to high maternal temperature.*
4. *Early decelerations in the fetal heart rate are the result of head compression, and are commonly seen throughout labor. They are associated with good neonatal outcome.*

90. The nurse notices that a two-year-old client who is receiving bleomycin (Blenoxane) IV is not voiding adequately, what action should be taken initially?

1. Stop the drug immediately.
2. Assess intake and output, be sure that the client is adequately hydrated.
3. Give a diuretic.
4. Do nothing; a decrease in urine is an expected side effect.

1. *The nurse must have the doctor's order to stop the drug. This would not be a wise move.*
2. *Great job! You remembered that the nurse should monitor renal function with Bleomycin and other antibiotic antineoplastic drugs. Monitoring includes checking lab values for BUN, and creatinine clearance, as well as intake and output.*
3. *Incorrect choice! The nurse must have a doctor's order to administer a diuretic, but first the nurse needs to check the hydration status.*
4. *No, doing nothing would not be a safe action as renal damage is a possible side effect of this drug.*

91. The physician ordered gr 3/4; on hand are 15 mg tablets. How many tablet(s) should the nurse give?

1. Three tablets.
2. One tablet.
3. Two tablets.
4. One and a half tablets.

1. *Right!! You have computed the dosage correctly: 3/4 gr x 60 mg/1 = 180 ÷ 4 = 45 mg. Then D/H x quantity is expressed as 45 mg/15 mg x 1 = 3 tablets.*
2. *Not correct. Go back and rethink the question. Did you convert the grains to milligrams?*
3. *No, this is incorrect. Did you first convert the grains to milligrams?*
4. *Incorrect. Is your equation upside down?*

92. If a client with thrombophlebitis is started on IV antibiotics, how should the nurse plan to administer the IV antibiotics?

1. Consult with the physician because another IV line will be needed since heparin is not compatible with most other IV medications.
2. Plan to piggyback the additional medications into the heparin line.
3. Refuse to give the additional medications as it would be unsafe practice.
4. Tell the client to watch for additional side effects, as heparin and other medications usually do not mix.

1. Correct. You remembered that many drugs inactivate heparin. The nurse also may need to consult with the pharmacist.
2. Incorrect response. Many drugs inactivate heparin, and piggybacking medications would not be a safe action.
3. Incorrect. Refusing to give medications would not be necessary. Just start another IV.
4. No, telling the client to watch for additional side effects would not be a professional response.

93. **A client diagnosed with TB has been taking isoniazid (INH) 300 mg p.o. daily for six weeks. He now complains of numbness and tingling in his hands and feet. Which of the following medications will most likely be ordered by the physician to decrease these symptoms?**

1. Isoxsuprine (Vasodilan).
2. Dipyridamole (Persantine).
3. Pyridoxine (Vitamin B6).
4. Cyclandelate (Cyclospasmol).

1. Incorrect. Vasodilan, a vasodilator, is used as adjunct for relief of symptoms associated with peripheral vascular disease. This is not the cause of the client's symptoms.
2. No, Persantine, a vasodilator, is used in coronary artery disease or the treatment of TIA's.
3. Excellent choice!! Pyridoxine is used to prevent Vitamin B6 deficiency secondary to INH therapy. The deficiency often manifests itself as peripheral neuropathies (numbness/tingling in the extremities, especially hands and feet).
4. Incorrect choice. Cyclospasmol, a vasodilator, is used to treat symptoms of peripheral vascular disease (PVD).

94. **A 33-year-old client is in counseling for generalized anxiety disorder. The psychiatrist prescribes buspirone (BuSpar) to control her extreme restlessness and irritability. The nurse knows that which of the following side effects is most common when taking buspirone?**

1. Drowsiness.
2. Sedation.
3. Ataxia.
4. Headaches.

1. This is not correct. Drowsiness is associated with the benzodiazepines but not BuSpar.
2. This is not correct. Sedation is a side effect of the benzodiazepines but not BuSpar.
3. This is not correct. Ataxia is a possible side effect of the benzodiazepines but is not associated with BuSpar.
4. Correct. Headaches are the most common side effect of BuSpar. Other common side effects are mild nausea and dizziness.

95. **A client is receiving magnesium sulfate for treatment of severe pregnancy induced hypertension (PIH). She begins to show symptoms of magnesium intoxication and the decision is made to administer calcium gluconate. Which of the following best describes the procedure the nurse should use for injection of calcium gluconate?**

1. Rapid IV administration via IV push.
2. Slow IV administration via piggyback IV drip.
3. Slow IV administration via IV push.
4. IM injection to provide for slow absorption.

1. No! Rapid IV push of calcium gluconate may result in cardiac arrest.
2. Wrong! IV piggyback will allow for slow administration, but in most situations this method is too slow.
3. That's right! Slow IV push is the correct procedure to achieve immediate, yet safe, treatment for magnesium intoxication.
4. Incorrect. IM injection is too slow to achieve the desired effects.

96. **A client is receiving ritodrine (Yutopar) for treatment of premature labor. Which clinical finding would warrant further assessments to evaluate this client?**

1. Maternal heart rate 124/minute for 10 minutes.
2. Fetal heart rate 174 bpm.
3. Blood pressure drop from 120/68 to 110/60.
4. Respiratory rate 34/minute for 10 minutes.

1. Wrong. Tachycardia is a common side effect of ritodrine therapy. The medication is not discontinued unless heart rate exceeds 140/min.
2. Incorrect choice! Fetal tachycardia is a common side effect of ritodrine therapy. Most texts agree that unless the rate exceeds 180 bpm there is no cause for concern.
3. Incorrect! This drop in BP is an expected response to magnesium sulfate and is not considered life-threatening hypotension.
4. Correct. This respiratory rate is excessive and may be a sign of impending pulmonary edema. The nurse needs to listen to lung sounds on this client.

97. **Ampicillin/sulbactam (Unasyn) 250 mg is diluted in 50 mL of D₅W. The antibiotic is to be delivered in 20 minutes though a soluset (set delivers 60 gtt per mL). Which is the correct rate for the nurse to set in order to deliver the medication in 20 minutes?**

1. 50 microgtt/min.
2. 17 microgtt/min.
3. 150 microgtt/min.
4. 38 microgtt/min.

1. *Incorrect. Remember, this is to be delivered in 20 minutes. (Hint—this means that to calculate the gtt/min, use 20 in the denominator instead of 60 as when calculating a rate/hour).*
2. *Not right. Is the equation set up incorrectly? Did you use mL x gtt/mL divided by total minutes? Go back and check your work.*
3. ***Excellent! Here's the math: 50 mL x 60 microgtt/ cc divided by 20 = 150 microgtt/min.***
4. *No, that's not it. These are microdrops, so use 60 in the equation where you plug in the gtt/mL.*

98. **Four days after admission, a client who is taking haloperidol (Haldol) is pacing up and down the hallway. The nurse observes him and assesses further by asking the client how he feels. He replies that he is very restless and can't seem to sit still. The nurse diagnoses the problem as the extrapyramidal side effect termed:**

1. Dystonia.
2. Parkinsonism.
3. Tardive dyskinesia.
4. Akathisia.

1. *This not correct. Dystonia, an extrapyramidal side effect, is characterized by muscle spasms, not motor restlessness. This cannot be the answer.*
2. *This is not correct. Parkinsonism, an extrapyramidal side effect, is characterized by symptoms that resemble those seen in Parkinson's disease. Look at the other options.*
3. *This is not correct. TD is an irreversible extrapyramidal effect characterized by stereotyped, involuntary movements.*
4. ***Correct! Akathisia is an EPS characterized by the client's complaint of a sense of inner restlessness, and observable behaviors, like pacing and fidgeting.***

99. **A client is being given an aminoglycoside for his bacterial infection. The nurse can aid in minimizing the risk of aminoglycoside toxicity through which of the following actions?**

1. Weighing the client daily.
2. Encouraging the client to drink at least 2000 mL of fluid daily.
3. Monitoring blood pressure prior to drug administration.
4. Instructing the client to take the medicine with food.

1. *Incorrect. Although daily weights are an assessment tool useful in monitoring fluid volume deficit or excess, the action doesn't directly address the major concern.*
2. ***Good choice! Aminoglycosides accumulate in the kidneys, which is their site of excretion. Hydration serves to reduce the extent to which these drugs will be concentrated in the renal tubules, which can lead to renal toxicity. Remember that this intervention may be contraindicated in clients with a history of decreased renal function.***
3. *No. Hypertension is not a symptom of aminoglycoside toxicity.*
4. *Wrong. Aminoglycosides are poorly absorbed from an intact intestinal tract, but are rapidly absorbed intramuscularly. The only oral uses of aminoglycosides are for surgical prophylaxis ("bowel sterilization") or treatment of gram-negative infections.*

100. **Which of the following clinical findings would indicate to the nurse that an antepartum client is experiencing an adverse reaction to betamethasone (Celestone)?**

1. Blood pressure 90/52.
2. Blood sugar 64.
3. Muscle weakness or cramping.
4. Temperature 103° F.

1. *Wrong choice! Hypertension, not hypotension, is a possible reaction to Celestone therapy.*
2. *Wrong! Hyperglycemia, not hypoglycemia, is a possible side effect of Celestone therapy.*
3. ***Good thinking! Muscle weakness or cramping is indicative of hypokalemia (low potassium), a possible adverse reaction to Celestone therapy.***
4. *No! Body temperature fluctuations are not related to Celestone therapy.*

NOTES

NCLEX-RN

Test 11
Management

NCLEX-RN TEST 11

1. A staff nurse is involved in the Continuous Quality Improvement program on the medical-surgical unit and is reviewing charting for the time of first postoperative ambulation of clients who have had abdominal surgery. The nurse knows this data collection represents a quality indicator that addresses:

   1. Structure.
   2. Process.
   3. Outcomes.
   4. Prospective time frame.

2. The nurse knows the specific expected and desired outcomes for clients with a particular diagnosis are:

   1. Established by legislation as law.
   2. Mandated by federal regulatory agencies.
   3. Based on predetermined standards of care.
   4. Arbitrarily established by each health care facility.

3. The nurse understands the overall goal of the process of continuous quality improvement is to:

   1. Improve the quality of client care.
   2. Meet federal guidelines.
   3. Ensure maintenance of Medicare and Medicaid reimbursement.
   4. Identify deficiencies in policies and procedures.

4. The nurse understands that the delivery of quality care to a specific client is primarily the responsibility of the:

   1. Institution providing the care.
   2. Joint Commission for Accreditation Healthcare Organizations.
   3. Individual care provider.
   4. Institution's medical staff and nursing administration.

5. It has been identified through quality monitoring tools that clients admitted to a hospital with a diagnosis of congestive heart failure have a length of stay that is two days longer than the established standard of three days. As a member of the continuous quality improvement committee addressing this issue, the nurse's next action will be to:

   1. Research the accuracy of the standard of care that has been accepted.

   2. Collect data regarding length of stay for these clients.
   3. Educate staff members on shortening the length of stay for these clients.
   4. Determine which actions can be instituted to correct this problem.

6. The nurse would define "standard of care" as a:

   1. Predetermined level of performance that is a model to be followed.
   2. Legally mandated requirement for minimal client care.
   3. Consumer-directed expectation for care delivery.
   4. Medically focused level of excellence for care delivery.

7. An adult client is transferred from a small rural hospital to the emergency department with a displaced fracture of the proximal femur that will require surgical intervention. The client has been medicated during transport with intravenous meperidine (Demerol). The nurse understands that consent for the surgical repair of the fracture:

   1. Is assumed since the client agreed to be transferred to another facility.
   2. Can be obtained from the client.
   3. Must be obtained from a relative or significant other of the client.
   4. Will be delayed until the Demerol is metabolized.

8. A nurse is are preparing a client for a cardiac catheterization. When asking if the client understands what will happen during the procedure, the client responds, "Something about my heart. I don't know. But I do trust my doctor to do what is best for me." This response reflects to the nurse that consent for this procedure was given:

   1. Involuntarily.
   2. Without an understanding of the proposed procedure.
   3. By a person who is mentally incompetent.
   4. With undue pressure.

9. A client has been involved in a motor vehicle collision and arrives at the hospital unconscious and in hypovolemic shock from internal hemorrhage. The client is rushed to surgery for an exploratory laparotomy for a ruptured spleen and lacerated liver. In this case, the nurse understands the signed consent for surgery:

1. Is waived due to the emergent, life-threatening condition of the client.
2. Must be obtained from a relative of the client.
3. Can be signed by a member of the hospital staff.
4. Requires a court order for treatment to occur.

10. **A nurse working on the ambulatory surgery unit frequently signs as a witness on consent for surgery forms. By signing as a witness, the nurse is:**

    1. Legally responsible to verify the client's understanding of the proposed procedure.
    2. Stating that the clients has been informed of the risks and benefits of the procedure.
    3. Verifying that the client signed the consent form.
    4. Verifying that the physician thoroughly informed the client about the risks and benefits of the procedure.

11. **The nurse knows that responsibility for obtaining an informed consent for a procedure rests with:**

    1. The person who will perform the procedure.
    2. The nurse who is caring for the client.
    3. Clerical staff in the facility.
    4. The hospital.

12. **The nurse knows informed consent is based in the ethical principles of:**

    1. Paternalism and fidelity.
    2. Veracity and nonmaleficence.
    3. Autonomy and beneficence.
    4. Justice and legal obligation.

13. **The American Nurses' Association's Code for Nurses with interpretive statements identifies the fundamental principle of:**

    1. Professional autonomy.
    2. Self-determination.
    3. Respect for persons.
    4. Nonmaleficence.

14. **A nurse is caring for a client with a chronic, debilitating condition who refuses any further treatment expresses a desire to die. Ethical decision-making about this client's care is best addressed by the nurse by:**

    1. Sharing the decision-making process.
    2. Performing treatments quickly to foster a peaceful death.
    3. Accepting the client's decision without discussion.
    4. Seeking intervention by family members.

15. **An ethical principle reflected by nursing actions that support a client's freedom of choice, self-determination, and independence is:**

    1. Basic human rights.
    2. Entitlement.
    3. Nonmaleficence.
    4. Autonomy.

16. **A nurse is considering accepting a job in a women's health clinic where abortions are performed as one of the services offered. Because of personal convictions, the nurse believes that abortion is wrong, but enjoys other aspects of women's healthcare. The nurse's decision to accept or decline this job:**

    1. Is an example of an ethical dilemma.
    2. Will be based on the potential economic benefits of the job.
    3. Is based on the nurse's professional duty to provide care to all clients.
    4. Is not impacted by the nurse's personal beliefs.

17. **The nurse's home-care client is returning from a skilled nursing care facility following rehabilitation from a cerebrovascular accident (CVA) and now walks with a walker. The nurse rearranges the furniture, removes throw rugs, and has grab bars installed in the client's bathroom. These actions reflect the nurse's attention to which ethical principle?**

    1. Beneficence.
    2. Nonmaleficence.
    3. Fidelity.
    4. Justice.

18. **Nurses encounter many ethical dilemmas in practice. The first step in ethical decision making requires the nurse to:**

    1. Collect, analyze, and interpret information.
    2. Be aware of the possible choices of action.
    3. List the advantages and disadvantages of both sides of the dilemma.
    4. Identify the institution's policy regarding the event that is presenting the dilemma.

19. **A client is asking the nurse about the cost of treatments at the healthcare facility where care is being received. The nurse should refer to which document when needing information about the client's right to this information.**

1. Code for Nurses.
2. Client's Bill of Rights.
3. Hospital policy manual.
4. Nurse Practice Act.

20. **A client is admitted to a teaching hospital by the primary care physician. The client's medical diagnosis and care provide an interesting case for medical and nursing students to be involved in and study. In this instance the nurse understands that the client:**

    1. Must accept care given by students.
    2. Has no control over who reviews the medical records.
    3. Can refuse to have students involved in care.
    4. Gave inferred consent for students to be involved in the care since care is being received at a teaching hospital.

21. **A mentally competent client refuses to be admitted to the hospital for treatment of pneumonia. What is an essential action that the nurse must perform?**

    1. Contact the physician after the client has left the hospital.
    2. Initiate legal measures to keep the client in the hospital.
    3. Ensure that the client understands the consequences of leaving the hospital.
    4. Delay the client's departure as long as possible.

22. **The nurse is caring for a client nearing the completion of rehabilitation for a spinal cord injury. The client asks for information about the Americans with Disabilities Act. Which response by the nurse contains the most accurate information about this legislation?**

    1. "It requires that all persons be treated equally regardless of their race, creed or other personal factors."
    2. "It requires that equal access and employment opportunities be available for people with disabilities in both the public and private sectors."
    3. "It establishes required employment quotas for disabled people in large companies."
    4. "It provides coverage of health care costs for people with disabilities."

23. **A client in a long-term care facility falls out of bed, fracturing the left hip. The side rails on the bed were not raised at bedtime, although this client had been identified to be at risk for falling. The nurse identifies this incident as an example of:**

1. Battery.
2. Negligence.
3. An intentional tort.
4. A criminal offense.

24. **A child is brought to the school nurse's office by a teacher who has noticed multiple bruises on the child's trunk and extremities in the last few days. The child reports "falling out of a tree". The nurse's assessment findings show patterns of bruising that would not be typically sustained from a fall from a tree. The nurse's legal responsibility is to:**

    1. Call the parents and further assess the causative event.
    2. Report the findings to the school principal and superintendent.
    3. Report the findings to local police and social service agencies.
    4. Reassess the child on a weekly basis for injuries.

25. **A nurse has recently started a new job with responsibilities and required skills that are different than those required in the past. The reference that will identify the legal parameters of the nurse's practice is:**

    1. The state's Nurse Practice Act.
    2. The Code for Nurses from the American Nurses' Association.
    3. The institution's policy manual.
    4. State Board of Nursing's licensing requirements.

26. **There are several types of laws that impact aspects of the delivery of healthcare. An example of a nursing issue that is addressed by constitutional law is:**

    1. Protection of privacy.
    2. Boundaries of nursing practice.
    3. Safety of drugs produced in the United States.
    4. Nursing licensing requirements.

27. **The nurse performs CPR on an adult who has suffered a cardiac arrest while at the grocery store. The Good Samaritan law provides civil immunity if the nurse:**

    1. Has advanced training in resuscitation of cardiac arrest clients.
    2. Is licensed to practice nursing in the state in which the event occurred.
    3. Has had training in basic life support.
    4. Continued to provide care until the client arrived at the hospital.

28. **The nurse is floated to a new nursing care unit and given a client assignment that necessitates the use of some unfamiliar skills and techniques. The nurse's best action in response to this assignment is to:**

    1. Do the best job possible during this shift.
    2. Absolutely refuse to provide any care for these clients.
    3. Make a formal complaint to the nursing manager.
    4. Ask to share a client assignment with an experienced nurse.

29. **In which situation would a nurse be protected from any legal action?**

    1. Stopping at an accident scene and providing first aid.
    2. Reporting suspected cases of abuse of dependent adults to the appropriate authorities.
    3. Teaching health maintenance practices to a group of women.
    4. Performing CPR on a drowning victim.

30. **A client receiving care from a home health agency asks the visiting nurse about a living will. The client is unsure about what is included in this document. The nurse's best answer is:**

    1. "It is a legally binding contract between a client and the physician."
    2. "It is a document that establishes who will make health care decisions for you if you are not able."
    3. "It is a document that verifies the client's wish for 'do not resuscitate' status while under the care of a health care provider."
    4. "It is a document that allows the client to express any wishes regarding health care decisions."

31. **In December 1991, the federal government placed a requirement on health care facilities to ensure client autonomy. The nurse understands this requirement involves:**

    1. An explanation of all institution policies regarding client care.
    2. An explanation of advanced directives.
    3. An explanation of financial arrangements for billing.
    4. Prohibition of use of physical restraints.

32. **The nurse is aware that a durable power of attorney for health care allows the designated decision-maker to:**

    1. Refuse treatment for the client.
    2. Access client's finances to assure payment for health care.

3. Be the executor of the client's estate.
4. Agree to active euthanasia when there is no chance of recovery for the client.

33. **What nursing action during the client admission process at any health care facility will help the healthcare team to understand the client's healthcare wishes?**

    1. Discussion of client's condition and needs with family members.
    2. Interviewing the client about health care decisions.
    3. Giving them a brochure regarding advanced directives.
    4. Ask if the client has a living will or durable power of attorney for health care decisions and place copies on the chart if one exists.

34. **A client needs a heart transplant due to severe cardiomyopathy. The nurse understands the biggest challenge for this client is:**

    1. Sufficient financial resources.
    2. High risk of transplant rejection.
    3. Finding a skilled transplant surgeon.
    4. Availability of a donor organ.

35. **Which condition would the nurse know would make a client an unsuitable organ or tissue donor?**

    1. HIV positive.
    2. Elderly.
    3. Diabetes.
    4. Advanced cardiovascular disease.

36. **The nurse has been caring for a young male client who has sustained extensive head injuries. The client is declared brain dead. Which statement would be best for the nurse to begin a conversation about the option of organ and tissue donation with the client's parents?**

    1. "I am legally required to inform you that if you want to, you can donate your son's organs for transplantation."
    2. "I want to talk to you about how important it is for you to consider donating your son's organs for transplantation. Many people die waiting for needed organs."
    3. "I want to give you some information about an option that you have regarding donating your son's organs to others who are in need."
    4. "Have you ever considered donating your organs for transplantation?"

37. **A client with end-stage cardiac diseases requires a heart transplant and expresses the fear to the nurse that "someone famous or with a lot of money**

will get it first". The nurse's best response to this client's concern is:

1. "Don't worry, your doctor will make sure that you get a heart when it is your turn."
2. "A national system determines who gets available organs based on how sick you are, how well the available organ matches, and how long you are sick. Money and fame are not criteria for choosing recipients."
3. "That's not something you need to worry about now. Concentrate on staying as healthy as possible. A positive attitude is so important to getting better."
4. "Famous and wealthy people shouldn't get a heart before you do, everyone has to wait the same amount of time."

38. **What is one way that nurses can participate in the donation process?**

1. Making sure that all clients have advanced directives.
2. Encouraging all clients to be tissue typed.
3. Discouraging do not resuscitate orders so that organs can be retrieved.
4. Presenting the option of organ donation to all suitable clients and families.

39. **As the nurse is discussing organ donation with a family, the spouse of the client asks you about the cost of donating organs. The nurse's best response is:**

1. "Your insurance company will cover all of the expenses."
2. "All costs are covered by the recipient and the transplant agency."
3. "The federal government covers the expenses under Medicare."
4. "The state will cover the expenses from a special Medicaid fund."

40. **Which statement does the nurse know to be accurate regarding the criteria for determination of death for purposes of organ donation?**

1. The primary care physician is solely responsible for determining when death has occurred.
2. Anencephalic babies are considered dead by federal standards.
3. Any person in a persistent vegetative state can be a potential source of organs for donation.
4. Death involves the complete and irreversible cessation of all function of the entire brain, including the brain stem.

41. **The nurse understands that the best person to discuss the option of organ donation with a family of a potential donor is:**

1. The nurse who has been caring for the client
2. Someone that the family knows personally.
3. Someone who is comfortable with discussing the organ donation process.
4. The primary care physician.

42. **The nurse is talking with a family of a client who is a potential organ donor. Which statement does the nurse understand to be true about families in this situation?**

1. If they donate organs it is because they want something positive to come from their loss.
2. They will find it easy to understand the concept of brain death.
3. Talking about donation with the family will increase their grief.
4. The time of death will not be important to them.

43. **The nurse is involved in the statewide organ procurement program as a transplant coordinator. Why is it important for the nurse to encourage members of all racial groups to become organ donors?**

1. All persons should be offered organ donation as an option because it is the fair thing to do.
2. Organ and tissue transplantation can only be successful within racial groups.
3. A better match of immunogenetic factors can be obtained within racial groups and increase the success of the transplantation.
4. Members of minority racial groups have a high incidence of organ failure.

44. **The mayor of the town has been admitted to the oncology unit. A local newspaper reporter phones the unit and is seeking information and states, "It is the public's right to know the health status of elected officials". The nurse's best action in response to inquiries from the news media is to:**

1. Only acknowledge that the person is a client on the unit, but give no specific details of the client's condition.
2. Refer any calls directly to the client's room so that the client and family can decide what to tell the press.
3. Refer all inquiries to the nursing supervisor.
4. Hang up on callers from the news media since the nurse is not required to speak to them.

45. **A client has been admitted to the substance abuse rehabilitation unit for alcohol detoxification. What**

information can the nurse release to callers inquiring about the client?

1. No information may be released, including whether the client is or was previously admitted to the unit.
2. The client's name and age may be released. No specific information about the condition may be released.
3. The client's doctor's name may be released so that the caller can contact the physician for information.
4. If the client has been discharged, this can be reported.

46. **What does the nurse understand to be the impact of computerized charting on the maintenance of confidentiality of client records?**

1. The same problems are associated with computerized and paper records.
2. Computers afford greater security of client records.
3. The use of computers presents different challenges to maintaining confidentiality of client records.
4. Technology is not at the advanced level needed to ensure security of client records.

47. **Maintaining confidentiality is an important aspect of a nurse's interaction with clients. In which situation would a nurse always be required to disclose information to an outside agency about the client or the client's situation?**

1. A client is admitted for pneumonia and has track marks from intravenous drug abuse.
2. A four-year-old child was left unsupervised for several hours at home and sustained a fractured leg after falling from a chair.
3. An elderly couple has been involved in a car accident.
4. A public official is admitted with depression and suicidal ideation.

48. **Case management involves several key elements. The nurse knows the development and implementation of a client's plan of care by an interdisciplinary team is an example of which key element?**

1. Efficient use of resources.
2. Collaborative health cares delivery.
3. Outcome orientation.
4. Focus on health maintenance.

49. **In 1992, the American Nurses' Association developed a proposal to address the needed changes in health care delivery. This proposal, "Nursing's Agenda for Health Care Reform," supports health care delivery that:**

1. Is based in hospital settings.
2. Is expanded and more expensive than the current system.
3. Focuses on highly specialized care for select clients.
4. Focuses on primary care delivered in community-based settings.

50. **The nurse is the case manager for a client who has been hospitalized for hip replacement surgery and will be moved to a skilled care facility for further physical therapy and rehabilitation. The nurse's responsibility as case manager in this situation is to:**

1. Coordinate the transfer and communicate the plan of care to staff at the skilled care facility.
2. Assist the family to transfer the client to the skilled care facility by private vehicle.
3. Ensure that the client is fully recovered and able to participate in therapy.
4. Submit client charges quickly to facilitate the billing process for hospital care.

51. **A nurse functioning in the role of case manager has many roles. One of these is to support all members of the case team in working toward mutual goals. The nurse functioning in this role is termed the:**

1. Educator.
2. Coordinator.
3. Facilitator.
4. Negotiator.

52. **Which client situation would the nurse know to be most likely handled by a case management approach to health care?**

1. Post-op care of a client following laparoscopic cholecystectomy.
2. Delivery of a full-term infant to a married woman.
3. A client with residual problems following a cerebrovascular accident.
4. A child with a fracture of his dominant arm.

53. **The nurse knows the best definition of a "critical path" that is used in the case management approach to the delivery of health care is a:**

1. Tool that outlines the important multidisciplinary actions that must occur to produce a desired outcome.
2. Tool that legally binds the health care facility to provide services as outlined.
3. Plan of care that focuses on nursing care only.
4. Plan to ensure that care is as inexpensive as possible.

54. A nurse new to the intensive care unit identifies a fellow staff nurse who is respected for exceptional knowledge and skill in delivering care to critically ill clients. This nurse is also respected by other nurses, physicians, and administration. What is the source of this nurse's power?

    1. Legitimacy.
    2. Coercive.
    3. Expert.
    4. Charismatic.

55. The nurse is a member of a hospital-wide committee that has developed new documentation forms to meet Joint Commission of Accreditation of Hospital standards. The nurse understands the greatest barrier to successful implementation of these new forms involves:

    1. Approval of forms by nursing administration.
    2. Staff resistance to learning new charting forms and standards.
    3. The cost of staff education.
    4. The development of quality monitoring tools for compliance with new documentation.

56. A group of nurses is discussing how they feel about nursing. One nurse expresses discomfort and confusion because of nursing administration's expectation that nursing staff be accountable and make independent decisions and one physician's expectation that orders will be followed without question. This nurse is experiencing role:

    1. Ambiguity.
    2. Conflict.
    3. Overload.
    4. Incompetence.

57. The nurse has interviewed for a position on a medical-surgical unit. The nurse's best action following the interview is to:

    1. Wait for the interviewer to contact you regarding a possible job offer.
    2. Seek input from staff members on the unit about your chances for getting the job.
    3. Send a note of thanks to the interviewer.
    4. Make daily phone calls to check if a decision has been made.

58. Which comment would be appropriate to make when attempting to resolve a conflict with a fellow nurse:

    1. "You are always late getting back from break and

    don't do your fair share of the work."
    2. "I don't want to discuss this now. I'm going to let the nurse manager know about it."
    3. "You are totally inconsiderate of my feelings about getting Christmas off."
    4. "I need to talk to you about the unit policies regarding break time."

59. A nurse is evaluating the performance of the nurse manager. Some of the behaviors that the nurse manager has displayed include establishment of staff nurse committees to address unit issues, an open-door policy for talking about concerns, and supportiveness of the professional development of all the staff. The nurse understands these behaviors reflect a management style that is:

    1. Autocratic.
    2. Laissez-faire.
    3. Democratic.
    4. Simplistic.

60. The nurse is interested in supporting a health-related bill that is due to be addressed by the state legislature. Which statement would be appropriate to include in a letter to the state legislator?

    1. "Although many nurses don't agree on how to improve client care, I think that we need more funds for hospital equipment."
    2. "As the president of my local nursing society, I can promise that all our members will vote for you in the next election."
    3. "I will expect to hear from you by the end of the week. I know that you will support this bill as I do."
    4. "I would like to request your support of State Bill 132 regarding appropriations for rural health clinic funding."

61. A nurse has recently noticed that one of the physicians makes suggestive comments whenever they are together. These comments make the nurse uncomfortable. The nurse's first action in this situation is to:

    1. Tell the physician that the comments create an uncomfortable environment and request that they be stopped.
    2. Report the complaint to the immediate nursing supervisor.
    3. To make a formal complaint to the medical board of the facility.
    4. To ignore the comments and try to stay away from this physician.

62. Negotiation is a technique used to manage con-

flict. The nurse recognizes the ultimate goal of the negotiation process is to:

1. Win all of the concessions desired from the other party.
2. Establish equality in the concessions that each party makes.
3. Make as many concessions as needed to make everyone happy.
4. Create a solution in which both parties are satisfied.

63. Many healthcare organizations expect nurses to function as a team member or leader in a variety of ways. Which behavior by the nurse would be detrimental to the formation of a team atmosphere?

1. Establishment of common goals with input from members of the team.
2. Clarifying the boundaries of the team when acting as leader.
3. Quickly deciding if member ideas have value or not.
4. Actively listening to each member's input.

64. The nurse is admitting a client with a medical diagnosis of lower gastrointestinal bleeding. Which task would be appropriate to delegate to a certified nursing assistant?

1. Taking vital signs.
2. Listening for bowel sounds.
3. Adjusting the rate of the intravenous infusion.
4. Explaining the plan of care to client and family.

65. The nurse has asked a nursing assistant to ambulate an elderly client. While walking, the client becomes dizzy and falls, fracturing a hip. The nurse understands that who is accountable for this injury to the client?

1. The client.
2. The hospital.
3. The nurse.
4. The nursing assistant.

66. The nurse wants to delegate a client care task to a nursing assistant. Which explanation by the nurse of the expectations for the completion of that task is most appropriate?

1. "Please do vital signs on all the clients we are caring for today."
2. "Please change the client's abdominal dressing before 10 am today."
3. "I have this medication for the client, would you

mind making sure that it is taken after breakfast? Let me know if the client's heart rate is above 100."
4. "The client will need to ambulate three times today and sit in the chair for 30 minutes during meal times. It requires two people to get the client out of bed and make sure the client uses a walker."

67. The R.N. has been working with a Licensed Practical Nurse who gives excellent nursing care to clients and is an effective team member. Which would be the best initial action by the R.N. to recognize the L.P.N.'s contributions to care?

1. Give feedback directly to the L.P.N.
2. Tell other staff how lucky you are to have the L.P.N. as part of your client care team.
3. Nominate the L.P.N. for Employee of the Month.
4. Detail the L.P.N.'s contributions to your nurse manager.

68. The nurse is working with a nursing assistant in a long-term care facility. What assessment must the nurse make before delegating an appropriate task to this nursing assistant?

1. The client's willingness to consent to the care of the nursing assistant.
2. The degree and frequency of supervision that the nursing assistant will require to complete the task.
3. Whether the task can be more efficiently completed yourself.
4. The federal regulations regarding functions of unlicensed assistive personnel in long term care facilities.

69. A nurse is being oriented to a new position as a staff nurse in the intensive care unit and would like feedback from the preceptor. What is the nurse's best action at this time?

1. Wait for the preceptor to initiate a performance review.
2. Request input from the preceptor on a regular basis.
3. Ask other staff what the preceptor has said.
4. Check with the nurse manager about a performance evaluation.

70. The nurse completed a variance report after administering an incorrect dose of a medication to a client. The client did not have any ill effects from the medication error. What is the purpose of the nurse completing a variance report in this situation?

1. To identify situations that contribute to the occurrence of medication errors.
2. To track employee performance for possible disci-

plinary action.

3. To alert hospital administration of a possible litigation situation.

4. To gather data for statistical analysis.

71. **A client who received a sedative-hypnotic medication at bedtime becomes confused during the night. The client gets out of bed and falls, sustaining a laceration that requires suturing. Which statement would be included as part of the nurse's documentation in the client's chart?**

1. "Client fell due to confusion caused by sleeping medication. "

2. "Client found lying on the floor in a pool of blood. Nursing assistant forgot to put siderails up at bedtime."

3. "Client found sitting on the floor. 3 cm laceration above left eyebrow. Oriented to name only."

4. "Client slipped in water on floor caused by leaking faucet that was reported to the maintenance department two days ago."

72. **Which situations would require the completion of a variance or incident report by the nurse?**

1. A disagree with the medical care ordered by the physician.

2. A dispute with a co-worker about client assignments.

3. The identification of a safety concern with a piece of equipment used on a regular basis.

4. The discovery that a pre-op client has received and eaten a breakfast tray.

73. **The nurse is notified by a hospital attorney that a client has filed a lawsuit against the hospital because of a fall sustained while in the hospital. The nurse was caring for the client at the time of the fall and completed a variance report about the incident. The nurse's variance report:**

1. Can be subpoenaed by the plaintiff's attorney.

2. Can only be used by the hospital attorneys as a privileged communication.

3. Will not be an important part of the case.

4. Is a part of the nurse's personnel file that cannot be subpoenaed.

74. **The focus of the advocate role of the professional nurse is on:**

1. Making decisions for clients when they are unable.

2. Placing a high priority on the client's rights.

3. Getting the most complete and complex care for the client.

4. Identifying the nurse's feelings about client situa-

tions.

75. **Communication is an essential skill for the nurse acting as an advocate. When the nurse says to the client, "Let me see if I understand what you mean....," the nurse is involved in the process of:**

1. Verification.

2. Amplification.

3. Clarification.

4. Affirming.

76. **One of the biggest challenges facing nurses who want to act as a client advocate is:**

1. Dealing with their own reactions to client decisions that conflict with the nurse's personal belief system.

2. A lack of reimbursement for activities involved in this role.

3. A lack of time to spend with clients.

4. Dealing with conflicts that can arise with other health care providers.

77. **Which statement is true regarding nurses' opportunities to act in an advocate role?**

1. Advocacy does not involve any personal or professional risks.

2. Advocacy is a new concept in nursing, becoming important in the last 20 years.

3. Power base has no impact on the effectiveness of the nurse in the advocate role.

4. Interpreting information for clients is an example of advocacy.

78. **The nurse's role in developing a continuum of care for a group of case managed clients involves:**

1. Ensuring that care the nurse personally delivers meets all standards of care.

2. Focusing on outcomes and the client's movement through various settings and services.

3. Making suggestions to other professions regarding the client's care.

4. Personally performing all aspects of the client's care.

79. **Maintaining a continuum of care is dependent on a variety of factors. Which factor does the nurse understand to be the most important?**

1. Development of a multidisciplinary and multi agency plan that addresses the desired outcomes for the client.

2. Assessing the client's progress on a monthly basis.

3. Accessing community resources early in the pro-

cess.

4. Keeping accurate assessments and documentation.

80. **Which statement does the nurse know to be true about the concept of continuum of care?**

1. It is a mandated standard of care that applies to all clients admitted to health care facilities.
2. It only involves members of the various health professions.
3. Each service is provided independent of other services.
4. It is a comprehensive, client-oriented system of care.

81. **A client presents to the neighborhood health clinic frequently with complaints of depression. The nurse discovers the client's involvement in an emotionally abusive relationship. The client feels trapped by the situation and does not know where to get help. The nurse's best action to meet this client's need is to:**

1. Continue to talk to the client about the manifestations of the depression.
2. Make a referral to the local organization that assists those in abusive relationships.
3. Make regular appointments for the client at the clinic.
4. Refer the client to the local emergency department for examination.

82. **A client has paraplegia and has become withdrawn and resistant to rehabilitative efforts of the staff. The best nursing intervention for this client would be:**

1. Allow the client to direct and control the timing and frequency of the therapy.
2. Limit visiting hours until the client begins to want to be social with others.
3. Consult with a staff psychologist or psychiatric clinical nurse specialist.
4. Inform the client that privileges are related to willingness to perform therapy.

83. **The nurse is discharging a client with congestive heart failure after making a referral for follow up with a community health agency. The ultimate goal for this client receiving care from a public health nursing agency will focus on:**

1. Assistance with personal care.
2. Adequate nutrition.
3. Proper immunization.
4. Client independence.

84. **The nurses working on the unit have identified** the need for updating the cardiac monitoring system so that arrhythmia detection can be increased for the safety of the clients. The nurse manager realizes this type of expenditure for equipment:

1. Is not feasible in the current cost-conscious era of health care.
2. Will need to be addressed in the capital budget plan for the unit.
3. Will result in a reduction in the personnel budget and possible loss of staff positions.
4. Is totally reimbursed by Medicare funds since these clients will benefit from the equipment.

85. **When asked to explain how a health maintenance organization charges for its services. The nurse's best answer is:**

1. Services are billed based on the client's ability to pay.
2. Clients are required to pay for all routine services completely out of their own pocket.
3. A predetermined set of services is provided for a fixed, prepaid charge.
4. Only charges incurred while an inpatient will be covered by an HMO.

86. **One way nurses can contribute to resource management is by:**

1. Discouraging clients from requesting extra personal services.
2. Taking heavier client assignments so that fewer staff members are needed.
3. Working extra shifts without accepting overtime pay.
4. Documenting care delivered and equipment used in the chart.

87. **The nurse is caring for a client who is openly homosexual and has contracted AIDS. Which action by the nurse help provide the best care possible for this client?**

1. Keep contact with the client very straightforward and businesslike.
2. Privately explore personal attitudes about sexuality.
3. Share care of this client with several other nurses to minimize the potential risk of contracting HIV.
4. Place the client in isolation to prevent transmission of the disease.

88. **The nurse is developing health promotion programs for clients in a community setting. Which of the following would be least appropriate for the nurse to include in these programs?**

1. Reducing genetic risk factors for illness.
2. Providing information about health maintenance choices.
3. Fostering of positive life-style changes.
4. Optimizing mental health.

89. **The nurse is planning interventions for a group of overweight teenage girls. What can the nurse do to best improve commitment to a long-term goal for weight loss for these clients?**

    1. Involve family members in the process.
    2. Keep detailed records of each girl's progress.
    3. Use a system of rewards for reinforcement of behavior.
    4. Attempt to develop self-motivation.

90. **As a nurse is developing a plan of care for a client, what consideration should be given to the spiritual aspects of the client?**

    1. Many clients are not receptive to spiritual support from health care providers.
    2. It should not be assumed that spiritual needs are important to every client.
    3. During illness or stress, clients and their families often have fewer spiritual needs.
    4. Spirituality is an essential need for humans.

91. **The nurse is caring for a client diagnosed with a terminal illness. The client asks several questions about the nurse's religious beliefs related to death and dying. The nurse's best response to this request is to:**

    1. Tell the client that religious beliefs are a personal matter.
    2. Change the topic since the client is obviously trying to divert attention from the illness.
    3. Encourage the client to express personal thoughts about death and dying.
    4. Offer to contact the client's minister or the hospital chaplain.

92. **A nursing diagnosis of spiritual distress has been made for a client with advanced acquired immune deficiency syndrome (AIDS). The nurse recognizes which behavior to be inconsistent with this diagnosis?**

    1. A desire to become closer to God and requests that you call a minister.
    2. Frequent crying and trouble sleeping at night.
    3. The client's statement that, "God has let me down.

I don't believe He hears me."
    4. Feeling apathetic about the disease and its progression.

93. **When caring for clients who practice Orthodox Judaism, the nurse would recognize all of the foods on the dinner tray sent from dietary to be appropriate except:**

    1. Macaroni and cheese, milk, and peas.
    2. Carrot sticks and cottage cheese.
    3. Kosher roast beef and ice cream.
    4. Kosher chicken breast and boiled potatoes.

94. **The nurse knows a client who is a devote Seventh Day Adventist will feel most comfortable if:**

    1. Allowed to have a crucifix in the room.
    2. A Bible is available for scripture readings.
    3. Assigned a room with a windows facing east.
    4. Assigned a private room.

95. **A female client presents to the emergency department following a motor vehicle collision and the nurse learns the client is a Jehovah's Witness. The nurse is aware that this causes a concern in this situation because the client will:**

    1. Insist on having family in the room at all times.
    2. Not consent to any surgical interventions for the sustained injuries.
    3. Not consent to any necessary blood transfusions.
    4. Not allow herself to be undressed and examined by a male physician.

96. **The nurse is talking to a resident of the long-term care facility who has returned from an overnight stay with his son and his wife. Which statement made by the resident would most warrant further investigation by the nurse for elder abuse?**

    1. "We had a nice visit. My grandchildren are a little unruly, but I enjoy that—in small doses!"
    2. "The food wasn't very good. My daughter-in-law never was a good cook."
    3. "Those bruises aren't anything. I get really clumsy at my son's house."
    4. "They needed a new TV, so we went out and I bought them a new one for Christmas."

97. **The nurse is interviewing an elderly client that may have been abused by a neighbor who provides much of the care for this person. The nurse's interview questions should:**

    1. Not directly ask if the client has ever been hurt by

someone.
2. Be confrontational.
3. Be nonthreatening and nonjudgmental.
4. Include as much information as possible.

98. **Which behavior indicates to the nurse a neglect of an elderly client by a caregiver?**

    1. A family member refuses to leave the nurse alone with the elderly client for an examination.
    2. An elderly client hasn't been taking necessary medications because the prescriptions have not been filled by the family member.
    3. An elderly client is brought to the clinic for a 3-month checkup by a family member.
    4. The caregiver speaks to the elderly client in an angry, berating way.

99. **The nurse recognizes that there is potential for physical and psychological abuse of elderly residents in nursing homes. The nurse's best action is to:**

    1. Ensure staff members who work on the nurse's shift are closely monitored for any inappropriate behavior towards residents.
    2. Keep staff members who tend to have a temper away from clients who suffer from conditions that put them at risk for being abused.
    3. Teach residents to behave in ways that do not provoke staff.
    4. Provide staff with education about elder abuse and stress management.

100. **The nurse knows that persons who abuse the elderly are often:**

    1. Financially dependency on the elderly person.
    2. Unrelated to the elderly person.
    3. Lacking in effective coping skills.
    4. Aware of the stressful nature of caring for an elderly family member.

NCLEX-RN

Test 11

Management Questions with Rationales

NCLEX-RN TEST 11 WITH RATIONALES

1. **A staff nurse is involved in the Continuous Quality Improvement program on the medical-surgical unit and is reviewing charting for the time of first postoperative ambulation of clients who have had abdominal surgery. The nurse knows this data collection represents a quality indicator that addresses:**

   1. Structure.
   2. Process.
   3. Outcomes.
   4. Prospective time frame.

   1. *INCORRECT. Structure indicators address organizational factors, such as financial support and physical/functional characteristics of the facility.*
   2. ***CORRECT. Process indicators measure nursing actions that are used to facilitate expected and desired outcomes in clients. Early ambulation is essential for the prevention of postoperative complications.***
   3. *INCORRECT. Outcome indicators look at client status at the time of discharge and compare it to desired outcomes for clients with the same diagnosis.*
   4. *INCORRECT. This relates to the choosing of clients from whom to collect data before the care is given. In this case, the nurse is looking at care that has already been given.*

2. **The nurse knows the specific expected and desired outcomes for clients with a particular diagnosis are:**

   1. Established by legislation as law.
   2. Mandated by federal regulatory agencies.
   3. Based on predetermined standards of care.
   4. Arbitrarily established by each health care facility.

   1. *INCORRECT. Although legislation may require that healthcare facilities address quality improvement, the specific outcomes are not established by law.*
   2. *INCORRECT. Reimbursement for Medicare and Medicaid may depend on having a quality improvement program in place in a healthcare facility, but the specific outcomes are not mandated by the federal government.*
   3. ***CORRECT. Standards of care are established by a variety of clinically oriented healthcare professional groups, such as the American Nurses' Association. These standards of care are based on the best information available from clinical practice and research.***

   4. *INCORRECT. Although each healthcare facility can identify and focus on specific client care issues, the expected and desired outcomes for each client diagnosis remain consistent across institutions.*

3. **The nurse understands the overall goal of the process of continuous quality improvement is to:**

   1. Improve the quality of client care.
   2. Meet federal guidelines.
   3. Ensure maintenance of Medicare and Medicaid reimbursement.
   4. Identify deficiencies in policies and procedures.

   1. ***CORRECT. The ultimate goal of continuous quality improvement is to improve the care and outcomes for clients.***
   2. *INCORRECT. Meeting federal guidelines is not the goal of continuous quality improvement. It is one of the mechanisms used to meet the overall goal.*
   3. *INCORRECT. Although maintaining certification for Medicare and Medicaid reimbursement payment is important, the overall goal of continuous quality improvement is to improve the quality of client care. If quality care is delivered, there is no difficulty with reimbursement.*
   4. *INCORRECT. Identifying deficiencies in policies and procedures can help in meeting the overall goal of continuous quality improvement.*

4. **The nurse understands that the delivery of quality care to a specific client is primarily the responsibility of the:**

   1. Institution providing the care.
   2. Joint Commission for Accreditation Healthcare Organizations.
   3. Individual care provider.
   4. Institution's medical staff and nursing administration.

   1. *INCORRECT. The institution is responsible for making resources available that make the delivery of quality care a possibility.*
   2. *INCORRECT. The Joint Commission for Accreditation of Healthcare Organizations monitors indicators of quality care for the purpose of accrediting healthcare organizations. This is an evaluative phase of care delivery.*
   3. ***CORRECT. The responsibility for the delivery of quality care rests with the person who directly provides the care. Nurses have a great impact on the quality of care provided in any healthcare organization.***
   4. *INCORRECT. The medical staff will monitor medi-*

cal care through a process of peer review that contributes to the delivery of quality care. The nursing administration's role is supportive of the processes and resource allocation that makes quality care delivery possible. The primary responsibility or delivery of quality care is not centralized.

5. **It has been identified through quality monitoring tools that clients admitted to a hospital with a diagnosis of congestive heart failure have a length of stay that is two days longer than the established standard of three days. As a member of the continuous quality improvement committee addressing this issue, the nurse's next action will be to:**

    1. Research the accuracy of the standard of care that has been accepted.
    2. Collect data regarding length of stay for these clients.
    3. Educate staff members on shortening the length of stay for these clients.
    4. Determine which actions can be instituted to correct this problem.

    1. *INCORRECT. Standards of care have been established following extensive research. These standards represent to best information available.*
    2. *INCORRECT. The data has already been collected regarding the length of stay for this client group. Collecting this data again will delay response to the problem.*
    3. *INCORRECT. Education is an important aspect of quality improvement; however, the content of the education must first be determined.*
    4. *CORRECT. Further analysis of data will identify factors that contribute to the longer length of stay. Actions to correct any problems identified is a subsequent step in the process.*

6. **The nurse would define "standard of care" as a:**

    1. Predetermined level of performance that is a model to be followed.
    2. Legally mandated requirement for minimal client care.
    3. Consumer-directed expectation for care delivery.
    4. Medically focused level of excellence for care delivery.

    1. *CORRECT. Standards of care are predetermined levels of performance established by an authority, such as the American Nurses' Association, and that are a model to be followed and practiced.*
    2. *INCORRECT. Standards of care are not legally mandated and represent more than minimal care delivery.*
    3. *INCORRECT. Standards of care are established by an authority such as the American Nurses' Association or other professional organizations.*
    4. *INCORRECT. Standards of care have been estab-*

lished for all aspects of care delivery and do not only focus on medical care.

7. **An adult client is transferred from a small rural hospital to the emergency department with a displaced fracture of the proximal femur that will require surgical intervention. The client has been medicated during transport with intravenous meperidine (Demerol). The nurse understands that consent for the surgical repair of the fracture:**

    1. Is assumed since the client agreed to be transferred to another facility.
    2. Can be obtained from the client.
    3. Must be obtained from a relative or significant other of the client.
    4. Will be delayed until the Demerol is metabolized.

    1. *INCORRECT. Consent for transfer to another facility for evaluation by a specialist does not assume consent for any further procedures or care.*
    2. *INCORRECT. This client has been given a narcotic that can alter the ability to understand the consent process.*
    3. *CORRECT. Consent cannot be obtained from a client who has received a medication, such as the Demerol, that can alter the ability to understand the consent process. Consent must be obtained from a relative or significant other in this case.*
    4. *INCORRECT. Delaying consent until the Demerol is metabolized would cause the client extra pain and may increase the chance of complications.*

8. **A nurse is preparing a client for a cardiac catheterization. When asking if the client understands what will happen during the procedure, the client responds, "Something about my heart. I don't know. But I do trust my doctor to do what is best for me." This response reflects to the nurse that consent for this procedure was given:**

    1. Involuntarily.
    2. Without an understanding of the proposed procedure.
    3. By a person who is mentally incompetent.
    4. With undue pressure.

    1. *INCORRECT. The client has voluntarily given consent. This response does not reflect an unwillingness to have the procedure done.*
    2. *CORRECT. The client's response reflects a lack of understanding about the proposed procedure. The nurse acts as a client advocate in this situation by requesting that the physician review the explanation with the client.*
    3. *INCORRECT. There is no evidence in this response that the client is not competent to make this decision.*
    4. *INCORRECT. There is nothing in this response*

that reflects that the client was pressured to give consent for this procedure.

9. **A client has been involved in a motor vehicle collision and arrives at the hospital unconscious and in hypovolemic shock from internal hemorrhage. The client is rushed to surgery for an exploratory laparotomy for a ruptured spleen and lacerated liver. In this case, the nurse understands the signed consent for surgery:**

   1. Is waived due to the emergent, life-threatening condition of the client.
   2. Must be obtained from a relative of the client.
   3. Can be signed by a member of the hospital staff.
   4. Requires a court order for treatment to occur.

   1. *CORRECT. Life-threatening situations in which the client cannot give consent allow care to be given without first obtaining consent from the client or relatives. To withhold care would constitute negligence on the part of the healthcare team.*
   2. *INCORRECT. Locating a relative quickly enough may not be possible in this life-threatening situation.*
   3. *INCORRECT. Hospital staff members cannot sign consents for clients who are not related to them.*
   4. *INCORRECT. Obtaining a court order to treat a client in this life-threatening situation would cause a delay that could result in the death of the client.*

10. **A nurse working on the ambulatory surgery unit frequently signs as a witness on consent for surgery forms. By signing as a witness, the nurse is:**

    1. Legally responsible to verify the client's understanding of the proposed procedure.
    2. Stating that the clients has been informed of the risks and benefits of the procedure.
    3. Verifying that the client signed the consent form.
    4. Verifying that the physician thoroughly informed the client about the risks and benefits of the procedure.

    1. *INCORRECT. The legal responsibility for explaining and ensuring the client's understanding of the procedure rests with the physician who will be performing that procedure.*
    2. *INCORRECT. This is the responsibility of the physician. The nurse may reinforce the information that was given by the physician.*
    3. *CORRECT. Signing as a witness on a procedural consent form means that the nurse verified the client was the one who signed the consent form.*
    4. *INCORRECT. It is not a nursing responsibility to monitor the thoroughness of the physician's explanation. If it is discovered that the client has questions or concerns, the nurse does have the responsibility to notify the physician of this need for further information.*

11. **The nurse knows that responsibility for obtaining an informed consent for a procedure rests with:**

    1. The person who will perform the procedure.
    2. The nurse who is caring for the client.
    3. Clerical staff in the facility.
    4. The hospital.

    1. *CORRECT. The person performing the procedure is legally responsible for obtaining informed consent. This is generally a physician, but a nurse in an advanced practice role would also be responsible if performing the procedure.*
    2. *INCORRECT. The nurse caring for the client is not responsible for obtaining informed consent. Verifying that a consent has been obtained before the procedure and witnessing the client's signature are typical nursing activities.*
    3. *INCORRECT. Clerical staff cannot obtain informed consent.*
    4. *INCORRECT. The hospital is often held responsible for making sure that informed consent has been obtained, but not for the obtaining the consent in the first place.*

12. **The nurse knows informed consent is based in the ethical principles of:**

    1. Paternalism and fidelity.
    2. Veracity and nonmaleficence.
    3. Autonomy and beneficence.
    4. Justice and legal obligation.

    1. *INCORRECT. Paternalism is a type of relationship between clients and healthcare providers in which the healthcare providers believe they know what is best for the client. Fidelity refers to the obligation to be faithful to commitments made to self and others.*
    2. *INCORRECT. Veracity refers to being truthful and not intentionally misleading the client. Nonmaleficence is the requirement that healthcare providers do no harm to their clients. Although these are important ethical principles in nursing practice, they are not the basis for informed consent.*
    3. *CORRECT. Informed consent is based in autonomy, or the right to self-determination, independence, and freedom of choice. Beneficence is the requirement that health care providers do "good" for the client.*
    4. *INCORRECT. Justice refers to treating everyone fairly. Healthcare providers who perform procedures do have a legal obligation to clients, which includes obtaining informed consent. These are important ethical principles, but are not the basis for informed consent.*

13. The American Nurses' Association's Code for Nurses with interpretive statements identifies the fundamental principle of:

    1. Professional autonomy.
    2. Self-determination.
    3. Respect for persons.
    4. Nonmaleficence.

    1. INCORRECT. *Professional autonomy is not addressed as the fundamental principle in the Code for Nurses.*
    2. INCORRECT. *Self-determination is an important aspect of client care, but it is not the fundamental principle addressed in the Code for Nurses.*
    3. CORRECT. *Respect for persons is the fundamental principle identified in the Code for Nurses. This respect for persons is the basis for all aspects of care delivery.*
    4. INCORRECT. *Nonmaleficence refers to the ethical principle "to do no harm". This is not the fundamental principle addressed in the Code for Nurses.*

14. A nurse is caring for a client with a chronic, debilitating condition who refuses any further treatment expresses a desire to die. Ethical decision-making about this client's care is best addressed by the nurse by:

    1. Sharing the decision-making process.
    2. Performing treatments quickly to foster a peaceful death.
    3. Accepting the client's decision without discussion.
    4. Seeking intervention by family members.

    1. CORRECT. *Ethical decisions about care should be discussed and shared between caregivers, the client, and the client's family. This is especially true when there appears to be no "right" or "wrong" answer.*
    2. INCORRECT. *Performing any act that fosters death, even a peaceful one, is illegal. The ethical aspects of this issue are hotly debated.*
    3. INCORRECT. *Ethical decisions should not be made in isolation without discussion. The client needs to understand the options and consequences of refused care.*
    4. INCORRECT. *Although family may be involved in the decision-making process, it would not be ethical to enlist the family in changing the client's mind. The degree of family involvement in the decision-making process depends on the wishes of the client.*

15. An ethical principle reflected by nursing actions that support a client's freedom of choice, self-determination, and independence is:

    1. Basic human rights.
    2. Entitlement.
    3. Nonmaleficence.
    4. Autonomy.

    1. INCORRECT. *This is a broad term for rights that all persons have. It is not an ethical principle, although it is one of the bases for these ethical principles.*
    2. INCORRECT. *Entitlement refers to the right to receive some service, support, or care from another.*
    3. INCORRECT. *Nonmaleficence refers to the ethical principle "to do no harm".*
    4. CORRECT. *Autonomy is supported by nursing actions that help clients to be independent, have freedom of choice, and determine their own life and future.*

16. A nurse is considering accepting a job in a women's health clinic where abortions are performed as one of the services offered. Because of personal convictions, the nurse believes that abortion is wrong, but enjoys other aspects of women's healthcare. The nurse's decision to accept or decline this job:

    1. Is an example of an ethical dilemma.
    2. Will be based on the potential economic benefits of the job.
    3. Is based on the nurse's professional duty to provide care to all clients.
    4. Is not impacted by the nurse's personal beliefs.

    1. CORRECT. *An ethical dilemma occurs when a situation occurs in which there are competing rules or principles. Abortion is legal, but may conflict with a nurse's personal belief system. It would be best to seek employment elsewhere or attempt to make an agreement with the clinic that participation in the performance of abortions will not be required.*
    2. INCORRECT. *Although the potential economic benefits of the job may be considered as part of the decision, it does not address the main issue of this situation.*
    3. INCORRECT. *The ANA Code for Nurses does state that nurses must provide services without consideration of social or economic status, personal attributes, or the nature of the health problem. However, nurse's can still choose not to take a position that conflicts with personal beliefs or seek an agreement that allows the nurse to not participate in the performance of abortions at this clinic.*
    4. INCORRECT. *An awareness of a personal value and belief system is important for nurses in any setting. Nurses will be happier in a job that is congruent with their own beliefs.*

17. The nurse's home-care client is returning from a skilled nursing care facility following rehabilitation from a cerebrovascular accident (CVA) and now walks with a walker. The nurse rearranges the furniture, removes throw rugs, and has grab bars installed in the client's bathroom. These actions reflect the nurse's attention to which ethical principle?

1. Beneficence.
2. Nonmaleficence.
3. Fidelity.
4. Justice.

1. *INCORRECT. Although beneficence refers to doing "good" for the client, there is another principle that is better reflected by these actions.*
2. **CORRECT. Nonmaleficence refers to the requirement to do no harm and to protect clients from harm if they cannot protect themselves. The actions taken in this situation are important for the prevention of injuries due to falling.**
3. *INCORRECT. Fidelity is the principle that accountability for our practice is based on. It refers to the obligation to be faithful to commitments that have been made to self and others.*
4. *INCORRECT. Justice is based in the obligation to be fair. These actions do not reflect this principle.*

18. Nurses encounter many ethical dilemmas in practice. The first step in ethical decision making requires the nurse to:

1. Collect, analyze, and interpret information.
2. Be aware of the possible choices of action.
3. List the advantages and disadvantages of both sides of the dilemma.
4. Identify the institution's policy regarding the event that is presenting the dilemma.

1. **CORRECT. Any decision requires the first step of getting more information that can be analyzed and interpreted. This is parallel to the assessment phase of the nursing process.**
2. *INCORRECT. The possible choices of action cannot be determined until all the information regarding the situation is gathered.*
3. *INCORRECT. It would be difficult to identify advantages and disadvantages without having all the information about the situation.*
4. *INCORRECT. Ethical decision-making is used when there are no clear right and wrong answers. The presence of an institutional policy regarding the situation may not relieve the ethical dilemma for the individual nurse.*

19. A client is asking the nurse about the cost of treatments at the healthcare facility where care is being received. The nurse should refer to which document when needing information about the client's right to this information.

1. Code for Nurses.
2. Client's Bill of Rights.
3. Hospital policy manual.
4. Nurse Practice Act.

1. *INCORRECT. This document directs how nurses approach client care. Although the Code for Nurses is based on respect for persons, another document directly addresses the client's right to this information.*
2. **CORRECT. The Client's Bill of Rights covers many aspects of care, including the right to explanation of treatment costs.**
3. *INCORRECT. Hospital policy manuals may outline the procedure for giving information to clients, but does not address the underlying right of the client to this information.*
4. *INCORRECT. The Nurse Practice Act establishes the legal parameters of nursing practice specific to each state.*

20. A client is admitted to a teaching hospital by the primary care physician. The client's medical diagnosis and care provide an interesting case for medical and nursing students to be involved in and study. In this instance the nurse understands that the client:

1. Must accept care given by students.
2. Has no control over who reviews the medical records.
3. Can refuse to have students involved in care.
4. Gave inferred consent for students to be involved in the care since care is being received at a teaching hospital.

1. *INCORRECT. Clients do not have to agree to having students involved in their care.*
2. *INCORRECT. Only those persons who are involved in the direct care or evaluation of care delivered are allowed access to client records. Unrestricted access constitutes a breach of confidentiality.*
3. **CORRECT. Clients have the legal right to refuse to have students involved in their care.**
4. *INCORRECT. It does not matter that the facility is a teaching hospital. The client's rights are no different in this setting than in a nonteaching hospital.*

21. A mentally competent client refuses to be admitted to the hospital for treatment of pneumonia. What is an essential action that the nurse must perform?

1. Contact the physician after the client has left the hospital.
2. Initiate legal measures to keep the client in the hospital.
3. Ensure that the client understands the consequences of leaving the hospital.
4. Delay the client's departure as long as possible.

1. INCORRECT. The physician should be contacted before the client leaves the hospital, if possible.

2. INCORRECT. This client is mentally competent and able to make this decision. Legal measures to force the client to stay would not be appropriate in this situation.

3. CORRECT. The client has the right to refuse any aspect of treatment. It is a nursing responsibility to make sure that the client understands the consequences of refusing treatment or admission that were explained to them by the physician.

4. INCORRECT. Delay the client's departure is inappropriate and could be interpreted as interfering with the client's right to refuse treatment.

22. **The nurse is caring for a client nearing the completion of rehabilitation for a spinal cord injury. The client asks for information about the Americans with Disabilities Act. Which response by the nurse contains the most accurate information about this legislation?**

1. "It requires that all persons be treated equally regardless of their race, creed or other personal factors."
2. "It requires that equal access and employment opportunities be available for people with disabilities in both the public and private sectors."
3. "It establishes required employment quotas for disabled people in large companies."
4. "It provides coverage of health care costs for people with disabilities."

1. INCORRECT. Although this is a basis for the development of the American with Disabilities Act, this is one of our basic human rights as Americans and is not directly addressed in the ADA.

2. CORRECT. The Americans with Disabilities Act legislates that access to public accommodations and services, telecommunication relay services, and employment be possible. This Act requires the private sector to be responsible for any costs associated with meeting the requirements of the Act.

3. INCORRECT. Quotas are not established by the Act. The focus of this Act is to remove barriers to employment for disabled persons.

4. INCORRECT. The Americans with Disabilities Act does not address economic reimbursement or entitlement for persons with disabilities.

23. **A client in a long-term care facility falls out of bed, fracturing the left hip. The side rails on the bed were not raised at bedtime, although this client had been identified to be at risk for falling. The nurse identifies this incident as an example of:**

1. Battery.
2. Negligence.
3. An intentional tort.
4. A criminal offense.

1. INCORRECT. Battery is defined as the touching with or without the intent to do harm.

2. CORRECT. Negligence refers to exposing a client to unreasonable risk of injury. In the case of a client who is identified as being at risk for falling, raised side rails help to decrease the risk for falling out of bed and is a standard of care for these clients.

3. INCORRECT. An intentional tort occurs when a person willfully and intentionally damages another in some way.

4. INCORRECT. This does not constitute a criminal offense. Negligence is a tort or violation of civil law. However, a serious tort can also be tried as a criminal offense.

24. **A child is brought to the school nurse's office by a teacher who has noticed multiple bruises on the child's trunk and extremities in the last few days. The child reports "falling out of a tree". The nurse's assessment findings show patterns of bruising that would not be typically sustained from a fall from a tree. The nurse's legal responsibility is to:**

1. Call the parents and further assess the causative event.
2. Report the findings to the school principal and superintendent.
3. Report the findings to local police and social service agencies.
4. Reassess the child on a weekly basis for injuries.

1. INCORRECT. The physical assessment findings point to abuse by someone. The nurse's legal responsibility is related to the safety of the child.

2. INCORRECT. Although the school principal will likely be notified as part of the school's procedure, this is not a legal responsibility.

3. CORRECT. All healthcare providers are mandatory reporters of child abuse. The nurse's primary concern is for the safety of the child. Procedures for reporting will differ in various locations, but most typically involves notification of police and social services personnel, who will then do an investigation.

4. *INCORRECT. If abuse is occurring in this child's home, waiting to intervene could put this child at risk for further abuse or serious injury.*

25. **A nurse has recently started a new job with responsibilities and required skills that are different than those required in the past. The reference that will identify the legal parameters of the nurse's practice is:**

1. The state's Nurse Practice Act.
2. The Code for Nurses from the American Nurses' Association.
3. The institution's policy manual.
4. State Board of Nursing's licensing requirements.

1. **CORRECT. Nursing practice is governed by the Nurse Practice Act in each state. There are variations in specifics of each Practice Act. It is the nurse's responsibility to understand the parameters of nursing practice. Questions about specific responsibilities and skills allowed by the Practice Act can be addressed by the State Board of Nursing.**
2. *INCORRECT. The Code for Nurses gives expectations for the professional conduct of nurses.*
3. *INCORRECT. Although the institution's policies should reflect legal nursing practice, the nurse's best reference is the original Nurse Practice Act.*
4. *INCORRECT. The licensing requirements establish the minimum criteria for obtaining a license to practice nursing, not specific aspects of nursing practice.*

26. **There are several types of laws that impact aspects of the delivery of healthcare. An example of a nursing issue that is addressed by constitutional law is:**

1. Protection of privacy.
2. Boundaries of nursing practice.
3. Safety of drugs produced in the United States.
4. Nursing licensing requirements.

1. **CORRECT. Constitutional law refers to the rights, privileges, and responsibilities that are derived from the United States Constitution, including the Bill of Rights.**
2. *INCORRECT. The boundaries of nursing practice are established by each state's Nurse Practice Act. This is an example of statutory law.*
3. *INCORRECT. The Food, Drug, and Cosmetic Act addressed safety of drugs produced in the United States. This is an example of statutory law.*
4. *INCORRECT. Licensing requirements are established by the State Boards of Nursing. This is an example of administrative law.*

27. **The nurse performs CPR on an adult who has suffered a cardiac arrest while at the grocery store. The Good Samaritan law provides civil immunity if the nurse:**

1. Has advanced training in resuscitation of cardiac arrest clients.
2. Is licensed to practice nursing in the state in which the event occurred.
3. Has had training in basic life support.
4. Continued to provide care until the client arrived at the hospital.

1. *INCORRECT. Performing CPR does not require advanced training in resuscitation.*
2. *INCORRECT. Being licensed is not a requirement of the provisions of the Good Samaritan laws.*
3. **CORRECT. Good Samaritan laws provide civil immunity when actions performed in an emergency are within the nurse's abilities and expertise.**
4. *INCORRECT. The nurse's relationship with the client in this situation legally ends when care is transferred to another qualified health provider. In this case, an EMT or paramedic on the ambulance that responds to the scene will assume care for the client.*

28. **The nurse is floated to a new nursing care unit and given a client assignment that necessitates the use of some unfamiliar skills and techniques. The nurse's best action in response to this assignment is to:**

1. Do the best job possible during this shift.
2. Absolutely refuse to provide any care for these clients.
3. Make a formal complaint to the nursing manager.
4. Ask to share a client assignment with an experienced nurse.

1. *INCORRECT. "Doing the best job possible" in a situation in which the nurse does not have the necessary skills may not meet the standard of care for this unit. It may not be possible to deliver safe care in this situation.*
2. *INCORRECT. There are aspects of care for these clients that the nurse is most likely competent to perform. It is appropriate to make any concerns about the appropriateness of the assignment clear to staff and the nursing supervisor.*
3. *INCORRECT. Complaining generally does not solve a problem. A discussion about necessary skills and orientation needs would be appropriate.*
4. **CORRECT. Make any concerns about the ability to provide safe care clear to the other staff. Working with an experienced nurse will provide an opportunity to learn some of these skills. Alter-**

nately, the nurse may divide the care tasks so that the less experienced nurse only does those skills and assessments that are within usual nursing practice. The experienced nurse would be responsible for the other aspects of care.

29. **In which situation would a nurse be protected from any legal action?**

    1. Stopping at an accident scene and providing first aid.
    2. Reporting suspected cases of abuse of dependent adults to the appropriate authorities.
    3. Teaching health maintenance practices to a group of women.
    4. Performing CPR on a drowning victim.

    1. *INCORRECT. In this situation the nurse would be held liable for providing first aid appropriately.*
    2. **CORRECT. The law protects nurses and other mandatory reporters from any civil or criminal action related to reporting of suspected cases of abuse. This is to remove this barrier to reporting.**
    3. *INCORRECT. The nurse still needs to ensure that the information provided is currently accurate and could be held liable for any misinformation and resulting injury.*
    4. *INCORRECT. Even though this is an emergency situation, the nurse is held to the standard of care for performing CPR correctly.*

30. **A client receiving care from a home health agency asks the visiting nurse about a living will. The client is unsure about what is included in this document. The nurse's best answer is:**

    1. "It is a legally binding contract between a client and the physician."
    2. "It is a document that establishes who will make health care decisions for you if you are not able."
    3. "It is a document that verifies the client's wish for 'do not resuscitate' status while under the care of a health care provider."
    4. "It is a document that allows the client to express any wishes regarding health care decisions."

    1. *INCORRECT. Living wills are not legally binding currently due to problems with agreement and understanding of terminology used in these documents.*
    2. *INCORRECT. This describes a durable power of attorney document.*
    3. *INCORRECT. Although "do not resuscitate" wishes may be part of the living will information, it is not a required part of this document. This answer is too narrow.*
    4. **CORRECT. The purpose of a living will is to allow the client an opportunity to decide what aspects of care and treatment is to be accepted or refused.**

31. **In December 1991, the federal government placed a requirement on health care facilities to ensure client autonomy. The nurse understands this requirement involves:**

    1. An explanation of all institution policies regarding client care.
    2. An explanation of advanced directives.
    3. An explanation of financial arrangements for billing.
    4. Prohibition of use of physical restraints.

    1. *INCORRECT. This would be a lengthy and unnecessary process. There are no federal regulations requiring this.*
    2. **CORRECT. The federal government enacted a law mandating that living wills and durable power of attorneys for health care, as well as the state laws governing these documents, must be explained to each client admitted to a health care facility.**
    3. *INCORRECT. This response does not address client autonomy.*
    4. *INCORRECT. The use of physical or pharmacological restraints is allowed and appropriate in specific situations.*

32. **The nurse is aware that a durable power of attorney for health care allows the designated decision-maker to:**

    1. Refuse treatment for the client.
    2. Access client's finances to assure payment for health care.
    3. Be the executor of the client's estate.
    4. Agree to active euthanasia when there is no chance of recovery for the client.

    1. **CORRECT. The durable power of attorney for health care designates someone to make decisions for a client who is unable to make decisions. This includes refusing or removing treatment.**
    2. *INCORRECT. This document only gives the designated decision-maker power to make decisions regarding health care for the client, not access to any assets of the client.*
    3. *INCORRECT. The executor of the client's estate is established in a last will and testament or by family relationship. This is not addressed by the durable power of attorney for health care.*
    4. *INCORRECT. Active euthanasia is not legal. It is viewed as commission of a homicide.*

33. **What nursing action during the client admission process at any health care facility will help the healthcare team to understand the client's healthcare wishes?**

    1. Discussion of client's condition and needs with family members.

2. Interviewing the client about health care decisions.
3. Giving them a brochure regarding advanced directives.
4. Ask if the client has a living will or durable power of attorney for health care decisions and place copies on the chart if one exists.

1. *INCORRECT. This action is appropriate as part of the admission process, but it is the client's right to determine what to receive unless physically or mentally unable to make those decisions.*
2. *INCORRECT. Although talking to clients about their wishes is a good idea, this response does not address how this information would be communicated with other members of the healthcare team.*
3. *INCORRECT. Information about advanced directives is appropriate to give to clients who have not already addressed this issue, but this does not give you information about their wishes now.*
4. ***CORRECT. It is a nursing responsibility to identify clients who do have advanced directives and ensure that copies are placed on the chart. Discussion of specific aspects of their wishes is also appropriate. The chart is the place where all members of the team can find this information.***

34. **A client needs a heart transplant due to severe cardiomyopathy. The nurse understands the biggest challenge for this client is:**

   1. Sufficient financial resources.
   2. High risk of transplant rejection.
   3. Finding a skilled transplant surgeon.
   4. Availability of a donor organ.

   1. *INCORRECT. Although this is a concern for many clients, it is not the biggest challenge.*
   2. *INCORRECT. Preventing transplant rejection is a concern after transplantation, but it is not the biggest challenge to the client at this time.*
   3. *INCORRECT. There are many skilled transplant surgeons around the country.*
   4. ***CORRECT. The biggest challenge to clients needing transplantation of any organ is finding a suitable donor organ. Many clients die before a matched organ is found.***

35. **Which condition would the nurse know would make a client an unsuitable organ or tissue donor?**

   1. HIV positive.
   2. Elderly.
   3. Diabetes.
   4. Advanced cardiovascular disease.

   1. ***CORRECT. The only clients that are generally excluded from organ or tissue donation are those with communicable diseases such as hepatitis and HIV. Persons with extracerebral malignancies are also typically excluded.***

2. *INCORRECT. Age is not an automatic exclusion criteria. The client's physical condition at time of death will determine the eligibility to be a donor.*
3. *INCORRECT. Diabetes is not an automatic exclusion criteria. The client's status must be evaluated. Always contact the local organ donation coordinator before ruling out a potential donor.*
4. *INCORRECT. Although advanced cardiovascular disease may preclude the donation of some organs, it is not an automatic exclusion criteria. Each client must be evaluated individually.*

36. **The nurse has been caring for a young male client who has sustained extensive head injuries. The client is declared brain dead. Which statement would be best for the nurse to begin a conversation about the option of organ and tissue donation with the client's parents?**

   1. "I am legally required to inform you that if you want to, you can donate your son's organs for transplantation."
   2. "I want to talk to you about how important it is for you to consider donating your son's organs for transplantation. Many people die waiting for needed organs."
   3. "I want to give you some information about an option that you have regarding donating your son's organs to others who are in need."
   4. "Have you ever considered donating your organs for transplantation?"

   1. *INCORRECT. This statement, with its focus on a legal requirement, may imply that the nurse does not support the idea of organ donation. Avoid statements that lead the family one way or the other.*
   2. *INCORRECT. This statement is a strong statement of the nurse's belief that organ donation is the right thing to do. It would not be appropriate to make statements that may make the family feel guilty if they choose not to donate.*
   3. ***CORRECT. This is the best statement to begin with. It makes the nurse's intention to give the family factual information clear and does not make any emotionally laden statements.***
   4. *INCORRECT. Asking the family members about their thoughts on donating their own organs shifts the focus away from the client's situation.*

37. **A client with end-stage cardiac diseases requires a heart transplant and expresses the fear to the nurse that "someone famous or with a lot of money will get it first". The nurse's best response to this client's concern is:**

   1. "Don't worry, your doctor will make sure that you get a heart when it is your turn."
   2. "A national system determines who gets available organs based on how sick you are, how well the

available organ matches, and how long you are sick. Money and fame are not criteria for choosing recipients."

3. "That's not something you need to worry about now. Concentrate on staying as healthy as possible. A positive attitude is so important to getting better."

4. "Famous and wealthy people shouldn't get a heart before you do, everyone has to wait the same amount of time."

1. INCORRECT. This does not address the client's concern. Individual physicians are not able to control the distribution of available organs.

2. CORRECT. This statement is factual and gives the client information about the selection of recipients for available organs and the criteria used.

3. INCORRECT. This statement does not address the client's concern.

4. INCORRECT. The information in this statement is incorrect. The amount of time on the transplant list is not standardized. A variety of criteria are used to determine recipient choice. Waiting time for an organ will vary greatly and is dependent on availability of organs.

38. What is one way that nurses can participate in the donation process?

1. Making sure that all clients have advanced directives.
2. Encouraging all clients to be tissue typed.
3. Discouraging do not resuscitate orders so that organs can be retrieved.
4. Presenting the option of organ donation to all suitable clients and families.

1. INCORRECT. Advanced directives address a client's wishes for life-sustaining measures to be used or not. They do not address organ donation.

2. INCORRECT. Tissue typing of all clients would not be feasible. It is a costly procedure that should be done only on suitable potential donors.

3. INCORRECT. This would be an unethical action to take. The decision for or against resuscitation should be made by the client or the client's family based on information about the client's condition, not because of potential donor suitability.

4. CORRECT. Nurses are often the best members of the healthcare team to address this issue with clients and families due to the relationship that has developed in the care process.

39. As the nurse is discussing organ donation with a family, the spouse of the client asks you about the cost of donating organs. The nurse's best response is:

1. "Your insurance company will cover all of the expenses."

2. "All costs are covered by the recipient and the transplant agency."
3. "The federal government covers the expenses under Medicare."
4. "The state will cover the expenses from a special Medicaid fund."

1. INCORRECT. The coverage of donor costs can vary widely between insurance companies. It would be wrong to make this assumption.

2. CORRECT. Once the donor has been declared dead, all expenses for the preservation and recovery of the organ(s) are covered by the recipient and the transplant agency.

3. INCORRECT. Although Medicare will cover a few selected organ transplants, this may not apply in this situation. The recipient may not be on Medicare.

4. INCORRECT. The coverage of transplant expenses for clients on Medicaid will vary widely from state to state. The recipient may not be on Medicaid.

40. Which statement does the nurse know to be accurate regarding the criteria for determination of death for purposes of organ donation?

1. The primary care physician is solely responsible for determining when death has occurred.
2. Anencephalic babies are considered dead by federal standards.
3. Any person in a persistent vegetative state can be a potential source of organs for donation.
4. Death involves the complete and irreversible cessation of all function of the entire brain, including the brain stem.

1. INCORRECT. The primary care physician typically must consult at least one other physician to confirm that the criteria of death have been met.

2. INCORRECT. Anencephalic babies have functioning brain stems. This does not meet the criteria of death.

3. INCORRECT. Persons in a persistent vegetative state have functioning brain stems and do not meet the criteria for death.

4. CORRECT. The Uniform Determination of Death Act defines death as the irreversible cessation of heart or respiratory function or the irreversible cessation of all function of the entire brain including the brain stem.

41. The nurse understands that the best person to discuss the option of organ donation with a family of a potential donor is:

1. The nurse who has been caring for the client.
2. Someone that the family knows personally.
3. Someone who is comfortable with discussing the organ donation process.

4. The primary care physician.

1. *INCORRECT. Although the primary care nurse would want to be involved in this process, it is not an automatic responsibility of the nurse.*
2. *INCORRECT. It is not necessary that the family know the person personally. In some situations this may present a barrier because of heightened emotions regarding the death.*
3. **CORRECT. A person who feels comfortable talking about organ donation is best suited for this task. If the nurse or physician is uncomfortable with the topic, this feeling could be transferred to the family and influence their decision. Knowledge about the process of donation is also important so the family's questions can be answered.**
4. *INCORRECT. Many physicians will want to participate in this process, but the fact of being the primary care physician does not automatically make the physician the best person to talk to the family.*

42. **The nurse is talking with a family of a client who is a potential organ donor. Which statement does the nurse understand to be true about families in this situation?**

1. If they donate organs it is because they want something positive to come from their loss.
2. They will find it easy to understand the concept of brain death.
3. Talking about donation with the family will increase their grief.
4. The time of death will not be important to them.

1. **CORRECT. Families often will state that the donation of organs was the only positive result of their loss.**
2. *INCORRECT. Families usually have a hard time understanding brain death and how it is determined.*
3. *INCORRECT. Presenting the option of organ donation is one way that the family can have control in a situation in which they feel they have no control. This can help ease the grief that the family is experiencing.*
4. *INCORRECT. The time of death is an important piece of information for the family. It is often confusing to the family because brain death and cessation of heartbeat do not occur at the same time. Be consistent in referring to the time of death as the time when brain death was declared.*

43. **The nurse is involved in the statewide organ procurement program as a transplant coordinator. Why is it important for the nurse to encourage members of all racial groups to become organ donors?**

1. All persons should be offered organ donation as an option because it is the fair thing to do.

2. Organ and tissue transplantation can only be successful within racial groups.
3. A better match of immunogenetic factors can be obtained within racial groups and increase the success of the transplantation.
4. Members of minority racial groups have a high incidence of organ failure.

1. *INCORRECT. Every person has the right to donate organs and it is mandated by law that every client is offered this option. Being "fair" is not the issue here.*
2. *INCORRECT. Although the race of the donor and recipient can impact success of transplantation, other factors have a greater impact.*
3. **CORRECT. Because there are genetic commonalties within races, it is more likely that a better match will be found. The closeness of the match between donor and recipient impacts the success of the transplant and minimizes the risk of rejection.**
4. *INCORRECT. The incidence of organ failure and needed transplantation within racial groups is not significantly different from other groups. The need for transplanted organs impacts all groups.*

44. **The mayor of the town has been admitted to the oncology unit. A local newspaper reporter phones the unit and is seeking information and states, "It is the public's right to know the health status of elected officials". The nurse's best action in response to inquiries from the news media is to:**

1. Only acknowledge that the person is a client on the unit, but give no specific details of the client's condition.
2. Refer any calls directly to the client's room so that the client and family can decide what to tell the press.
3. Refer all inquiries to the nursing supervisor.
4. Hang up on callers from the news media since the nurse is not required to speak to them.

1. *INCORRECT. Since the unit is a specialized care setting for oncology clients, acknowledging that the mayor is a client can lead to speculation about the mayor's condition. It is not the public's right to know who has been hospitalized.*
2. *INCORRECT. It would put undue stress on the client and family to speak to the news media without preparation.*
3. **CORRECT. Give no information about the client. If the reporter persists after being told that, due to confidentiality issues, no information can be given out about any clients, refer these calls to the nursing supervisor or follow established procedure in the institution.**
4. *INCORRECT. Although the frustration with news reporters may tempt the nurse to hang up on these callers, doing so would be rude and reflect poorly*

on the nurse as a professional and the institution for which the nurse works. Follow the institution's policies for release of client information.

45. **A client has been admitted to the substance abuse rehabilitation unit for alcohol detoxification. What information can the nurse release to callers inquiring about the client?**

   1. No information may be released, including whether the client is or was previously admitted to the unit.
   2. The client's name and age may be released. No specific information about the condition may be released.
   3. The client's doctor's name may be released so that the caller can contact the physician for information.
   4. If the client has been discharged, this can be reported.

   1. *CORRECT. Federal regulations address the confidentiality of alcohol and drug abuse client records. No information may be released regarding these clients, including whether or not they are or ever were a client in a substance abuse rehabilitation program.*
   2. *INCORRECT. Federal regulations prohibit the release of clients' information when they are involved in substance abuse rehabilitation.*
   3. *INCORRECT. This would put undue expectations on a physician to field calls about a client's status. Because physicians often specialize in caring for clients with substance abuse problems, telling who the physician is can lead to speculation about the client's reason for admission.*
   4. *INCORRECT. Federal regulations prohibit the release of any information regarding clients in substance abuse rehabilitation programs, including whether they were discharged.*

46. **What does the nurse understand to be the impact of computerized charting on the maintenance of confidentiality of client records?**

   1. The same problems are associated with computerized and paper records.
   2. Computers afford greater security of client records.
   3. The use of computers presents different challenges to maintaining confidentiality of client records.
   4. Technology is not at the advanced level needed to ensure security of client records.

   1. *INCORRECT. Because of the different formats of the client record, the problems associated with maintaining confidentiality will differ.*
   2. *INCORRECT. This is not necessarily true. Computers can be accessed by outside sources, such as computer hackers who have accessed even the most secure computer systems.*
   3. *CORRECT. Computers do present different chal-*

lenges to maintaining confidentiality. These include access control using passwords and restricted access, limited screen time, and secure locations for computer terminals.
   4. *INCORRECT. Technology is a tool for human use. There are security measures that can minimize problems with security of client records. No technology would be foolproof and absolutely secure.*

47. **Maintaining confidentiality is an important aspect of a nurse's interaction with clients. In which situation would a nurse always be required to disclose information to an outside agency about the client or the client's situation?**

   1. A client is admitted for pneumonia and has track marks from intravenous drug abuse.
   2. A four-year-old child was left unsupervised for several hours at home and sustained a fractured leg after falling from a chair.
   3. An elderly couple has been involved in a car accident.
   4. A public official is admitted with depression and suicidal ideation.

   1. *INCORRECT. Although it is illegal to use street drugs, track marks may be present from scarring from previous use. The nurse would not be required to report this finding to law enforcement.*
   2. *CORRECT. This situation reflects child neglect and endangerment. Nurses are mandatory reporters of any client situation in which children or the elderly are being abused or neglected.*
   3. *INCORRECT. Motor vehicle accidents do not have to be reported in every state. Be aware of what the regulations are in your state.*
   4. *INCORRECT. Regardless of the fact that this is a public official, this type of information is never shared outside of the healthcare team caring for this client.*

48. **Case management involves several key elements. The nurse knows the development and implementation of a client's plan of care by an interdisciplinary team is an example of which key element?**

   1. Efficient use of resources.
   2. Collaborative health cares delivery.
   3. Outcome orientation.
   4. Focus on health maintenance.

   1. *INCORRECT. Efficient use of resources is important, but this is not the best answer.*
   2. *CORRECT. A plan of care that integrates all care providers necessary for the client's care is an example of collaboration and cooperation between health professionals.*
   3. *INCORRECT.. A focus on planned outcomes for clients is part of case management, but this is not the best answer. The example focuses on the use of*

a team approach to care.

4. *INCORRECT. The example given focuses on the process of using a team approach to client care.*

49. **In 1992, the American Nurses' Association developed a proposal to address the needed changes in health care delivery. This proposal, "Nursing's Agenda for Health Care Reform," supports health care delivery that:**

    1. Is based in hospital settings.
    2. Is expanded and more expensive than the current system.
    3. Focuses on highly specialized care for select clients.
    4. Focuses on primary care delivered in community-based settings.

    1. *INCORRECT. Nursing proposes moving away from the high cost setting of the hospital.*
    2. *INCORRECT. Nursing proposes improving access to primary care with the hope of decreasing the use and expense of hospitalization for clients.*
    3. *INCORRECT. Nursing proposes the improvement of access to primary care. Highly specialized care is tertiary care that is highly expensive.*
    4. **CORRECT. *Nursing's Agenda for Health Care Reform proposes increased access to primary care in community based settings. Health maintenance and disease prevention are two aspects of primary care that can minimize the use of more expensive services.***

50. **The nurse is the case manager for a client who has been hospitalized for hip replacement surgery and will be moved to a skilled care facility for further physical therapy and rehabilitation. The nurse's responsibility as case manager in this situation is to:**

    1. Coordinate the transfer and communicate the plan of care to staff at the skilled care facility.
    2. Assist the family to transfer the client to the skilled care facility by private vehicle.
    3. Ensure that the client is fully recovered and able to participate in therapy.
    4. Submit client charges quickly to facilitate the billing process for hospital care.

    1. **CORRECT. *Case managers coordinate, communicate, and manage care across healthcare settings.***
    2. *INCORRECT. It would not be appropriate for someone with a recent hip replacement to be transferred from one facility to another by private vehicle. Getting in and out of the car and sitting with hips flexed at 90 degrees could cause dislocation of the artificial hip joint and be painful for the client.*

3. *INCORRECT. It is important to know that the client is capable of participation in therapy since this is the purpose of the skilled care, however full recovery will not occur in the hospital setting.*
4. *INCORRECT. Charges for care are generated from a variety of sources within the hospital setting. As case manager, the nurse's primary responsibility is the coordination of the care of the client.*

51. **A nurse functioning in the role of case manager has many roles. One of these is to support all members of the case team in working toward mutual goals. The nurse functioning in this role is termed the:**

    1. Educator.
    2. Coordinator.
    3. Facilitator.
    4. Negotiator.

    1. *INCORRECT. The educator role involves teaching the client, family, and other providers about the process of case management.*
    2. *INCORRECT. In the coordinator role, the nurse arranges for, monitors, and organizes the services that are needed by clients.*
    3. **CORRECT. *The facilitative role involves supporting all the members of the care team in setting and achieving mutual goals.***
    4. *INCORRECT. The negotiator role involves making negotiations for the plan of care, services and arrangements for payment for services.*

52. **Which client situation would the nurse know to be most likely handled by a case management approach to health care?**

    1. Post-op care of a client following laparoscopic cholecystectomy.
    2. Delivery of a full-term infant to a married woman.
    3. A client with residual problems following a cerebrovascular accident.
    4. A child with a fracture of his dominant arm.

    1. *INCORRECT. This procedure does not typically require the degree of management used in the case management approach to health care as long as no complications occur.*
    2. *INCORRECT. If no complications or social concerns exist, the delivery of an infant does not require case management.*
    3. **CORRECT. *A client with ongoing needs for care or rehabilitation is very likely to receive care that is directed by a case manager due to the complexity and cost of the client's needs.***
    4. *INCORRECT. This problem alone will not necessitate a case management approach.*

53. The nurse knows the best definition of a "critical path" that is used in the case management approach to the delivery of health care is a:

    1. Tool that outlines the important multidisciplinary actions that must occur to produce a desired outcome.
    2. Tool that legally binds the health care facility to provide services as outlined.
    3. Plan of care that focuses on nursing care only.
    4. Plan to ensure that care is as inexpensive as possible.

    1. *CORRECT. A critical path outlines the actions that all members of the health care team must complete in a timely manner in order to achieve desired client outcomes and an appropriate length of stay.*
    2. *INCORRECT. Critical paths do establish the standard of care in the institution, but variances from the path do occur due to a variety of reasons. Documentation of these variances is important, along with the revised plan to correct or address the variance. Critical paths are not "legal" documents.*
    3. *INCORRECT. Critical paths address appropriate nursing care, but also actions that other disciplines are responsible for. It is a holistic approach to the plan of care.*
    4. *INCORRECT. Control of cost is part of the reason for the development of critical paths, however this definition does not address the most important reasons for the use of critical paths.*

54. A nurse new to the intensive care unit identifies a fellow staff nurse who is respected for exceptional knowledge and skill in delivering care to critically ill clients. This nurse is also respected by other nurses, physicians, and administration. What is the source of this nurse's power?

    1. Legitimacy.
    2. Coercive.
    3. Expert.
    4. Charismatic.

    1. *INCORRECT. Legitimate power is related to the position that an individual holds within an organization.*
    2. *INCORRECT. Coercive power is used when fear of punishment from a superior occurs.*
    3. *CORRECT. This nurse is demonstrating expert power that is based on expertise in critical-care nursing practice.*
    4. *INCORRECT. Charismatic power is related to personal characteristics of an individual.*

55. The nurse is a member of a hospital-wide committee that has developed new documentation forms to meet Joint Commission of Accreditation of Hospital standards. The nurse understands the greatest barrier to successful implementation of these new forms involves:

    1. Approval of forms by nursing administration.
    2. Staff resistance to learning new charting forms and standards.
    3. The cost of staff education.
    4. The development of quality monitoring tools for compliance with new documentation.

    1. *INCORRECT. Approval for new documentation forms occurs as part of the process of development. In this situation, it is likely that administration will be supportive of the committee's work.*
    2. *CORRECT. Resistance to change is a frequently encountered problem when introducing new policies or procedures. Planning for change is an important part of this committee's work.*
    3. *INCORRECT. Staff education can be costly, but can be minimized by using various approaches to the educational process. This is not the biggest challenge.*
    4. *INCORRECT. Although it is important to monitor compliance with documentation standards, this is not the biggest challenge to successful implementation. It is part of the evaluation phase.*

56. A group of nurses is discussing how they feel about nursing. One nurse expresses discomfort and confusion because of nursing administration's expectation that nursing staff be accountable and make independent decisions and one physician's expectation that orders will be followed without question. This nurse is experiencing role:

    1. Ambiguity.
    2. Conflict.
    3. Overload.
    4. Incompetence.

    1. *INCORRECT. Role ambiguity occurs when roles are vague or inadequately defined.*
    2. *CORRECT. A conflict exists between the expected behaviors for the staff nurse from two sources of authority - nursing administration and the physician.*
    3. *INCORRECT. Role overload occurs when a role demands too much for an individual's resources.*
    4. *INCORRECT. Role incompetence occurs when the nurse does not have the knowledge or skills for the task or expectation.*

57. The nurse has interviewed for a position on a medical-surgical unit. The nurse's best action following the interview is to:

1. Wait for the interviewer to contact you regarding a possible job offer.
2. Seek input from staff members on the unit about your chances for getting the job.
3. Send a note of thanks to the interviewer.
4. Make daily phone calls to check if a decision has been made.

1. *INCORRECT. Waiting without making any further contact may be viewed as a lack of interest.*
2. *INCORRECT. This would be inappropriate, and staff members may only be able to OFFER speculation. There is nothing to be gained by bypassing the person who makes the decision.*
3. **CORRECT. Send a note of thanks. Include comments about continued interest in the position and any other information that needs to be reinforced or relayed to the nurse manager.**
4. *INCORRECT. This would be annoying to the nurse manager. Try to establish at the end of the interview what time frame exists for the decision.*

58. **Which comment would be appropriate to make when attempting to resolve a conflict with a fellow nurse:**

1. "You are always late getting back from break and don't do your fair share of the work."
2. "I don't want to discuss this now. I'm going to let the nurse manager know about it."
3. "You are totally inconsiderate of my feelings about getting Christmas off."
4. "I need to talk to you about the unit policies regarding break time."

1. *INCORRECT. This is an inflammatory statement that, although it might be true, will only cause more barriers to the resolution of the conflict.*
2. *INCORRECT. Delaying conflict resolution or involving superiors without first attempting to resolve the problem can set up adversarial feelings. It is best to attempt to resolve most problems first before going to the nurse manager.*
3. *INCORRECT. This statement is based from one perspective only. It is accusatory and would erect barriers to discussion of the problem of holiday staffing.*
4. **CORRECT. This statement opens the conversation in a non-threatening way. The focus is on the issue of length of break time rather than on any personal characteristic of the individual.**

59. **A nurse is evaluating the performance of the nurse manager. Some of the behaviors that the nurse manager has displayed include establishment of staff nurse committees to address unit issues, an open-door policy for talking about concerns, and supportiveness of the professional development of all the staff. The nurse understands these behaviors reflect a management style that is:**

1. Autocratic.
2. Laissez-faire.
3. Democratic.
4. Simplistic.

1. *INCORRECT. An autocratic management style is characterized by behaviors such as making all decisions without staff input, focus on completion of tasks, and limited access to communication with the manager.*
2. *INCORRECT. The laissez-faire manager provides little structure or direction to the group.*
3. **CORRECT. These behaviors represent a manager who values the professional status and input of the members of the staff. This does not mean that all decisions are made by committee. There are situations that will be identified as being within the nurse manager's domain for decision making.**
4. *INCORRECT. This is not a recognized style of management.*

60. **The nurse is interested in supporting a health-related bill that is due to be addressed by the state legislature. Which statement would be appropriate to include in a letter to the state legislator?**

1. "Although many nurses don't agree on how to improve client care, I think that we need more funds for hospital equipment."
2. "As the president of my local nursing society, I can promise that all our members will vote for you in the next election."
3. "I will expect to hear from you by the end of the week. I know that you will support this bill as I do."
4. "I would like to request your support of State Bill 132 regarding appropriations for rural health clinic funding."

1. *INCORRECT. Regardless of disagreements within the nursing profession, it is best to not point this out to legislators. It makes it seem that there is not unified support of a particular issue.*
2. *INCORRECT. Do not make promises that you haven't any power to keep.*
3. *INCORRECT. This places a demand on a busy legislator. It is better to express a willingness to talk further with the legislator without placing an expectation.*
4. **CORRECT. This is a very appropriate opening sentence for the letter. Make sure to refer to the bill by number and topic. Keep the letter concise and to the point. Be sure to give reasons why the bill should or should not be passed and what the impact of the bill is on the legislator's constituency.**

61. **A nurse has recently noticed that one of the physicians makes suggestive comments whenever they are together. These comments make the nurse uncomfortable. The nurse's first action in this situation is to:**

    1. Tell the physician that the comments create an uncomfortable environment and request that they be stopped.
    2. Report the complaint to the immediate nursing supervisor.
    3. To make a formal complaint to the medical board of the facility.
    4. To ignore the comments and try to stay away from this physician.

    1. CORRECT. The first step in dealing with any behavior from another person that makes you uncomfortable is to tell them that you find this inappropriate and that you expect them to stop that behavior. Share how you are dealing with this problem with friends or family. You may want to put this statement in writing also and make sure to keep a copy.
    2. INCORRECT. This may be a step in the formal process of filing a complaint about someone's behavior, but it is not the first action that should be taken.
    3. INCORRECT. This could result in punitive action against the physician. It is best to give the physician the opportunity to realize the comments are not welcomed and to correct the behavior before making a formal complaint.
    4. INCORRECT. Trying to avoid the physician is likely to be difficult.

62. **Negotiation is a technique used to manage conflict. The nurse recognizes the ultimate goal of the negotiation process is to:**

    1. Win all of the concessions desired from the other party.
    2. Establish equality in the concessions that each party makes.
    3. Make as many concessions as needed to make everyone happy.
    4. Create a solution in which both parties are satisfied.

    1. INCORRECT. It is generally a good idea to have some "expendable" items that can be conceded without endangering the basic goal. Going into a negotiation with the attitude that you must win all the desired concessions will set you up for disappointment and can lead to a breakdown in the communication process that is essential for negotiation.
    2. INCORRECT. It is not necessary for balance or

    equality in concessions made by the parties during a negotiation. Often this is unrealistic or impossible.
    3. INCORRECT. Trying to please everyone by making concessions may leave you in a worse position than when you started.
    4. CORRECT. The goal of negotiation is to create a "win-win" situation in which both parties are satisfied with results.

63. **Many healthcare organizations expect nurses to function as a team member or leader in a variety of ways. Which behavior by the nurse would be detrimental to the formation of a team atmosphere?**

    1. Establishment of common goals with input from members of the team.
    2. Clarifying the boundaries of the team when acting as leader.
    3. Quickly deciding if member ideas have value or not.
    4. Actively listening to each member's input.

    1. INCORRECT. This is an essential aspect of team building. All members must understand and commit to the goals that have been established by the group.
    2. INCORRECT. When acting in the leader role, this is one of the actions or behaviors that may be necessary in order to keep the team on course.
    3. CORRECT. Every idea generated by the team should be given consideration as a possible solution or action to be taken. Dismissing ideas quickly without consideration can result in a member feeling devalued and, therefore, less likely to present their ideas in the future. Open communication and respect are essential for team function.
    4. INCORRECT. Team building is supported by active listening skills.

64. **The nurse is admitting a client with a medical diagnosis of lower gastrointestinal bleeding. Which task would be appropriate to delegate to a certified nursing assistant?**

    1. Taking vital signs.
    2. Listening for bowel sounds.
    3. Adjusting the rate of the intravenous infusion.
    4. Explaining the plan of care to client and family.

    1. CORRECT. Taking vital signs is a task that is appropriate for a certified nursing assistant to perform. It is a task that is included in the education necessary for certification.
    2. INCORRECT. This is an essential assessment for a client with this diagnosis. This requires the nurse's own attention.

3. INCORRECT. *Dealing with intravenous lines and fluids is a task that should be done by the nurse. There are a variety of assessments and techniques that are necessary for this task.*

4. INCORRECT. *Education of clients and their families is a primary nursing function. The nursing assistant will not have adequate information or ability to explain the plan of care.*

65. **The nurse has asked a nursing assistant to ambulate an elderly client. While walking, the client becomes dizzy and falls, fracturing a hip. The nurse understands that who is accountable for this injury to the client?**

    1. The client.
    2. The hospital.
    3. The nurse.
    4. The nursing assistant.

    1. INCORRECT. *The client is not accountable for falling.*

    2. INCORRECT. *Although the hospital might be held accountable for injuries if litigation occurs because of this injury, this accountability is primarily related to having ensured staff competency and adequacy for client care.*

    3. CORRECT. *The nurse is responsible and accountable for correct delegation. This includes the right task delegated to the right person with adequate communication about specific expectations for performance. The nurse's assessment of the client's condition and ability to ambulate would guide what information would be conveyed to the nursing assistant.*

    4. INCORRECT. *Although the nursing assistant does carry some accountability, it is the nurse's primary responsibility for the care delivered by assisting personnel.*

66. **The nurse wants to delegate a client care task to a nursing assistant. Which explanation by the nurse of the expectations for the completion of that task is most appropriate?**

    1. "Please do vital signs on all the clients we are caring for today."
    2. "Please change the client's abdominal dressing before 10 am today."
    3. "I have this medication for the client, would you mind making sure that it is taken after breakfast? Let me know if the client's heart rate is above 100."
    4. "The client will need to ambulate three times today and sit in the chair for 30 minutes during meal times. It requires two people to get the client out of bed and make sure the client uses a walker."

    1. INCORRECT. *This gives very vague direction about the frequency for each client and parameters for reporting findings.*

2. INCORRECT. *Changing an abdominal dressing will also require the assessment of the wound. This task should not be delegated to the nursing assistant.*

3. INCORRECT. *This would violate a basic principle of medication administration. Medications can only be administered by a licensed caregiver. This task is not appropriate for the nursing assistant.*

4. CORRECT. *These directions give the type of task to be done, the frequency and duration, and information about the mechanics of ambulating the client.*

67. **The R.N. has been working with a Licensed Practical Nurse who gives excellent nursing care to clients and is an effective team member. Which would be the best initial action by the R.N. to recognize the L.P.N.'s contributions to care?**

    1. Give feedback directly to the L.P.N.
    2. Tell other staff how lucky you are to have the L.P.N. as part of your client care team.
    3. Nominate the L.P.N. for Employee of the Month.
    4. Detail the L.P.N.'s contributions to your nurse manager.

    1. CORRECT. *The best way to recognize someone's abilities and contributions is through direct feedback to that person. Direct communication of both positive and negative feedback fosters teamwork.*

    2. INCORRECT. *Although this is not inappropriate, the other staff members are not the ones who need to hear feedback on the L.P.N.'s performance.*

    3. INCORRECT. *It may be that this would be a well-deserved honor for the L.P.N., but would not be the initial action.*

    4. INCORRECT. *The nurse manager will likely welcome positive comments about staff members and even seek input as part of the employee evaluation process. However, this is not the initial action.*

68. **The nurse is working with a nursing assistant in a long-term care facility. What assessment must the nurse make before delegating an appropriate task to this nursing assistant?**

    1. The client's willingness to consent to the care of the nursing assistant.
    2. The degree and frequency of supervision that the nursing assistant will require to complete the task.
    3. Whether the task can be more efficiently completed yourself.
    4. The federal regulations regarding functions of unlicensed assistive personnel in long term care facilities.

    1. INCORRECT. *The types of tasks that should be delegated to the nursing assistant would not require the client's consent.*

2. *CORRECT. Any time that a task is delegated, the nurse must assess how much supervision or periodic inspection the individual requires based on the task, their individual abilities and experience, and the client situation. Successful delegation involves the right task to the right person with the right communication of expectations and the right feedback on performance.*

3. *INCORRECT. One of the barriers to successful delegation is the belief that you are the only one that can do a task efficiently and effectively.*

4. *INCORRECT. The choice of tasks to delegate will be impacted by regulations for accreditation and licensing of long term care facilities. The right task is only part of the process of appropriate delegation.*

69. **A nurse is being oriented to a new position as a staff nurse in the intensive care unit and would like feedback from the preceptor. What is the nurse's best action at this time?**

1. Wait for the preceptor to initiate a performance review.
2. Request input from the preceptor on a regular basis.
3. Ask other staff what the preceptor has said.
4. Check with the nurse manager about a performance evaluation.

1. *INCORRECT. Waiting for feedback will hinder the ability to correlate performance with appropriate corrections or to reinforce positive performance. Feedback is most effective when it is given frequently and timely.*

2. *CORRECT. If uncomfortable with the amount of feedback being received, initiate a discussion with the preceptor. This helps to open lines of communication and may lead to a plan for regular, scheduled feedback to occur.*

3. *INCORRECT. This could undermine the relationship with the preceptor and can lead to misunderstandings due to other staff's interpretation of the nurse's performance or comments that have been made.*

4. *INCORRECT. The preceptor is supervising the orientation and is responsible for giving feedback. Going to the nurse manager may undermine the relationship with the preceptor.*

70. **The nurse completed a variance report after administering an incorrect dose of a medication to a client. The client did not have any ill effects from the medication error. What is the purpose of the nurse completing a variance report in this situation?**

1. To identify situations that contribute to the occurrence of medication errors.

2. To track employee performance for possible disciplinary action.
3. To alert hospital administration of a possible litigation situation.
4. To gather data for statistical analysis.

1. *CORRECT. The purpose of completing variance reports is to identify factors that contributed to the occurrence of the problem. This is part of quality improvement efforts in health care facilities.*

2. *INCORRECT. Using variance reports as a means for employee discipline will hinder reporting of problems and inhibit the finding of solutions to improve quality of client care.*

3. *INCORRECT. It is not likely that litigation will occur in a situation in which no injury occurred. This is not the primary purpose of variance reports.*

4. *INCORRECT. Much of the information on variance reports can be analyzed using statistics, but this is not the primary purpose of variance reports. The data is a tool for a bigger purpose.*

71. **A client who received a sedative-hypnotic medication at bedtime becomes confused during the night. The client gets out of bed and falls, sustaining a laceration that requires suturing. Which statement would be included as part of the nurse's documentation in the client's chart?**

1. "Client fell due to confusion caused by sleeping medication."
2. "Client found lying on the floor in a pool of blood. Nursing assistant forgot to put siderails up at bedtime."
3. "Client found sitting on the floor. 3 cm laceration above left eyebrow. Oriented to name only."
4. "Client slipped in water on floor caused by leaking faucet that was reported to the maintenance department two days ago."

1. *INCORRECT. This statement draws a conclusion about why the client fell. Although sedative-hypnotics can cause confusion, it would be inappropriate to make the assumption that the medication is the cause.*

2. *INCORRECT. This statement includes an imprecise comment "pool of blood" that is open to interpretation. It also places blame on the nursing assistant. This is not appropriate.*

3. *CORRECT. This statement presents some of the facts and assessments related to this event. The nurse would also include vital signs, further assessments, notification of physician, treatments or procedures done per physician orders, and client's response.*

4. *INCORRECT. This statement draws a conclusion about the cause of the client's fall and includes an inflammatory statement about the maintenance department's response. Remember that the chart*

should focus on the client's condition, not institutional / departmental problems.

72. **Which situations would require the completion of a variance or incident report by the nurse?**

    1. A disagree with the medical care ordered by the physician.
    2. A dispute with a co-worker about client assignments.
    3. The identification of a safety concern with a piece of equipment used on a regular basis.
    4. The discovery that a pre-op client has received and eaten a breakfast tray.

    1. *INCORRECT. A variance report would not address this problem in a timely manner. Be aware of the proper procedure in your institution for pursuing concerns about adequacy and appropriateness of medical care.*
    2. *INCORRECT. This is a staff problem that should be resolved between the co-workers if possible with possible mediation by the nurse manager.*
    3. *INCORRECT. If a safety concern with a piece of equipment is identified, remove that piece of equipment from use and follow the facility's procedure for placing a work order for repair of the equipment. If equipment actually causes an injury to a person, then a variance report would be appropriate.*
    4. **CORRECT. This situation represents a variation from the standard of care and will cause a change in the plan of care for this client due to the need to delay the surgical procedure.**

73. **The nurse is notified by a hospital attorney that a client has filed a lawsuit against the hospital because of a fall sustained while in the hospital. The nurse was caring for the client at the time of the fall and completed a variance report about the incident. The nurse's variance report:**

    1. Can be subpoenaed by the plaintiff's attorney.
    2. Can only be used by the hospital attorneys as a privileged communication.
    3. Will not be an important part of the case.
    4. Is a part of the nurse's personnel file that cannot be subpoenaed.

    1. *INCORRECT. As long as the variance report was not placed in the client record, it is not a document that can be subpoenaed.*
    2. **CORRECT. Variance reports are a privileged communication between an employee and the administration of the institution. It supplies the hospital attorney with information regarding the incident in question. The general purpose of variance reports is for quality improvement.**

    3. *INCORRECT. The variance report is an important for the hospital attorney. This report gives pertinent information about the incident.*
    4. *INCORRECT. Variance reports should not be placed in the employee's personnel file, which may be subpoenaed by the plaintiff's lawyer.*

74. **The focus of the advocate role of the professional nurse is on:**

    1. Making decisions for clients when they are unable.
    2. Placing a high priority on the client's rights.
    3. Getting the most complete and complex care for the client.
    4. Identifying the nurse's feelings about client situations.

    1. *INCORRECT. A member of the health care team cannot legally make decisions for clients under most circumstances.*
    2. **CORRECT. Advocacy involves actions that support maintenance or development of client's rights.**
    3. *INCORRECT. As advocates, nurses work to provide care that supports clients' wishes for their own care. This may not always be the most complex or complete care that is possible in a given client situation.*
    4. *INCORRECT. As an advocate, the nurse focuses on the client, not personal feelings about the client's situation.*

75. **Communication is an essential skill for the nurse acting as an advocate. When the nurse says to the client, "Let me see if I understand what you mean....," the nurse is involved in the process of:**

    1. Verification.
    2. Amplification.
    3. Clarification.
    4. Affirming.

    1. *INCORRECT. The process of verification involves establishing the accuracy and reality of the information the client has been given.*
    2. *INCORRECT. Amplification involves an exploration of the needs and demands of the client that will impact the decision process.*
    3. **CORRECT. Clarification is a communication process that strives to ensure that the nurse and client understand the same meanings for events and processes.**
    4. *INCORRECT. Affirming is the process of validating that the client's decision or behavior is congruent with the client's belief system.*

76. **One of the biggest challenges facing nurses who want to act as a client advocate is:**

1. Dealing with their own reactions to client decisions that conflict with the nurse's personal belief system.
2. A lack of reimbursement for activities involved in this role.
3. A lack of time to spend with clients.
4. Dealing with conflicts that can arise with other health care providers.

1. *CORRECT. An essential attribute of the nurse acting in the advocate role is being open-minded. The focus is on supporting the client's decisions regardless of the nurse's personal beliefs about what the decision should be. Client self-determination is the priority.*
2. *INCORRECT. The advocate role should not be viewed as separate from other aspects of nursing care.*
3. *INCORRECT. Time management problems can lead to barriers to acting as an advocate. This isn't the biggest challenge to the nurse's success as a client advocate.*
4. *INCORRECT. Although dealing with the reactions of other health care providers can be a challenge, it is an expected part of the advocacy role. This is not the biggest challenge to the nurse's success as an advocate.*

77. **Which statement is true regarding nurses' opportunities to act in an advocate role?**

1. Advocacy does not involve any personal or professional risks.
2. Advocacy is a new concept in nursing, becoming important in the last 20 years.
3. Power base has no impact on the effectiveness of the nurse in the advocate role.
4. Interpreting information for clients is an example of advocacy.

1. *INCORRECT. Advocacy does involve some personal and professional risk. Advocates can sometimes be viewed as troublemakers by others. Personal risk involves conflicts with the nurse's personal belief system and a need to be well informed.*
2. *INCORRECT. Advocacy has been part of nursing since the early 1900's. Some of the issues and settings have changed, but the essence of nursing's commitment has not changed.*
3. *INCORRECT. Power and authority of the individual nurse and of the nursing staff in a particular institution directly impacts the success and effectiveness of the nurse's advocacy attempts.*
4. *CORRECT. As an advocate, nurses interpret information for clients and their families so that they can make informed decisions. This is a good example of a nursing action that is based in the advocate role.*

78. **The nurse's role in developing a continuum of care for a group of case managed clients involves:**

1. Ensuring that care the nurse personally delivers meets all standards of care.
2. Focusing on outcomes and the client's movement through various settings and services.
3. Making suggestions to other professions regarding the client's care.
4. Personally performing all aspects of the client's care.

1. *INCORRECT. The care delivered by an individual nurse is one part of the continuum. A focus on this alone will not address continuity.*
2. *CORRECT. Nurses focus on outcomes and the client's "journey" through services and settings when addressing continuity of care.*
3. *INCORRECT. Communication is an essential part of maintaining continuity of care, but it is only one part. The nursing focus is broader.*
4. *INCORRECT. This would not be realistic and would not provide the best possible service to the client.*

79. **Maintaining a continuum of care is dependent on a variety of factors. Which factor does the nurse understand to be the most important?**

1. Development of a multidisciplinary and multi agency plan that addresses the desired outcomes for the client.
2. Assessing the client's progress on a monthly basis.
3. Accessing community resources early in the process.
4. Keeping accurate assessments and documentation.

1. *CORRECT. The most important factor in the successful maintenance of continuity of care is to have a plan that includes all disciplines and agencies that are appropriate to this client's care and that are needed to achieve desired outcomes.*
2. *INCORRECT. Frequency of client progress assessments will vary depending on the stage of care that is being delivered and the individual needs of the client.*
3. *INCORRECT. Awareness and communication with community resources will enable caregivers to plan effectively for the care of the client, but will be accessed when needed within the broader framework of that plan.*
4. *INCORRECT. It is important to keep accurate assessments and documentation, but this does not necessarily ensure that continuity is maintained.*

80. **Which statement does the nurse know to be true about the concept of continuum of care?**

1. It is a mandated standard of care that applies to all clients admitted to health care facilities.
2. It only involves members of the various health professions.
3. Each service is provided independent of other services.
4. It is a comprehensive, client-oriented system of care.

1. *INCORRECT. The continuum of care is not mandated and it involves more than care delivered in health care facilities.*
2. *INCORRECT. Continuity of care integrates services from a variety of sources, both within health professions and community organizations and volunteers.*
3. *INCORRECT. Services across the continuum of care are integrated and interdependent.*
4. **CORRECT. Continuum of care is an integrated, client-oriented system of care that includes comprehensive services from health care, mental health, social services, and community resources.**

81. **A client presents to the neighborhood health clinic frequently with complaints of depression. The nurse discovers the client's involvement in an emotionally abusive relationship. The client feels trapped by the situation and does not know where to get help. The nurse's best action to meet this client's need is to:**

1. Continue to talk to the client about the manifestations of the depression.
2. Make a referral to the local organization that assists those in abusive relationships.
3. Make regular appointments for the client at the clinic.
4. Refer the client to the local emergency department for examination.

1. *INCORRECT. Although this is appropriate to do, it does not address the client's need for help with the abusive relationship, which may be part of the cause of the depression.*
2. **CORRECT. Battered spouse's groups have special training and support networks for assisting those involved in abusive relationships.**
3. *INCORRECT. Although the client may need further appointments for counseling for the depression, this does not address the need for specific help with the abusive relationship.*
4. *INCORRECT. If there are physical injuries, this would be appropriate. The health clinic is able to refer to appropriate agencies. An emergency room visit is not necessary.*

82. **A client has paraplegia and has become withdrawn and resistant to rehabilitative efforts of the staff.**

The best nursing intervention for this client would be:

1. Allow the client to direct and control the timing and frequency of the therapy.
2. Limit visiting hours until the client begins to want to be social with others.
3. Consult with a staff psychologist or psychiatric clinical nurse specialist.
4. Inform the client that privileges are related to willingness to perform therapy.

1. *INCORRECT. This would be harmful if the client elects to minimize or eliminate aspects of the therapy.*
2. *INCORRECT. Limiting visiting hours may only increase the client's withdrawn affect. Imposing social isolation is not appropriate.*
3. **CORRECT. It is a good idea to access someone with a greater knowledge about the psychological impact of such a life-changing injury for evaluation and development of a plan of care for the client.**
4. *INCORRECT. This response does not address the holistic need of the client. This statement made in isolation of a complete plan of care would not be enforceable and may be interpreted as punitive.*

83. **The nurse is discharging a client with congestive heart failure after making a referral for follow up with a community health agency. The ultimate goal for this client receiving care from a public health nursing agency will focus on:**

1. Assistance with personal care.
2. Adequate nutrition.
3. Proper immunization.
4. Client independence.

1. *INCORRECT. Assistance with personal cares may occur, but this is not the goal of a public health nursing agency.*
2. *INCORRECT. Adequate nutrition will likely be assessed and interventions planned, but this is not the ultimate goal in public health nursing.*
3. *INCORRECT. Immunizations are one of the services that public health agencies often supply, but this is not the focus in this situation.*
4. **CORRECT. Client independence is the ultimate goal in public health nursing. Interventions are planned that support this goal.**

84. **The nurses working on the unit have identified the need for updating the cardiac monitoring system so that arrhythmia detection can be increased for the safety of the clients. The nurse manager realizes this type of expenditure for equipment:**

1. Is not feasible in the current cost-conscious era of health care.
2. Will need to be addressed in the capital budget plan for the unit.
3. Will result in a reduction in the personnel budget and possible loss of staff positions.
4. Is totally reimbursed by Medicare funds since these clients will benefit from the equipment.

1. *INCORRECT. Although cost is a concern, if the equipment currently being used does not meet current standards of providing care, it is likely that the institution will not resist this expenditure as long as it is included in the budget.*
2. **CORRECT. The capital budget plans for the expenditure of monies for equipment and major purchases that have a long life of use.**
3. *INCORRECT. Personnel budgets are separate from the budget for expenditures for equipment or other major purchases. If the entire budget is managed well, there should be no need for reductions in any one budget.*
4. *INCORRECT. Medicare funds do not reimburse institutions for equipment purchases, regardless if clients on Medicare use the equipment or not. Charges for use of equipment are submittable to Medicare.*

85. **When asked to explain how a health maintenance organization charges for its services. The nurse's best answer is:**

1. Services are billed based on the client's ability to pay.
2. Clients are required to pay for all routine services completely out of their own pocket.
3. A predetermined set of services is provided for a fixed, prepaid charge.
4. Only charges incurred while an inpatient will be covered by an HMO.

1. *INCORRECT. Ability to pay does not factor into the billing practices of HMO's.*
2. *INCORRECT. Participants in an HMO are encouraged to access routine health screenings and maintenance care. These are typically covered by the plan.*
3. **CORRECT. The HMO establishes the specific services that are covered at a fixed level of reimbursement to the provider and cost to the participant.**
4. *INCORRECT. HMO's focus on preventative services and health maintenance and will pay for these services and inpatient costs.*

86. **One way nurses can contribute to resource management is by:**

1. Discouraging clients from requesting extra personal services.

2. Taking heavier client assignments so that fewer staff members are needed.
3. Working extra shifts without accepting overtime pay.
4. Documenting care delivered and equipment used in the chart.

1. *INCORRECT. This could have a negative impact on quality of client care and public image of the institution. These actions are counterproductive in resource management.*
2. *INCORRECT. This acceptance of heavier client loads could jeopardize client safety and decrease the quality of care.*
3. *INCORRECT. Personal sacrifice does not equate with effective resource management and may maintain a paternalistic relationship between the facility and the nursing staff.*
4. **CORRECT. Reimbursement for care and equipment is linked to the appropriate documentation of care delivered and what equipment was used.**

87. **The nurse is caring for a client who is openly homosexual and has contracted AIDS. Which action by the nurse help provide the best care possible for this client?**

1. Keep contact with the client very straightforward and businesslike.
2. Privately explore personal attitudes about sexuality.
3. Share care of this client with several other nurses to minimize the potential risk of contracting HIV.
4. Place the client in isolation to prevent transmission of the disease.

1. *INCORRECT. This approach to the client will inhibit the nurse's ability to care for the client in a holistic manner. Being "businesslike" can limit discussion of the emotional, spiritual, and psychological impact of this client's condition.*
2. **CORRECT. Being aware of personal attitudes and feelings about homosexuality as a sexual choice is important to providing care for this client. The personal belief system of the nurse may affect the way that care is delivered.**
3. *INCORRECT. The use of universal precautions is the nurse's best defense against contracting any illness from a client. Sharing the care of this client for the reason of minimizing exposure to the client impedes the development of a nurse-client therapeutic relationship.*
4. *INCORRECT. Universal precautions are the best way to decrease the chance of transmission of HIV. Some clients with AIDS may need to be placed in protective isolation to prevent infections due to an impaired immune response.*

88. The nurse is developing health promotion programs for clients in a community setting. Which of the following would be least appropriate for the nurse to include in these programs?

    1. Reducing genetic risk factors for illness.
    2. Providing information about health maintenance choices.
    3. Fostering of positive life-style changes.
    4. Optimizing mental health.

    1. *CORRECT. Many genetic risk factors for illness cannot be reduced. Identification of genetic risk factors is a focus of disease prevention.*
    2. *INCORRECT. This is one of the focuses of health promotion—providing information, skills, services, and support to people so that they can make positive life-style changes.*
    3. *INCORRECT. This is a focus of health promotion—life-style changes that positively impact the quality of physical, mental, and social health.*
    4. *INCORRECT. This is a focus of health promotion—a holistic perspective of health.*

89. The nurse is planning interventions for a group of overweight teenage girls. What can the nurse do to best improve commitment to a long-term goal for weight loss for these clients?

    1. Involve family members in the process.
    2. Keep detailed records of each girl's progress.
    3. Use a system of rewards for reinforcement of behavior.
    4. Attempt to develop self-motivation.

    1. *INCORRECT. Although family support can be important, this will not necessarily improve commitment to long-term goals.*
    2. *INCORRECT. This will help each girl to track her progress, but is not the best way to increase commitment.*
    3. *INCORRECT. Rewards can be used and may be helpful, extrinsic rewards do not help with long-term goal commitment.*
    4. *CORRECT. Long-term commitment to life-style changes is based in intrinsic motivation. The individual must choose to take the actions necessary for health changes.*

90. As a nurse is developing a plan of care for a client, what consideration should be given to the spiritual aspects of the client?

    1. Many clients are not receptive to spiritual support from health care providers.
    2. It should not be assumed that spiritual needs are important to every client.
    3. During illness or stress, clients and their families often have fewer spiritual needs.
    4. Spirituality is an essential need for humans.

    1. *INCORRECT. Don't confuse religion and spirituality. Spiritual support focuses on the values and meanings of the client's experiences.*
    2. *INCORRECT. Spiritual needs are not the same as religious affiliation. Spiritual needs address the values, meanings, and purposes that are important to the client.*
    3. *INCORRECT. Spiritual needs will vary between clients but will often be greater during times of stress or when there are challenges to the client's spirituality.*
    4. *CORRECT. Spirituality refers to the values, meanings, and purposes that clients and families attach to events in their lives. Spirituality should not be confused with religion. All humans have a spiritual component. A failure to address the spiritual aspects of the client would be a failure to address the holistic nature of the person.*

91. The nurse is caring for a client diagnosed with a terminal illness. The client asks several questions about the nurse's religious beliefs related to death and dying. The nurse's best response to this request is to:

    1. Tell the client that religious beliefs are a personal matter.
    2. Change the topic since the client is obviously trying to divert attention from the illness.
    3. Encourage the client to express personal thoughts about death and dying.
    4. Offer to contact the client's minister or the hospital chaplain.

    1. *INCORRECT. This type of response will erect a barrier to communication with this client about a topic of concern. What could the nurse say to open communication without sharing personal information?*
    2. *INCORRECT. This response does not address the underlying concern of this client and will erect barriers to development of open communication between the nurse and the client.*
    3. *CORRECT. Depending on the situation, the nurse may want to share some thoughts on this topic. Self-disclosure is a communication skill that can help to open lines of communication. If the nurse does not want to share personal beliefs, this client's need to talk about impending death can still be recognized, and the client can be encouraged to discuss any thoughts on the subject.*
    4. *INCORRECT. It may be appropriate to offer this to the client, but the client has initiated a communication with the nurse that needs to be attended to. The opportunity to discuss such an important issue to the client should not be delayed. This response could also cause barriers to communication between the nurse and the client.*

92. A nursing diagnosis of spiritual distress has been made for a client with advanced acquired immune deficiency syndrome (AIDS). The nurse recognizes which behavior to be inconsistent with this diagnosis?

   1. A desire to become closer to God and requests that you call a minister.
   2. Frequent crying and trouble sleeping at night.
   3. The client's statement that, "God has let me down. I don't believe He hears me."
   4. Feeling apathetic about the disease and its progression.

   1. *CORRECT. This statement reflects that the client is aware of her spiritual needs and an action to address that need.*
   2. *INCORRECT. Spiritual distress is sometimes manifested by difficulty sleeping and bouts of crying.*
   3. *INCORRECT. This statement reflects anger at God. This is one of the behaviors exhibited by clients experiencing spiritual distress.*
   4. *INCORRECT. Apathy is a manifestation of spiritual distress that clients can exhibit.*

93. When caring for clients who practice Orthodox Judaism, the nurse would recognize that all of the foods on the dinner tray sent from dietary to be appropriate except:

   1. Macaroni and cheese, milk, and peas.
   2. Carrot sticks and cottage cheese.
   3. Kosher roast beef and ice cream.
   4. Kosher chicken breast and boiled potatoes.

   1. *INCORRECT. This combination of foods would be appropriate for a client practicing kosher dietary restrictions.*
   2. *INCORRECT. This would be an appropriate combination of foods.*
   3. *CORRECT. Kosher dietary restrictions prohibit mixing of meat and milk products at the same meal.*
   4. *INCORRECT. These are appropriate foods. Any meat must be slaughtered according to kosher regulations.*

94. The nurse knows a client who is a devote Seventh Day Adventist will feel most comfortable if:

   1. Allowed to have a crucifix in the room.
   2. A Bible is available for scripture readings.
   3. Assigned a room with a windows facing east.
   4. Assigned a private room.

   1. *INCORRECT. A crucifix depicts the body of Jesus Christ on the cross. This is a religious symbol of the Catholic faith.*

   2. *CORRECT. Having a Bible available for scripture reading is important to members of this faith.*
   3. *INCORRECT. The direction the room faces is not important to members of this faith.*
   4. *INCORRECT. Although individuals may prefer to be in a private room, it is not related to the religious orientation of the person.*

95. A female client presents to the emergency department following a motor vehicle collision and the nurse learns the client is a Jehovah's Witness. The nurse is aware that this causes a concern in this situation because the client will:

   1. Insist on having family in the room at all times.
   2. Not consent to any surgical interventions for the sustained injuries.
   3. Not consent to any necessary blood transfusions.
   4. Not allow herself to be undressed and examined by a male physician.

   1. *INCORRECT. This isn't a behavior that is related to the client's faith.*
   2. *INCORRECT. Jehovah Witnesses will consent to surgical procedures as needed for injuries.*
   3. *CORRECT. As a Jehovah's Witness, this client will believe that blood transfusions violate God's laws and will not be likely to consent to a transfusion if needed.*
   4. *INCORRECT. This behavior is not related to the fact that the client is a Jehovah's Witness.*

96. The nurse is talking to a resident of the long-term care facility who has returned from an overnight stay with his son and his wife. Which statement made by the resident would most warrant further investigation by the nurse for elder abuse?

   1. "We had a nice visit. My grandchildren are a little unruly, but I enjoy that—in small doses!"
   2. "The food wasn't very good. My daughter-in-law never was a good cook."
   3. "Those bruises aren't anything. I get really clumsy at my son's house."
   4. "They needed a new TV, so we went out and I bought them a new one for Christmas."

   1. *INCORRECT. This statement is a fairly typical response of grandparents to behavior of grandchildren.*
   2. *INCORRECT. Being a bad cook does not constitute abuse. Inadequate or inappropriate food can be a sign of neglect in some situations in which the elderly person is dependent on a caregiver for supplying food.*
   3. *CORRECT. The presence of bruises that were not present before the client left the nursing home could indicate abuse. The elderly who are physi-*

cally abused will often refer to themselves as "clumsy" or "accident prone". Assess and interview this client. Make sure to document any findings.

4. *INCORRECT. Although financial abuse does occur, buying a gift for family members is something that the anyone may do. If the nurse sees a pattern of spending in a resident without the financial resources, or if the resident does not have money for their own personal needs because of spending money on family members, then the nurse should do further assessments of the situation.*

97. The nurse is interviewing an elderly client that may have been abused by a neighbor who provides much of the care for this person. The nurse's interview questions should:

1. Not directly ask if the client has ever been hurt by someone.
2. Be confrontational.
3. Be nonthreatening and nonjudgmental.
4. Include as much information as possible.

1. *INCORRECT. Interview questions should be direct. Although this is not the first question that should be asked, at some point in the interview the nurse will need to directly ask if the client has been hurt by someone.*
2. *INCORRECT. Being confrontational can set up defensive barriers to further discussion.*
3. ***CORRECT. This tone to the nurse's questions will give offer the best chance of keeping communication open with the client and getting the information needed to make an accurate assessment of this client's situation.***
4. *INCORRECT. Making questions too complex or information loaded can confuse the client and make the questions difficult to answer.*

98. Which behavior indicates to the nurse a neglect of an elderly client by a caregiver?

1. A family member refuses to leave the nurse alone with the elderly client for an examination.
2. An elderly client hasn't been taking necessary medications because the prescriptions have not been filled by the family member.
3. An elderly client is brought to the clinic for a 3-month checkup by a family member.
4. The caregiver speaks to the elderly client in an angry, berating way.

1. *INCORRECT. This type of behavior is most often noted in persons who have physically abused an elderly member of the family.*
2. ***CORRECT. Neglect occurs when a need of the client is not being met by the caregiver. In this***

case, it would be expected that the caregiver would ensure that the prescriptions be filled. This can occur due to ignorance or inattention on the part of the caregiver.

3. *INCORRECT. This behavior would reflect that the family member is assisting the client with transportation.*
4. *INCORRECT. This behavior would indicate that psychological abuse is occurring.*

99. The nurse recognizes that there is potential for physical and psychological abuse of elderly residents in nursing homes. The nurse's best action is to:

1. Ensure staff members who work on the nurse's shift are closely monitored for any inappropriate behavior towards residents.
2. Keep staff members who tend to have a temper away from clients who suffer from conditions that put them at risk for being abused.
3. Teach residents to behave in ways that do not provoke staff.
4. Provide staff with education about elder abuse and stress management.

1. *INCORRECT. Although it is good to be aware of the behaviors of staff, this is a reactive approach to the problem. Abusive behavior must occur to be observed. What action could decrease the likelihood that abuse will occur?*
2. *INCORRECT. This is not a realistic possibility in the majority of situations. It does not address the problem of staff's aggressive, abusive tendencies.*
3. *INCORRECT. This would constitute psychological abuse to expect residents to modify behavior to afford being abused. The responsibility for prevention of abuse lies with the staff and administration of the facility.*
4. ***CORRECT. This is a proactive intervention that will give staff the information and skills that are necessary to prevent abuse in this setting. The stress management component recognizes that caring for the elderly can be stressful and frustrating at times. Giving the staff training for stress management skills addresses this aspect of potential abuse.***

100. The nurse knows that persons who abuse the elderly are often:

1. Financially dependency on the elderly person.
2. Unrelated to the elderly person.
3. Lacking in effective coping skills.
4. Aware of the stressful nature of caring for an elderly family member.

1. ***CORRECT. Abuse is more likely to occur when a caregiver is financially dependent on the elderly person.***

2. *INCORRECT. Abuse most often occurs within a family. Typically a spouse or parent is the victim of the abuse.*

3. *INCORRECT. People who exhibit effective coping skills are less likely to abuse an elderly person that they are caring for.*

4. *INCORRECT. Awareness of the potential stress in caring for an elderly family member is the first step in prevention of abuse.*

NCLEX-RN

Alternate Test Item Formats

OVERVIEW

A. NCLEX Item Types
1. Standard Multiple Choice Question
   a. Traditionally, the format of NCLEX questions
   b. Still the most commonly seen type of question on the NCLEX
   c. Has four options, only one of which is correct ("one best option")
   d. Mastering this format is critical to your success on the NCLEX.
2. As of April 2003, the NCLEX started including items other than standard multiple choice questions. These items are known as Alternate Test Item Formats.
   a. Fill-in-the-Blank
      1) Calculation
      2) Sequence
   b. Multiple Response
   c. Hot Spot
   d. Charts, Tables, Graphic Images
3. The average standard question takes 60 to 70 seconds to answer.
4. The average candidate will be administered only one or two of these alternate items.

POINTS TO REMEMBER:
You should allot a slightly longer time for alternate test items.

SECTION II

FILL-IN-THE-BLANK

A. Overview
1. Definition: Fill-in-the-blank items are a type of alternate item that will be primarily numerical. This type of question typically involves either solving a math problem or putting a list of options into the correct sequence.
2. Method of Answer: To answer these questions, you will need to type a number into the answer box on the screen.
B. Types
1. Calculation item
   a. This type of fill-in-the-blank question typically involves solving a math problem.

   b. Method of Answer: To answer these questions, you will need to type a number into the answer box on the screen.
   c. Read the question carefully. If you see the question is asking for the answer in a specific unit amount, it is not necessary to put units in your answer.

POINTS TO REMEMBER:
1. Write equation down on your scrap paper.
2. Be certain you are solving for the correct unit value!
3. Show all of your work.
4. Bring up drop-down calculator.
5. Double-check your work

GRAPHIC 1
FILL-IN-THE-BLANK CALCULATION ITEM

There are 13 clients being seen in the emergency room and 5 clients in the waiting room. What is the total number of clients?

Type your answer in the box below.

| 18 |

2. Sequence item
   a. This type of fill-in-the-blank question requires you to put a list of options into the correct order.
   b. Method of Answer: To answer these questions, you will need to type a series of numbers into the answer box on the screen.
   c. Read the question carefully. Sequence items on the NCLEX may require you to put the options in the order that you would perform them, or in order of priority.
   d. It is not necessary to separate the numbers in any way, so do not insert spaces, dashes, commas, slashes or any other spacing device between the numbers.

POINTS TO REMEMBER:

Remember that there is only one correct sequence that preserves the client's safety at all stages during the procedure.

GRAPHIC 2
FILL-IN-THE-BLANK SEQUENCE ITEM

Put the following words in alphabetical order.

1. Pizza
2. Apples
3. Onion
4. Bacon
5. Rice

Type your answer in the box below.

24315

SECTION III

MULTIPLE RESPONSE

A. Overview
   1. Definition: Multiple response items are a type of alternate item that require you to choose more than one answer from up to six options. Any number of the options may be correct.
   2. Method of Answer: To answer these questions, you will need to click on all the answers that apply.
   3. On the NCLEX, you will receive credit only for completely correct answers; there is no "partial credit" given for these item types.

GRAPHIC 3
MULTIPLE RESPONSE ITEM

Which of the following are types of vegetables?

Select all that apply.

☑ 1. Broccoli
☑ 2. Cucumber
☐ 3. Peach
☐ 4. Orange
☐ 5. Grape

POINTS TO REMEMBER:

Consider each response as you would a true-false question; is that statement true about the question or false? Click on all that you determine are true.

SECTION IV

HOT SPOT

A. Overview
   1. Definition: Hot spot items are a type of alternate item that will be a "point and click" exercise. Hot spot items will usually require you to identify an anatomical location on a figure.
   2. Method of Answer: To answer these questions, you will need to point at an area on the screen with your cursor and click on the correct spot. As you move your mouse around the screen, you will see an arrow. Once you select a spot and click, the arrow will change into a circle with an "X" in it.
   3. Read the question carefully, then analyze the image.
   4. The NCLEX will allow you to reclick as many times as necessary.

POINTS TO REMEMBER:

It is very important to remember that the screen is NOT a mirror image! If you see that the question is asking for an answer on the right or left side of the body, make sure you are clicking on the correct side.

GRAPHIC 4
HOT SPOT ITEM

The nurse is performing a cardiac assessment. Identify where the nurse will place the stethoscope to best auscultate the apical pulse.

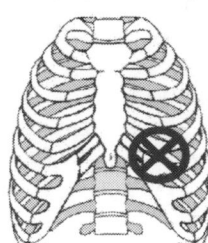

SECTION V

CHARTS, TABLES, & GRAPHIC IMAGES

A. Overview
1. Any of the NCLEX standard multiple choice or alternate items may also include charts, tables or other graphic images that you must analyze and understand in order to correctly answer the question.
2. It is important that you read the question carefully first, then analyze the image.

GRAPHIC 5
CHARTS, TABLES, GRAPHIC IMAGES ITEM

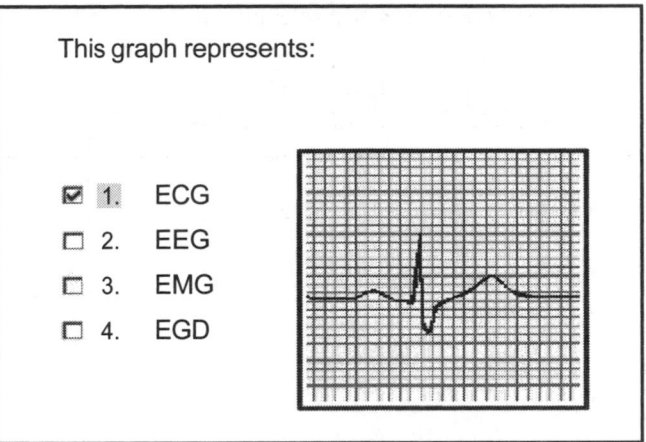

This graph represents:

☑ 1. ECG
☐ 2. EEG
☐ 3. EMG
☐ 4. EGD

NOTES

NCLEX-RN

INDEX

Pediatric Nursing

Women's Health Nursing

Psychiatric Nursing

Communication Theory

Geriatrics

Nursing Management

Continuous Quality Improvement

Informed Consent

Ethical Practice

Client Rights

Legal Responsibilities

Organ Donation

Confidentiality

Case Management

Concepts of Management

Advocacy

Consultation and Referrals

Resource Management

Health Promotion

Religious and Spiritual Influences on Health

✓Elder Abuse or Neglect

Teaching/Learning Theory

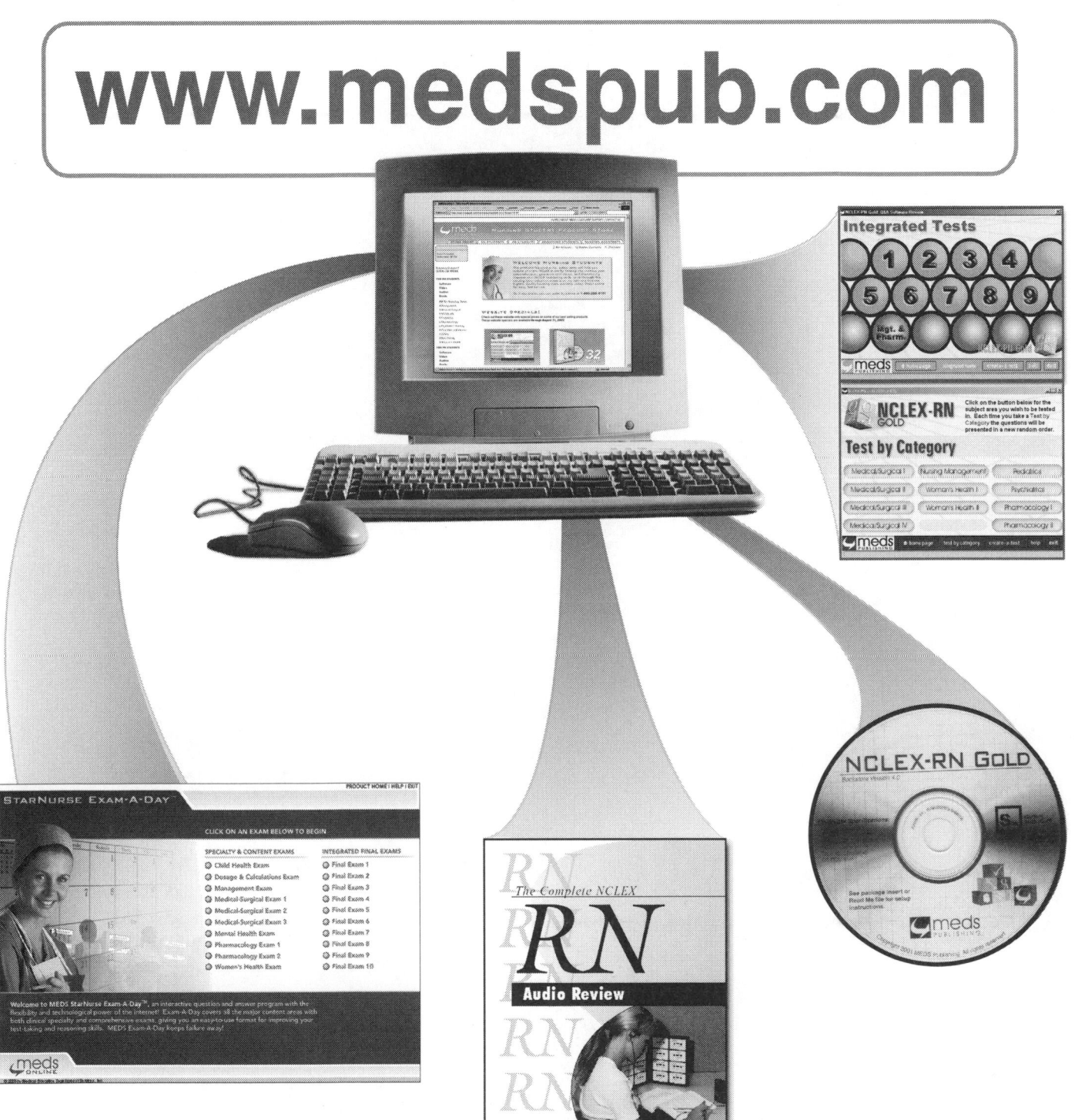